Assessment

A 2-in-1 Reference for Nurses

Assessment

A 2-in-1 Reference for Nurses

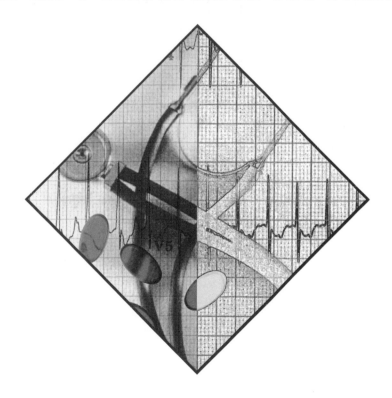

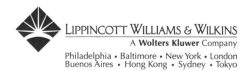

LIPPINCOTT WILLIAMS & WILKINS
A **Wolters Kluwer** Company

Philadelphia • Baltimore • New York • London
Buenos Aires • Hong Kong • Sydney • Tokyo

STAFF

Executive Publisher
Judith A. Schilling McCann, RN, MSN

Editorial Director
H. Nancy Holmes

Clinical Director
Joan M. Robinson, RN, MSN

Senior Art Director
Arlene Putterman

Editorial Project Manager
Jennifer Pierce Kowalak

Clinical Project Manager
Beverly Ann Tscheschlog, RN, BS

Editor
Julie Munden

Clinical Editor
Lisa Morris Bonsall, RN, MSN, CRNP

Copy Editors
Kimberly Bilotta (supervisor),
Scotti Cohn, Tom DeZego, Joy Epstein,
Dona Hightower Perkins, Lisa Stockslager,
Dorothy P. Terry, Pamela Wingrod

Designers
Lesley Weissman-Cook (project manager)

Digital Composition Services
Diane Paluba (manager), Joyce Rossi Biletz,
Donna S. Morris

Manufacturing
Patricia K. Dorshaw (director),
Beth Janae Orr

Editorial Assistants
Megan L. Aldinger, Tara L. Carter-Bell,
Linda K. Ruhf

Librarian
Wani Z. Larsen

Indexer
Barbara Hodgson

**Library of Congress
Cataloging-in Publication Data**

Assessment : a 2-in-1 reference for nurses.
   p. ; cm.
Includes index.
  1. Nursing assessment—Handbooks, manuals, etc. I. Lippincott Williams & Wilkins.
  [DNLM: 1. Nursing Assessment—methods—Handbooks. 2. Nursing Assessment—methods—Nurses' Instruction. WY 49 A8455 2004]
RT48.A873 2004
616.07'5—dc22
ISBN 1-58255-319-X (alk. paper)   2003024955

Contents

Contributors and consultants

Deborah A. Andris, RN, CS, MSN, APNP
Nurse Practitioner, Bariatric Surgery Program
Medical College of Wisconsin
Milwaukee

Jemma Bailey-Kunte, RN, MS, APRN-BC, FNP
Clinical Lecturer
Binghamton (N.Y.) University
Nurse Practitioner
Lourdes Hospital
Binghamton, N.Y.

Cheryl A. Bean, RN, DSN, ANP, AOCN, APRN, BC
Associate Professor
Indiana University School of Nursing
Indianapolis

Natalie Burkhalter, RN, MSN, ACNP, CS, FNP
Associate Professor
Texas A&M International University
Laredo

Catherine B. Holland, RN, PhD, ANP, APRN, BC, CNS
Associate Professor
Southeastern Louisiana University
Baton Rouge

Julia Anne Isen, RN, MS, FNP-C
Nurse Practitioner — Internal Medicine
Veteran Administration Medical Center
San Francisco
Assistant Clinical Professor
University of California San Francisco
    School of Nursing

Nancy Banfield Johnson, RN, MSN, ANP (inactive)
Nurse Manager
Kendal at Ithaca (N.Y.)

Gary R. Jones, RN, MSN, CNS, FNP
ARNP, Disease Management Program
Mercy Health Center
Fort Scott, Kans.

Vanessa C. Kramasz, RN, MSN, FNP-C
Nursing Faculty & Family Nurse Practitioner
Gateway Technical College
Kenosha, Wis.

Priscilla A. Lee, RN, MN, FNP
Instructor in Nursing
Moorpark (Calif.) College

Ann S. McQueen, RNC, MSN, CRNP
Family Nurse Practitioner
Healthlink Medical Center
Southampton, Pa.

William J. Pawlyshyn, RN, MN, MS, APRN, BC
Nurse Practitioner Consultant
New England Geriatrics
West Springfield, Mass.

Regina Reed, RN, MSN, FNP
Associate Professor
Washington State Community College
Marrietta, Ohio

Foreword

Competence in assessment is the foundation of clinical practice. Today, more than ever, nurses face multiple challenges in their daily practice. Demands, including preparing for physical examinations, collecting the proper tools, performing the assessments, recording the findings, and decision making, all require skill, efficiency, and rapid turnaround. Nurses are also faced with utilizing all available data in determining the needs of a growing, ever-changing, multiproblem patient population. The ultimate challenge is balancing these tasks with total competence, all the while keeping patient care in the forefront.

As your daily practice demands that you handle multiple decisions in patient care, it's evident that more resources are needed to increase your competency level. *Assessment: A 2-in-1 Reference for Nurses* was designed with this thought in mind. The ability to assess abnormal systems is essential in the care of patients. Too often, nurses find themselves ill-equipped for this critical step. Shorter patient hospital stays, combined with the increased complexity in health problems, result in added stressors for nurses, which can be eased with resources to aid in decision-making.

Assessment: A 2-in-1 Reference for Nurses presents information in a two-in-one review format that quickly points you to needed information. Practical information, such as assessment techniques and specific disorders, is presented in the main text while a review of this information is featured in an easy-to-access bulleted format in the margins of the book — lending to enhanced readability and accessibility. Normal findings are addressed in each area of assessment, inspection, palpation, percussion, and auscultation. More in-depth information is highlighted by special icons that point the nurse in the direction of the care necessary for each assessment, including:

- *Abnormal findings* — that address individual assessments.
- *Special points* — that identify lifespan, gender, and racial differences in assessment findings.
- *Clinical alerts* — that identify emergency situations found during assessments and how to intervene.
- *Know-how* — that describes specific techniques vital to the best assessment.

The presentation of subjective data — an essential component of all assessments — is the cornerstone of this incredible resource. The first four chapters are devoted to a detailed collection of subjective data, including health history, assessment techniques, mental health status, and nutritional assessment. Each system chapter thereafter refocuses the reader on the information that must be obtained before the patient is physically touched during the examination, including chief complaint, related problems, current and past health, and family and psychosocial history.

Additional features of this book include full-color inserts that aid in the understanding of assessment techniques, such as identifying cardiovascular landmarks and sites for heart sounds, distinguishing respiratory landmarks, and recognizing disorders of the skin, ears, and eyes. Also included are numerous illustrations that specify what to look for and what to do during your assessments. Furthermore, the appendices, *Quick-reference guide to laboratory test results, Quick guide to head-to-toe assess-*

ment, *Laboratory value changes in elderly patients,* and *Resources for professionals, patients, and caregivers* are a perfect complement to this valuable resource.

Assessment: A 2-in-1 Reference for Nurses can be used as a supplemental text as well as a ready reference in any clinical setting. It offers a practical approach to identifying assessment needs based on the symptoms presented by the patient and then provides the nurse with the information needed to determine and interpret the clinical findings.

Because health care information is growing at a staggering rate, it's almost impossible for the novice, or even the skilled nurse, to keep abreast of the knowledge base needed to maintain competency in patient care. As we are expected to see more and more multiproblem patients in our complex health care environments, resources such as *Assessment: A 2-in-1 Reference for Nurses* will help nurses, in any patient care setting, gain the competency level necessary to assess and determine the needed actions to support their patients.

Saundra L. Turner, RN, BA, MSN, EdD, CS, FNP
Interim Chair of Advanced Practice Nursing
Acting Director of Faculty Practice
Medical College of Georgia
Augusta

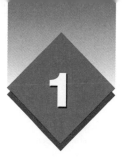

Health history

OBTAINING A HEALTH HISTORY

Obtaining a health history is the first of two essential steps in the nursing assessment process. Although these steps can be time-consuming, it's important to complete these tasks accurately and thoroughly. Doing so will help you uncover significant problems and establish an appropriate care plan for your patient.

The health history organizes physiologic, psychological, cultural, and psychosocial information. It relates to the patient's current health status and accounts for such influences as lifestyle, family relationships, and cultural influences. This chapter will tell you what you need to know to get the most out of an assessment interview and what to look for when collecting health history data.

PREPARING TO TAKE THE HISTORY

Before beginning the assessment interview, take time to self-reflect, read the chart, and set goals.

SELF-REFLECTION

Nurses have the unique opportunity to develop relationships with people from a broad spectrum of ages, classes, races, and ethnicities. It can be challenging at times to be respectful of individual differences. Self-reflection can help to deepen your own personal awareness and allow you to be open to these differences.

CHART REVIEW

Before speaking with the patient, review his medical chart. This will allow you to gather information and develop ideas of what to focus on during your interview. Remember, however, that data may not be complete and that information comes from different observers. Don't let the chart prevent you from developing new ideas or approaches.

Nursing assessment
+ Two parts: Health history and physical assessment
+ Helps set appropriate care plan

Health history
+ Physiologic, psychological, cultural, and psychosocial information
+ History of current complaint
+ Lifestyle, family, and cultural influences

Preparation

Self-reflection
+ Aids appreciation of diversity in others

Chart review
+ Helps set the focus for interview

Considering communication barriers

This diagram shows the components of nurse-patient communication. Note the factors that affect communication, such as orientation, preconceptions, and language. Your sensitivity to these influences makes the difference between effective and ineffective communication.

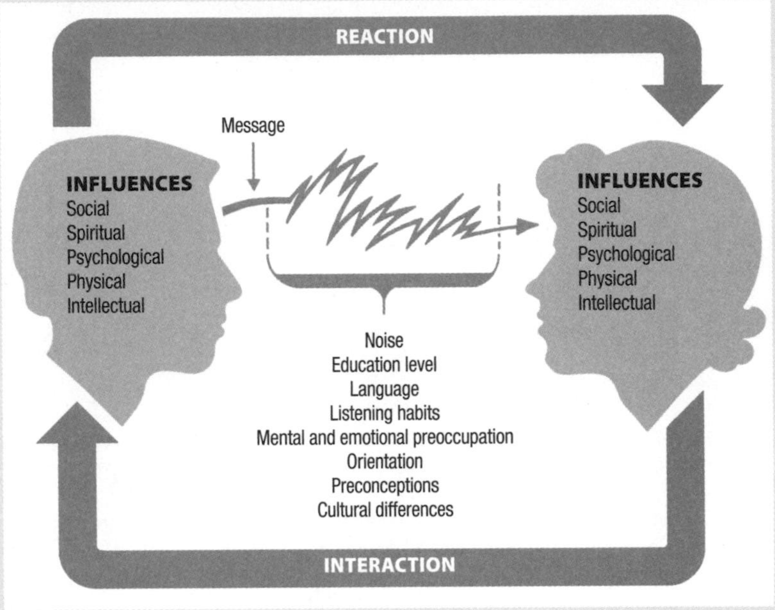
REACTION
Message
INFLUENCES
Social
Spiritual
Psychological
Physical
Intellectual
INFLUENCES
Social
Spiritual
Psychological
Physical
Intellectual
Noise
Education level
Language
Listening habits
Mental and emotional preoccupation
Orientation
Preconceptions
Cultural differences
INTERACTION

Preparation

Set goals
- Helps to stay focused and organized

Set goals

Clarify your own goals for the interview. You may need to complete a certain form for insurance purposes, or you may want to validate the information in the medical chart. Your goals will differ from patient to patient. Clarifying goals before beginning the interview will help you to stay focused and organized.

The accuracy and completeness of the patient's answers largely depend on your skill as an interviewer. Before you start asking questions, review the communication guidelines in the following sections.

Communicating effectively

- Encourage a dialogue
- Watch for nonverbal gestures
- Be aware of your own body language
- Overcome emotional and cultural barriers

COMMUNICATING EFFECTIVELY

Effective health interviews require good communication and interpersonal skills. The interview is a dialogue with the patient, not a simple question-and-answer session. An effective communication style helps eliminate mannerisms—yours or the patient's—that may hinder the candid exchange of information. By developing self-awareness and acceptance of different lifestyles, you can overcome barriers to effective communication, such as emotional or cultural biases. (See *Considering communication barriers.*)

Effective interview skills rely on nonverbal and verbal communication. The patient can manipulate conversation to create a desired impression but rarely can manipulate nonverbal communication. Observe his body language for clues to unstated feelings or behaviors. In addition, be aware of your own body language to ensure optimal communication. Your posture, gestures, eye contact, and tone of voice can express interest and understanding. Your appearance can also affect your relationship with the patient. A patient is reassured by a nurse who's clean, neat, and wearing conservative clothes and a name tag.

THERAPEUTIC USE OF SELF

Using interpersonal skills in a healing way to help the patient is called therapeutic use of self. Three important techniques enhance therapeutic use of self, including exhibiting empathy, demonstrating acceptance, and giving recognition.

To show empathy, use phrases that address the patient's feelings such as "That must have upset you." To show acceptance, use neutral statements such as "I hear what you're saying" and "I see." Nonverbal behaviors, such as nodding or making momentary eye contact, also provide encouragement without indicating agreement or disagreement. To give recognition, listen actively to what the patient says, occasionally providing verbal or nonverbal acknowledgment to encourage him to continue speaking.

PATIENT'S EXPECTATIONS

Personal values and previous experiences with the health care system can affect the patient's health history expectations. Help him clarify expectations, concerns, and questions. If possible, provide answers that appropriately address the patient's misconceptions. A patient may be uncomfortable providing personal information; reassure him that the information is confidential and accessible only to authorized health care professionals.

TAKING NOTES

No one can remember all the details of a health history without taking notes, although you'll remember more as your experience increases. Write down short phrases, dates, and words, rather than trying to write a narrative. Don't let note taking distract you from the patient, and put down your pen when a sensitive subject is being discussed.

COLLECTING OBJECTIVE AND SUBJECTIVE DATA

An assessment involves collecting two kinds of data: objective and subjective.

Objective data is obtained through observation and is verifiable. For instance, a red, swollen arm in a patient who's complaining of arm pain is an example of data that can be seen and verified by someone other than the patient. Subjective data, on the other hand, can't be verified by anyone other than the patient; it's based solely on the patient's own account — for example, "My head hurts" or "I have trouble sleeping at night."

A health history is used to gather subjective data about the patient and to explore past and present problems. First, ask the patient about his general physical and emotional health, and then ask him questions about specific body systems and structures.

Therapeutic use of self
✦ Use interpersonal skills in a healing way
✦ Exhibit empathy
✦ Demonstrate acceptance
✦ Give recognition

Patient's expectations
✦ Clarify expectations, concerns, and questions
✦ Correct misconceptions

Taking notes
✦ Jot down phrases, important dates, and key words

Collecting objective and subjective data
✦ Collect objective data (observation that's verifiable) and subjective data (verifiable only by patient)

Interviewing the patient

Before you perform a patient interview, keep in mind these tips:
+ Select a quiet, private setting.
+ Choose terms carefully and avoid using jargon.
+ Use appropriate body language.
+ Confirm patient statements to avoid misunderstanding.
+ Use open-ended questions.

Key interview components

+ Physical surroundings
+ Patient comfort
+ Confidentiality
+ Interview structure
+ Patient's concerns and goals
+ Language assessment
+ Hearing assessment
+ Respect

Special points: Interpreters

+ Available in most facilities
+ Can be a family member
+ Sign-language interpreter for hearing-impaired patients

INTERVIEWING THE PATIENT

Physical surroundings, psychological atmosphere, interview structure, and questioning style can affect the interview flow and outcome; so can your ability to adopt a communication style to fit each patient's needs and situation. Before asking your first question, you'll need to set the stage, explain what you'll cover during the interview, and establish rapport with the patient. (See *Interviewing the patient*.) In addition, take these steps when interviewing a patient:

+ Choose a quiet, private, well-lit interview setting away from distractions. Such a setting will make it easier for you and the patient to interact and will help the patient feel more at ease. Take the time to make adjustments to the location and seating as needed.

+ Make sure that the patient is comfortable. Sit facing him, 3′ to 4′ (1 to 1.5 m) away.

+ Introduce yourself and explain that the purpose of the health history and assessment is to identify the patient's problem and provide information for planning his care.

+ Reassure the patient that everything he says will be kept confidential.

+ Tell the patient how long the interview will last and ask him what he expects from the interview. Identifying the patient's concerns and goals at the beginning of the interview will help you to use time effectively and address all of the issues.

+ Use touch sparingly. Many people aren't comfortable with strangers hugging, patting, or touching them.

+ Assess the patient to see if language barriers exist. For instance, does he speak and understand English? Can he hear you clearly?

 SPECIAL POINTS *Most facilities have language interpreters available to assist with English translations, or a member of the patient's family may also be helpful for interpretation. If your patient is hearing impaired, make sure the area is well-lit, face him and speak clearly, so that he can read your lips. If needed, have the patient use an assistive device, such as a hearing aid or an amplifier. If the patient uses sign language, you'll need to check with your facility for a sign-language interpreter.*

+ Speak slowly and clearly, using easy-to-understand language. Avoid medical terms and jargon.

+ Address the patient by a formal name, such as Mr. Jones or Ms. Carter. Don't call him by his first name unless he asks you to. Treating the patient with respect encourages him to trust you and provides more accurate and complete information. If you're unsure how to pronounce the patient's name, don't be afraid to ask. You can say, "I'm not sure how to pronounce your name. Could you say it for me?" Then repeat it back to him to make sure you heard it correctly.

KNOW-HOW

Asking questions

Questions can be characterized as either open-ended or closed.

OPEN-ENDED QUESTIONS
Open-ended questions require the patient to express feelings, opinions, and ideas. They also help you gather more information than can be gathered with closed questions. Open-ended questions encourage a good nurse-patient rapport because they show that you're interested in what the patient has to say. Examples of such questions include:
◆ Why did you come to the hospital tonight?
◆ How would you describe the problems you're having with your breathing?
◆ What lung problems, if any, do other members of your family have?

CLOSED QUESTIONS
Closed questions elicit yes-or-no answers or one- to two-word responses. They limit the development of nurse-patient rapport. Closed questions can help you "zoom in" on specific points but they don't provide the patient with an opportunity to elaborate. Examples of closed questions include:
◆ Do you ever get short of breath?
◆ Are you the only one in your family with lung problems?

◆ Listen attentively and make eye contact frequently.

 SPECIAL POINTS *Remember that the patient's cultural behaviors and beliefs may differ from your own. Be aware that people in a number of cultures — including Native Americans, Asians, and people from Arab-speaking countries — may find eye contact disrespectful or aggressive.*

◆ Use reassuring gestures, such as nodding your head, to encourage the patient to keep talking.

◆ Watch for nonverbal cues that indicate the patient is uncomfortable or unsure about how to answer a question. For example, he might lower his voice or glance around uneasily.

◆ Be aware of your own nonverbal cues that might cause the patient to "clam up" or become defensive. For example, if you cross your arms, you might appear "closed off" from him. If you stand while he's sitting, you might appear superior. If you glance at your watch, you might appear bored or rushed, which could keep the patient from answering questions completely.

Observe the patient closely to see if he understands each question. If he doesn't appear to understand, repeat the question using different words or familiar examples. For instance, instead of asking, "Did you have respiratory difficulty after exercising?" ask, "Did you have to sit down after walking around the block?"

You might also use a different type of question. An open-ended question such as "How did you fall?" lets the patient respond more freely. His response can provide answers to many other questions.

For instance, from the patient's answer, you might learn that he has fallen before, that he was unsteady on his feet, and that he fell before dinner. Armed with this information, you might deduce that he had a syncopal episode caused by hypoglycemia.

You can also ask closed questions, which are unlikely to provide extra information but might encourage the patient to give clear, concise feedback. (See *Asking questions*.)

Asking questions
◆ **Open-ended questions** require the patient to express his feelings, opinions, and ideas — encouraging nurse-patient rapport
◆ **Closed questions** require yes-no or one- to two-word responses — limiting nurse-patient rapport

Key interview components
(continued)
◆ Reassuring gestures
◆ Nonverbal cues
◆ Assessment of patient comprehension

Special points: Cultural behaviors
◆ Eye contact may be considered disrespectful or aggressive in some cultures

Communicating effectively

Communicating effectively can make or break an interview. Follow these tips for effective communication:

◆ Use silence effectively.
◆ Encourage responses.
◆ Use repetition and reflection to help clarify meaning.
◆ Use clarification to make ambiguous information clearer.
◆ Summarize and conclude with, "Is there anything else?"

Communication strategies

◆ Select strategies for specific situations
◆ Your attitude and patient's interpretation can vary
◆ Individualize your style for each patient

Silence

◆ Leads the patient to continue talking
◆ Lets you assess his ability to organize thoughts
◆ Gets easier with practice

Active listening

◆ Concentrates solely on the patient
◆ Senses the patient's emotional state
◆ Encourages patient to continue through verbal and nonverbal communication

Types of adaptive questions

◆ Directed and open-ended
◆ Graded response
◆ Series
◆ Multiple-choice

USING COMMUNICATION STRATEGIES

In addition to the tips listed above, some special communication techniques—silence, active listening, adaptive questioning, facilitation, confirmation, reflection, clarification, observation, validation, highlighting transitions, summarizing, and conclusion—can help you make the most of your patient interview. Remember, however, that successful techniques in one situation may not be effective in another. Your attitude and the patient's interpretation of your questions can vary. So be sure to individualize your style for each patient, as needed. (See *Communicating effectively*.)

Silence

Moments of silence during the interview encourage the patient to continue talking and give you a chance to assess his ability to organize thoughts. You may find this technique difficult (most people are uncomfortable with silence), but the more often you use it, the more comfortable you'll become.

Active listening

Active listening involves:
◆ fully attending to the patient
◆ being aware of the patient's emotional state
◆ using verbal and nonverbal communication to encourage the patient to continue to speak.

Active listening takes practice. It's easy to become distracted and begin to think ahead to your next question or something else. You must concentrate and focus your attention on what's being communicated by the patient.

Adaptive questioning

A goal of the interview process is to facilitate the flow of the interview while asking the right questions to add detail to the patient's story. Use the following adaptive questioning techniques to help you do this:
◆ directed questioning
◆ questioning to elicit a graded response
◆ asking a series of questions, one at a time
◆ offering multiple-choice answers.

Directed questioning should flow from the general to the specific. Directed questions shouldn't be leading questions that require a yes-or-no answer. Examples:
◆ "Tell me about your chest pain."
◆ "Where did you feel it?"
◆ "Did you feel pain anywhere else?"
◆ "Where?"

Questions that require a graded response rather than a single answer will allow you to elicit more information from the patient. For example, instead of asking "Do you get short of breath while climbing stairs?" ask "What physical activities make you short of breath?" Also, be sure to ask questions one at a time. When asking, "Do you have a history of asthma, hypertension, diabetes, or heart disease?" the patient may become confused. Instead, ask, "Do you have a history of any of the following?" and then list them one at a time, pausing after each problem to give the patient time to think and respond.

Sometimes it's difficult for patients to respond to questions without some guidance. Offer multiple choices in order to limit bias. "Is your pain aching, dull, throbbing, pressing, burning, or what?" This gives the patient an idea of what you're looking for, and also gives permission to describe the pain in his own words.

Facilitation

Facilitation encourages the patient to continue with his story. Using such phrases as "please continue," "go on," or even "uh-huh" shows him that you're interested in what he's saying. Leaning forward and maintaining eye contact are also examples of facilitation.

Confirmation

Confirmation ensures that both you and the patient are on the same track. You might say, "If I understand you correctly, you said…" and then repeat the information the patient gave. This technique helps to clear up misconceptions you or the patient might have.

Reflection

Reflection — repeating something that the patient has just said — can help you obtain more specific information. For example, a patient with a stomachache might say, "I know I have an ulcer." You might repeat, "You know you have an ulcer?" And the patient might then say, "Yes. I had one before and the pain is the same."

When appropriate, give him an opportunity to reconsider a response and to add information. For example, if the patient says he has provided complete information about his meals, a question that encourages reflection is, "Do you think you've covered all the important things about your nutrition?"

Stating what's implied or unspoken sometimes helps interpret a patient's statement accurately or yields additional insight into the patient's symptoms or concerns. Start by asking, "What events led to this?"

Clarification

Clarification is used to clear up confusing, vague, or misunderstood information. For example, if your patient says, "I can't stand this," your response might be, "What can't you stand?" or "What do you mean by 'I can't stand this?'" This gives the patient an opportunity to explain his statement.

Observation

Observe the patient to interpret and validate nonverbal behavior. For example, the statement, "I notice that you're rubbing your eyes a lot. Do they bother you?" may lead to a discussion of other health concerns.

Validation

Validating the patient's emotional experiences will make him feel accepted and more willing to communicate openly with you. A patient who has been involved in a trauma may experience distress even if no physical injuries occurred. Stating "A

Facilitation
+ Encourages patient to continue story

Confirmation
+ Clears up misconceptions or misinformation

Reflection
+ Repeats information to get more specific information
+ Provides patient opportunity to reconsider response and add information

Clarification
+ Reaffirms patient's statements

Observation
+ Interprets nonverbal behavior

Validation
+ Helps patient to feel that his emotions are legitimate

Highlighting transitions

♦ Allows patient to feel more in control

Summarizing

♦ Restates data that you've collected from the patient
♦ Aids with transitions during interview
♦ Enhances nurse-patient collaboration

Conclusion

♦ Signals end of interview
♦ Gives the patient an opportunity to add final thoughts

Health history content

♦ Biographic data
♦ Chief complaint
♦ Medical history
♦ Family history
♦ Psychosocial history
♦ Stress level
♦ ADLs

Key biographic data

♦ Name, address, phone number
♦ Birth date and age
♦ Marital status
♦ Religion (optional)
♦ Nationality
♦ Living arrangements
♦ Emergency contact person
♦ Primary physician
♦ Prior treatment for complaint

car accident can remind us of our own mortality. That must have been scary for you." helps the patient feel that his emotions are legitimate.

Highlighting transitions

Be sure to tell the patient when you're changing directions during the interview. It allows the patient to feel more in control. Transition with phrases such as "Now I'd like to ask you some questions about your family history." Make clear what the patient should expect or do next.

Summarizing

Summarizing is restating the information the patient gave you. It ensures that the data you've collected is accurate and complete. Summarizing also signals that the interview is about to end. You can also use summarization at different points in the interview to structure the interview and aid with transitions. It also allows you to organize your thinking and convey it to the patient. This adds to a more collaborative relationship.

Conclusion

Signaling the patient that you're ready to conclude the interview provides him the opportunity to gather his thoughts and make any final statements. You can do this verbally by saying, "I think I have all the information I need now. Is there anything you'd like to add?"

Techniques to avoid

Some interview techniques create communication problems between the nurse and the patient. Techniques to avoid include asking "why" or "how" questions, asking probing or persistent questions, using inappropriate language, giving advice, giving false reassurance, and changing the subject or interrupting. Also avoid using clichés or stereotyped responses, giving excessive approval or agreement, jumping to conclusions, and using defensive responses.

SPECIFIC QUESTIONS TO ASK

Asking the right questions is a critical part of an interview. Be sure to routinely document the date and time that the interview is occurring. To obtain a complete health history, gather information from each of the following categories, in sequence:

1. biographic data
2. chief complaint
3. medical history
4. family history
5. psychosocial history
6. stress level
7. activities of daily living (ADLs).

Biographic data

Begin the health history by obtaining biographic information from the patient. Do this first so you don't forget about this information after you become involved in details of the patient's health. Ask the patient for his name, address, telephone number, birth date, age, marital status, religion, and nationality. Find out whom he lives with and the name and telephone number of a person to contact in case of an emergency.

Also ask the patient about his health care, including who his primary physician is and how he gets to the physician's office. Ask if he has ever been treated before for his present problem.

Using the PQRST device

Use the PQRST mnemonic device to fully explore your patient's chief complaint. When you ask the questions below, you'll encourage him to describe his symptoms in greater detail.

PROVOCATIVE OR PALLIATIVE
Ask the patient:
◆ What provokes or relieves the symptom?
◆ Do stress, anger, certain physical positions, or other things trigger the symptom?
◆ What makes the symptom worsen or subside?

QUALITY OR QUANTITY
Ask the patient:
◆ What does the symptom feel like, look like, or sound like?
◆ Are you having the symptom right now? If so, is it more or less severe than usual?
◆ To what degree does the symptom affect your normal activities?

REGION OR RADIATION
Ask the patient:
◆ Where in the body does the symptom occur?
◆ Does the symptom appear in other regions? If so, where?

SEVERITY
Ask the patient:
◆ How severe is the symptom? How would you rate it on a scale of 1 to 10, with 10 being the most severe?
◆ Does the symptom seem to be diminishing, intensifying, or staying about the same?

TIMING
Ask the patient:
◆ When did the symptom begin?
◆ Was the onset sudden or gradual?
◆ How often does the symptom occur?
◆ How long does the symptom last?

Your patient's answers to basic questions can provide important clues about his personality, medical problems, and reliability. If he can't furnish accurate information, ask him for the name of a friend or relative who can. Document who gave you the information.

Chief complaint

Try to pinpoint why the patient is seeking health care at this time. Document this information in the patient's exact words to avoid misinterpretation. Ask how and when the symptoms developed, what led the patient to seek medical attention, and how the problem has affected his life and ability to function.

To ensure you don't omit pertinent data, use the PQRST mnemonic device, which provides a systematic approach to obtaining information. (See *Using the PQRST device.*)

Exploring the chief complaint

◆ Document the patient's exact words
◆ Ask how and when symptoms developed
◆ Find out what led him to seek care
◆ Ask how the problem affects ADLs
◆ Find out about recent minor illnesses or health concerns
◆ For comprehensive data gathering, use PQRST device

Key points in the medical history

✦ Past and current health history
✦ Past hospitalizations, childhood illnesses, and immunizations
✦ Current treatment, problem, and physician's name
✦ Environmental and medication allergies
✦ Medication history
✦ Alternative therapies

Key questions about family history

✦ Are mother, father, and siblings living?
✦ If not, what were their ages and causes of death?
✦ Do any family members have diabetes, high blood pressure, heart disease, or other diseases?

Key psychosocial history points

✦ Occupation
✦ Education
✦ Financial status
✦ Responsibilities
✦ Coping strategies
✦ Support systems
✦ Exercise

The patient may present for health maintenance assessment, health counseling, or health education. In this case, ask the patient about recent minor illnesses or health concerns.

Medical history

Ask the patient about past and current medical problems, such as hypertension, diabetes, or back pain. Typical questions include:

✦ Have you ever been hospitalized? If so, when and for what reason?
✦ What childhood illnesses did you have? Did you receive all of your childhood immunizations?
✦ Are you under treatment for any problem? If so, what's the problem and who's your physician?
✦ Have you ever had surgery? If so, when and for what reason?
✦ Are you allergic to anything in the environment or to any medications? If so, what kind of allergic reaction do you have?
✦ Are you taking medications, including over-the-counter preparations, such as aspirin, vitamins, and cough syrup? If so, how much do you take and how often do you take it? Do you use home remedies such as homemade ointments? Do you use herbal preparations or take dietary supplements? Do you use other alternative therapies, such as acupuncture, therapeutic massage, or chiropractic therapy?

Family history

Questioning the patient about his family's health is a good way to uncover his risk of having certain illnesses. Some diseases may be genetically linked, such as cardiovascular disease, alcoholism, depression, and cancer. Others, such as hemophilia, cystic fibrosis, sickle cell anemia, and Tay-Sachs disease are genetically transmitted. Typical questions include:

✦ Are your mother, father, and siblings living? If not, how old were they when they died? What was the cause of death?
✦ If they're alive, do they have diabetes, high blood pressure, heart disease, asthma, cancer, sickle cell anemia, hemophilia, cataracts, glaucoma, or other illnesses?

Use a genogram to organize family data. (See *Developing a genogram*.)

Psychosocial history

Find out how the patient feels about himself, his place in society, and his relationships with others. Ask about his occupation, education, financial status, and responsibilities. Typical questions include:

✦ How have you coped with medical or emotional crises in the past? (See *Asking about abuse*, page 12.)
✦ Has your life changed recently? What changes in your personality or behavior have you noticed?
✦ How adequate is the emotional support you receive from family and friends?
✦ How often do you exercise? What types of things do you do to exercise? Do you walk, use a stationary bike, or lift weights? How often do you eat a healthful diet?
✦ How close do you live to health care facilities, and can you get to them easily?
✦ Do you have health insurance?
✦ Are you on a fixed income with no extra money for health care?

Developing a genogram

A genogram provides a visual family health summary. It includes the patient and his spouse, children, and parents. To develop a genogram, first draw the relationships of family members to the patient, as shown, and then fill in the ages of living members and note deceased members and the ages at which they died. Also, record diseases that have a familial tendency (such as Huntington's chorea) or an environmental cause (such as lung cancer from exposure to coal tar).

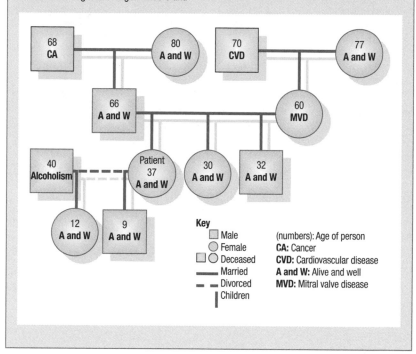

Key
- ☐ Male
- ○ Female
- ☐○ Deceased
- — Married
- - - Divorced
- | Children

(numbers): Age of person
CA: Cancer
CVD: Cardiovascular disease
A and W: Alive and well
MVD: Mitral valve disease

Visualizing your patient's family

+ Develop a genogram that provides a visual family health summary
+ First, draw the relationships of the family members to the patient
+ Next, fill in the ages of living members
+ Note deceased members and ages at which they died
+ Finally, record diseases that have a familial tendency or an environmental cause

Stress level

Emotional, social, and physical demands on the body cause stress. The amount of stress the patient experiences affects physiologic and psychological health. These questions can help assess stress and coping strategies:

+ How do you know when you're feeling stressed?
+ What situations are stressful to you?
+ How do you respond physically to stress? For example, do you sweat, get butterflies in your stomach, develop a headache, or become nauseated?
+ What do you do when you're feeling stressed?
+ Does stress ever affect your family relationships or your work? If so, how?
+ What stresses have you experienced during the past year?
+ How did you deal with these stresses?
+ Did these stresses cause significant changes for you?
+ Do you think stress affects your health?

Key points about stress

+ Awareness of stress
+ Situations that cause stress

Factors affecting stress level

+ Emotional demands
+ Social pressures
+ Physical strains
+ Reactions to stress
+ Recent stress management

Exploring abuse

✦ Ask open-ended questions
✦ Watch for reactions
✦ Assess how the patient interacts with you and others
✦ If the patient reports abuse or if you have reason to suspect abuse, you must report it

Exploring ADLs

✦ Reveals what's normal for patient
✦ Assists in developing care plan

Asking about diet and elimination

✦ Appetite, special diets, food allergies
✦ Person who shops and cooks
✦ Frequency of bowel movements and laxative use

Asking about exercise and sleep

✦ Exercise program
✦ Activities
✦ Sleep patterns

Asking about work and leisure

✦ Occupation
✦ Leisure activities
✦ Hobbies

Asking about tobacco, alcohol, and drugs

✦ Tobacco use, including forms
✦ Alcohol and illicit drug use

KNOW-HOW

Asking about abuse

Abuse is a tricky subject. Anyone can be a victim of abuse: a boyfriend or girlfriend, a spouse, an elderly patient, a child, or a parent. Also, abuse can come in many forms: physical, psychological, emotional, and sexual. So when taking a health history, ask two open-ended questions: When do you feel safe at home? When don't you feel safe?

WATCH THE REACTION
Even when you don't immediately suspect an abusive situation, be aware of how your patient reacts to open-ended questions. Is the patient defensive, hostile, confused, or frightened? Assess how he interacts with you and others. Does he seem withdrawn or frightened or show other inappropriate behavior? Keep his reactions in mind when you perform your physical assessment.

Remember, if the patient reports abuse of any kind to you, you are a mandated reporter. Inform the patient that you are obligated to report the incident to the appropriate authorities.

ADLs

Find out what's normal for the patient by asking him to describe his typical day. Areas to include in your assessment are diet and elimination; exercise and sleep; work and leisure; use of tobacco, alcohol, and other drugs; and religious observances.

Diet and elimination

Ask the patient about his appetite, special diets, and food allergies. Can he afford to buy enough food? Who cooks and shops at his house? Ask about the frequency of bowel movements and laxative use.

Exercise and sleep

Ask the patient if he has a special exercise program and, if so, why? Have him describe it. What activities does he perform and for how long? Is he satisfied with his current activity and exercise levels? Ask how many hours he sleeps at night, what his sleep pattern is like, and whether he feels rested after sleep.

Work and leisure

Ask the patient what he does for a living and what he does during his leisure time. Does he have hobbies?

Use of tobacco, alcohol, and other drugs

Ask the patient if he smokes cigarettes. Also, inquire about use of other forms of tobacco, such as pipes, cigars, and chewing tobacco. How much tobacco is consumed daily? How long has he used tobacco? Does he drink alcohol? If so, what kind and how much each day? How long has he consumed alcohol? Ask if he uses illicit drugs, such as marijuana or cocaine. If so, how often?

Patients may understate the amount they drink because of embarrassment. If you're having trouble getting what you believe are honest answers to such questions, you might try overestimating the amount. For example, you might say, "You told me you drink beer. Do you drink about a six-pack per day?" The patient's response might be, "No, I drink about half that."

Religious observances

Ask the patient if he has religious beliefs that affect diet, dress, or health practices. Patients will feel reassured when you make it clear that you understand these points.

DISCUSSING ADVANCE DIRECTIVES

The patient has the right to make his own decisions regarding his health care. It's recommended to discuss advance directives with all patients and document their wishes. Ask the patient if he has a living will. Has he thought about who should be the person to make decisions for him if he can't? Ask him about what "quality of life" means to him. What types of medical treatment would he want if his death is imminent?

ADAPTING TO SPECIFIC SITUATIONS

Your skills at handling difficult interviews will evolve throughout your career. The following situations may be especially challenging.

The silent patient

Periods of silence may be uncomfortable, especially for the novice interviewer. Try not to feel obligated to keep the conversation going. Silence has many meanings and purposes. It allows the patient to collect thoughts, remember details, and decide whether he would like to discuss certain information with you. You should appear attentive and give encouragement when appropriate. Watch the patient closely for nonverbal cues.

Silence could be a response to your approach at asking questions. Could the patient be overwhelmed or even offended? Ask the patient directly if something is wrong by saying, "Have I done something to upset you?"

Some patients are just naturally quiet. Be accepting and ask the patient for other ways that you can gather the necessary information. Perhaps he'll give you permission to talk with family or friends or access other sources of information.

The talkative patient

The patient who rambles can be just as difficult. You probably have limited time to conduct the interview and need to gather much information during that time. Several techniques can be helpful in this situation.

Give the patient 5 to 10 minutes of free rein and listen closely to the conversation. What clues is the patient giving you? Perhaps he has lacked a good listener and is expressing pent-up concerns. Does he seem anxious or display disorganized thought processes?

Try to focus on what seems most important to the patient. Show your interest in those areas. Interrupt if needed, but do so courteously. It's acceptable to be direct and set limits if needed. Use the techniques of transitioning and summarization to help you do this.

If possible, set up a time for a second interview. Say, "I know we have much more to talk about. Can you come in again next week?"

The anxious patient

Anxiety is an emotion commonly experienced during sickness, treatment, or the health care system itself. Watch for verbal and nonverbal clues of anxiety. These may include:

✦ sitting tensely
✦ fidgeting

Asking about religion
✦ Religious observances
✦ Affect on diet, dress, or health practices

Discussing advance directives
✦ Ask about a living will
✦ Ask patient to define "quality of life"
✦ Find out what medical treatments he does and doesn't want

Adapting to specific situations
✦ Poses a challenge
✦ Hones your skills
✦ Involves diverse patient groups

The silent patient
✦ Allow time for the patient to collect his thoughts
✦ Give encouragement and watch for nonverbal cues

The talkative patient
✦ Listen for clues
✦ Focus on what seems most important to patient
✦ Use transitioning and summarizing to control timeframe
✦ Set up a second interview if necessary

The anxious patient
✦ Watch for verbal and nonverbal clues
✦ Ask about anxiety
✦ Encourage patient to share

The crying patient
+ Reassure patient that crying is okay
+ Use supportive remarks

The confusing patient
+ Focus on the patient's symptoms
+ Perform mental status examination if you suspect a psychiatric or neurologic disorder

The angry patient
+ Don't waste time arguing
+ Listen without showing disapproval
+ Use a firm, quiet voice and a nonthreatening manner
+ Call for assistance if necessary

Language barriers
+ Beware of using friends and family members as interpreters
+ Stress the need for exact translation to the interpreter
+ Include interpreter in the interview, but address the patient

Assessing reading ability
+ Assess patient's reading and writing ability
+ Respond sensitively to the illiterate patient

+ sighing frequently
+ licking lips
+ sweating
+ trembling
+ silence.

   When you detect anxiety, express your impressions to the patient, and encourage him to talk about any underlying concerns. Be cautious not to transmit your own anxiety about completing the interview.

The crying patient
Crying is usually therapeutic and can signal strong emotions, such as sadness, anger, or frustration. Allow the patient to cry and respond with empathy. If the patient is on the verge of tears, pausing or gentle probing may give the signal that it's okay to cry. Offer a tissue and wait while the patient composes himself. Use supportive remarks, such as "I'm glad you got that out," to put the patient at ease. It's unusual for crying to escalate and become uncontrollable.

The confusing patient
Patients with multiple symptoms can be confusing. Focus on the meaning or the function of the symptoms and guide the interview appropriately. Multiple medical illnesses may be the cause of a positive review of systems, but a somatization disorder could also be the cause.

   In some instances, you may become confused by the patient. This may occur if the history is vague and difficult to understand, if language is hard to follow, or ideas are poorly related to one another. Use appropriate communication strategies to get the information you're looking for.

   If you suspect a psychiatric or neurologic disorder, don't spend too much time trying to get a detailed history. Shift to the mental status examination and focus on level of consciousness, orientation, and memory.

The angry patient
Encounters with a hostile or angry patient occur occasionally. To maintain control of the interview, don't waste time or energy arguing with the patient or feeling insulted. Rather, listen without showing disapproval. Try to relax. Speak in a firm, quiet voice, and use short sentences. A composed, unobtrusive, and nonthreatening manner usually soothes the patient. However, if this technique fails, postpone the interview and, if necessary, call for assistance.

The patient with a language barrier
When the patient speaks a different language, make every attempt to get an interpreter. The ideal interpreter is an objective person who's familiar with the language and culture of the patient. Beware of using friends and family members as interpreters; confidentiality may be violated or meanings may be distorted.

   Establish a rapport with the interpreter and review what information would be most useful. Tell the interpreter that you need her to interpret exactly what you're saying. Seat the interpreter next to you and allow the patient to establish a rapport with her as well. Address the patient directly and keep sentences short and simple. Be patient and allow more time for this interview.

The patient with reading difficulty
Always assess the patient's reading ability before giving written instructions. Ask "I understand this may be difficult to discuss, but do you have problems reading?" Respond sensitively and remember that illiteracy isn't synonymous with lack of intelligence.

The patient with impaired hearing

Communicating with a hearing-impaired patient presents many of the same challenges as communicating with those who speak a different language. Ask the patient what his preferred method of communication is. If he prefers sign language, make every effort to find an interpreter.

If the patient can read lips, follow these guidelines:
+ Face him directly, in good light.
+ Speak at a normal tone and rate.
+ Don't let your voice trail off at the ends of sentences.
+ Avoid covering your mouth or looking down.
+ Have him repeat what you said back to you.

If the patient has unilateral hearing loss, sit on the hearing side. If he has a hearing aid, make sure he's using it and that it's functioning properly. Eliminate background noise as much as possible. Supplement instructions with written copies.

The patient with impaired vision

Use the following suggestions when interviewing a blind patient:
+ Shake hands to establish contact.
+ Explain who you are and why you're there.
+ Orient him to the room and tell him if anyone else is present.
+ Remember to use words in response because postures and gestures are unseen.

MAINTAINING A PROFESSIONAL OUTLOOK

Don't let your personal opinions interfere with your assessment. Maintain a professional, neutral approach and don't offer advice. For example, don't suggest that the patient enter a drug rehabilitation program. That type of response puts him on the defensive and may make him reluctant to answer subsequent questions honestly.

Also, avoid saying such things as, "The physician knows what's best for you." Such statements make the patient feel inferior and break down communication. Finally, don't use leading questions such as "You don't do drugs, do you?" to get the answer you're hoping for. This type of question, based on your own value system, will make the patient feel guilty and might prevent him from responding honestly.

REVIEWING STRUCTURES AND SYSTEMS

The final part of the health history is a systematic assessment of the patient's body structures and systems. Always start at the top of the head and work your way down the body. This helps ensure that you cover every area.

SPECIAL POINTS *When questioning an elderly patient, remember that he may have difficulty hearing or communicating. He may have sensory impairment, impaired memory, or a decreased attention span. If your patient is confused or has trouble communicating, you may need to rely on a family member for some or all of the health history.*

ASKING THE RIGHT QUESTIONS

Information gained from a health history forms the basis for your care plan, enabling you to distinguish physical changes and devise a holistic approach to treatment. As with other nursing skills, you can improve your interviewing technique only with practice, practice, and more practice. (See *Evaluating a symptom*, page 16.)

The hearing-impaired patient

+ Provide a sign-language interpreter, if requested
+ Sit on the patient's hearing side
+ Face patient directly and speak at a normal tone and rate
+ Have patient repeat what you say
+ Supplement oral instructions with written copies

The vision-impaired patient

+ Shake hands to establish contact
+ Identify yourself and why you're there
+ Orient patient to the room
+ Use words instead of postures and gestures

Tips for maintaining a professional outlook

+ Don't let your personal opinions interfere
+ Don't offer advice
+ Maintain a professional, neutral approach
+ Don't use leading questions

Reviewing structures and systems

+ Final part of the health history
+ Assess patient from head to toe

Asking the right questions

+ Forms basis for your care plan
+ Improves with practice

Evaluating a symptom

- Identify problem
- Form a first impression
- Take a brief or thorough history, depending on urgency
- Perform a focused physical examination
- Perform a full physical examination if time permits
- Evaluate your findings
- Intervene appropriately
- After patient is stabilized, review your findings again
- Devise your care plan

KNOW-HOW

Evaluating a symptom

The patient is vague in describing his chief complaint. Using your interviewing skills, you discover his problem is related to abdominal distention. Now what? This flowchart will help you decide what to do next, using abdominal distention as the patient's chief complaint.

Question the patient to identify the symptom bothering him. He tells you, "My stomach gets bloated."

Form a first impression. Does the patient's condition alert you to an emergency? For example, does he say the bloating developed suddenly? Does he mention that other signs or symptoms occur with it, such as sweating or light-headedness? (Both are indicators of hypovolemia.)

Yes

Take a brief history to gather more clues. For example, ask the patient if he has severe abdominal pain or difficulty breathing or if he has ever had an abdominal injury.

Perform a focused physical examination to quickly determine the severity of the patient's condition. Check for bruising, lacerations, changes in bowel sounds, or abdominal rigidity.

No

Now, take a thorough history to get an overview of the patient's condition. Ask him about associated signs or symptoms. Note especially GI disorders that can lead to abdominal distention.

Now, thoroughly examine the patient to evaluate the chief sign or symptom and to detect additional signs and symptoms. Place the patient in a recumbent position and observe him for abdominal asymmetry. Inspect the skin, auscultate for bowel sounds, percuss and palpate the abdomen, and measure his abdominal girth.

Evaluate your findings. Are emergency signs or symptoms present, such as abdominal rigidity or abnormal bowel sounds?

Yes

Based on your findings, intervene appropriately to stabilize the patient. Notify the physician immediately, place the patient in a supine position, administer oxygen, and start an I.V. line. GI or nasogastric tube insertion and emergency surgery may be needed.

After the patient's condition is stabilized, review your findings to consider possible causes, such as trauma, large-bowel obstruction, mesenteric artery occlusion, or peritonitis.

No

Review your findings to consider possible causes, such as cancer, bladder distention, cirrhosis, heart failure, or gastric dilation.

Evaluate your findings and devise an appropriate care plan. Position the patient comfortably, administer analgesics, and prepare the patient for diagnostic tests.

Here are some key questions to ask your patient about each body structure and system. You may need to alter your history taking if the patient is in pain or unable to answer your questions.

General health

What's your usual weight? Have you noticed that your clothes fit more loosely or tightly than usual? Do you suffer from excessive fatigue? How many colds or other minor illnesses do you have each year? Do you ever have unexplained episodes of fevers, weakness, or night sweats? Do you ever have trouble carrying out ADLs?

Skin, hair, and nails

Do you have any known skin diseases such as psoriasis? Do you have rashes, scars, sores, or ulcers? Do you have any skin growths, such as warts, moles, tumors, or masses? Do you experience skin reactions to hot or cold weather? Have you noticed any changes in the amount, texture, or character of your hair? Have you noticed any changes in your nails? Do you have excessive nail splitting, cracking, or breaking?

Head

Do you get headaches? If so, where is the pain located and how intense is it? How often do the headaches occur, and how long do they last? Does anything trigger them, and how do you relieve them? Have you ever had a head injury? Do you have lumps or bumps on your head?

Eyes, ears, and nose

When was your last eye examination? Do you wear glasses or contact lenses? Do you have glaucoma, cataracts, or color blindness? Does light bother your eyes? Do you have excessive tearing, blurred vision, double vision, or dry, itchy, burning, inflamed, or swollen eyes?

Do you have loss of balance, ringing in your ears, deafness, or poor hearing? Have you ever had ear surgery? If so, why and when? Do you wear a hearing aid? Are you having pain, swelling, or discharge from your ears? If so, has this problem occurred before and how frequently?

Have you ever had nasal surgery? If so, why and when? Have you ever had sinusitis or nosebleeds? Do you have nasal problems that cause breathing difficulties, frequent sneezing, or discharge?

Mouth and throat

Do you have mouth sores, a dry mouth, loss of taste, a toothache, or bleeding gums? Do you wear dentures, and do they fit? Do you have a sore throat, fever, or chills? How often do you get a sore throat, and have you seen a physician for this?

Do you have difficulty swallowing? If so, is the problem with solids or liquids? Is it a constant problem or does it accompany sore throat or another problem? What, if anything, makes it go away?

Neck

Do you have swelling, soreness, lack of movement, stiffness, or pain in your neck? If so, did something specific cause it to happen such as too much exercise? How long have you had this symptom? Does anything relieve it or aggravate it?

Respiratory system

Do you have shortness of breath on exertion or while lying in bed? How many pillows do you use at night? Do you have pain or wheezing when breathing? Do you have a productive cough? If so, do you cough up blood-tinged sputum? Do you have night sweats?

Key questions about general health
+ Usual weight
+ Clothing fit
+ Fatigue, minor illnesses, fevers, weakness, or night sweats
+ Inability to perform ADLs

Key questions about skin, hair, and nails
+ Skin diseases, rashes, scars, sores, or ulcers
+ Skin growths, warts, or moles
+ Changes in amount, texture, or character of hair
+ Nail splitting or breaking

Key questions about the head
+ Headache location, incidence, duration, and relief
+ Lumps or bumps on head

Key questions about eyes, ears, and nose
+ Date of last eye examination and findings
+ Glasses, color blindness, inflammation, other eye disorders
+ Ear disorders or surgery
+ Nasal problems or surgery

Key questions about the mouth and throat
+ Mouth or gum problems, dryness, dentures
+ Swallowing problems

Key questions about the neck
+ Swelling, soreness, or immobility
+ Stiffness or pain

Key respiratory questions
+ Shortness of breath, pain, wheezing, cough, night sweats
+ History of pneumonia or other respiratory infections

Have you ever been treated for pneumonia, asthma, emphysema, or frequent respiratory tract infections? Have you ever had a chest X-ray or a tuberculin skin test? If so, when, and what were the results?

Cardiovascular system

Do you have chest pain, palpitations, irregular heartbeat, fast heartbeat, shortness of breath, or a persistent cough? Have you ever had an electrocardiogram? If so, when?

Do you have high blood pressure, peripheral vascular disease, swelling of the ankles and hands, varicose veins, cold extremities, or intermittent pain in your legs?

Breasts

Ask women these questions: Do you perform monthly breast self-examinations? Have you noticed a lump, a change in breast contour, breast pain, or discharge from your nipples? Did you breast-feed? If so, when and for how long? Have you ever had breast cancer? If not, has anyone else in your family had it? Have you ever had a mammogram? When, and what were the results?

Ask men these questions: Do you have pain in your breast tissue? Have you noticed lumps or a change in contour?

GI system

Have you had nausea, vomiting, loss of appetite, heartburn, abdominal pain, frequent belching, or passing of gas? Have you lost or gained weight recently? How often do you have a bowel movement, and what color, odor, and consistency are your stools? Have you noticed a change in your regular pattern? Do you use laxatives frequently? Have you had hemorrhoids, rectal bleeding, hernias, gallbladder disease, or a liver disease such as hepatitis?

Urinary system

Do you have urinary problems, such as burning during urination, incontinence, frequency, urgency, retention, reduced urinary flow, or dribbling? Do you get up during the night to urinate? If so, how many times? What color is your urine? Have you ever noticed blood in it? Have you been treated for kidney stones?

Reproductive system

Ask women these questions: How old were you when you started menstruating? How often do you get your period, and how long does it usually last? Do you notice any premenstrual tension or changes in your mood? Do you have clots or pain? If you're postmenopausal, at what age did you stop menstruating? If you're perimenopausal, what symptoms are you experiencing? Have you ever been pregnant? If so, how many times? Did you ever have problems with infertility? Did you have complications with pregnancy or delivery? What was the method of delivery? How many pregnancies resulted in live births? How many resulted in miscarriages? Have you ever had an abortion?

Are you sexually active? With men, women, or both? Are you involved in a long-term, monogamous relationship? What's your method of birth control? Have you had frequent vaginal infections or a sexually transmitted disease? Do you have vaginal discharge, itching, sores, or lumps? When was your last gynecologic examination and Papanicolaou test? What were the results?

Ask men these questions: Do you perform monthly testicular self-examinations? Have you ever had a prostate examination and, if so, when? Have you noticed penile pain, discharge, or lesions or testicular lumps? Are you sexually active? With men, women, or both? Which form of birth control do you use? Have you ever had a hernia? If so, when and how was it treated? Have you had a vasectomy? Are you

---

Key cardiovascular questions

- Chest pain, palpitations, cough
- High blood pressure, swelling, varicose veins, cold extremities

Key questions about the breasts

- Lumps, pain, discharge, contour
- History of breast cancer
- Mammogram, breast-feeding

Key GI questions

- Nausea, vomiting, appetite loss
- Heartburn, abdominal pain, gas
- Elimination pattern, laxative use, bleeding
- Hernia, gallbladder disease, hepatitis

Key urinary questions

- Burning during urination
- Incontinence, frequency, urgency, retention, reduced flow
- Urine color or kidney stones

Key reproductive questions

Women
- Start of menses, duration, and character; menopause
- Premenstrual mood changes
- Pregnancy and deliveries
- Sexual activity, birth control methods, STDs

Men
- Testicular self-examinations, prostate examinations
- Penile pain, discharge, lesions, testicular lumps, vasectomy
- Sexual activity, birth control methods, STDs

involved in a long-term, monogamous relationship? Have you ever had a sexually transmitted disease?

Musculoskeletal system

Do you have difficulty walking, sitting, or standing? Are you steady on your feet, or do you lose your balance easily? Do you have arthritis, gout, a back injury, muscle weakness, or paralysis?

Neurologic system

Have you ever had seizures? Do you ever experience tremors, twitching, numbness, tingling, or loss of sensation in a part of the body? Are you less able to get around than you think you should be?

Endocrine system

Have you been unusually tired lately? Do you feel hungry or thirsty more than usual? Have you lost weight for unexplained reasons? How well can you tolerate heat or cold? Have you noticed changes in your hair texture or color? Have you been losing hair? Do you take hormone medications?

Hematologic system

Have you ever been diagnosed with anemia or blood abnormalities? Do you bruise easily or become fatigued quickly? Have you ever had a blood transfusion? If so, did you have any transfusion reactions?

Emotional status

Do you ever experience mood swings or memory loss? Do you ever feel anxious, depressed, or unable to concentrate? Are you feeling unusually stressed? Do you ever feel unable to cope? Have you ever attempted suicide or contemplated it?

Conclude the health history by summarizing all findings. For the well patient, list the patient's health promotion strengths and resources along with defined health education needs. If the interview points out a significant health problem, tell the patient what it is and begin to address the problem. This may involve referral to a physician, education, or plans for further investigation.

Key musculoskeletal questions
- ✦ Trouble walking, sitting, standing
- ✦ Arthritis, gout, back injury, muscle weakness, paralysis

Key neurologic questions
- ✦ Seizures, tremors, twitching
- ✦ Numbness, tingling, loss of sensation

Key endocrine questions
- ✦ Fatigue, hunger, thirst, weight loss
- ✦ Heat and cold intolerance
- ✦ Changes in hair texture or color

Key hematologic questions
- ✦ Anemia or blood abnormalities
- ✦ Bruising easily or quickly fatigued
- ✦ Blood transfusions or reactions.

Key questions about emotional status
- ✦ Mood swings, anxiety, or depression
- ✦ Memory loss or inability to concentrate
- ✦ Stress, inability to cope, suicide attempt

Fundamental physical assessment techniques

Physical assessment

+ Measures vital signs, height, and weight
+ Assesses all organs and body systems
+ Allows for patient teaching
+ Hones critical thinking skills
+ Guides your care plan

A LOOK AT PHYSICAL ASSESSMENT

After you've taken the patient's health history, proceed to the hands-on part of the assessment. During the physical assessment, you'll use all of your senses and a systematic approach to collect information about your patient's health. A complete physical examination—appropriate for periodic health checks—includes a general survey, vital sign measurements, height and weight measurements, and assessment of all organs and body systems. At times, a modified physical examination, based on the patient's history and complaints, may be warranted.

As you proceed through the physical examination, you can also teach your patient about his body. For instance, you can explain how to do a testicular self-examination or why the patient should monitor the appearance of a mole.

More than anything else, successful assessment requires critical thinking. How does one finding fit in with the big picture? An initial assessment guides your whole care plan.

Preparation

+ Take time to prepare
+ Plan your approach and demeanor
+ Start by washing your hands in front of the patient

PREPARING FOR THE EXAMINATION

Take the time to prepare for the examination before beginning. Think about how you'll approach the patient, your demeanor, and how you'll make the patient comfortable. Make sure you wash your hands before beginning and that you do this in front of the patient—it's a subtle way to show concern for the patient's welfare.

APPROACHING THE PATIENT

When first examining a patient, feelings of anxiety are inevitable. Let the patient know if you're new at doing physical assessments and try to appear calm, competent, and organized. You may need to go back and assess certain things that you've forgotten. This isn't uncommon. Even though you may be doing certain items out of order, try to do so smoothly, without causing too much discomfort to the patient.

If you're a beginner at physical assessments, certain tasks may take you longer than experienced clinicians. Explain to the patient ahead of time if you anticipate taking a long time for certain aspects of the examination. State "I'll be spending a little extra time listening to your lungs, but this doesn't mean that I hear anything wrong."

Over time, as you become more comfortable doing physical assessments, you'll become quicker and more efficient. You may begin sharing your findings with the patient as you go along. Be selective, however, of what you share. You may want to finish your complete assessment before making conclusions. If you find an unexpected abnormality, such as a suspicious lesion or a wound, avoid showing alarm or other negative reaction.

Scope of the examination

How complete should your assessment be? This question has no definite answer. As a rule, a new patient should have a complete physical examination, regardless of his reason for seeking care or the type of setting in which you practice. A more limited or problem-focused assessment may be appropriate for the patient requiring urgent care or a patient you know well.

A comprehensive examination is more than an assessment of body systems. It also:
+ is a source of knowledge about the patient
+ helps to identify or rule out physical cause for the patient's concerns
+ serves as a baseline for future comparisons
+ provides important opportunities for health promotion
+ increases the credibility of your reassurance and advice.

If you'll be performing a focused examination, choose the methods for assessing the problem carefully. The scope of your examination should be determined by:
+ the patient's symptoms
+ the patient's age
+ the patient's health history
+ your knowledge of disease patterns.

For example, if a patient presents with a sore throat, you'll need to decide if he needs careful palpation of the liver and spleen to assess for mononucleosis, or if he has a cold and this examination isn't necessary.

Periodic physical assessment for screening and prevention is recommended for several areas. These include:
+ blood pressure measurement
+ cardiac assessment
+ breast examination
+ assessment for splenic and hepatic enlargement
+ pelvic examination with a Papanicolaou test.

Planning some logistics

The examination sequence should be planned to maximize patient comfort, avoid frequent position changes, and enhance your efficiency. As a rule, move from "head to toe." (See *Suggested physical examination sequence,* page 22.)

Approaching the patient

+ Act calm, competent, and organized
+ Assess patient in a certain order
+ Assure patient there isn't necessarily anything wrong if you take extra time
+ Be selective of what you share
+ Finish assessment before making any conclusions

Scope of the examination

+ Determined by patient's symptoms, age, and health history
+ Based on your knowledge of disease patterns

Comprehensive examination
+ Provides a source of knowledge about your patient
+ Helps identify or rule out physical cause
+ Serves as a baseline for future comparisons
+ Provides opportunity for health promotion
+ Increases your credibility

Periodic physical assessment
+ Helps with screening and prevention

Planning some logistics

+ Plan examination sequence
+ Avoid frequent position changes
+ Move from "head to toe"
+ Stand on the patient's right side for better assessment of jugular vein distention, apical pulse, and right kidney

Suggested physical examination sequence

You'll develop your own personal sequence for physical assessments as you gain more experience. Use the suggested sequence below as a guide.

In the sitting position:
✦ General survey
✦ Vital signs
✦ Skin of upper torso (anterior and posterior)
✦ Head and neck, including thyroid and lymph nodes
✦ Mental status, cranial nerves, upper extremity strength and tone, cerebellar function
✦ Thorax and lungs
✦ Breasts
✦ Musculoskeletal assessment of upper extremities

In the supine position, turned to the left side, with the head of the bed raised 30 degrees:
✦ Cardiovascular assessment

Sitting, leaning forward:
✦ Cardiovascular assessment (for murmur of aortic insufficiency)
Lying supine:
✦ Thorax and lungs
✦ Breasts and axillae
✦ Abdomen
✦ Peripheral vascular and skin of the lower extremities and lower torso
✦ Lower extremity strength and tone, reflexes
Standing:
✦ Gait
✦ Musculoskeletal examination
Lithotomy position:
✦ Pelvic and rectal examinations of women
Supine, turned to left side:
✦ Prostate and rectal examinations of men

It's recommended that you perform the physical assessment while standing at the patient's right side and moving to different positions as necessary. This technique has several advantages compared to the left side:
✦ It's more reliable to assess jugular vein distention from the right.
✦ The palpating hand rests easier on the apical impulse.
✦ The right kidney can be palpated more frequently than the left kidney.

ADJUSTING THE ENVIRONMENT

Adjusting the environment
✦ Position patient for mutual comfort
✦ Adjust height of bed or table as needed
✦ Adjust lighting level as needed for inspection
✦ Arrange a quiet environment to facilitate auscultation

The reliability of your assessment depends on several factors, including your comfort, lighting, and noise. Take the time to adjust the examination area for your comfort. Raise the bed or table, if needed, being sure to lower it again at the end of the examination. You may need to ask the patient to move closer to you at times to make it easier for you to reach certain areas of the body. Awkward positions will impair the quality of your assessments.

Good lighting is important for the inspection aspect of your assessment. When a light source is perpendicular to the patient, shadows are minimized and subtle changes in the surface you're examining may be lost. Tangential lighting casts light across the surfaces of the body and will make contours, elevations, and depressions easier and sharper to visualize. Tangential lighting is optimal for evaluating the jugular venous pulse, the thyroid gland, and the apical impulse.

A quiet environment is optimal during the assessment. Background noise can interfere with auscultation and can be distracting throughout the examination. Try to adjust the environment as best you can. Ask those nearby to lower the volume on their televisions or radios, or to lower their voices. Be courteous and thank them when the examination is completed.

PROMOTING COMFORT

Remain professional during the entire examination and show concern for the patient's privacy and modesty. This will help the patient to feel respected and more at ease. Close doors and curtains before beginning the examination.

You'll learn the methods for draping the patient with a gown or sheet as you assess each of the different organ systems. Indeed, the goal should be to visualize only one area of the body at a time. This preserves the patient's modesty and allows you to better focus on what you're doing. For example, during the abdominal examination, only the abdomen should be exposed. Cover the patient's chest with his gown and place a sheet or drape over the inguinal area and lower extremities.

Before beginning parts of the assessment that may be awkward or stressful for the patient, briefly tell the patient what you'll be doing. Keep the patient informed as you proceed.

Be clear in your instructions at each step of the examination. Say "I'd like to listen to your heart now. Please lie down." Be sensitive to his feelings and comfort. Assess nonverbal cues such as facial expression. Ask "Are you okay?" Rearrange pillows or blankets as needed for comfort and warmth throughout the assessment.

When you're finished, tell the patient your impressions as appropriate. Tell him what to expect next, whether it will be making a follow-up appointment (for an outpatient), or assessing laboratory values (for an inpatient). Leave the hospitalized patient in a comfortable and safe position, with the bed in the low position and the side rails raised.

COLLECTING THE TOOLS

Generally, for a physical examination, a nurse will need a thermometer, stethoscope, sphygmomanometer, visual acuity chart, penlight or flashlight, measuring tape and pocket ruler, marking pencil, and a scale.

A complete collection of equipment will also include these items:
♦ a wooden tongue blade to help assess the gag reflex and reveal the pharynx
♦ safety pins to test how well a patient differentiates between dull and sharp pain
♦ cotton balls to check fine-touch sensitivity
♦ test tubes filled with hot and cold water to assess temperature sensitivity
♦ common, easily identified substances, such as ground coffee and vanilla extract, to evaluate smell and taste sensations
♦ a water-soluble lubricant and disposable gloves for rectal and vaginal examinations.

Certain steps in the physical examination may require such equipment as an ophthalmoscope, a nasoscope, an otoscope, and a tuning fork. Other equipment may include a reflex hammer, skin calipers, vaginal speculum, goniometer, and transilluminator. (See *Reviewing assessment equipment,* pages 24 to 27.)

PERFORMING A GENERAL SURVEY

After assembling the necessary equipment, begin the first part of the physical assessment: forming your initial impressions of the patient, preparing him for the assessment, and obtaining his baseline data, including height, weight, and vital signs. This information will direct the rest of your assessment.

(Text continues on page 27.)

Promoting patient comfort

Privacy
♦ Remain professional and show concern
♦ Close doors and curtains

Modesty
♦ Drape patient with a gown or sheet
♦ Visualize one area at a time

Communication
♦ Explain each step of the examination
♦ Tell patient what to expect when you're finished

The tools
♦ Thermometer
♦ Stethoscope
♦ Sphygmomanometer
♦ Visual acuity chart
♦ Penlight or flashlight
♦ Measuring tape and pocket ruler
♦ Marking pencil
♦ Scale

General survey
♦ Form your initial impressions
♦ Prepare patient for assessment
♦ Obtain height, weight, and vital signs

Reviewing assessment equipment

Physical examination usually requires the following equipment: thermometer, stethoscope, sphygmomanometer, visual acuity charts, and a scale. It may also require an ophthalmoscope, otoscope, nasoscope, tuning forks, reflex hammer, skin calipers, transilluminator, or a goniometer. The ophthalmoscope comes with various apertures; the otoscope, with specula of various sizes. Nasoscopes, tuning forks, reflex hammers, skin calipers, transilluminators, and goniometers are available in several types.

THERMOMETER

Several types of thermometers measure body temperature, such as chemical dot, digital, electronic digital, and infrared. Each type provides accurate readings when used properly.

CHEMICAL DOT THERMOMETER

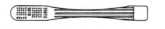

DIGITAL THERMOMETER

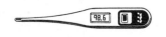

INFRARED THERMOMETER

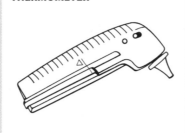

ELECTRONIC DIGITAL THERMOMETER

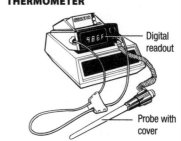

STETHOSCOPE

All stethoscopes have earpieces, binaurals, tubing, and a chest piece (head). However, some have several removable chestpieces suitable for adult and pediatric patients. Others, designed specifically for use on an adult or a child, have only one chestpiece.

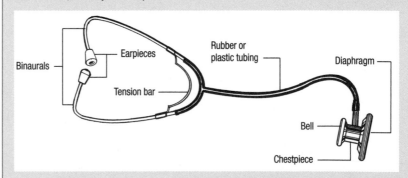

Reviewing assessment equipment *(continued)*

OTOSCOPE

Used to assess the ear, the otoscope consists of a handle and battery housing, a head with a light source and magnifying lens, and removable specula of varying sizes.

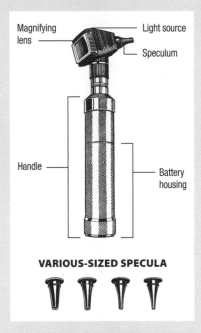

Magnifying lens

Light source

Speculum

Handle

Battery housing

VARIOUS-SIZED SPECULA

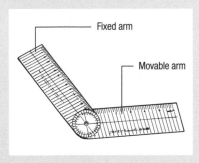

GONIOMETER

Used to assess joint motion, this device is a protractor with a movable arm and a fixed arm (axis). The center, or zero point, is placed on the patient's joint; the fixed arm is placed perpendicular to the plane of motion. As the patient moves the joint, the movable arm indicates the angle in degrees.

Fixed arm

Movable arm

TUNING FORK

Used to assess touch and hearing, tuning forks produce specific frequencies when struck. A low-frequency fork, such as a 256-Hz device, can test vibration sensation; a high-frequency fork, such as a 512-Hz device, can test hearing.

256-HZ FORK

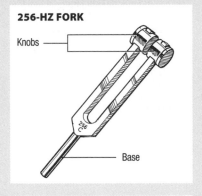

Knobs

Base

512-HZ FORK

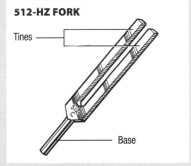

Tines

Base

SKIN CALIPERS

Used to assess a patient's nutritional status, skin calipers measure the thickness in millimeters of subcutaneous tissue.

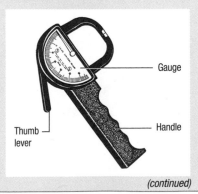

Gauge

Handle

Thumb lever

(continued)

Reviewing assessment equipment *(continued)*

SPHYGMOMANOMETER

Most hospitals have aneroid manometers, with a needle gauge that shows the pressure; others may have sphygmomanometers with mercury manometers but many are phasing this out.

MERCURY MANOMETER

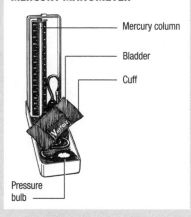

- Mercury column
- Bladder
- Cuff
- Pressure bulb

ANEROID MANOMETER

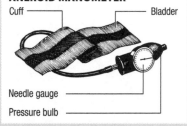

- Cuff
- Bladder
- Needle gauge
- Pressure bulb

REFLEX HAMMER

Used to evaluate deep tendon reflexes during the neurologic assessment, this small, rubber-tipped hammer is also called a *percussion hammer.*

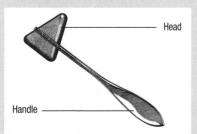

- Head
- Handle

OPHTHALMOSCOPE

Used to assess the eyes, the ophthalmoscope consists of a handle, which holds batteries, and a head, which twists into place. The head contains a system of mirrors and lenses and a light source. Various apertures fit over the lenses.

FRONT VIEW

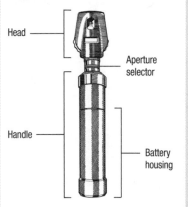

- Head
- Aperture selector
- Handle
- Battery housing

BACK VIEW

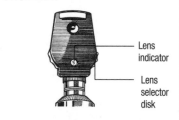

- Lens indicator
- Lens selector disk

APERTURES

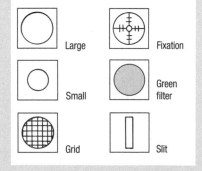

- Large
- Fixation
- Small
- Green filter
- Grid
- Slit

Reviewing assessment equipment *(continued)*

NASOSCOPE

Used to assess the nostrils, the nasoscope consists of a short, narrow head fitted with a light. A metal nasal speculum used with a penlight, or an ophthalmoscope fitted with a special nasal tip may also be used to examine the nasal interior.

OPHTHALMOSCOPE WITH NASAL TIP

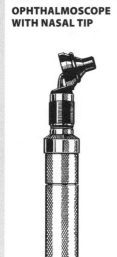

NASOSCOPE WITH LIGHT

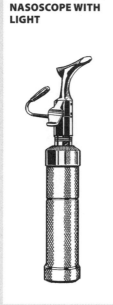

NASAL SPECULUM

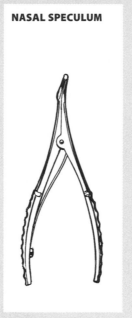

TRANSILLUMINATOR

Used to assess sinus contents, identify hydrocephalus in a child, or detect a scrotal hydrocele, this battery-operated device consists of an ophthalmoscope handle and a transilluminator head (light source with a narrowed light beam). When pressed against the body in a darkened room, the light produces a red glow that can detect air, tissues, or fluid. Electric transilluminators are also available. (*Note:* a flashlight can be converted to a transilluminator by placing a rubber adaptor over its lamp).

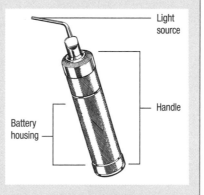

Light source

Handle

Battery housing

During your first contact with the patient, be prepared to receive a steady stream of impressions, mostly visual. The patient's gender, race, and approximate age will be obvious. Because some health concerns may relate to these factors, be sure to note them. Also be sure to note less obvious factors that can contribute to an overall impression, including signs of distress; facial characteristics; body type, posture, and movements; speech; dress, grooming, and personal hygiene; and psychological state. (See *Observing the patient,* page 28.)

First-contact impressions

✦ Gender, race, approximate age
✦ Signs of distress
✦ Facial and body characteristics
✦ Posture and movements
✦ Speech
✦ Dress, grooming, personal hygiene
✦ Psychological state

Observing the patient

The patient's behavior and appearance can offer subtle clues about his health. Carefully observe him for unusual behavior or signs of illness. Use this mnemonic checklist — SOME TEAMS — to help you remember what to look for:

S **SYMMETRY**
Are his face and body symmetrical?

O **OLD**
Does he look his age?

M **MENTAL ACUITY**
Is he alert, confused, agitated, or inattentive?

E **EXPRESSION**
Does he appear ill, in pain, or anxious?

T **TRUNK**
Is he lean, stocky, obese, or barrel-chested?

E **EXTREMITIES**
Are his fingers clubbed? Does he have joint abnormalities or edema?

A **APPEARANCE**
Is he clean and appropriately dressed?

M **MOVEMENT**
Are his posture, gait, and coordination normal? Does he move around in a normal fashion?

S **SPEECH**
Is his speech relaxed, clear, strong, understandable, and appropriate? Does it sound stressed?

Preparing the patient

+ Introduce yourself before assessment
+ Keep in mind that patient may be apprehensive
+ Explain what you'll do
+ Tell him about position changes and equipment
+ Maintain a professional attitude

PREPARING THE PATIENT

If possible, introduce yourself to the patient before the assessment, preferably when he's dressed. Meeting him under less-threatening circumstances will decrease his anxiety when you actually perform the assessment. (See *Tips for assessment success*.)

Keep in mind that the patient may be worried that you'll find a problem. He may also consider the assessment an invasion of his privacy because you're observing and touching sensitive, private and, perhaps, painful body areas.

Before you start, briefly explain what you're planning to do, why you're doing it, how long it will take, what position changes it will require, and what equipment you'll use. As you perform the assessment, explain each step in detail. A well-prepared patient won't be surprised or feel unexpected discomfort, so he'll trust you more and cooperate better.

Put your patient at ease but know where to draw the line. Maintain professionalism during the examination. Humor can help put the patient at ease but avoid sarcasm and keep jokes in good taste.

When you're finished with your assessment, allow the patient to get dressed. Document your findings in a short, concise paragraph. Include only essential information that communicates your overall impression of the patient. For example, if your patient has a lesion, simply note it now. You'll describe the lesion in detail when you complete the physical assessment.

Tips for assessment success

Before starting the physical assessment, review this checklist.

- ✦ Eliminate as many distractions and disruptions as possible.
- ✦ Ask your patient to void.
- ✦ Wash your hands before and after the assessment—preferably in the patient's presence.
- ✦ Have all the necessary equipment on hand and in working order.
- ✦ Make sure the examination room is well-lit and warm.
- ✦ Warm your hands and equipment before touching the patient.
- ✦ Be aware of your nonverbal communication and of possible negative reactions from the patient.

OBTAINING BASELINE DATA

Accurate measurements of your patient's height, weight, and vital signs provide critical information about his body functions.

The first time you assess a patient, record his baseline vital signs and statistics. Afterward, take measurements at regular intervals, depending on the patient's condition and your facility's policy. A series of readings usually provide more valuable information than a single set. If you obtain an abnormal value, take the vital sign again to make sure it's accurate. Remember that normal readings vary with the patient's age and from patient to patient (an abnormal value for one patient may be a normal value for another).

Height and weight

For every patient in any setting, record height and weight (anthropometric measurements) as part of your assessment profile. Although the general survey gives an overall impression of body size and type, height and weight measurements provide more-specific information about a patient's general health and nutritional status. These measurements should be taken periodically throughout the patient's life to help evaluate normal growth and development and to identify abnormal patterns of weight gain or loss (frequently an early sign of acute or chronic illness). (See *Measuring height and weight*, page 30.)

 SPECIAL POINTS *Accurate height and weight measurements also serve other important purposes. In children, they guide dosage calculations for various drugs; in adults, they help guide cancer chemotherapy and anesthesia administration, and they help evaluate the response to I.V. fluids, drugs, or nutritional therapy.*

Vital signs

Assessing vital signs—blood pressure, pulse rate, respirations, and temperature—is a basic nursing responsibility and an important method for monitoring essential body functions. Vital signs give insight into the function of specific organs—especially the heart and the lungs—as well as entire body systems. You obtain vital signs to establish baseline measurements, observe for trends, identify physiologic problems, and monitor a patient's response to therapy.

When assessing vital signs, keep in mind that a single measurement usually proves far less valuable than a series of measurements, which can substantiate a trend. In most cases, look for a change—from the normal range, from the patient's normal measurement, or from previous measurements. Because vital signs reflect basic body functions, significant changes warrant further investigation.

Obtaining baseline data

- ✦ Helps to gain critical information about body functions
- ✦ Involves measuring height, weight, and vital signs

Height and weight

- ✦ Reveals general health and nutritional status
- ✦ Helps evaluate normal growth and development
- ✦ Identifies abnormal patterns of weight gain or loss

Special points

- ✦ Guides dosage calculations for drugs in children
- ✦ Guides cancer and anesthetic administration and response to treatments in adults

Vital signs

- ✦ Gives insight into organs and body system functions
- ✦ Establishes baseline measurements
- ✦ Helps observe for trends
- ✦ Identifies physiologic problems
- ✦ Monitors response to therapy

KNOW-HOW

Measuring height and weight

Ask the patient to remove his clothes and shoes and to dress in a hospital gown. Then use these techniques to measure his height and weight.

BALANCING THE SCALE
Slide both weight bars on the scale to zero. The balancing arrow should stop in the center of the open box. If the scale has wheels, lock them before the patient gets on.

MEASURING HEIGHT
Ask the patient to get on the scale and turn his back to it. Move the height bar over his head and lift the horizontal arm. Then lower the bar until the horizontal arm touches the top of his head. Now read the height measurement from the height bar.

MEASURING WEIGHT
Slide the lower weight into the groove representing the largest increment below the patient's estimated weight. For example, if you think the patient weighs 145 lb (65.8 kg), slide the weight into the groove for 100 lb (45.4 kg).

Slide the upper weight across until the arrow on the right stops in the middle of the open box. If the arrow hits the bottom, slide the weight to a lower number. If the arrow hits the top, slide the weight to a higher number.

The patient's weight is the sum of these numbers. For example, if the lower weight is on 150 lb (68 kg) and the upper weight is on 12 lb (5.4 kg), the patient weighs 162 lb (73.5 kg).

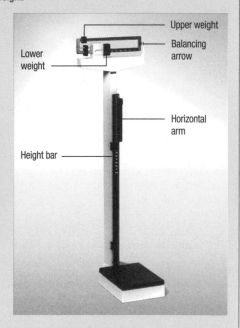

Labels on figure: Lower weight; Upper weight; Balancing arrow; Horizontal arm; Height bar

Blood pressure

Blood pressure measurements are helpful in evaluating cardiac output, fluid and circulatory status, and arterial resistance. Blood pressure measurements consist of systolic and diastolic readings. The systolic reading reflects the maximum pressure exerted on the arterial wall at the peak of left ventricular contraction. Normal systolic pressure is less than 120 mm Hg.

The diastolic reading reflects the minimum pressure exerted on the arterial wall during left ventricular relaxation. This reading is generally more significant than the systolic reading because it evaluates arterial pressure when the heart is at rest. Normal diastolic pressure is less than 80 mm Hg.

The sphygmomanometer, a device used to measure blood pressure, consists of an inflatable cuff, a pressure manometer, and a bulb with a valve. To obtain a blood pressure measurement, center the cuff over an artery, inflate the cuff, and then deflate it. (See *Choosing the right blood pressure cuff,* and *Using a sphygmomanometer,* page 32.)

Choosing the right blood pressure cuff

When choosing a blood pressure cuff, keep these points in mind:
✦ The width of the bladder of the cuff should be about 40% of the circumference of the patient's upper arm.

✦ The length of the bladder of the cuff should be about 80% of the circumference of the patient's arm.
✦ A cuff that's too short or too narrow will give a falsely high reading.

As the cuff deflates, listen with a stethoscope for Korotkoff's sounds, which indicate the systolic and diastolic pressures. Blood pressure can be measured from most extremity pulse points. The brachial artery is used for most patients because of its accessibility. (See *Tips for hearing Korotkoff's sounds,* page 33.)

 ABNORMAL FINDINGS *When assessing a patient's blood pressure for the first time, take measurements in both arms. Consider a slight pressure difference (5 to 10 mm Hg) between arms to be normal; a difference of 15 mm Hg or more may indicate cardiac disease, especially coarctation of the aorta or arterial obstruction.*

In some cases, you may want to assess orthostatic (postural) blood pressure by taking readings with the patient lying down, sitting, and standing, then checking for differences with each position change. Normally, blood pressure rises or falls slightly with a position change. A drop of 20 mm Hg or more, however, indicates orthostatic hypotension.

In a patient with venous congestion or hypertension, you may detect a silent period between systolic and diastolic sounds, when you can't hear intervening pulse sounds. Known as the auscultatory gap, *this phenomenon may cause you to underestimate the systolic or overestimate the diastolic significantly. To avoid either error, be sure to inflate the blood pressure cuff at least 20 mm Hg over the point at which the palpated pulse first disappeared. (See* Assessing hypertension, *page 34.)*

Blood pressure measurement considerations
Anxiety
High blood pressure is frequently caused by anxiety, especially during an initial visit. Try to relax the patient and repeat the procedure later in the examination. If possible, have the patient take his blood pressure at home or in a community setting to rule out "white coat hypertension."

Obese or thin arm
It's important to use a wide cuff for an obese patient's arm. If the patient's arm circumference is greater than 16″ (40.6 cm), use a thigh cuff. For the patient with a very thin arm, you may need to use a pediatric cuff.

Hypertensive patient
To rule out coarctation of the aorta, the following two assessments should be performed for every patient with hypertension:
✦ Comparison of the strength and timing of the radial and femoral pulses
✦ Comparison of the blood pressures in the arm and leg.

To assess the blood pressure in the leg, use a wide, long thigh cuff that has a bladder size of 7″ × 16½″ (17.5 × 42 cm), and apply it to the midthigh. Center the bladder over the posterior surface and listen over the popliteal artery. Ideally, the patient should be in a prone position, but you can also do this with the patient

Blood pressure
(continued)
✦ Use wide cuff or pediatric cuff as necessary

Abnormal findings
✦ Hypertension: may be caused by anxiety
✦ Cardiac disease: difference of 15 mm Hg or more between arms
✦ Orthostatic hypotension: drop of 20 mm Hg or more from sitting to standing position
✦ Venous congestion or hypertension: silent period (auscultatory gap) between systolic and diastolic sounds (avoid by inflating cuff at least 20 mm Hg over point when palpated pulse first disappeared)

Blood pressure measurement considerations

Anxious patient
✦ Try to relax patient and repeat procedure later

Obese or thin-arm patient
✦ Requires use of specialized cuff (thigh cuff for obese patient; pediatric cuff for thin-arm patient)

Hypertensive patient
✦ Compare pulses and blood pressures to rule out aortic coarctation

KNOW-HOW

Using a sphygmomanometer

Follow the guidelines below to use a sphygmomanometer properly:

✦ For accuracy and consistency, position your patient with his upper arm at heart level and his palm turned up.

✦ Apply the cuff snugly, 1″ (2.5 cm) above the brachial pulse, as shown in the top photo.

✦ Position the manometer in line with your eye level.

✦ Palpate the brachial or radial pulse with your fingertips while inflating the cuff.

✦ Inflate the cuff to 30 mm Hg above the point where the pulse disappears.

✦ Place the bell of the stethoscope over the point where you felt the pulse, as shown in the bottom photo. Using the bell will help you better hear Korotkoff's sounds, which indicate pulse.

✦ The sounds will become muffled and then disappear. The last Korotkoff's sound you hear is the diastolic pressure.

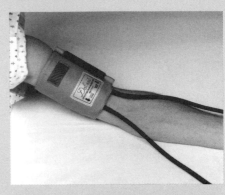

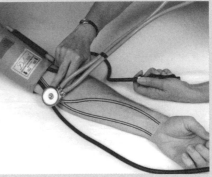

Blood pressure measurement considerations

Abnormal findings

✦ coarctation of the aorta and occlusive aortic disease (femoral pulse weaker and later, and blood pressure lower in legs than arms)

Pulse

✦ Reflects amount of blood ejected with each heartbeat
✦ Note rate, rhythm, and amplitude
✦ Normal: 60 to 100 beats/minute
✦ Radial pulse is the most easily accessible
✦ In cardiovascular emergencies, palpate for femoral or carotid pulse

in a supine position with his leg flexed slightly and his heel resting on the bed or table. When an appropriate-sized cuff is used for the arm and leg, blood pressure measurements should be equal.

 ABNORMAL FINDINGS *Coarctation of the aorta or occlusive aortic disease is suggested by a femoral pulse that's weaker and later than the radial pulse. Also, blood pressure is lower in the legs than in the arms in these conditions.*

Pulse

The patient's pulse reflects the amount of blood ejected with each heartbeat. To assess the pulse, palpate one of the patient's arterial pulse points and note the rate, rhythm, and amplitude (strength) of the pulse. By assessing heartbeat characteristics, you can determine how well the heart handles its blood volume and, indirectly, how well it perfuses organs with oxygenated blood. A normal pulse for an adult is between 60 and 100 beats/minute.

The radial pulse is the most easily accessible. However, in cardiovascular emergencies, you may palpate for the femoral or carotid pulse. The vessels where you palpate for these pulses are larger and closer to the heart and more accurately reflect the heart's activity. (See *Locating pulse sites,* page 35.)

Tips for hearing Korotkoff's sounds

If you have difficulty hearing Korotkoff's sounds, try to intensify them by increasing vascular pressure below the cuff. Here are two techniques you can use.

HAVE THE PATIENT RAISE HIS ARM
Palpate the brachial pulse and mark its location with a pen to avoid losing the pulse spot. Apply the cuff and have the patient raise his arm above his head. Then inflate the cuff about 30 mm Hg above the patient's systolic pressure. Have him lower his arm until the cuff reaches heart level, deflate the cuff, and take a reading.

HAVE THE PATIENT MAKE A FIST
Position the patient's arm at heart level. Inflate the cuff to 30 mm Hg above the patient's systolic pressure and ask him to make a fist. Have him rapidly open and close his hand about 10 times; then deflate the cuff and take the reading.

To palpate for a pulse, use the pads of your index and middle fingers. Press the area over the artery until you feel pulsations. If the rhythm is regular, count the beats for 30 seconds and then multiply by two to get the number of beats per minute. However, when taking the patient's pulse for the first time (or when obtaining baseline data) count the beats for 1 minute.

Avoid using your thumb to count the pulse because the thumb has a strong pulse of its own. If you need to palpate the carotid artery, avoid exerting a lot of pressure, which can stimulate the vagus nerve and cause reflex bradycardia. Also, don't palpate both carotid pulses at the same time. Putting pressure on both sides of the patient's neck can impair cerebral blood flow and function.

 ABNORMAL FINDINGS *If the pulse rhythm is irregular or the patient has a pacemaker, count the beats for 60 seconds. If an irregular pattern is palpated, atrial fibrillation should be suspected. Irregular rhythms should be investigated using an electrocardiogram.*

When you note an irregular pulse, take these steps:
✦ Evaluate whether the irregularity follows a pattern.
✦ Auscultate the apical pulse while palpating the radial pulse. You should feel the pulse every time you hear a heartbeat.
✦ Measure the difference between the apical pulse rate and radial pulse rate, a measurement called the *pulse deficit*.

A pulse deficit occurs when a premature heartbeat can't produce the wave of blood needed to fill the arteries; thus, peripheral radial artery pressure is too low to palpate every heartbeat. To calculate a pulse deficit, have another nurse record one pulse rate while you record the other for 60 seconds. Usually, you must obtain an electrocardiogram to confirm findings.

You also need to assess the pulse amplitude. To do this, use a numerical scale or a descriptive term to rate or describe the strength. Numerical scales differ slightly among facilities but the following scale is commonly used.
✦ Absent pulse — not palpable, measured as 0
✦ Weak or thready pulse — difficult to feel, easily obliterated by slight finger pressure, measured as +1
✦ Normal pulse — easily palpable, obliterated by strong finger pressure, measured as +2
✦ Bounding pulse — readily palpable, forceful, not easily obliterated by pressure from the fingers, measured as +3.

Pulse

Abnormal findings
✦ Irregular pulse rhythm (atrial fibrillation)

Assessing hypertension

The seventh report of the Joint National Committee on Detection, Evaluation, and Treatment of High Blood Pressure recommends that hypertension be diagnosed when a higher than normal level has been found on at least two readings after initial screening. The chart below outlines the classification for adults ages 18 and older.

CATEGORY	SYSTOLIC BLOOD PRESSURE (mm Hg)		DIASTOLIC BLOOD PRESSURE (mm Hg)
Normal	< 120	and	< 80
Prehypertension	120 to 139	or	80 to 89
Stage 1 hypertension	140 to 159	or	90 to 99
Stage 2 hypertension	≥ 160	or	≥ 100

You can also evaluate a patient's heart rate by auscultating at the heart's apex with a stethoscope. This method is superior for assessing heart rhythm (regularity).

Respirations

Along with counting respirations, be aware of the depth and rhythm of each breath. To determine the respiratory rate, count the number of respirations for 60 seconds. A rate of 16 to 20 breaths/minute is normal for an adult. If the patient knows you're counting how often he breathes, he may subconsciously alter the rate. To avoid this, count his respirations while you take his pulse.

Pay attention as well to the depth of the patient's respirations by watching his chest rise and fall. Is his breathing shallow, moderate, or deep? Observe the rhythm and symmetry of his chest wall as it expands during inspiration and relaxes during expiration. If respirations are too shallow to see a rise and fall of the chest wall, hold the back of your hand next to the patient's nose and mouth to feel expirations. Be aware that skeletal deformity, broken ribs, and collapsed lung tissue can cause unequal chest expansion.

 ABNORMAL FINDINGS *Use of accessory muscles can enhance lung expansion when oxygenation drops. Patients with chronic obstructive pulmonary disease (COPD) or respiratory distress may use neck muscles, including the sternocleidomastoid muscles, and abdominal muscles for breathing. The patient's position during normal breathing may also suggest problems such as COPD. Prolonged expiration suggests narrowing in the bronchioles. Normal respirations are quiet and easy, so note abnormal sounds, such as wheezing or stridor.*

Body temperature

Temperature can be measured and recorded in degrees Fahrenheit (° F) or degrees Celsius (° C). You can take a patient's temperature by several routes, including tympanic (infrared), oral, rectal, or axillary. Unless a specific route is ordered, choose the one that seems most appropriate for the patient's age and physical condition. Whichever route you choose, document it on the patient's chart.

Respirations

+ Normal: 16 to 20 breaths/minute
+ Determine if breathing is shallow, moderate, or deep
+ Observe rhythm and symmetry
+ Be aware that skeletal deformity, broken ribs, and collapsed lung tissue can cause unequal chest expansion

Abnormal findings

+ Use of neck, sternocleidomastoid, and abdominal muscles for breathing
+ Prolonged expiration suggesting narrowing in bronchioles
+ Wheezing or stridor

Body temperature

+ Measured and recorded in Fahrenheit (° F) or Celsius (° C)
+ Routes include tympanic (infrared), oral, rectal, or axillary

Locating pulse sites

This illustration shows the locations of the major peripheral arterial pulses and the apical pulse.

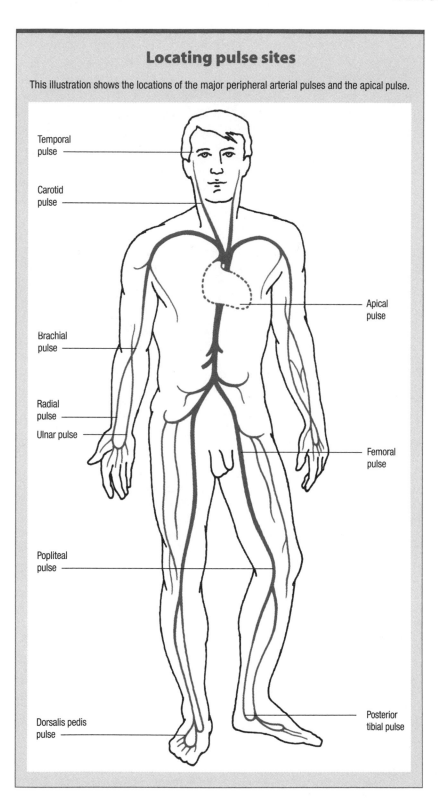

Temporal pulse

Carotid pulse

Brachial pulse

Radial pulse

Ulnar pulse

Popliteal pulse

Dorsalis pedis pulse

Apical pulse

Femoral pulse

Posterior tibial pulse

How temperature readings compare

You can take the patient's temperature four different ways. The chart below compares each route.

ROUTE	NORMAL TEMPERATURE	READING TIME	USED FOR
Oral	97.7° to 99.5° F (36.5° to 37.5° C)	3 to 5 minutes	Adults and older children who are awake, alert, oriented, and cooperative
Axillary (armpit)	96.7° to 98.5° F (35.9° to 36.9° C)	11 minutes	Neonates, patients with impaired immune systems when infection is a concern; less accurate because it can vary with blood flow to the skin
Rectal	98.7° to 100.5° F (37° to 38° C)	2 minutes	Infants, young children, and confused or unconscious patients; wear gloves and lubricate the thermometer
Tympanic (ear)	98.2° to 100° F (36.8° to 37.8° C)	No set time; responds to subtle thermal changes and is unaffected by mouth breathing or patient movement	Adults and children, conscious and cooperative patients, and confused or unconscious patients; provides automatic timing through a push-button device

Temperature routes

Tympanic (infrared)
◆ Causes little or no discomfort to ear canal
◆ Results obtained in seconds

Oral
◆ Interfering factors: mouth breathing, hot or cold beverages, smoking

Rectal
◆ Ideal for hypothermic patients or in children after febrile seizures
◆ Contraindicated in patients with anal lesions, bleeding hemorrhoids, or history of recent rectal surgery

Axillary (armpit)
◆ Ideal for alert patients who have had oral surgery, can't close lips around a thermometer, or with an oxygen mask

Use of the tympanic (infrared) thermometer has become increasingly popular. There's little or no discomfort when it's placed in the ear canal, and the results are obtained in a matter of seconds, providing maximum convenience for the nurse and the patient. Follow the manufacturer's directions for the most accurate results.

The oral route is another convenient method. Ideal for an alert adult, make sure the patient doesn't breathe through his mouth and hasn't had a hot or cold beverage or smoked a cigarette in the past 15 minutes; these factors can cause an inaccurate reading. Avoid taking an oral temperature in a patient who has an oral deformity or who has undergone recent oral surgery. Because of possible breakage, avoid using an oral glass-mercury thermometer in a young child, a confused patient, or a patient with a frequent cough, seizure disorder, or shaking chills.

When absolute accuracy is required, such as with hypothermic patients or with children after febrile seizures, take a temperature rectally. Avoid the rectal route in a patient with anal lesions, bleeding hemorrhoids, or history of recent rectal surgery. Also avoid the rectal route in a patient with a cardiac disorder because it may stimulate the vagus nerve, possibly leading to vasodilation and a decreased heart rate.

You can also measure a temperature by the axillary route if a tympanic thermometer is unavailable. You can use this technique with an alert patient who has had oral surgery, a patient who can't close his lips around a thermometer because of a deformity, or a patient who's wearing an oxygen mask.

Normal body temperature ranges from about 96.8° F to 99.5° F (36° C to 37.5° C). When evaluating temperature, keep in mind that some people have a higher or lower baseline temperature.

Effects of age on vital signs

Vital-sign ranges vary from neonate to older adult, as shown in the chart below.

AGE	TEMPERATURE		PULSE RATE (beats/ minute)	RESPIRATORY RATE (breaths/ minute)	BLOOD PRESSURE (mm Hg)
	°*Fahrenheit*	°*Celsius*			
Neonate	98.6 to 99.8	37 to 37.7	100 to 190	30 to 40	Systolic: 39 to 90 Diastolic: 16 to 60
3 years	98.5 to 99.5	36.9 to 37.5	80 to 125	20 to 30	Systolic: 78 to 114 Diastolic: 46 to 78
10 years	97.5 to 98.6	36.4 to 37	70 to 110	16 to 22	Systolic: 90 to 132 Diastolic: 56 to 86
16 years	97.6 to 98.8	36.4 to 37.1	55 to 100	15 to 20	Systolic: 104 to 142 Diastolic: 60 to 92
Adult	96.8 to 99.5	36 to 37.5	60 to 100	12 to 20	Systolic: 95 to 140 Diastolic: 60 to 90
Older adult	96.5 to 97.5	35.8 to 36.4	60 to 100	15 to 25	Systolic: 140 to 160 Diastolic: 70 to 90

 ABNORMAL FINDINGS *Hyperthermia describes an oral temperature above 106° F (41.1° C). Causes of hyperthermia include:*
✦ *infection*
✦ *trauma*
✦ *malignancy*
✦ *blood disorders*
✦ *drug reactions*
✦ *immune disorders.*

Hypothermia describes a rectal temperature below 95° F (35° C). The main cause of hypothermia is exposure to cold.

To convert Celsius to Fahrenheit, multiply the Celsius temperature by 1.8 and add 32. To convert Fahrenheit to Celsius, subtract 32 from the Fahrenheit temperature and divide by 1.8. (See *How temperature readings compare,* and *Effects of age on vital signs.*)

Body temperature

Abnormal findings
✦ Hyperthermia — oral temperature above 106° F (41.1° C) caused by infection, trauma, malignancy, blood disorders, drug reactions, and immune disorders
✦ Hypothermia — rectal temperature below 95° F (35° C) caused by exposure to cold

Physical assessment techniques

✦ Inspection
✦ Palpation
✦ Percussion
✦ Auscultation

Facts about inspection

✦ Yields false or misleading findings if done hastily
✦ Direct inspection: Relies on sight, hearing, and smell
✦ Indirect inspection: Uses equipment to expose internal tissues or to enhance view of a specific body area
✦ Covers landmarks, color, size, location, movement, texture, symmetry, odors, and sounds

Facts about palpation

✦ Feels pulsations and vibrations
✦ Locates body structures
✦ Assesses size, texture, warmth, mobility, and tenderness
✦ Detects pulse, muscle rigidity, enlarged lymph nodes, skin or hair dryness, organ tenderness, or breast lumps
✦ Measures chest expansion and contraction with each respiration

PHYSICAL ASSESSMENT TECHNIQUES

During the physical assessment, use drapes so only the area being examined is exposed. Develop a pattern for your assessment, starting with the same body system and proceeding in the same sequence. Organize your steps to minimize the number of times the patient needs to change position. By using a systematic approach, you'll also be less likely to forget an area.

No matter where you start your physical assessment, you'll use four techniques: inspection, palpation, percussion, and auscultation. The techniques are used in sequence, except when performing an abdominal assessment. Because palpation and percussion can alter bowel sounds, the sequence for assessing the abdomen is: inspection, auscultation, percussion, and palpation.

INSPECTION

Critical observation or inspection is the most commonly used assessment technique. It begins when you first meet the patient and continues throughout the health history and physical examination. Performed correctly, it also reveals more than the other techniques. However, an incomplete or hasty inspection may neglect important details or even yield false or misleading findings. To ensure accurate, useful information, approach inspection in a careful, unhurried manner, pay close attention to details, and try to draw logical conclusions from the findings.

Inspection can be direct or indirect. During direct inspection, rely totally on sight, hearing, and smell. During indirect inspection, use equipment such as a nasal or vaginal speculum or an ophthalmoscope to expose internal tissues or to enhance the view of a specific body area.

To inspect a specific body area, first make sure the area is sufficiently exposed and adequately lit. Then survey the entire area, noting key landmarks and checking the overall condition. Next, focus on specifics, such as color, size, location, movement, texture, symmetry, odors, and sounds.

PALPATION

Palpation requires you to touch the patient with different parts of your hand, using varying degrees of pressure. To do this, you need short fingernails and warm hands. It involves touching the body to feel pulsations and vibrations, to locate body structures (particularly in the abdomen), and to assess such characteristics as size, texture, warmth, mobility, and tenderness. Palpation allows you to detect a pulse, muscle rigidity, enlarged lymph nodes, skin or hair dryness, organ tenderness, or breast lumps as well as measure the chest's expansion and contraction with each respiration. Always palpate tender areas last. Tell the patient the purpose of your touch and what you're feeling with your hands.

Usually, palpation follows inspection. For example, if a rash is present on inspection, determine through palpation if the rash has a raised surface or feels tender or warm. However, during an abdominal or urinary system examination, palpation should be performed last to avoid causing the patient discomfort and stimulating peristalsis (smooth muscle contractions that force food through the GI tract, bile through the bile duct, and urine through the ureters).

Correct palpation requires a highly developed sense of touch. Learn to use the various parts of the fingers and hands for different purposes; also expect to learn several palpation techniques. (See *Understanding palpation techniques.*)

KNOW-HOW

Understanding palpation techniques

To perform thorough assessments, you'll need to learn the four palpation techniques described below. *Light palpation* involves using the tips and pads of the fingers to apply light pressure to the skin surface. *Deep palpation* requires the use of both hands and heavier pressure. *Light ballottement* involves gentle, repetitive bouncing of tissues against the hand (think of bouncing a small ball gently). *Deep ballottement* requires heavier pressure to assess deeper structures.

LIGHT PALPATION
For light palpation, press gently on the skin, indenting it ½″ to ¾″ (1 to 2 cm). Use the lightest touch possible because too much pressure blunts your sensitivity. To concentrate on what you're feeling, close your eyes.

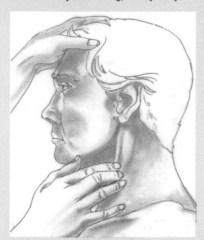

DEEP PALPATION (BIMANUAL PALPATION)
For deep palpation, increase your fingertip pressure, indenting the skin about 1½″ (3.8 cm). Place your other hand on top of the palpating hand to control and guide your movements. To perform a variation of deep palpation that allows pinpointing an inflamed area, press firmly with one hand, and then lift your hand away quickly. If the patient complains of increased pain as you release the pressure, you've identified rebound tenderness. (Suspect peritonitis if you elicit rebound tenderness when examining the abdomen.)

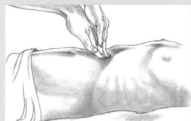

LIGHT BALLOTTEMENT
To perform light ballottement, apply light, rapid pressure from quadrant to quadrant on the patient's abdomen. Keep your hand on the skin surface to detect any tissue rebound.

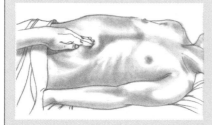

DEEP BALLOTTEMENT
To perform deep ballottement, apply abrupt, deep pressure, then release the pressure, but maintain fingertip contact with the skin.

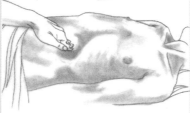

Key techniques for palpation
✦ Light palpation — involves using tips and pads of fingers to apply light pressure to skin's surface
✦ Deep palpation — requires use of both hands and heavier pressure
✦ Light ballottement — involves gentle, repetitive bouncing of tissues against the hand
✦ Deep ballottement — requires heavier pressure to assess deeper structures

Key features to palpate
✦ Texture
✦ Temperature
✦ Moisture
✦ Motion
✦ Consistency of structures

Don't forget to wear gloves when palpating, especially when palpating mucous membranes or other areas where you might come in contact with body fluids.

As you palpate each body system, evaluate these features:
✦ *Texture* — rough or smooth?
✦ *Temperature* — warm, hot, or cold?
✦ *Moisture* — dry, wet, or moist?
✦ *Motion* — still or vibrating?
✦ *Consistency of structures* — solid or fluid-filled?

The patient may react to palpation with anxiety, embarrassment, or discomfort. This, in turn, can lead to muscle tension or guarding, possibly interfering with palpation and causing misleading results. To put the patient at ease and thus enhance the accuracy of palpation findings, follow these guidelines:
✦ Warm your hands before beginning.
✦ Explain what you'll do and why, and describe what the patient can expect, especially in sensitive areas.
✦ Encourage the patient to relax by taking several deep breaths while concentrating on inhaling and exhaling.
✦ Stop palpating immediately if the patient complains of pain.

Facts about percussion
✦ Tapping fingers or hands quickly and sharply against body surfaces to detect tenderness or assess reflexes
✦ Locating organ borders to identify shape and position and determine if solid or filled

PERCUSSION

Percussion involves tapping the fingers or hands quickly and sharply against body surfaces (usually the chest and abdomen) to produce sounds, to detect tenderness, or to assess reflexes. Percussing for sound (the most common percussion goal) helps locate organ borders, identify shape and position, and determine if an organ is solid or filled with fluid or gas.

Three basic percussion methods include indirect (mediate), direct (immediate), and blunt (fist) percussion. In indirect percussion, the examiner taps one finger against an object — usually the middle finger of the other hand — held against the skin surface. Although indirect percussion commonly produces clearer, crisper sounds than direct or blunt percussion, this technique requires practice to achieve good sound quality. (See *Percussion: Three techniques.*)

Percussing for sound — perhaps the most difficult assessment method to master — requires a skilled touch and an ear trained to detect slight sound variations. Organs and tissues produce sounds of varying loudness, pitch, and duration, depending on their intensity. For instance, air-filled cavities such as the lungs produce markedly different sounds from those produced by the liver and other dense tissues.

When percussing for sound with the direct or indirect method, use quick, light blows to create vibrations that penetrate about 1½″ to 2″ (4 to 5 cm) under the skin surface. The returning sounds reflect the contents of the percussed body cavity. (See *Types of percussion sounds,* page 42.)

Normal percussion sounds over the chest and abdomen include:
✦ *resonance* — the long, low hollow sound heard over an intercostal space lying above healthy lung tissue
✦ *tympany* — the loud, high-pitched, drumlike sound heard over a gastric air bubble or gas-filled bowel
✦ *dullness* — the soft, high-pitched thudding sound normally heard over more solid organs, such as the liver and heart.

 CLINICAL ALERT Dullness heard in a normally resonant or tympanic area points to the need for further investigation.

KNOW-HOW

Percussion: Three techniques

To assess patients completely, you'll need to use three percussion techniques: indirect, direct, and blunt.

INDIRECT PERCUSSION

To perform indirect percussion, use the second finger of your nondominant hand as the pleximeter (the mediating device used to receive the taps) and the middle finger of your dominant hand as the plexor (the device used to tap the pleximeter). Place the pleximeter finger firmly against a body surface such as the upper back. With your wrist flexed loosely, use the tip of your plexor finger to deliver a crisp blow just beneath the distal joint of the pleximeter. Be sure to hold the plexor perpendicular to the pleximeter. Tap lightly and quickly, removing the plexor as soon as you have delivered each blow.

BLUNT PERCUSSION

To perform blunt percussion, strike the ulnar surface of your fist against the body surface. Alternatively, you may use both hands by placing the palm of one hand over the area to be percussed, then making a fist with the other hand and using it to strike the back of the first hand. Both techniques aim to detect tenderness — *not* to create a sound — over such organs as the kidneys, gallbladder, or liver. (Another blunt percussion method, used in a neurologic examination, involves tapping a rubber-tipped reflex hammer against a tendon to create a reflexive muscle contraction.)

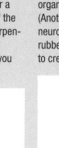

DIRECT PERCUSSION

To perform direct percussion, tap your hand or fingertip directly against the body surface. This method helps assess an adult's sinuses for tenderness or elicit sounds in a child's thorax.

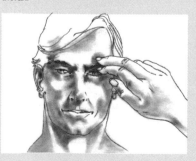

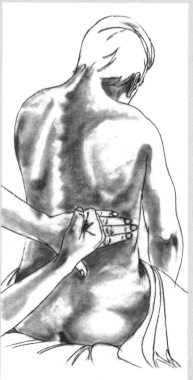

Percussion techniques

Indirect percussion
- Use second finger of your nondominant hand as pleximeter (mediating device used to receive taps)
- Use middle finger of your dominant hand as plexor (device used to tap pleximeter)
- Tap lightly and quickly, removing plexor as soon as you have delivered each blow

Direct percussion
- Tap your hand or fingertip directly against body surface

Blunt percussion
- Strike ulnar surface of your fist against body surface
- Detect possible tenderness over organs

Percussion sounds

Normal
+ Resonance
+ Tympany
+ Dullness

Abnormal
+ Hyperresonance
+ Flatness

Facts about percussion

Abnormal findings
+ Hyperresonance: emphysema
+ Flatness: pleural fluid accumulation or pleural thickening

Auscultation techniques

+ Use diaphragm of stethoscope to detect high-pitched sounds (breath and bowel sounds)
+ Use bell side to listen to low-pitched sounds (abnormal heart sounds and bruits)
+ Provide a quiet environment
+ Be aware that gown and bed linens can cause interference

Types of percussion sounds

Percussion produces sounds that vary according to the tissue being percussed. This chart shows important percussion sounds along with their characteristics and typical sources.

SOUND	INTENSITY	PITCH	DURATION	QUALITY	SOURCE
Resonance	Moderate to loud	Low	Long	Hollow	Normal lung
Tympany	Loud	High	Moderate	Drumlike	Gastric air bubble; intestinal air
Dullness	Soft to moderate	High	Moderate	Thudlike	Liver; full bladder; pregnant uterus
Hyper-resonance	Very loud	Very Low	Long	Booming	Hyperinflated lung (as in emphysema)
Flatness	Soft	High	Short	Flat	Muscle

ABNORMAL FINDINGS *Abnormal percussion sounds may be heard over body organs. Consider hyperresonance — a long, loud, low-pitched sound — to be a classic sign of lung hyperinflation, which can occur in emphysema. Flatness, similar to dullness but shorter in duration and softer in intensity, may also be heard over pleural fluid accumulation or pleural thickening.*

To enhance percussion technique and improve results, keep your fingernails short and warm your hands before starting. Have the patient void before you begin; otherwise, you could mistake a full bladder for a mass or cause the patient discomfort. Make sure the examination room is quiet and distraction free. Remove any jewelry or other items that could clatter and interfere with the ability to hear returning sounds.

Before performing percussion, briefly explain to the patient what you'll do and why. This technique may startle and upset an unprepared patient. In an obese patient, expect percussion sounds to be muffled by a thick subcutaneous fat layer. To help overcome this problem, use the lateral aspect of the thumb as the pleximeter and tap sharply on the last thumb joint with your plexor finger.

As you percuss, move gradually from areas of resonance to those of dullness and then compare sounds. Also compare sounds on one side of the body to sounds on the other side.

AUSCULTATION

Auscultation — usually the last step — involves listening for various breath, heart, and bowel sounds with a stethoscope. Most auscultated sounds result from air or fluid movement, such as the rush of air through respiratory pathways, the turbulent flow of blood through blood vessels, and the movement of gas (agitated by peristalsis) through the bowels.

You can hear pronounced body sounds, such as the voice, loud wheezing, or stomach growls, fairly easily, but you'll need a stethoscope to hear softer sounds.

Using a stethoscope

Even if using a stethoscope is second nature to you, it might still be a good idea to brush up on your technique. For starters, your stethoscope should have these features:

- snug-fitting ear plugs, which you'll position toward your nose
- tubing no longer than 15″ (38 cm) and an internal diameter not greater than ⅛″ (0.3 cm)
- a diaphragm and a bell.

HOW TO AUSCULTATE

Hold the diaphragm firmly against the patient's skin, enough to leave a slight ring afterward. Hold the bell lightly against the patient's skin, just enough to form a seal. Holding the bell too firmly causes the skin to act as a diaphragm, obliterating low-pitched sounds.

Hair on the patient's chest may cause friction on the end piece, which can mimic abnormal breath sounds such as crackles. You can minimize this problem by lightly wetting the hair before auscultating.

A FEW MORE TIPS

Also keep these points in mind:
- Provide a quiet environment.
- Make sure the area to be auscultated is exposed. Don't try to auscultate over a gown or bed linens because they can interfere with sounds.
- Warm the stethoscope head in your hand.
- Close your eyes to help focus your attention.
- Listen to and try to identify the characteristics of one sound at a time.

Use the diaphragm of the stethoscope to detect high-pitched sounds, such as breath sounds and bowel sounds, and use the bell side to listen to low-pitched sounds, such as abnormal heart sounds and bruits (abnormal blowing sound heard when auscultating an artery). Use a high-quality, properly fitting stethoscope, provide a quiet environment, and make sure the body area to be auscultated is sufficiently exposed. Remember that a gown or bed linens can interfere with sound transmission.

Instruct the patient to remain quiet and still. Before starting, warm the stethoscope head (diaphragm and bell) in your hand; otherwise, the cold metal may cause the patient to shiver, possibly causing unwanted sounds. Next, place the diaphragm or bell over the appropriate area. Closing your eyes to help focus your attention, listen intently to individual sounds, and try to identify their characteristics. Determine the intensity, pitch, and duration of each sound, and check the frequency of recurring sounds. To prevent the spread of infection among patients, clean the heads and end pieces with alcohol or a disinfectant. (See *Using a stethoscope*.)

RECORDING YOUR FINDINGS

Begin your documentation with general information, including the patient's age, race, gender, general appearance, height, weight, body mass, vital signs, communication skills, behavior, awareness, orientation, and level of cooperation. Next, precisely record all information you obtained using the four physical assessment techniques. (See *Documenting your findings*, page 44.)

Just as you followed an organized sequence in your examination, you should also follow an organized pattern for recording your findings. Document all information about one body system, for example, before proceeding to another.

Use anatomic landmarks in your descriptions so other people caring for the patient can compare their findings to yours. For instance, you might describe a wound as "3.8 × 6.4 cm, located 2½″ (6.4 cm) below the umbilicus at the midclavicular line."

Using a stethoscope

- Instruct patient to remain quiet and still
- Warm stethoscope head in your hand
- Place diaphragm or bell over appropriate body area
- Close your eyes to help focus your attention
- Listen intently to individual sounds
- Attempt to identify sounds' characteristics
- Determine intensity, pitch, and duration of each sound
- Check for frequency of recurring sounds

Recording your findings

- Age, race, and gender
- General appearance
- Height, weight, and body mass
- Vital signs
- Communication skills, behavior, level of awareness

How to document

- Precisely record all physical assessment findings
- Include all information about one body system before proceeding to another
- Use descriptions, such as anatomic landmarks and positions on a clock, to record your findings
- Use an appropriate form

Documenting your findings

Whether documenting an initial assessment on a patient admitted to your unit or writing a routine assessment note after a home visit, you'll need to document your findings using the appropriate form. The example below is part of an initial assessment form similar to one you might use.

GENERAL INFORMATION

Age _55_   Sex _M_   Height _163 cm_   Weight _57 kg_

T _37°C_   P _76_   R _14_   B/P (R) _150/90 sitting_   (L) _____

Room _328_

Admission time _0800_

Admission date _5-09-04_

Doctor _Manzel_

Admitting diagnosis
Pneumonia

Patient's stated reason for hospitalization
To get rid of pneumonia

Allergies _penicillin, codeine_

Current medications _None_

Name	Dosage	Last taken

GENERAL SURVEY

In no acute distress, slender, appears younger than stated age. Is alert and well-groomed. Communicates well. Makes eye contact and expresses appropriate concern throughout exam.

— _C. Smith, RN_

With some structures, such as the tympanic membrane or breast, you can pinpoint a finding by its position on a clock. For instance, you might write "breast mass at 3 o'clock." If you use this method, however, make sure others recognize the same landmark for the 12 o'clock reference point.

Mental health assessment

A LOOK AT MENTAL HEALTH ASSESSMENT

Effective patient care requires consideration of both psychological and physiologic aspects of health. A patient who seeks medical help for chest pain, for example, may also need to be assessed for anxiety or depression. Knowing the basic function and structures of the brain will help you perform a comprehensive mental health assessment and recognize any abnormalities. (See chapter 8, Neurologic system, for a review.)

The mental health assessment refers to the scientific process of identifying a patient's psychosocial problems, strengths, and concerns. Besides serving as the basis for treating psychiatric patients, mental health assessment has broad nursing applications. Recognizing psychosocial problems and how they affect a person's health is important in any clinical setting. On a medical-surgical unit, for example, you may encounter a patient who experiences depression, has a thought disorder, or has attempted suicide—recognizing these psychosocial problems is key to providing effective treatment.

OBTAINING A HEALTH HISTORY

Begin your assessment by obtaining a health history. For this assessment to be effective, you need to establish a therapeutic relationship with the patient that's built on trust. You must communicate to him that his thoughts and behaviors are important. Effective communication involves both sending and receiving messages, in the form of words and in the form of nonverbal communication. Eye contact, posture, facial expressions, gestures, clothing, affect, and even silence can convey a powerful message. (See *Therapeutic communication techniques,* page 46.)

Mental health assessment
- ✦ Helps to recognize any abnormalities
- ✦ Identifies psychosocial problems, strengths, and concerns
- ✦ Recognizes how psychosocial problems affect health

Obtaining a health history
- ✦ Establishes patient's trust
- ✦ Affirms patient's thoughts and behaviors
- ✦ Involves effective verbal and nonverbal communication

Therapeutic communication techniques

+ Listening
+ Rephrasing
+ Broad openings and general statements
+ Clarification
+ Focusing
+ Silence
+ Suggesting collaboration
+ Sharing impressions

Therapeutic communication techniques

Therapeutic communication is the foundation for developing a successful nurse-patient relationship. Here are some techniques that are effective in developing that relationship.

LISTENING

Listening intently to the patient enables the nurse to hear and analyze everything the patient is saying, alerting the nurse to the patient's communication patterns.

REPHRASING

Succinct rephrasing of key patient statements helps ensure the nurse understands and emphasizes important points in the patient's message. For example, the nurse might say, "You're feeling angry and you say it's because of the way your friend treated you yesterday."

BROAD OPENINGS AND GENERAL STATEMENTS

Using broad openings and general statements to initiate conversations encourages the patient to talk about any subject that comes to mind. These openings allow the patient to focus the conversation and demonstrate the nurse's willingness to interact. An example of this technique is: "Is there something you'd like to talk about?"

CLARIFICATION

Asking the patient to clarify a confusing or vague message demonstrates the nurse's desire to understand what the patient is saying. It can also elicit precise information crucial to the patient's recovery. An example of clarification is: "I'm not sure I understood what you said."

FOCUSING

In the technique called focusing, the nurse assists the patient in redirecting attention toward something specific. It fosters the patient's self-control and helps avoid vague generalizations, thereby enabling the patient to accept responsibility for facing problems. "Let's go back to what we were just talking about," would be one example of this technique.

SILENCE

Refraining from comment can have several benefits: Silence gives the patient time to talk, think, and gain insight into problems, and it allows the nurse to gather more information. The nurse must use this technique judiciously, however, to avoid seeming uninterested or judgmental.

SUGGESTING COLLABORATION

When used correctly, suggesting collaboration gives the patient the opportunity to explore the pros and cons of an approach. It must be used carefully to avoid directing the patient. An example of this technique is: "Perhaps we can meet with your parents to discuss the matter."

SHARING IMPRESSIONS

In the technique called sharing impressions, the nurse attempts to describe the patient's feelings and then seeks corrective feedback from the patient. This allows the patient to clarify misperceptions and gives the nurse a better understanding of the patient's true feelings. For example, the nurse might say, "Tell me if my perception of what you're telling me agrees with yours."

Key techniques for a systematic interview

+ Describe patient's behavioral disturbances
+ Assess emotional and social history
+ Assess mental status
+ Assess psychological functioning
+ Listen objectively and respond with empathy

A systematic interview helps you acquire broad information about the patient. The interview should include a description of the patient's behavioral disturbances, a thorough emotional and social history, and mental status tests.

Using this information, you'll be able to assess the patient's psychological functioning, understand his coping methods and their effect on his psychosocial growth, and build a therapeutic alliance that encourages the patient to talk openly. The information you gather along the way will enable you to develop an effective care plan.

The success of the health history hinges on your ability to listen objectively and respond with empathy. Keep in mind these guidelines when interviewing patients:

✦ Have clearly set goals in mind. Remember, the assessment interview isn't a random discussion. Your purpose may be to obtain information from a patient, to screen for abnormalities, or to further investigate an identified psychiatric condition, such as depression, paranoia, or suicidal thoughts.

✦ Don't let personal values obstruct your professional judgment. For example, when assessing appearance, judge attire on its appropriateness and cleanliness, not on whether it suits your taste.

✦ Pay attention to unspoken signals. Throughout the interview, listen carefully for indications of anxiety or distress. What topics do the patient pass over vaguely? You may find important clues in the patient's method of self-expression and in the subjects he avoids.

SPECIAL POINTS   A patient's background and values can affect how he responds to illness and adapts to care. Certain questions and behaviors considered acceptable in one culture may be inappropriate in another. A person who blames bad luck on a power called "juju" would be considered delusional in the United States. Neighbors in Nigeria, however, would consider this quite normal. When dealing with a patient from an unfamiliar culture, consult with an outside resource before drawing conclusions about his mental state.

✦ Don't make assumptions about how past events affected the patient emotionally. Try to discover what each event meant to the patient. Don't assume, for example, that the death of a loved one provoked a mood of sadness in a patient. A death by itself doesn't cause sadness, guilt, or anger. What matters is how the patient perceives the loss.

✦ Monitor your own reactions; the mental health patient may provoke an emotional response strong enough to interfere with your professional judgment. A depressed patient may make you depressed and a hostile patient may provoke your anger. An anxious patient may cause you to develop anxiety after the interview. A violent, psychotic patient who has lost touch with reality may easily induce fear.

You may find yourself identifying with a patient. Perhaps the patient has similar interests or experiences or is close to your age. Such feelings pose a real threat to establishing a therapeutic relationship; they may disrupt your objectivity or cause you to avoid or reject the patient. Consult with a psychiatric clinical specialist if you recognize within yourself strong prejudices toward a patient. Develop self-awareness as a tool to monitor patients and to further your own professional growth.

CREATE A SUPPORTIVE ATMOSPHERE

Choose a quiet, private setting for the assessment interview. Interruptions and distractions threaten confidentiality and interfere with effective listening. If you're meeting the patient for the first time, introduce yourself and explain the purpose of the interview. Sit a comfortable distance from the patient and give him your undivided attention.

The patient must feel comfortable enough to discuss his problems. You'll encounter patients who are angry and argumentative. Other patients will be too withdrawn to even say why they're seeking help. You'll have to deal with diverse cultural norms. Some patients may come from cultural backgrounds that frown on discussing intimate details with a stranger, even a nurse. Adolescents may refuse to discuss sexual activity in front of their parents. Listen carefully to the patient and respond with sensitivity. Reassure the patient that you respect his need for privacy. Ask privately who should be present at the interview and how the patient wants to be addressed. Attempt to make the immediate environment calm and quiet, to calm the patient. Reassure him that he's safe, if necessary.

During the interview, adopt a professional but friendly attitude, and maintain eye contact. A calm, nonthreatening tone of voice encourages the patient to talk more openly. Avoid value judgments. Don't rush through the interview; building a trusting therapeutic relationship takes time. Remember to allow the patient to carry the conversation and redirect him as necessary.

PATIENT INTERVIEW

A patient interview establishes a baseline and provides clues to the underlying or precipitating cause of the patient's current problem. Remember the patient may not be a reliable source of information, particularly if he has a mental illness or other mental impairment. If possible, verify his responses with family members, friends, or health care personnel. Also, check hospital records for previous admissions, if possible, and compare his past and present behavior, symptoms, and circumstances.

Use the following guidelines for conducting a patient interview. (See *Guidelines for an effective interview.*)

Demographic data

Determine the patient's age, ethnic origin, primary language, birthplace, religion, and marital status. Use this information to establish a baseline and validate the patient's record.

 SPECIAL POINTS *Age-related losses may take a toll on the mental functioning of elderly patients. These may include:*
- *deaths of friends and family*
- *retirement*
- *decrease in income*
- *decreased physical capabilities*
- *impairments in vision and hearing*
- *decreased stimulation*
- *growing isolation.*

Chief complaint

Ask what the patient expects to accomplish through treatment. A person with low self-esteem may seek a better self-image. A patient with schizophrenia may want to be rid of hallucinations. Some patients may not understand the purpose of the interview and subsequent therapy. Help such patients identify the benefits of dealing with problems openly.

Include in your assessment a statement of the patient's chief complaint in his own words. Some patients don't have an overriding concern, whereas others insist that nothing is wrong. Patients enmeshed in a medical problem may fail to recognize their own depression or anxiety. Carefully observe such patients for signs of disturbed mental health.

The patient may not voice his chief complaint directly. Instead, you or others may note that he's having difficulty coping or that he's exhibiting unusual behavior. If this occurs, determine whether the patient is aware of the problem. When documenting the patient's response, write it down word for word and enclose it in quotation marks. Be sure to note his corresponding physical behavior as well.

When possible, fully discuss the patient's chief complaint. Ask about when symptoms began, their severity and persistence, and whether they occurred abruptly or insidiously. If discussing a recurrent problem, ask the patient what prompted him to seek help at this time.

Key features of the patient interview
- Demographic data
- Chief complaint
- History of psychiatric illness
- Socioeconomic data
- Family history
- Medication history
- Physical illnesses

Key demographic data
- Age
- Ethnic origin
- Primary language
- Birthplace
- Religion
- Marital status

Special points
- Age-related loss can affect mental function in elderly patients

Exploring the chief complaint
- When symptoms began
- Symptom severity and persistence
- Whether symptom occurred abruptly or insidiously
- What prompted patient to seek help

Guidelines for an effective interview

+ Begin the interview with a broad, empathetic statement: "You look distressed; tell me what's bothering you today."
+ Explore normal behaviors before discussing abnormal ones: "What do you think has enabled you to cope with the pressures of your job?"
+ Phrase inquiries sensitively to lessen the patient's anxiety: "Things were going well at home and then you became depressed. Tell me about that."
+ Ask the patient to clarify vague statements: "Explain to me what you mean when you say, 'They're all after me.'"

+ Help the patient who rambles to focus on his most pressing problem: "You've talked about several problems. Which one bothers you the most?"
+ Interrupt nonstop talkers as tactfully as possible: "Thank you for your comments. Now let's move on."
+ Express empathy toward tearful, silent, or confused patients who have trouble describing their problem: "I realize that it's difficult for you to talk about this."

History of psychiatric illnesses

Discuss past psychiatric disturbances—such as episodes of delusions, violence, attempted suicides, drug or alcohol abuse, or depression. Ask the patient if he has ever undergone psychiatric treatment. Did treatment help? Even though the patient may be reluctant to respond, such questions may elicit early warnings of depression, dementia, suicide risk, psychosis, or adverse reactions to drug therapy.

Socioeconomic data

A patient suffering hardships is more likely to show symptoms of distress during an illness. Information about your patient's educational level, housing conditions, income, employment status, and family may provide clues to his current problem.

Family history

Questions about family customs, child-rearing practices, and emotional support received during childhood may give important insights into the environmental influences on the patient's development.

How does the patient react while disclosing his family history? For example, when a patient tells you about his parents divorce, can you detect feelings of jealousy, hostility, or unresolved grief?

Ask about the emotional health of relatives. Is there a family history of substance abuse, alcoholism, suicide, psychiatric hospitalization, child abuse, or violence? Is there a history of psychological disorders? Ask about physical disorders as well. A family history of diabetes mellitus or thyroid disorders, for instance, can point to the need to investigate whether the patient's problem has an organic basis.

If the patient can't provide answers to important questions or appears unreliable, ask for permission to interview family members or friends.

Medication history

Certain drugs can cause symptoms of mental illness. Review medications the patient is taking, including over-the-counter (OTC) and herbal preparations, and check for interactions. If he's taking a psychiatric drug, ask if his symptoms have improved, if he's taking the medication as prescribed, and if he has had adverse reactions.

Past psychiatric illnesses

+ Episodes of delusions
+ Violence
+ Attempted suicides
+ Drug or alcohol abuse
+ Depression

Socioeconomic data

+ Educational level
+ Housing conditions
+ Income
+ Employment status
+ Family

Family history

+ Substance abuse and alcoholism
+ Suicide and psychiatric hospitalization
+ Child abuse and violence
+ Psychosocial disorders
+ Diabetes mellitus
+ Thyroid disorders

Medication history

+ Prescription medications
+ OTC and herbal preparations
+ Psychiatric drug use and reactions

Physical illnesses
✦ History of medical disorders that cause distorted thought processes, disorientation, or depression.

Assessing mental status
✦ LOC
✦ Posture and motor behaviors
✦ Appearance
✦ Speech
✦ Mood and affect
✦ Intellectual performance and judgment
✦ Insight and perception
✦ Coping mechanisms
✦ Thought content
✦ Sexual drive
✦ Competence

Assessing LOC
✦ Intensity of verbal and tactile stimulation needed to arouse the patient
✦ Quality of patient's response

Assessing posture and movement
✦ Character of posture
✦ Pace, range, and character of movements
✦ Changes in posture and motor behavior with certain topics of discussion

Abnormal findings
✦ Slumped posture (depression, fatigue, suspiciousness)
✦ Tense posture (anxiety)
✦ Unsteady gait (physical abnormalities, drug and alcohol influence)
✦ Swinging, dancing, expansive movements (manic episode)

Physical illnesses
Find out if the patient has a history of medical disorders that may cause distorted thought processes, disorientation, depression, or other symptoms of mental illness. For instance, does he have a history of renal or hepatic failure, infection, thyroid disease, increased intracranial pressure, or a metabolic disorder?

ASSESSING MENTAL STATUS

Most of your mental status assessment can be done during your interview. As you take a health history, you'll quickly learn the patient's level of alertness and orientation, mood, attention, and memory. As his history unfolds, you'll pick up clues regarding his insight, judgment, and recurring or unusual thoughts or perceptions.

The mental status assessment is a tool for assessing psychological dysfunction and for identifying the causes of psychopathology. You should try to integrate certain parts of the mental status assessment with other parts of the examination. This will make the complete assessment more efficient.

Understanding the components of this examination will enable you to plan appropriate interventions. Assess the patient's level of consciousness (LOC), posture and motor behaviors, appearance, behavior, speech, mood and affect, intellectual performance, judgment, insight, perception, coping mechanisms, thought content, sexual drive, and competence.

LEVEL OF CONSCIOUSNESS

Begin by assessing the patient's LOC, a basic brain function. Identify the intensity of stimulation needed to arouse the patient. Does the patient respond when called in a normal conversational tone, or in a loud voice? Does it take a light touch, vigorous shaking, or painful stimulation to rouse the patient?

Describe the patient's response to stimulation, including the degree of quality of movement, content and coherence of speech, and level of eye opening and eye contact. Finally, describe the patient's actions once the stimulus is removed.

 ABNORMAL FINDINGS *An impaired LOC may indicate the presence of tumor, abscess, hematoma, hydrocephalus, electrolyte or acid-base imbalance, or toxicity from liver or kidney failure, alcohol, or drugs. A lethargic patient is drowsy but arousable and able to respond to you. An obtunded patient may open his eyes and look at you, but is slow to respond and somewhat confused. If you discover an alteration in consciousness, refer the patient for a more complex medical examination.*

POSTURE AND MOTOR BEHAVIOR

Is the patient lying in bed or walking around? Note his posture and ability to relax. Observe the pace, range, and characteristics of his movements. Are they under voluntary control? Are certain parts immobile? Do his posture and motor behavior change with certain topics of discussion?

 ABNORMAL FINDINGS *A slumped posture may indicate depression, fatigue, or suspiciousness, whereas an uneven or unsteady gait might suggest physical abnormalities or the influence of drugs or alcohol. A tense posture and restlessness could indicate anxiety. A patient experiencing a manic episode may display swinging, dancing, or expansive movements.*

Appearance

The patient's appearance helps to indicate his emotional and mental status. Describe the patient's weight, coloring, skin condition, odor, body build, and obvious physical impairments. Note discrepancies between the patient's feelings about his health and your observations. Answer these questions:

- Is the patient's appearance appropriate for his age, gender, and situation?
- Are his skin, hair, nails, and teeth clean?
- Is his manner of dress appropriate?
- If the patient wears cosmetics, are they appropriately applied?
- Does the patient maintain direct eye contact? Does he stare at you for long periods?
- Is the patient's posture erect or slouched? Is his head lowered?
- Observe his gait—is it brisk, slow, shuffling, or unsteady? Does he walk normally?

 ABNORMAL FINDINGS A disheveled appearance may indicate self-neglect or a preoccupation with other activities. Excessive fastidiousness may be seen in obsessive-compulsive disorder. A pale, emaciated, sad appearance may indicate depression.

Behavior

Describe the patient's demeanor and way of relating to others. When entering the room, does the patient appear sad, joyful, or expressionless? Does he use appropriate gestures? Does he acknowledge your initial greeting and introduction? Does he keep an appropriate distance between himself and others? Does he have distinctive mannerisms, such as tics or tremors? Does he gaze directly at you, at the floor, or around the room?

When responding to your questions, is the patient cooperative, mistrustful, embarrassed, hostile, or overly revealing? Describe the patient's activity level. Is he tense, rigid, restless, or calm? Also, note any extraordinary behavior.

 ABNORMAL FINDINGS An inability to sit still may indicate anxiety. Disconnected gestures may indicate that the patient is hallucinating. A patient who experiences auditory hallucinations may speak to a person who isn't there and tilt his head to listen. Pressured, rapid speech and a heightened level of activity may indicate the manic phase of a bipolar disorder.

Speech

Observe the content and quality of the patient's speech, noting:
- illogical choice of topics
- irrelevant or illogical replies to questions
- speech defects such as stuttering
- excessively fast or slow speech
- sudden interruptions
- excessive volume
- barely audible speech
- altered voice tone and modulation
- slurred speech
- an excessive number of words (overproductive speech)
- minimal, monosyllabic responses (underproductive speech).

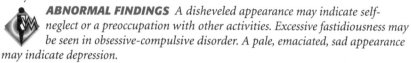

Assessing appearance
- Weight
- Coloring
- Skin, hair, nails, teeth condition
- Odor
- Appropriate dress and cosmetics
- Eye contact
- Posture and gait
- Obvious physical impairments

Abnormal findings
- Disheveled appearance (self-neglect)
- Excessive fastidiousness (obsessive-compulsive disorder)
- Emaciated appearance (depression)

Assessing behavior
- Demeanor and relation to others
- Sadness, joyfulness, or lack of expression
- Distance between patient and others
- Tics or tremors
- Cooperative, mistrustful, embarrassed, hostile, or overly revealing responses

Abnormal findings
- Inability to sit still (anxiety)
- Disconnected gestures (hallucination)
- Pressured, rapid speech and higher level of activity (manic phase of bipolar disorder)

Assessing speech
- Observe content and quality

Abnormal findings
- Illogical topic choice, replies to questions
- Sudden interruptions
- Excessive volume
- Altered tone, modulation, speed, volume
- Slurring
- Overproductive, underproductive
- Speech defects

Assessing mood and affect

✦ Ask the patient about his current feelings
✦ Observe his facial expression and posture
✦ Ask if he's able to keep mood changes under control
✦ Note lability of affect, flat affect, inappropriate affect

Abnormal findings

✦ Mood swings (medications, substance abuse, stress, dehydration, electrolyte imbalance, disease, childbirth, menopause)
✦ Labile, flat, or inappropriate affect

Assessing intellectual performance

Orientation

✦ Ask the patient about time, date, place, and circumstances as well as his name

Immediate and delayed recall

✦ Ask the patient to recall something that just occurred and to remember events after a reasonable amount of time passes

Recent memory

✦ Ask the patient about an event experienced in the past few hours or days

Notice how much time elapses before the patient reacts to your questions. If the patient communicates only with gestures, determine whether this is an isolated behavior or part of a pattern of diminished responsiveness.

 ABNORMAL FINDINGS *Slowed speech could be a sign of depression. Rapid, loud speech could indicate a manic episode.*

MOOD AND AFFECT

Mood refers to a person's pervading feeling or state of mind. Usually, the patient will project a prevailing mood, although this mood may change in the course of a day. For example, depressed patients may smile occasionally but will revert to their prevailing mood of sadness.

Affect refers to a person's expression of his mood. Variations in affect are referred to as range of emotion.

To assess mood and affect, begin by asking the patient about his current feelings. Also, look for indications of mood in facial expression and posture. Does the patient seem able to keep mood changes under control?

 ABNORMAL FINDINGS *Mood swings may indicate a physiologic disorder. Medications, illicit drug or alcohol use, stress, dehydration, electrolyte imbalance, or disease may all induce mood changes. After childbirth and during menopause, many women experience profound depression.*

Other indications of a mood disorder include:

✦ *lability of affect—rapid, dramatic fluctuation in the range of emotion*
✦ *flat affect—unresponsive range of emotion, possibly an indication of schizophrenia or Parkinson's disease*
✦ *inappropriate affect—inconsistency between expression (affect) and mood (for example, a patient who smiles when discussing an anger-provoking situation).*

INTELLECTUAL PERFORMANCE

An emotionally distressed patient may show an inability to reason abstractly, make judgments, or solve problems. To develop a picture of his intellectual abilities, use the following series of simple tests. Note that these tests screen for organic brain syndrome as well. If organic brain syndrome is suspected, follow up with additional physical, neurobehavioral, and psychological testing.

Orientation

Ask the patient the time, date, place, and circumstance as well as his name. Disorientation occurs when memory or attention is impaired such as in delirium.

Immediate and delayed recall

Assess the patient's ability to recall something that just occurred and to remember events after a reasonable amount of time passes.

For example, to test immediate recall say, "I want you to remember three words: apple, house, and umbrella. What are the three words I want you to remember?" Tell the patient to remember these words for future recall. To test delayed recall, ask the patient to repeat the same words in 5 to 10 minutes.

Recent memory

Ask the patient about an event experienced in the past few hours or days. For example, when was he admitted to the hospital? You should know the correct re-

Testing attention

Tests for attention that are commonly used are digit span, serial 7's, and spelling backward.

DIGIT SPAN
The digit span test involves reciting a series of numbers and having the patient repeating them back to you. Start with two numbers at a time and increase the number of digits in the series as tolerated. If the patient makes a mistake, try again with another series of the same length. Stop after a second failure.

Next, start again with a series of two digits and have the patient repeat the numbers backward. Again, increase the number of digits in the series as tolerated.

Normally, the patient can repeat at least five digits forward and at least four digits backward.

SERIAL 7'S
Starting from 100, have the patient subtract 7 and keep subtracting 7.

SPELLING BACKWARD
Say a five-letter word to the patient, spell it, and then have the patient spell it backward to you.

---

sponse or be able to validate it with a family member. A patient may confabulate plausible answers to mask memory deficits. Impairment of recent memory is seen in the patient with dementia or delirium.

Remote memory
Assess the patient's ability to remember events in the more distant past, such as where he was born or where he attended high school. Remote memory is impaired in the late stage of dementia. Recent memory loss with intact remote memory may indicate an organic disorder.

Attention level
Assess the patient's ability to concentrate on a task for an appropriate length of time. If the patient has a poor attention level, remember to provide simple, written instructions for health care. (See *Testing attention*.)

Comprehension
Assess the ability of the patient to understand material, retain it, and repeat the content. Ask the patient to read part of a news article and explain it. Evaluate his thought processes and cognitive function. (See *Abnormal thought processes*, page 54.)

Concept formation
To test the patient's ability to think abstractly, ask the meaning of common proverbs. Interpreting the proverb, "People in glass houses shouldn't throw stones" to mean that glass is breakable shows concrete thinking. Interpreting the proverb as saying, "Don't criticize others for what you do yourself" shows abstract thinking. You may use other well-known proverbs, such as "A stitch in time saves nine" or, "Don't count your chickens before they hatch."

Tests for attention
+ Digit span — recite a series of numbers and have the patient repeat them back to you
+ Serial 7's — have the patient subtract 7 from 100 and keep subtracting 7
+ Spelling backward — say a 5-letter word, spell it, then have the patient spell it backward to you

Assessing intellectual performance

Remote memory
+ Ask the patient to remember distant events such as where he was born

Attention level
+ Evaluate ability to concentrate on a task for an appropriate length of time

Comprehension
+ Evaluate ability to understand material, retain it, and repeat the content such as a newspaper article

Concept formation
+ Evaluate understanding and interpretation of common proverbs

Assessing intellectual performance

Special points: Concept formation
+ Abstract thinking abilities usually develop around age 12
+ Some American expressions may confuse people from foreign countries

Abnormal findings: Concept formation
+ Concrete answers (mental retardation, severe anxiety, organic brain syndrome, schizophrenia)
+ Inability to give answer (low intellect, brain damage)

Assessing judgment
+ Assess ability to evaluate choices and draw conclusions

Assessing insight
+ Evaluate the patient's view of himself and his illness
+ Evaluate his degree of insight: full, partial, or lacking

Abnormal thought processes

During your interview, you may identify some of the following abnormalities in the patient's thought processes.

+ *Derailment*—speech vacillates from one subject to another; the subjects are unrelated; ideas slip off track between clauses
+ *Flight of ideas*—continuous flow of speech in which the patient jumps abruptly from topic to topic
+ *Neologisms*—distorted or invented words
+ *Confabulation*—fabrications of facts or events to fill in the gaps where memory loss has occurred
+ *Clanging*—the patient chooses a word based on sound rather than meaning
+ *Echolalia*—repeating words or phrases that others say
+ *Incoherence*—incomprehensible speech
+ *Circumstantiality*—indirection and delay in reaching the point due to unnecessary detail
+ *Blocking*—sudden interruption of speech
+ *Perseveration*—persistent repetition of words or ideas

 SPECIAL POINTS *People normally develop abstract thinking abilities around age 12.*

 ABNORMAL FINDINGS *Concrete answers may indicate mental retardation, severe anxiety, organic brain syndrome, or schizophrenia. Patients with schizophrenia may also give elaborate or bizarre answers. Inability to give any answer may indicate low intellectual ability or brain damage.*

 SPECIAL POINTS *Keep in mind that some familiar American sayings may confuse people from foreign cultures.*

General knowledge
To determine the patient's store of common knowledge, ask questions appropriate to his age and level of learning; for example, "Who is the president?" or "Who is the vice president?"

JUDGMENT
Assess the patient's ability to evaluate choices and to draw appropriate conclusions. Ask the patient, "What would you do if you found a stamped, addressed, sealed airmail letter lying on the sidewalk?" An answer such as "Track down the recipient" would indicate impaired judgment.

Questions that emerge naturally during conversation (for example, "What would you do if you ran out of medication?") may also help to evaluate the patient's judgment.

Defects in judgment may also become apparent while the patient tells his history. Pay attention to how the patient handles interpersonal relationships and occupational and economic responsibilities. Judgment may be poor in a patient with delirium, dementia, mental retardation, or psychotic state.

INSIGHT
Some of your questions at the beginning of the interview will give you valuable information about insight. For example, "What brings you here today?"

Is the patient able to see himself realistically? Is he aware of his illness and its circumstances? To assess insight, ask "What do you think has caused your anxiety?" or "Have you noticed a recent change in yourself?"

Expect patients to show varying degrees of insight. For example, an alcoholic patient may admit to having a drinking problem but blame it on his job.

Severe lack of insight may indicate a psychotic state.

PERCEPTION

Perception refers to interpretation of reality as well as use of the senses. Psychologists are placing increasing importance on perception in understanding psychological disorders. For example, psychoanalysts have long said that depression results from internal, unresolved conflicts that became activated after a real or perceived loss. Recently, proponents of the cognitive theory of depression have suggested that depression arises from distorted perception. Depressed patients perceive themselves as worthless, the world as barren, and the future as bleak.

 ABNORMAL FINDINGS *The patient with a disorder of sensory perception may experience hallucinations, in which he perceives nonexistent external stimuli, or illusions in which he misinterprets external stimuli. Tactile, olfactory, and gustatory hallucinations usually indicate organic disorders.*

Not all visual and auditory hallucinations are associated with psychological disorders. For example, heat mirages, visions of a recently deceased loved one, and illusions evoked by environmental effects or experienced just before falling asleep don't indicate abnormalities. A patient may also experience mild and transitory hallucinations. Constant visual and auditory hallucinations may, however, give rise to strange or bizarre behavior. Disorders associated with hallucinations include schizophrenia and acute organic brain syndrome after withdrawal from alcohol or barbiturate addiction.

COPING MECHANISMS

The patient who's faced with a stressful situation may adopt coping, or defense, mechanisms — behaviors that operate on an unconscious level to protect the ego. Examples include denial, displacement, fantasy, identification, projection, repression, rationalization, reaction formation, and regression. Look for an excessive reliance on these coping mechanisms. (See *Exploring coping mechanisms,* page 56.)

THOUGHT CONTENT

Assess the patient's thought patterns as expressed throughout the examination. Are the patient's thoughts well-connected to reality? Are the patient's ideas clear, and do they progress in a logical sequence? Observe for indications of morbid thoughts and preoccupations, or abnormal beliefs.

 ABNORMAL FINDINGS *Delusions and obsessions are abnormalities in thought content. Usually associated with schizophrenia, delusions are false beliefs without a firm basis in reality. Grandiose and persecutory delusions are most common. Other types are somatic, nihilistic, and control. Ideas of reference (misinterpreting acts of others in a highly personal way) are closely related to delusions but don't represent the same level of ego disintegration.*

Some patients suffer intense preoccupations, also called obsessions *that interfere with daily living. Patients may constantly think about hygiene, for example. A compulsion is a preoccupation that's acted out such as constantly washing one's hands. Most compulsive patients must exert great effort to control their compulsions. (See* Abnormal thought content, *page 57.)*

Assessing perception
✦ Assess ability to interpret reality and use senses

Abnormal findings
✦ Hallucinations (visual, auditory, tactile, olfactory, gustatory)

Assessing coping
✦ Identify the patient's coping mechanisms

Assessing thought content
✦ Assess the patient's thought patterns
✦ Observe him for morbid thoughts and preoccupations, or abnormal beliefs

Abnormal findings
✦ Delusions — false beliefs without firm basis in reality (misinterpreting acts of others)
✦ Obsessions — intense preoccupations that interfere with daily living (constantly thinking about hygiene)
✦ Compulsions — preoccupations that are acted out constantly (washing one's hands)

Exploring coping mechanisms

Coping, or defense mechanisms, help to relieve anxiety. Common coping mechanisms include:

✦ *Denial*—refusal to admit truth or reality
✦ *Displacement*—transferring emotion from its original object to a substitute
✦ *Fantasy*—creation of unrealistic or improbable images to escape from daily pressures and responsibilities
✦ *Identification*—unconscious adoption of the personality characteristics, attitudes, values, and behavior of another person
✦ *Projection*—displacement of negative feelings onto another person

✦ *Rationalization*—substitution of acceptable reasons for the real or actual reasons motivating behavior
✦ *Reaction formation*—behaving in a manner opposite from the way the person feels
✦ *Regression*—return to behavior of an earlier, more comfortable time
✦ *Repression*—exclusion of unacceptable thoughts and feelings from the conscious mind, leaving them to operate in the subconscious.

 ABNORMAL FINDINGS *Compulsions, phobias, and anxieties are commonly associated with neurotic disorders. Delusions and feelings of unreality or depersonalization are more commonly associated with psychotic disorders. Delusions may also occur in delirium, severe mood disorders, and dementia.*

Also observe the patient for suicidal, self-destructive, violent, or superstitious thoughts; recurring dreams; distorted perceptions of reality; and feelings of worthlessness.

Assessing sexual drive
✦ Assess changes in sexual desire and level of pleasure
✦ Be prepared for a patient who feels uncomfortable
✦ Be tactful but direct
✦ Avoid language that implies heterosexual orientation

SEXUAL DRIVE

Changes in sexual drive provide valuable information in psychological assessment, but you may have to sharpen your skills in assessing sexual activity. Prepare yourself for patients who are uncomfortable discussing their sexuality. Avoid language that implies a heterosexual orientation. Introduce the subject tactfully but directly. For example, say to the patient, "I'm going to ask you a few questions about your sexual activity because it's an important part of almost everyone's life." Follow-up questions might include:
✦ Are you sexually active?
✦ Do you usually have relations with men or women?
✦ Have you noticed any recent changes in your interest in sexual intercourse?
✦ Do you have the same pleasure from sexual intercourse now as before?
✦ What form of protection did you use during your last sexual encounter?

Assessing competence
✦ Assess the patient's understanding of reality and consequences of actions
✦ Assess his comprehension of illness and treatment and consequences of avoiding treatment
✦ Assume competence unless patient behavior strongly suggests otherwise

COMPETENCE

Can the patient understand reality and the consequences of his actions? Does the patient understand the implications of his illness, its treatment, and the consequences of avoiding treatment? Use extreme caution when assessing changes in competence. Unless behavior strongly indicates otherwise, assume that the patient is competent. Remember that legally, only a judge has the power or right to declare a person incompetent to make decisions regarding personal health and safety or financial matters.

Abnormal thought content

With careful questioning, you may detect abnormalities in thought content during your interview. Make sure you follow the patient's lead. For example, "You told me a few minutes ago that your mother was responsible for your illness; would you please elaborate?" With this type of questioning, you can find abnormalities in thought content, which may include:

✦ *Obsessions*—intrusive and inappropriate thoughts, images, or impulses that the patient feels are unacceptable

✦ *Compulsions*—repetitive behaviors that result from attempts to alleviate an obsession

✦ *Phobias*—irrational and disproportionate fears of objects or situations

✦ *Depersonalization*—feeling that one has become detached from one's mind or body or has lost his identity

✦ *Delusions*—false, fixed beliefs that others don't share

✦ *Feelings of unreality*—sense that things in the environment are strange, unusual, or remote.

ASSESSING SELF-DESTRUCTIVE BEHAVIOR

Healthy, adventurous people may intentionally take death-defying risks, especially during youth. The risks taken by self-destructive patients, however, aren't death-defying, but death-seeking.

Suicide—intentional, self-inflicted death—may be carried out with guns, drugs, poisons, rope, automobiles, or razor blades. It may also be carried out through drowning, jumping, or refusing food, fluids, or medications. In a subintentional suicide, a person has no conscious intention of dying but nevertheless engages in self-destructive acts that could easily become fatal.

Risk factors for suicide include:
✦ history of psychiatric illness
✦ substance abuse
✦ personality disorder
✦ prior suicide attempt
✦ family history of suicide.

Not all self-destructive behavior is suicidal in intent. Some patients engage in self-destructive behavior because it helps them to feel alive. A patient who has lost touch with reality may cut or mutilate body parts to focus on physical pain, which may be less overwhelming than emotional distress. Such behavior may indicate a borderline personality disorder.

Assess depressed patients for suicidal tendencies. Not all such patients want to die, but a higher percentage of depressed patients commit suicide than patients with other diagnoses. Patients who are chemically dependent and those who are schizophrenic also present a high suicide risk as well as people experiencing intolerably high levels of anxiety.

SPECIAL POINTS *Suicide rates are highest among men older than age 65, but are increasing among teenagers and young adults.*

People with suicidal schizophrenia may become agitated instead of depressed. Voices may tell them to kill themselves. Alarmingly, some people with schizophrenia provide only vague behavioral clues before taking their lives.

On perceiving signals of hopelessness, perform a direct suicide assessment. Protect the patient from self-harm during a suicidal crisis. After treatment, the pa-

Assessing self-destructive behavior

✦ Assess the patient for risk-taking, death-seeking behaviors
✦ Note that patient may or may not be intentionally suicidal

Risk factors for suicide
✦ History of psychiatric illness
✦ Substance abuse
✦ Personality disorder
✦ Prior suicide attempt
✦ Family history of suicide
✦ Being male older than age 65
✦ High anxiety
✦ Depression
✦ Chemical dependence
✦ Schizophrenia

Special points: Suicide
✦ Highest among men older than age 65
✦ Increasing among teenagers and young adults

Key factors in spotting suicidal patients

✦ Withdrawn personality
✦ Social isolation
✦ Signs of depression
✦ Farewells to friends and family
✦ Organizing personal affairs
✦ Giving away possessions
✦ Covert or obvious suicide messages

Recognizing and responding to suicidal patients

Watch for these warning signs of impending suicide:
✦ withdrawal
✦ social isolation
✦ signs of depression, which may include constipation, crying, fatigue, helplessness, hopelessness, poor concentration, reduced interest in sex and other activities, sadness, and weight loss
✦ farewells to friends and family
✦ putting affairs in order
✦ giving away prized possessions
✦ expression of covert suicide messages and death wishes
✦ obvious suicide messages such as "I'd be better off dead."

ANSWERING A THREAT

If a patient shows signs of impending suicide, assess the seriousness of the intent and the immediacy of the risk. Consider a patient with a chosen method who plans to commit suicide in the next 48 to 72 hours a high risk.

Tell the patient that you're concerned. Then urge him to avoid self-destructive behavior until the staff has an opportunity to help him. You may specify a time for the patient to seek help.

Next, consult with the treatment team about arranging for psychiatric hospitalization or a safe equivalent such as having someone watch the patient at home. Initiate safety precautions for those at high suicide risk:

✦ Provide a safe environment. Check and correct conditions that could be dangerous for the patient. Look for exposed pipes, windows without safety glass, and access to the roof or open balconies.
✦ Remove dangerous objects, such as belts, razors, suspenders, light cords, glass, knives, nail files, and clippers.
✦ Make the patient's specific restrictions clear to staff members, plan for observation of the patient, and clarify day- and night-staff responsibilities.

Patients may ask you to keep their suicidal thoughts confidential. Remember, such requests are ambivalent; suicidal patients want to escape the pain of life, but they also want to live. A part of them wants you to tell other staff so they can be kept alive. Tell patients that you can't keep secrets that endanger their lives or conflict with their treatment. You have a duty to keep them safe and to ensure the best care.

Be alert when the patient is shaving, taking medication, or using the bathroom. Besides observing the patient, maintain personal contact with him. Encourage continuity of care and consistency of primary nurses. Helping the patient build emotional ties to others is the ultimate technique for preventing suicide.

---

tient will think more clearly and, hopefully, find reasons for living. (See *Recognizing and responding to suicidal patients.*)

Psychological and mental status testing

✦ Specific tests augment interview assessment
✦ Measures orientation, registration, recall, calculation, language, and graphomotor function
✦ Assesses cognitive function and loss

PSYCHOLOGICAL AND MENTAL STATUS TESTING

Although most of your mental status assessment can be done during your interview, you'll also need to evaluate other aspects of your patient's mental status. These aspects can be assessed using psychological and mental status tests.

SPECIAL POINTS *Most elderly patients do well on mental health examinations, but functional impairments may become evident as they get older. Elderly people are slower to retrieve and process data, and they take more time to learn new material. Motor responses may be slow and the ability to perform complex tasks may be impaired.*

MINI-MENTAL STATE EXAMINATION

The Mini-Mental State Examination measures orientation, registration, recall, calculation, language, and graphomotor function. This test offers a quick and simple way to quantify cognitive function and screen for cognitive loss. Each section of the test involves a related series of questions or commands. The patient receives one point for each correct answer.

To give the examination, seat the patient in a quiet, well-lit room. Ask him to listen carefully and to answer each question as accurately as he can.

Don't time the test but score it right away. To score, add the number of correct responses. The patient can receive a maximum score of 30 points.

 ABNORMAL FINDINGS *Usually, a score below 24 indicates cognitive impairment, although this may not be an accurate cutoff for highly or poorly educated patients. A score below 20 usually appears in patients with delirium, dementia, schizophrenia, or affective disorder, and not in normal elderly people or in patients with neurosis or personality disorder.*

COGNITIVE CAPACITY SCREENING EXAMINATION

The Cognitive Capacity Screening Examination measures orientation, memory, calculation, and language. It's an interviewer-administered test of 30 items that's used to assess dementia and delirium.

COGNITIVE ASSESSMENT SCALE

The Cognitive Assessment Scale measures orientation, general knowledge, mental ability, and psychomotor function. It's used as a screening tool for the diagnosis of cognitive impairments associated with advancing age.

It takes approximately 45 minutes to administer and is composed of 103 items grouped into 10 categories:
+ temporal orientation
+ spatial orientation
+ attention-concentration and calculation
+ immediate recall
+ language
+ remote memory
+ judgment and abstraction
+ agnosia
+ apraxia
+ recent memory.

BECK DEPRESSION INVENTORY

The Beck Depression Inventory (BDI) helps diagnose depression, determine its severity, and monitor the patient's response during treatment. A self-administered, self-scored test, the BDI asks patients to rate how often they experience symptoms of depression, such as poor concentration, suicidal thoughts, guilt feelings, and crying. Questions focus on both cognitive symptoms such as impaired decision making, and on physical symptoms such as loss of appetite. Elderly and physically ill patients commonly score high on questions regarding their physical symptoms; their scores may stem from aging, physical illness, or depression.

 ABNORMAL FINDINGS *The sum of 21 items gives the total, with a maximum score of 63. A score of 10 to 18 indicates mild depression; 19 to 29, moderate to severe depression; 30 to 63, severe depression.*

Mini-Mental State Examination
+ Involves 30 related questions or commands worth one point each

Abnormal findings
+ Score below 24: Cognitive impairment
+ Score below 20: Delirium, dementia, schizophrenia, or affective disorder

Cognitive Capacity Screening Examination
+ Measures orientation, memory, calculation, and language to assess dementia and delirium

Cognitive Assessment Scale
Screens for age-induced impairment by testing:
+ Temporal orientation
+ Spatial orientation
+ Attention-concentration and calculation
+ Immediate recall
+ Language
+ Remote memory
+ Judgment and abstraction
+ Agnosia
+ Apraxia
+ Recent memory

Beck Depression Inventory
+ Assesses severity of depression
+ Monitors patient's response to treatment
+ Has patient rate symptoms, such as poor concentration, suicidal thoughts, and guilty feelings
+ Evaluates both cognitive symptoms and physical symptoms

Abnormal findings
+ Score of 10 to 18: Mild depression
+ Score of 19 to 29: Moderate to severe depression
+ Score of 30 to 63: Severe depression

You may help patients complete the BDI by reading the questions, but be careful not to influence their answers. Instruct patients to choose the answer that describes them most accurately.

If you suspect depression, a BDI score above 17 may provide objective evidence for the need for treatment. To monitor the patient's depression, repeat the BDI during the course of treatment.

GLOBAL DETERIORATION SCALE

Global Deterioration Scale

+ Assesses and stages primary degenerative dementia such as Alzheimer's disease
+ Evaluates orientation, memory, and neurologic function

The Global Deterioration Scale (GDS) assesses and stages primary degenerative dementia based on orientation, memory, and neurologic function. It provides caregivers with an overview of the stages of cognitive function for those suffering from a primary degenerative dementia such as Alzheimer's disease. The results are broken down into seven stages:
+ Stages 1 to 3 are the predementia stages.
+ Stages 4 to 7 are the dementia stages.

Beginning in stage 5, an individual can no longer survive without assistance. Caregivers can get an idea of where an individual is at in the disease process by observing that individual's behavioral characteristics and comparing them to the GDS.

MINNESOTA MULTIPHASIC PERSONALITY INVENTORY

Minnesota Multiphasic Personality Inventory

+ Assesses personality traits and ego function
+ Reveals coping strategies, defenses, strengths, gender identification, and self-esteem
+ May suggest risk for suicide or violence, hypochondria, emotional distress
+ Interpretation based on 1930s personality profiles; may be faulty

Made up of 566 items, the Minnesota Multiphasic Personality Inventory test is a structured paper-and-pencil test that provides a practical technique for assessing personality traits and ego function in adolescents and adults. Most patients who read English require little assistance in completing this test.

Psychologists translate a patient's answers into a psychological profile. Use caution in interpreting profiles. Patient answers are compared with diagnostic criteria established and standardized in the 1930s. Critics charge that the personality profile models developed in the 1930s were based on studies of small groups (30 people) and may no longer provide a valid basis for diagnosis.

Test results include information on coping strategies, defenses, strengths, gender identification, and self-esteem. The psychologist combines the patients' profile with data gathered from the interview and explains the test results to the patient.

The test pattern may strongly suggest a diagnostic category. If results indicate a risk for suicide or violence, monitor the patient's behavior. If results show frequent somatic complaints indicating possible hypochondria, evaluate the patient's physical status. If complaints lack medical confirmation, help the patient explore how these symptoms may signal emotional distress.

DRAW-A-PERSON TEST

Draw-a-person test

+ Patient's drawing of a human figure of each sex
+ Interpreted in relation to patient's diagnosis
+ Estimates a child's developmental level

In the draw-a-person test, the patient draws a human figure of each sex. The psychologist interprets the drawing systematically and correlates his interpretation with diagnosis. This test also provides an estimate of a child's developmental level.

SENTENCE COMPLETION TEST

Sentence completion test

+ Reveals patient's fantasies, fears, aspirations, or anxieties

In the sentence completion test, the patient completes a series of partial sentences. A sentence might begin, "When I get angry, I…." The response may reveal the patient's fantasies, fears, aspirations, or anxieties.

The Rorschach test: What do you see?

The illustration depicts two of ten inkblots shown to patients during a Rorschach test. The patient describes his impressions of each inkblot and the psychologist analyzes the content of the responses as an aid in personality evaluation.

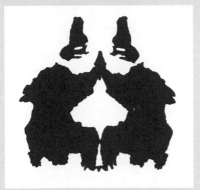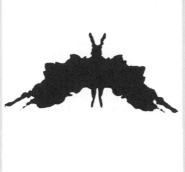

THEMATIC APPERCEPTION TEST

With the thematic apperception test, the patient views a series of pictures depicting ambiguous situations, he then tells a story describing each picture. The psychologist evaluates these stories systematically to obtain insights into the patient's personality, particularly regarding interpersonal relationships and conflicts.

THE RORSCHACH TEST

During a Rorschach test, the patient is asked to describe his impressions of 10 inkblots. The psychologist analyzes the content of the responses as an aid in personality evaluation. (See *The Rorschach test: What do you see?*)

PHYSICAL ASSESSMENT

Because mental health problems may stem from organic causes or medical treatment, a physical assessment is also warranted. Observe the patient for key signs and symptoms and examine him by using inspection, palpation, percussion, and auscultation.

CLASSIFICATION OF MENTAL DISORDERS

Mental status disorders are classified according to the American Psychiatric Association's *Diagnostic and Statistical Manual of Mental Disorders,* Fourth Edition, Text Revision (*DSM-IV-TR*). The classification emphasizes observable data and de-emphasizes subjective and theoretical impressions. This manual offers a standardized interdisciplinary system for all members of the mental health care team to use. It includes a complete description of psychiatric disorders and other conditions,

The Rorschach test
+ Depicts inkblots for patient interpretation
+ Aids in personality evaluation

Thematic apperception test
+ Lends insight into personality, relationships, and conflicts through story completion exercises

Physical assessment
+ Reveals organic causes and medical treatments as possible roots of a mental health problem
+ Includes observation, inspection, palpation, percussion, and auscultation

Classification of mental disorders
+ Uses APA's *DSM-IV-TR*
+ Includes complete description of psychiatric disorders and their required diagnostic criteria
+ Emphasizes observable data and de-emphasizes subjective and theoretical impressions

Understanding the *DSM-IV-TR*

When evaluating a psychiatric patient, considering factors that may have influenced his condition, such as life stresses or physical illness is an important part in arriving at a diagnosis. To help health care providers accomplish this, the *American Psychiatric Association's Diagnostic and Statistical Manual of Mental Disorders,* Fourth Edition, Text Revision (*DSM-IV-TR*) offers a more flexible approach to diagnosis and a more realistic picture of the patient, which should improve treatment. The key? The *DSM-IV-TR* multiaxial evaluation requires that every patient be assessed on each of five axes.

AXIS I
Clinical syndromes; conditions not attributable to a mental disorder that are a focus of attention or treatment; additional codes

AXIS II
Personality disorders; specific developmental disorders

AXIS III
Physical disorders and conditions, general medical conditions

AXIS IV
Psychosocial and environmental problems

AXIS V
Global Assessment and Functioning; highest level of adaptive functioning during the past year.

For example, a patient's diagnosis might read as follows:
Axis I: adjustment disorder with anxious mood
Axis II: obsessive-compulsive personality
Axis III: Crohn's disease, acute bleeding episode
Axis IV: 5 to 6 (moderately severe); recent remarriage, death of father
Axis V: very good; patient has been a successful single parent, new wife, schoolteacher, part-time journalist.

and describes diagnostic criteria that must be met to support each diagnosis. (See *Understanding the* DSM-IV-TR.)

Psychiatric disorders

Facts about schizophrenia

✦ Signs and symptoms of distortion of normal function or a loss of normal function for 1 month
✦ Marked inability to function in social settings or at work
✦ Positive signs: Delusions, hallucinations, disorganized speech, disorganized or catatonic behavior
✦ Negative signs: Flat or inappropriate affect, inability to speak, poor eye contact, distant and unresponsive facial expression, limited body language

PSYCHIATRIC DISORDERS

Here's a list of psychiatric disorders according to the *DSM-IV-TR* and the assessment findings you can expect.

SCHIZOPHRENIA

Schizophrenia is characterized by both positive and negative signs and symptoms that have been present for a significant time during a 1-month period, with some signs and symptoms lasting for at least 6 months. These signs and symptoms are associated with marked inability to function in social settings or at work.

The positive signs and symptoms focus on a distortion of normal function, whereas the negative signs and symptoms indicate a loss of normal functions. Positive signs and symptoms include delusions, hallucinations, disorganized speech, and grossly disorganized or catatonic behavior.

The negative signs and symptoms of schizophrenia include flat affect, inability to speak, and lack of self-initiating behaviors. The patient typically shows a flat or inappropriate affect, exhibits poor eye contact, a distant and unresponsive facial expression, and limited body language.

OBSESSIVE-COMPULSIVE DISORDER

Obsessive-compulsive disorder is characterized by recurrent obsessions or compulsions that are severe enough to be time consuming (they take more than 1 hour per day) or they cause significant distress or impairment.

Obsessions may focus on anything, but patients commonly obsess about contamination, religion, repeated doubts, violence, sexuality, and obscenities. The obsessions are typically unrelated to real-life problems.

Compulsions are repetitive behaviors such as hand washing or mental acts such as silently repeating words to prevent or reduce anxiety or distress. They aren't performed for pleasure or gratification; the patient is typically driven to perform the compulsion to reduce the distress that accompanies the obsession.

MAJOR DEPRESSIVE DISORDER

Major depressive disorder occurs when the patient experiences a depressed mood or decreased interest or pleasure in all or almost all activities for at least 2 weeks' duration. These symptoms must occur almost every day and must be present for most of each day. For many patients, their social, occupational, and general functioning is greatly impaired.

Typical symptoms of depression include severe fatigue, inability to concentrate or make decisions, and feelings of sadness, worthlessness, or extreme guilt. The patient may also experience significant appetite changes with either weight loss or gain, and sleep disturbances, decreased libido, slowed movements, and recurrent thoughts of death.

BIPOLAR I DISORDER

Bipolar I disorder is characterized by the occurrence of one or more manic (extreme euphoria with loss of reality testing) episodes or mixed (both depressed and manic) episodes. Some patients may also have one or more major depressive episode.

During a manic episode, the patient is euphoric or irritable. Typical signs and symptoms include delusions of grandeur, flight of ideas, and extreme talkativeness. The patient may also be easily distracted and overindulge in pleasurable activities to the extent of causing negative consequences. It isn't uncommon for the patient to spend money recklessly or engage in high-risk sexual activities. He may require little sleep and may fail to meet his self-care needs.

GENERALIZED ANXIETY DISORDER

A patient with generalized anxiety disorder worries excessively and experiences tremendous anxiety almost daily. The worry lasts for longer than 6 months and is usually disproportionate to the situation. Patients typically worry about everyday, routine experiences, such as job responsibilities, finances, household chores, and misfortune to their children.

The patient may exhibit trembling and twitching. He may complain of muscle aches or soreness and shakiness. He may also experience signs and symptoms such as dry mouth, sweating, nausea, urinary frequency, or diarrhea.

Facts about obsessive-compulsive disorder

- ✦ Recurrent obsessions unrelated to real-life problems
- ✦ Typical obsessions: contamination, religion, doubts, violence, sexuality, obscenities
- ✦ Time-consuming, compulsive behaviors the patient is driven to perform to reduce the anxiety of the obsession
- ✦ Typical compulsions: Hand washing or reciting words

Facts about major depressive disorder

- ✦ Depressed mood or decreased interest or pleasure in activities for 2 weeks
- ✦ Impairs social, occupational, and general functioning
- ✦ Typical symptoms: fatigue, inability to concentrate or make decisions, sadness, feelings of worthlessness, guilt, appetite change, weight loss or gain, sleep disturbance, and thoughts of death

Facts about bipolar I disorder

- ✦ One or more manic or mixed episodes
- ✦ Mania: Euphoria or irritability, delusions of grandeur, flight of ideas, talkativeness, focus on pleasure, self-care neglect

Facts about generalized anxiety disorder

- ✦ Excessive worry and anxiety almost daily for 6 months
- ✦ Worry over everyday, routine experiences
- ✦ Typical complaints: trembling, twitching, muscle aches

Nutritional assessment

EVALUATING NUTRITIONAL STATUS

A healthy and balanced nutritional status should be the goal for every individual. This goal is met when nutrient supply, or intake, meets the demand, or requirement. An imbalance occurs when there's overnutrition (supply exceeds demand) or undernutrition (demand exceeds supply).

A patient's nutritional status is evaluated by examining information from several sources, including a nutritional screening as well as his medical history, physical assessment findings, and laboratory results, in order to detect potential imbalances. The sources used depend on the patient and setting. A comprehensive nutritional assessment may then be conducted to set goals and determine interventions to correct actual or potential imbalances.

Based on the information gathered in the comprehensive nutritional assessment, the patient may require restrictions in diet, such as a reduction in calories, fat, saturated fat, cholesterol, sodium, or other nutrients. Other diet plans involve therapeutic correction of imbalances, such as by increasing or decreasing certain minerals or vitamins.

NORMAL NUTRITION

Nutrition refers to the sum of the processes by which a living organism ingests, digests, absorbs, transports, uses, and excretes nutrients. For nutrition to be adequate, a person must receive the proper nutrients, including carbohydrates, proteins, lipids, vitamins, minerals, and water. Also, his digestive system must function properly for his body to make use of these nutrients.

The body breaks down nutrients mechanically and chemically into simpler compounds for absorption in the stomach and intestines. The mechanical breakdown of food begins with chewing and then continues in the stomach and intestine as food is churned in the GI tract. The chemical processes start with the salivary enzymes in the mouth and continue with acid and enzyme action throughout the rest of the GI tract.

Anabolism and catabolism

Anabolism is a "building up" process that occurs when simple substances, such as nutrients, are converted into more complex compounds to be used for tissue growth, maintenance, and repair.

Catabolism is a "breaking down" process that occurs when complex substances are converted into simple compounds and stored or used for energy.

Carbohydrates

Composed of carbon, hydrogen, and oxygen, carbohydrates provide the primary source of energy, yielding 4 kcal/g. Experts recommend that carbohydrates make up 50% to 60% of an individual's daily dietary intake.

Ingested as starches (complex carbohydrates) and sugars (simple carbohydrates), carbohydrates are the chief protein-sparing ingredients in a nutritionally sound diet. Carbohydrates are absorbed primarily as glucose; some are absorbed as fructose and galactose and converted to glucose by the liver. A body cell may metabolize glucose to produce the energy needed to maintain cell life or may store it in the muscles and liver as glycogen. It can be converted quickly when the body needs energy fast. If glucose is unavailable, the body breaks down stored fat, a source of energy during periods of starvation. (See *Anabolism and catabolism.*)

 ABNORMAL FINDINGS *Excessive carbohydrate intake — especially of simple carbohydrates — can cause obesity, predisposing the patient to many disorders, including hypertension.*

Proteins

Proteins, which consist of amino acids joined by peptide bonds, are complex organic compounds containing carbon, hydrogen, oxygen, and nitrogen atoms. One gram of protein yields 4 kcal. Proteins are necessary for growth, maintenance, and repair of body tissues. Cells of the body can't survive without protein.

Different proteins contain different amino acids. Not all protein food sources are identical in quality. Complete proteins — such as those found in poultry, fish, meat, eggs, milk, and cheese — can maintain body tissue and promote a normal growth rate; incomplete proteins, such as vegetables and grains, lack essential amino acids. Essential amino acids are organic proteins that the body needs for nitrogen balance but can't produce itself.

The body doesn't store protein. This nutrient has a limited life span and constantly undergoes change. The rate of protein turnover varies in different tissues. When the usual sources (carbohydrates and fat) can't meet the body's energy demands, the body uses protein precursors to generate energy.

In a healthy individual with adequate caloric and protein intake, nitrogen intake should equal nitrogen excretion (nitrogen balance). Positive nitrogen balance occurs when nitrogen intake exceeds its output — for example, during pregnancy or growth periods. Negative nitrogen balance occurs when nitrogen output exceeds intake.

ABNORMAL FINDINGS *In a patient with inadequate protein intake, negative nitrogen balance occurs, resulting in tissue wasting; insufficient quality of digested dietary protein; or excessive tissue breakdown after stress, injury, immobilization, or disease.*

Facts about carbohydrates
+ Composed of carbon, hydrogen, and oxygen
+ Primary source of energy
+ 50% to 60% of dietary intake
+ Ingested as starches and sugars; absorbed as glucose, fructose, and galactose
+ Convert quickly when body needs energy fast

Abnormal findings
+ Excessive carbohydrate intake — can lead to obesity and hypertension

Facts about proteins
+ Consist of amino acids joined by peptide bonds
+ Contain carbon, hydrogen, oxygen, and nitrogen
+ Vital for cell growth, maintenance, and repair
+ Complete protein foods — maintain body tissue and promote a normal growth rate
+ Incomplete protein foods — lack essential amino acids needed for nitrogen balance
+ Aren't stored by the body
+ Maintain nitrogen balance through adequate caloric and protein intake
+ Positive nitrogen balance — nitrogen intake exceeds output
+ Negative nitrogen balance — nitrogen output exceeds intake

Abnormal findings
+ Inadequate protein intake — results in tissue wasting, insufficient quality of digested protein, or excessive tissue breakdown

Five types of lipoproteins

+ Chylomicrons
+ Very-low-density lipoproteins
+ Low-density lipoproteins
+ Intermediate-density lipoproteins
+ High-density lipoproteins

Understanding lipoproteins

Synthesized primarily in the liver, lipoproteins consist of lipids combined with plasma proteins. The five types of lipoproteins are chylomicrons, very-low-density lipoproteins (VLDLs), low-density lipoproteins (LDLs), intermediate-density lipoproteins (IDLs), and high-density lipoproteins (HDLs).

CHYLOMICRONS

Chylomicrons are the lowest-density lipoproteins, consisting mostly of triglycerides derived from dietary fat, with small amounts of protein and other lipids. In the form of chylomicrons, long-chain fatty acids and cholesterol move from the intestine to the blood and storage areas. Researchers haven't found a connection between an above-normal level of circulating chylomicrons (type I hyperlipoproteinemia) and coronary artery disease (CAD).

VLDLs

VLDLs contain mostly triglycerides with some phospholipids and cholesterol. Produced in the liver and small intestine, VLDLs transport glycerides. Obese patients and those with diabetes and, less commonly, young patients with CAD, may have above-normal VLDL levels (type IV hyperlipoproteinemia).

LDLs

LDLs consist mainly of cholesterol, with comparatively few triglycerides. By-products of VLDL breakdown, LDLs have the highest atherogenic potential (conducive to forming plaques containing cholesterol and other lipid material in the arteries). An elevated LDL level (type II hyperlipoproteinemia) commonly accompanies an elevated VLDL level.

IDLs

IDLs are short-lived and contain almost equal amounts of cholesterol and triglycerides and smaller amounts of phospholipids and protein. IDLs are converted to LDLs by lipase.

HDLs

HDLs, which are about 50% protein and 50% phospholipids, cholesterol, and triglycerides, may help remove excess cholesterol. Because patients with high HDL levels have a lower incidence of CAD, many researchers believe HDLs may help protect against CAD.

Facts about lipids

+ Chemically similar to carbohydrates
+ Consist of carbon, hydrogen, and oxygen
+ Essential for normal functioning
+ Combine with plasma proteins to form lipoproteins for transport
+ Should be 30% of daily caloric intake

Facts about vitamins

+ Essential for normal metabolism, growth, and development
+ Contribute to enzyme reactions
+ A, D, E, K—fat-soluble vitamins

Lipids

Chemically similar to carbohydrates, lipids consist of carbon, hydrogen, and oxygen. However, they have a smaller proportion of oxygen than carbohydrates, and also differ in their structure and properties.

Lipids and other fats are essential for normal functioning. To be transported throughout the body, they must combine with plasma proteins to form lipoproteins. (See *Understanding lipoproteins*.) Similarly, free fatty acids combine with albumin; and cholesterol, triglycerides, and phospholipids bind to globulin.

One gram of fat yields 9 kcal. Fats should make up about 30% of the daily caloric intake—5% to 10% less than the amount ingested by the average person. Saturated fats should account for only about one-third of total fat consumption, and an individual should consume no more than 300 mg of cholesterol per day.

Vitamins and minerals

Essential for normal metabolism, growth, and development, vitamins and minerals are biologically active organic compounds that contribute to enzyme reactions that facilitate the metabolism of amino acids, fats, and carbohydrates. Although the body requires relatively small amounts of vitamins, inadequate vitamin intake leads to deficiency states and disorders.

Water-soluble vitamins include vitamins C and B complex. Fat-soluble vitamins include vitamins A, D, E, and K. Surgery, disease, medication, metabolic disorders,

---

Role of minerals in metabolism

Dietary intake of minerals is essential for these physiologic functions:
- maintenance of acid-base balance and osmotic pressure
- membrane transfer of essential compounds
- metabolism of enzymes
- muscle contractility
- nerve impulse transmission
- growth.

---

and trauma affect the activity of vitamins in the body. Because readily observable changes don't occur until the late stages of vitamin deficiency, you must assess the patient's dietary intake and observe for subtle changes that provide an early warning of vitamin depletion.

Minerals are equally essential to good nutrition and participate in various physiologic activities. (See *Role of minerals in metabolism.*)

Water

Essential to sustain life, water transports nutrients throughout the body and may contribute minerals when consumed.

NUTRITIONAL SCREENING

Nutritional screening looks at certain variables to determine the risk of nutritional problems in certain populations. A screening may target pregnant women, elderly people, or those with particular conditions (such as cardiac disorders) to detect deficiencies or potential imbalances. A dietitian, diet technician, or other qualified health care professional may perform this type of screening. Routine screening takes place during the initial history and physical assessment.

The most commonly examined values include:
- height and weight history
- unintentional weight loss (more than 5% in 30 days)
- laboratory values
- skin integrity
- appetite
- present illness or diagnosis
- medical history
- diet
- functional status
- advanced age (age 80 and older).

WELLNESS SCREEN

A wellness screen has been developed by the Nutritional Screening Initiative, a project of the American Academy of Family Physicians, the American Dietetic Association, and the National Council on the Aging, Inc. This screening tool also assesses body mass index (BMI), which evaluates height in relationship to weight as well as eating habits, living environment, and functional status. (See *Using a wellness screen,* page 68.)

Facts about minerals
- Maintain acid-base balance and osmotic pressure
- Aid membrane transfer of essential compounds
- Essential for enzyme metabolism, muscle contraction, nerve impulse transmission, growth

Facts about water
- Essential to sustain life
- Transports nutrients
- May contribute minerals

Nutritional screening
- Height and weight history
- Unintentional weight loss (more than 5% in 30 days)
- Laboratory values
- Skin integrity
- Present illness or diagnosis
- Medical history
- Diet and appetite
- Functional status
- Advanced age (age 80 and older)

Wellness screen
- Assesses BMI
- Evaluates eating habits
- Looks at living environment
- Assesses functional status
- Indicates risk and need for further assessment

Using a wellness screen

A wellness screen is an effective assessment tool for evaluating nutritional status. It provides useful information about the patient's body mass index (BMI), eating habits, living environment, and functional status. A checkmark next to any statement indicates that the patient is at risk and requires further assessment. If indicated, contact the appropriate resources who can provide additional help.

Patient's name: _Robert Harrison_   **Date** _5/30/04_

BODY MASS INDEX
The BMI measures total body fat based on height and weight. To calculate your patient's BMI, first obtain his height to the nearest inch and his weight to the nearest pound. Calculate his BMI by dividing the body weight in kilograms by height in meters squared or by dividing the weight in pounds by height in inches squared and multiplying that result by 703.

Height (in): ___71___
Weight (lb): ___220___
BMI: ___31___

Check whether:
- ☐ the patient lost or gained 10 lb or more in the past 6 months.
- ☐ the BMI is less than 18.5.
- ☑ the BMI is greater than 24.9.

EATING HABITS
Check whether the patient:
- ☐ doesn't have enough food to eat each day.
- ☐ usually eats alone.
- ☐ doesn't eat anything on one or more days each month.
- ☐ has a poor appetite.
- ☐ is on a special diet.
- ☑ eats vegetables two or fewer times per day.
- ☑ drinks milk or eats milk products once or less per day.
- ☐ eats fruit or drinks fruit juice once or less daily.
- ☐ eats breads, cereals, pasta, rice, or other grains five or fewer times daily.
- ☐ has difficulty chewing or swallowing.
- ☑ has more than one alcoholic drink per day (if a woman); more than two drinks per day (if a man).
- ☐ has pain in the mouth, teeth, or gums.

LIVING ENVIRONMENT
Check whether the patient:
- ☐ lives on an income of less than $6,000 per year (per individual in the household).
- ☑ lives alone.
- ☐ is housebound.
- ☐ is concerned about home security.
- ☐ lives in a home with inadequate heating or cooling.
- ☐ doesn't have a stove or refrigerator.
- ☐ can't or prefers not to spend money on food (less than $25 per person spent on food each week).

FUNCTIONAL STATUS
Check whether the patient needs help with:
- ☐ bathing.
- ☐ dressing.
- ☐ grooming.
- ☐ toileting.
- ☐ eating.
- ☐ walking or moving about.
- ☐ traveling (outside of the home).
- ☑ preparing food.
- ☑ shopping for food or other necessities.

Measuring BMI

- ◆ Obtain patient's height to nearest inch and weight to nearest pound
- ◆ Divide weight in kilograms by height in meters squared
- ◆ Or, divide weight in pounds by height in inches squared and multiply that result by 703

Levels of risk for malnutrition

A patient may be assigned a risk level according to protocols established by your facility. An example of such a risk table is shown here. Even if a patient is determined to be at low risk or no risk at all, periodic evaluations should be done to detect changes in his nutritional status.

RISK FACTOR	LOW	MILD	MODERATE	HIGH
Weight (% ideal body weight)	> 90	80 to 90	70 to 80	< 70
Serum albumin (g/dl)	> 3.4	3.0 to 3.3	2.5 to 2.9	< 2.5
Intake	Adequate	Fair to good	Poor to fair	Poor to fair
Skin (pressure ulcers)	Intact	Stage I or stage II	Stage III or stage IV	Stage III or stage IV
Diet	Solid	Solid, stable enteral nutrition	Nothing by mouth (NPO), clear liquid, unstable enteral nutrition, parenteral nutrition	NPO, clear liquid, unstable enteral nutrition, parenteral nutrition
Actions	Monitor; provide basic nutrition care	Provide supplements; assist with food choices; teach and counsel	Refer to dietitian	Refer to dietitian

Risk for malnutrition
+ Ranges from low to mild to moderate to high
+ Factors include weight, serum albumin levels, intake, skin integrity, diet, and actions
+ Assigned to patient based on protocols established by facility
+ Higher-risk patients require comprehensive nutritional assessment
+ Lower- to moderate-risk patients require periodic reevaluation

RISK ASSESSMENT

Once the wellness screening is complete, a level of risk for nutritional problems is assigned. Those individuals at higher risk should be given a comprehensive nutritional assessment, whereas those at lower to moderate risk should be periodically reevaluated. (See *Levels of risk for malnutrition*.)

COMPREHENSIVE NUTRITIONAL ASSESSMENT

When the nutritional screening has identified a patient at risk, a comprehensive nutritional assessment is conducted to examine additional factors and better determine the degree of malnutrition. Using this assessment, a baseline nutritional status is determined and effective nutritional care is planned. Because of the extensive training required and the need for accuracy, a registered dietitian is usually responsible for conducting this assessment.

The comprehensive assessment is commonly performed on moderate- to high-risk patients with some degree of protein-calorie malnutrition. Major parameters examined include:
+ health (medical) history
+ physical examination findings
+ laboratory test results.

Comprehensive nutritional assessment
+ Medical history
+ Physical examination findings
+ Laboratory test results

Multiple criteria must be examined to provide an accurate evaluation of the patient's nutritional status. No single criterion can be used to evaluate a patient, and it may not be necessary to gather all possible information for every patient. The decision to consider what information to evaluate is left to the dietitian's discretion.

OBTAINING A HEALTH HISTORY

A past and current health history is usually gathered from the patient's medical record or through an interview with the patient.

Past health history

In the history, it's important to identify an existing condition that might affect nutritional status. The condition's impact on nutritional status depends on the severity of the existing condition and how long the patient has been afflicted. (See *Tips for detecting nutritional problems.*)

Ask the patient if he has ever experienced any major illnesses, trauma, extensive dental work, hospitalizations, or chronic medical conditions. Any of these can alter nutritional intake.

Poor nutritional status may reveal:
+ chewing and swallowing problems resulting from ill-fitting dentures, missing teeth, or mechanical problems, such as an obstruction, inflammation, or edema
+ neurologic problems, such as dysphagia, Parkinson's disease, stroke, or traumatic brain injury
+ anorexia
+ cognitive impairments
+ paralysis or physical disabilities, which may impair the patient's ability to feed himself.

Obtain information about food allergies. By causing the patient to eliminate certain foods, allergies increase the risk of nutritional deficiencies. Use information about food allergies to help the patient plan safe, balanced meals and to prevent the hospitalized patient from being served foods that can cause allergic reactions.

Other conditions that compromise nutritional status include eating disorders, such as anorexia nervosa and bulimia, and substance abuse. Ask the patient if he has ever had (or been told he has) any of these conditions.

Other problems may also be detected that result in impairment in digestion and absorption, resulting in altered nutritional status. These problems include inflammatory, obstructive, or functional disorders of the GI tract, such as:
+ lactose intolerance
+ cystic fibrosis
+ pancreatic disorders
+ inflammatory bowel diseases
+ minimal function in the small intestine due to a disorder, such as Crohn's disease or surgical excision (short-gut syndrome)
+ radiation enteritis
+ liver disorders.

Nutrition may also be affected by conditions known to accelerate metabolism. These conditions include:
+ pregnancy
+ fever
+ sepsis
+ thermal injuries
+ pressure ulcers
+ cancer

Past health history
+ May reveal major illnesses, trauma, dental work, hospitalizations, chronic medical conditions, food allergies, weight changes

Causes of poor nutrition
+ Chewing and swallowing problems
+ Neurologic problems
+ Anorexia and other eating disorders
+ Cognitive impairments
+ Paralysis or physical disabilities
+ Food allergies
+ Substance abuse
+ Inflammatory, obstructive, or functional disorders of Gi tract
+ Conditions that accelerate metabolism
+ Conditions that alter nutrient metabolism, absorption, or excretion
+ Poorly balanced weight-loss or weight-gain programs

Tips for detecting nutritional problems

Nutritional problems may stem from physical conditions, drug use, diet, or lifestyle factors. Use this list to help determine if your patient is at risk for a nutritional problem.

PHYSICAL CONDITION
- ◆ Chronic illnesses (diabetes, cystic fibrosis, malabsorption syndromes, or neurologic, cardiac, pulmonary, renal, hepatic, or thyroid problems)
- ◆ Family history of diabetes or heart disease
- ◆ Draining wounds or fistulas
- ◆ Obesity or a weight gain of 20% above normal body weight
- ◆ Unplanned weight loss of 20% below normal body weight
- ◆ History of or recent GI disturbances
- ◆ Anorexia nervosa or bulimia
- ◆ Depression or anxiety
- ◆ Severe trauma
- ◆ Recent chemotherapy, radiation therapy, or bone marrow transplantation
- ◆ Physical limitation (paresis or paralysis)

- ◆ Recent major surgery
- ◆ Pregnancy, especially teen or multiple birth
- ◆ Elderly or very young patients
- ◆ Burns

DRUG USE AND DIET
- ◆ Fad diets
- ◆ Steroid, diuretic, immunosuppressant, or antacid use
- ◆ Mouth, tooth, or denture problems
- ◆ Excessive alcohol intake
- ◆ Strict vegetarian diet
- ◆ Liquid diet or nothing by mouth for more than 3 days

LIFESTYLE
- ◆ Lack of support from family and friends
- ◆ Financial problems

- ◆ acquired immunodeficiency syndrome (AIDS)
- ◆ major surgery
- ◆ trauma
- ◆ burns.

Some conditions, such as diabetes mellitus, hormonal imbalances, and starvation, alter nutrient metabolism. In addition, diarrhea and malabsorption syndromes, such as celiac disease, cause increased nutrient excretion, whereas other conditions, such as renal insufficiency, impair nutrient excretion.

Ask the patient if he has followed a planned weight-loss or weight-gain program within the past 6 months. If so, have him describe the program. Is the program well-balanced?

Current health history

In the health history, it's relevant to also obtain information about the patient's current nutritional status. Ask the patient if he has changed his diet recently. If so, ask him to describe specific changes and their duration. Has his caloric intake increased or decreased? A decreased intake contributes to weight loss and may lead to nutritional deficiency. An increased intake may lead to weight gain but doesn't rule out nutritional deficiency.

Has the patient experienced any unusual stress or trauma, such as surgery, change in employment, or family illness? Stress and trauma magnify the body's need for essential nutrients.

Ask the patient if he has gained or lost a significant amount of weight or undergone a change in appetite, bowel habits, mobility, physical exercise, or lifestyle. Significant changes may indicate underlying disease.

Current health history
- ◆ Reveals recent diet and caloric intake changes
- ◆ Uncovers experiences of unusual stress or trauma, change in employment, or family illness
- ◆ Reveals weight gain or loss
- ◆ Shows change in appetite, bowel habits, mobility, physical exercise, or lifestyle

---

Caffeine content of common beverages

Use this chart to estimate the amount of caffeine your patient consumes daily.

BEVERAGE	CAFFEINE CONTENT
Coffee (brewed), 1 cup	85 mg
Coffee (instant), 1 cup	60 mg
Black tea (brewed), 1 cup	50 mg
Cola, 12 oz	32 to 65 mg
Green tea (brewed), 1 cup	30 mg
Cocoa, 1 cup	8 mg
Decaffeinated coffee, 1 cup	3 mg

Current health history
(continued)

Abnormal findings
+ Weight gain — endocrine imbalance causing Cushing's syndrome or hypothyroidism
+ Weight loss — cancer, GI disorders, diabetes mellitus, or hyperthyroidism

ABNORMAL FINDINGS *Weight gain in a patient may indicate an endocrine imbalance, such as Cushing's syndrome or hypothyroidism. Weight loss may result from cancer, GI disorders, diabetes mellitus, or hyperthyroidism.*

Does the patient take prescription or over-the-counter (OTC) drugs, especially vitamin or mineral supplements or appetite suppressants? If so, what's the purpose, starting date, dose, and frequency of each? Does he use any "natural" or "health" foods? If so, which ones and how much does he use, and why? Does he avoid certain foods such as meat? Answers here may reveal a nutritional deficiency requiring supplementation. The patient himself may perceive a nutritional deficiency and self-prescribe a supplement. In other cases, the response may reveal routine drug use that can cause nutritional deficiencies or related problems.

Other questions to ask the patient include:
+ Do you drink alcohol? If so, how much per day or week and what kind? How long have you been drinking alcohol?
+ Do you smoke or use chewing tobacco or snuff?
+ How much coffee, tea, cola, and cocoa do you drink each day?

Alcohol intake provides calories (7 kcal/g) but no essential nutrients. Chronic alcohol abuse leads to malnutrition. Use of tobacco products may affect taste, which in turn affects appetite. Coffee, tea, cola, and cocoa contain caffeine, a habit-forming stimulant that increases heart rate, respiratory rate, blood pressure, and secretion of stress hormones. In moderate amounts of 50 to 200 mg/day, caffeine is relatively harmless. Intake of greater amounts can cause sensations of nervousness and intestinal discomfort. (See *Caffeine content of common beverages.*)

Patients who drink eight or more cups of coffee per day may complain of insomnia, restlessness, agitation, palpitations, and recurring headaches. Sudden abstinence after long periods of even moderate daily caffeine intake can cause withdrawal symptoms such as headache.

Family history

Next, explore possible genetic or familial disorders that may affect the patient's nutritional status. Find out if the family history includes cardiovascular disease,

Crohn's disease, diabetes mellitus, cancer, GI tract disorders, sickle cell anemia, allergies, food intolerance (for example, lactose intolerance), or obesity. These disorders may affect digestion or metabolism of food and alter the patient's nutritional status.

Stress and coping mechanisms

How much stress does the patient encounter in his daily life? What's his usual method of coping? Responses to earlier questions on patterns of activity and nutrition may provide clues to how the patient handles stress.

Ask him if stress, from his job or elsewhere, influences his eating patterns. Daily schedules commonly interfere with mealtimes, predisposing the patient to nutritional deficiencies.

Does the patient use food or drink to get through stressful times? Individuals undergoing stress may increase or decrease food intake or change the type of food they eat. Keep in mind that the patient may not be fully aware of his behavior or may be reluctant to discuss it.

Socioeconomic factors

Economic, cultural, and socioeconomic factors can markedly affect a patient's nutritional health. Ask the following questions:
+ Where and how is your food prepared?
+ Do you have access to adequate storage and refrigeration?
+ Do you receive welfare payments, Social Security payments, Supplemental Security Income, food stamps, or assistance from the Women, Infants, and Children Program?

If the patient doesn't cook his own food, his nutritional health depends on whether others are available to help him. Inadequate food storage and refrigeration can lead to nutritional problems. A change in economic status or the loss of a food program may also disrupt the patient's nutritional well-being.

Self-concept

Ask the patient, "Do you like the way you look?" and "Are you content with your present weight?" Society's focus on thinness and physical prowess may cause children to become overweight and adults to feel uncomfortable. Many weight-reduction plans guarantee success; if the patient fails to lose weight or maintain weight loss, he may perceive himself as a failure. Poor self-image may cause these patients to avoid settings that require vigorous exercise or body exposure. To make matters worse, advertisements constantly remind these individuals of the pleasures of food and drink.

Misconception about ideal weight and poor self-image can also lead to eating disorders, such as anorexia nervosa or bulimia.

Social support

Find out if the patient eats alone or with others. Single adults and isolated elderly patients may neglect their nutrition. A person grieving over the recent loss of a loved one may also lose interest in food.

Ask the patient to rate the importance of mealtimes on a scale of 1 to 10, with 10 being the most important. This rating will help determine if meals are enjoyed or endured. The patient who merely endures his meals may develop an eating disorder.

Intake information

Intake information helps you assess what and how much your patient eats. This information can help identify problems in nutritional status and behaviors that need improvement.

Family history
+ Cardiovascular disease, Crohn's disease, diabetes mellitus, cancer, GI tract disorders, sickle cell anemia, allergies, food intolerance, obesity

Stress and coping mechanisms
+ Daily stressors
+ Methods of coping
+ Eating patterns

Socioeconomic factors
+ Food preparation
+ Adequate storage and refrigeration
+ Financial assistance

Self-concept
+ Comfort with personal appearance, including weight
+ Possibility of eating disorder

Social support
+ Preference to dine alone or with others
+ Importance of meals on scale of 1 to 10

Intake information
+ Nutritional behaviors, such as food choices and amount of food consumed

Observing what the patient eats provides an objective measurement of the kinds and amount of foods consumed. Of course, close observation of a patient is rarely possible. A screening, commonly a questionnaire geared to nutritional problems, can help fill in this information gap. Open-ended questions are more useful than closed, "yes-or-no" questions for obtaining accurate information. Important areas for questioning include:

✦ number of meals and snacks eaten in a 24-hour period
✦ unusual food habits
✦ time of day most of the calories are consumed
✦ skipped meals
✦ meals eaten away from home
✦ number of fruits and vegetables eaten daily
✦ number of servings (and types) of grains eaten daily
✦ how often red meat, poultry, and fish are eaten, including type and amount
✦ how often meatless meals are consumed
✦ number of hours of television watched daily while eating snacks or meals
✦ types and amount of dairy products consumed daily
✦ how often desserts and sweets are eaten
✦ types and amount of beverages (including alcohol) consumed
✦ food allergies or intolerances
✦ dietary supplements and why they are taken
✦ medications, including OTC products and herbal supplements.

 SPECIAL POINTS What your patient eats depends on various cultural and economic influences. Understanding these influences can give you more insight into the patient's nutritional status:

✦ *Socioeconomic status may affect a patient's ability to afford healthful foods in the quantities needed to maintain proper nutrition.*
✦ *Work schedule can affect the amount and type of food a patient eats, especially if he works full-time at night.*
✦ *Religion can influence food choices. For example, some Jews and Muslims don't eat pork products, and many Roman Catholics avoid meat on Ash Wednesday and Fridays during Lent.*
✦ *Ethnic background influences food choices. For example, fish and rice are staple foods for many Asians.*

Diet history tools

More formal tools for taking a patient's diet history have been developed. The 24-hour food recall and the food frequency record are tools that you can use to examine what, how much, and how often a patient typically eats to determine his nutritional status.

The 24-hour recall

A quick and easy method of evaluating a patient's intake is through the 24-hour recall. In order to complete this, the patient must be able to recount all the types and amounts of foods and beverages he has consumed during a 24-hour period.

The time period may be the past 24 hours or a typical 24-hour period. To help the patient identify portion sizes, food models or pictures of typical portions can be used. Specific details may be necessary in some recall situations, such as food preparation (for example, frying versus dry roasting meat). Open-ended questions also reveal more information than typical "yes-or-no" questions. When the information is obtained, recall data is evaluated to see if the patient's nutritional needs are being met.

Intake information

Special points: Cultural and economic influences on eating

✦ Socioeconomic status — affects ability to afford healthful foods in quantities needed to maintain proper nutrition
✦ Work schedule — affects amount and type of food eaten, especially if working full-time at night
✦ Religion and ethic background — influence food choices

Diet history tools

✦ Determines what, when, and how often patient eats to assess nutritional status

The 24-hour recall

✦ Records foods and beverages consumed in 24-hours
✦ Uses food models or pictures to help identify portion sizes
✦ Reveals food preparation techniques, such as frying
✦ Asks open-ended questions to reveal more information

Food frequency record

The food frequency record is a checklist of particular foods that helps you determine what the patient is specifically consuming and how often. The checklist may list the foods in one column, and the patient marks off how often they're eaten in another column. The choices may include time periods, how often the food is consumed (such as per day, per week, or per month), or if the food is eaten frequently, seldom, or never. The data doesn't typically include the serving size, and it may only include specific foods or nutrients suspected of being deficient or excessive in the patient's diet.

Another method of gathering information for the food frequency record is to use a questionnaire that lists food items organized by food groups. In this document, the patient records the type of food consumed and how often.

Either checklist provides a more complete dietary picture when used in conjunction with the 24-hour recall. When deficiencies or excesses are identified, goals may be developed to address nutritional and educational needs.

Psychosocial factors

Other factors could be uncovered during the history that may influence the patient's nutritional habits, including:

+ illiteracy
+ language barriers
+ knowledge of nutrition and food safety
+ cultural or religious influences
+ social isolation
+ limited or low income
+ inadequate cooking resources, such as major appliances or kitchen access
+ limited access to transportation
+ physical inactivity or illness
+ use of tobacco or illicit drugs
+ limited community resources.

When psychosocial factors have been identified, the patient teaching plan will need to incorporate these elements as appropriate. For example, if you identify that your patient can't read or doesn't read well, a picture guide on which foods are appropriate and which should be avoided may be more helpful to the patient than written words alone.

DETERMINING PHYSICAL FINDINGS

Physical examinations help determine your patient's health status and identify any illnesses. Physical factors discovered during the comprehensive nutritional assessment may be related to an alteration in nutritional status and malnutrition. However, such findings as height and weight reflect chronic changes in nutritional status rather than acute processes.

Assessing body systems

When performing your head-to-toe assessment, remember that clinical signs are seen late. Nutritional deficiencies are most readily detected in the area of rapid turnover of the epithelial tissues.

Skin, hair, and nails

When assessing the patient's skin, hair, and nails, ask yourself these questions: Is his hair shiny and full? Is his skin free from blemishes and rashes? Is it warm and dry, with normal color for that particular patient? Are his nails firm with pink nail beds?

Diet history tools
(*continued*)

Food frequency record
+ Records food likes and dislikes
+ Reveals frequency and times when foods are eaten
+ Lists suspected deficient or excessive foods in diet
+ Sets goals for nutritional and educational needs

Psychosocial factors
+ Illiteracy and language barriers
+ Knowledge of nutrition and food safety
+ Cultural or religious influences
+ Social isolation
+ Limited or low income and inadequate cooking resources
+ Limited access to transportation
+ Physical inactivity or illness
+ Use of tobacco or illicit drugs
+ Limited community resources

Body system assessment
+ Clinical signs seen late
+ Nutritional deficiencies detected in epithelial tissues

Skin, hair, and nails
+ Appearance and fullness of hair
+ Blemish- and rash-free skin
+ Normal skin color for that patient
+ Firm nails and pink nail beds

Body system assessment

Eyes, nose, throat, and neck
+ Eyes — color and clearness
+ Nose — moist and pink-colored mucous membranes
+ Throat — pink tongue with papillae present; moist, pink gums
+ Neck — possible masses interfering with swallowing

Cardiovascular system
+ Regular heart rhythm
+ Normal heart rate and blood pressure for patient's age
+ Swelling of extremities

Pulmonary system
+ Clear lungs on auscultation
+ Ability to clear own secretions
+ Normal lung excursion

GI system
+ Appetite and GI problems
+ Elimination patterns and regularity
+ Absence of abdominal masses on palpation

Neuromuscular system
+ Alertness and responsiveness
+ Reflexes
+ Paresthesia of legs and feet
+ Muscle wasting, calf pain

Height
+ Measured using fixed measuring stick, with patient standing straight, without shoes, against a wall

Weight
+ Measured on a beam-balance scale, or bed scale for bedridden patient
+ Helpful if weight is measured on same scale at same time of day

KNOW-HOW

Overcoming height measurement problems

A patient confined to a wheelchair or one who can't stand straight because of scoliosis poses a challenge in measuring accurate height. An approximate measurement of height can be obtained by measuring "wingspan."

Have the patient hold his arms straight out from the sides of his body. Children may be told to hold their arms out "like bird wings." Measure from the tip of one middle finger to the tip of the other; this distance is the patient's approximate height.

Eyes, nose, throat, and neck

Are the patient's eyes clear and shiny? Are the mucous membranes in his nose moist and pink? Is his tongue pink with papillae present? Are his gums moist and pink? Is his mouth free from ulcers or lesions? Is his neck free from masses that would impede swallowing?

Cardiovascular system

Is the patient's heart rhythm regular? Are his heart rate and blood pressure normal for his age? Are his extremities free from swelling?

Pulmonary system

Are the patient's lungs clear to auscultation? Can he clear his own secretions? Is lung excursion normal?

GI system

Is the patient's appetite satisfactory, with no reported GI problems? Are his elimination patterns regular? Is his abdomen free from abnormal masses on palpation?

Neuromuscular system

Is the patient alert and responsive? Are his reflexes normal? Is his behavior appropriate? Are his legs and feet free from paresthesia? Is there any evidence of muscle wasting? Does the patient experience calf pain?

Assessing other physical features
Height

Height should be measured with the patient standing as straight as possible, without shoes, against a wall using a fixed measuring stick. Adaptations may be needed if the patient can't stand or cooperate. (See *Overcoming height measurement problems*.)

 SPECIAL POINTS *When measuring height, it's important to note the growth of children as well as diminishing height in older adults. Growth of children may be noted on standardized charts, such as those developed by the American Academy of Pediatrics, to assess growth patterns for possible abnormalities. Diminishing height in older adults may be related to osteoporotic changes and should be investigated.*

Weight

Weight may be measured on a beam-balance scale, or a bed scale if the patient is bedridden. The information gathered is more helpful if the weight is measured on the same scale at the same time of day (typically before breakfast and after voiding), in the same amount of clothing, and without shoes.

KNOW-HOW

Interpreting BMI

Currently, the most widely accepted classification of weight status is the body mass index (BMI). The BMI can be used as a measure of obesity, protein-calorie malnutrition as well as an indicator of health risk. All measures other than normal place the patient at a higher health risk, and nutritional needs should be assessed accordingly.

CLASSIFICATION	BMI
Underweight	≤ 18.5
Normal	18.5 to 24.9
Overweight	25 to 29.9
Obesity class 1	30 to 34.9
Obesity class 2	35 to 39.9
Obesity class 3	≥ 40

Body mass index

A useful measurement for assessing nutritional status is the body mass index (BMI), which uses a patient's weight and height to help classify him as underweight, normal, or obese. The BMI is calculated by dividing the body weight in kilograms by height in meters squared or by dividing the weight in pounds by height in inches squared and multiplying that result by 703. (See *Interpreting BMI*.)

Ideal body weight

Ideal body weight (IBW), also helpful in assessing nutritional status, is a reference standard for clinical use. For men, this measurement is 106 lb (48.1 kg) for a height of 5′ (1.5 m), plus an additional 6 lb (2.7 kg) for each inch over 5′. For women, IBW is 100 lb (45.4 kg) for a height of 5′, plus 5 lb (2.3 kg) for each inch over 5′. (See *Height and weight table,* page 78.)

IBW range can be 10% higher or lower depending on body size. The percentage of IBW is obtained by dividing the patient's true weight by the IBW and then multiplying that number by 100. This percentage can be used to determine the patient's weight status and accompanying health risk:

✦ An obese person is greater than 120% of IBW.
✦ An overweight person is 110% to 120% of IBW.
✦ A person whose weight is normal is 90% to 110% of IBW.
✦ A mildly underweight person is 80% to 90% of IBW.
✦ A moderately underweight person is 70% to 79% of IBW.
✦ A severely underweight person is less than 70% of IBW.

Body composition measurements

Measurements of body composition include the triceps skinfold measurement, the midarm circumference, and the midarm muscle circumference. These measure-

Body mass index
✦ Calculated by dividing weight in kilograms by height in meters squared or by dividing weight in pounds by height in inches squared and multiplying that result by 703

Ideal body weight
✦ Helpful in assessing nutritional status
✦ Serves as a reference standard
✦ For men, measurement is 106 lb for a height of 5′, plus an additional 6 lb for each inch over 5′
✦ For women, measurement is 100 lb for a height of 5′, plus 5 lb for each inch over 5′

Body composition measurements
✦ Include triceps skinfold measurement and midarm and midarm muscle circumference.

Height and weight table

Ongoing research suggests that people can carry more weight as they age, without added health risk. Because people of the same height may differ in muscle and bone makeup, a range of weights is shown for each height in this table. The higher weights in each category apply to men, who typically have more muscle and bone than women. Height measurements are without shoes; weight measurements are without clothes.

HEIGHT	WEIGHT	
	Ages 19 to 34	*Ages 35 and older*
5'0"	97 to 128	108 to 138
5'1"	101 to 132	111 to 143
5'2"	104 to 137	115 to 148
5'3"	107 to 141	119 to 152
5'4"	111 to 146	122 to 157
5'5"	114 to 150	126 to 162
5'6"	118 to 155	130 to 167
5'7"	121 to 160	134 to 172
5'8"	125 to 164	138 to 178
5'9"	129 to 169	142 to 183
5'10"	132 to 174	146 to 188
5'11"	136 to 179	151 to 194
6'0"	140 to 184	155 to 199
6'1"	144 to 189	159 to 205
6'2"	148 to 195	164 to 210
6'3"	152 to 200	168 to 216
6'4"	156 to 205	172 to 222
6'5"	160 to 211	177 to 228
6'6"	164 to 216	182 to 234

Facts about height and weight

+ People carry more weight as they age, without added health risk
+ People of the same height differ in muscle and bone makeup; therefore, a range of weights is used when assessing a patient
+ Men typically have more muscle and bone than women; therefore, they usually weight more

ments provide quantitative information about body composition made up of fat or muscle tissue. Measurements may be compared with reference standards or may be used to evaluate changes. If measurements are less than 90% of the reference value, nutritional intervention is indicated. Keep in mind that the patient and technical variations may limit the use of anthropometric measurements.

Triceps skinfold measurements

Triceps skinfold measures subcutaneous fat stores and is an index of total body fat. To measure the skinfold, the patient's arm hangs freely and a fold of skin located slightly above midpoint is grasped between the thumb and forefinger. As the skin is pulled away from underlying muscle, calipers are applied and the measurement is read to the nearest millimeter. (See *Taking anthropometric arm measurements,* page 80.)

Three readings are taken. These readings may be from the same site or other appropriate sites (biceps, thigh, calf, subscapular, or suprailiac skinfolds). The readings are then added together and divided by three to record the average. For men, 11.3 mm is 90% of standard; for women, 14.9 mm.

Midarm circumference

Midarm circumference measures muscle mass and subcutaneous fat. This value is taken from the midpoint of the individual's nondominant arm using a measuring tape. The forearm is flexed at 90 degrees and placed in a dependent position while a tape measure is placed around the mid-upper arm between the top of the acromion process of the scapula and olecranon process of the ulna. Readings are taken while the tape is held firmly—but not too tightly—and recorded to the nearest millimeter.

Midarm muscle circumference

Midarm muscle circumference provides an index of muscle mass and is an indication of somatic protein stores. The value is calculated by multiplying the triceps skin fold measurement by 3.14, then multiplying that value by the midarm circumference measurement. The value is recorded in centimeters. This value is minimally affected by edema and provides a quick estimation.

Overall appearance

Physical examination, which includes observing the patient's general appearance, may reveal signs of malnutrition that are related to a nutritional deficiency. However, signs may also be due to other conditions or disorders and can't be considered indicative, but only suggestive of a nutritional deficiency. In addition, remember that physical signs and symptoms may vary among populations because of genetic and environmental differences. (See *Evaluating nutritional disorders,* page 81.)

EVALUATING LABORATORY DATA

Laboratory test results can detect nutritional problems in early stages before physical signs and symptoms appear. Most of the routine tests assess protein-calorie information, with serum albumin used most commonly to screen for nutritional problems. Tests are done to help determine adequacy of protein stores. Some tests measure by-products of protein catabolism (such as creatinine) and others measure products of protein anabolism (such as albumin level, transferrin level, hemoglobin level, hematocrit, prealbumin, retinol binding protein, and total lymphocyte count).

(Text continues on page 82.)

Skinfold measurements

+ Measure subcutaneous fat stores
+ Serve as an index of total body fat
+ Performed by grasping patient's skin and measuring with calipers to nearest millimeter

Midarm circumference

+ Measures muscle mass and subcutaneous fat
+ Performed by reading measuring tape around mid-upper arm and recording to the nearest millimeter

Midarm muscle circumference

+ Provides an index of muscle mass
+ Gives an indication of somatic protein stores
+ Measured by multiplying triceps skin fold measurement by 3.14, then multiplying that value by the midarm circumference measurement
+ Value recorded in centimeters

Laboratory data

+ Serum albumin level
+ Creatinine height index
+ Transferrin level
+ Hemoglobin level
+ Hematocrit
+ Prealbumin
+ Retinol binding protein
+ Total lymphocyte count

Taking anthropometric arm measurements

- ◆ Patient and technical variations may limit the use of anthropometric measurements
- ◆ Three readings are taken
- ◆ The readings may be from biceps, thigh, calf, subscapular, or suprailiac skinfolds
- ◆ Add readings together and divide by 3 to record average
- ◆ For men, 11.3 mm is 90% of standard; for women, 14.9 mm
- ◆ A measurement of less than 90% of standard indicates caloric deprivation
- ◆ A measurement over 90% indicates adequate or more than adequate energy reserves

Taking anthropometric arm measurements

Follow these steps to determine triceps skinfold thickness, midarm circumference, and midarm muscle circumference.

TRICEPS SKINFOLD THICKNESS

1. Find the midpoint circumference of the arm by placing the tape measure halfway between the axilla and the elbow. Grasp the patient's skin with your thumb and forefinger, about ⅜" (1 cm) above the midpoint, as shown below.
2. Place the calipers at the midpoint and squeeze for 3 seconds.
3. Record the measurement to the nearest millimeter.
4. Take two more readings and use the average of all three.

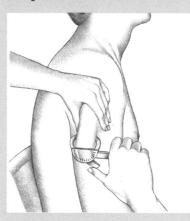

MIDARM CIRCUMFERENCE AND MIDARM MUSCLE CIRCUMFERENCE

1. At the midpoint measure the midarm circumference, as shown below. Record the measurement in centimeters.
2. Calculate the midarm muscle circumference by multiplying the triceps skinfold thickness — measured in millimeters — by 3.14.
3. Subtract this number from the midarm circumference.

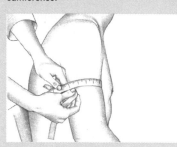

Recording the measurements
Record all three measurements as a percentage of the standard measurements (see chart below), using this formula:

$$\frac{\text{Actual measurement}}{\text{Standard measurement}} \times 100\%$$

After taking and recording the measurements above, consult the chart below to determine your patient's caloric status. Remember, a measurement of less than 90% of the standard indicates caloric deprivation. A measurement over 90% indicates adequate or more than adequate energy reserves.

MEASUREMENT	STANDARD	90%
Triceps skinfold thickness	Men: 12.5 mm Women: 16.5 mm	Men: 11.3 mm Women: 14.9 mm
Midarm circumference	Men: 29.3 cm Women: 28.5 cm	Men: 26.4 cm Women: 25.7 cm
Midarm muscle circumference	Men: 25.3 cm Women: 23.3 cm	Men: 22.8 cm Women: 20.9 cm

Evaluating nutritional disorders

Use this chart to determine the implications of the signs and symptoms revealed in the patient's nutritional assessment.

BODY SYSTEM OR REGION	SIGN OR SYMPTOM	IMPLICATIONS
General	✦ Weakness and fatigue ✦ Weight loss	✦ Anemia or electrolyte imbalance ✦ Decreased calorie intake or increased calorie use or inadequate nutrient intake or absorption
Skin, hair, and nails	✦ Dry, flaky skin ✦ Dry skin with poor turgor ✦ Rough, scaly skin with bumps ✦ Petechiae or ecchymoses ✦ Sore that won't heal ✦ Thinning, dry hair ✦ Spoon-shaped, brittle, or ridged nails	✦ Vitamin A, vitamin B-complex, or linoleic acid deficiency ✦ Dehydration ✦ Vitamin A deficiency or essential fatty acid deficiency ✦ Vitamin C or K deficiency ✦ Protein, vitamin C, or zinc deficiency ✦ Protein deficiency ✦ Iron deficiency
Eyes	✦ Night blindness; corneal swelling, softening, or dryness; Bitot's spots (gray triangular patches on the conjunctiva) ✦ Red conjunctiva	✦ Vitamin A deficiency ✦ Riboflavin deficiency
Throat and mouth	✦ Cracks at the corner of mouth ✦ Magenta-colored tongue ✦ Beefy, red tongue ✦ Soft, spongy, bleeding gums ✦ Swollen neck (goiter)	✦ Riboflavin or niacin deficiency ✦ Riboflavin deficiency ✦ Vitamin B_{12} deficiency ✦ Vitamin C deficiency ✦ Iodine deficiency
Cardiovascular	✦ Edema ✦ Tachycardia, hypotension	✦ Protein deficiency and zinc deficiency ✦ Fluid volume deficit
GI	✦ Ascites	✦ Protein deficiency
Musculoskeletal	✦ Bone pain and bow leg ✦ Muscle wasting ✦ Pain in calves and thighs	✦ Vitamin D or calcium deficiency ✦ Protein, carbohydrate, and fat deficiency ✦ Thiamine deficiency
Neurologic	✦ Altered mental status ✦ Paresthesia	✦ Dehydration and thiamine or vitamin B_{12} deficiency ✦ Vitamin B_{12}, pyridoxine, or thiamine deficiency

Serum albumin

+ Indicates protein levels in the body
+ Makes up more than 50% of total proteins in blood
+ Helps maintain osmotic pressure
+ Requires functioning liver cells and an adequate supply of amino acids

Abnormal findings

+ Decreased level — may be due to serious protein deficiency

Creatinine height index

+ Involves 24-hour urine collection
+ Measures urinary excretion of creatinine
+ Helps define body protein mass
+ Evaluates protein completion

Transferrin

+ Carrier protein that transports iron
+ Synthesized mainly in the liver
+ Decrease indicates depletion of protein stores
+ Normal value is greater than 200 mg/dl

Abnormal findings

+ Decreased values may indicate inadequate protein production; elevated levels may indicate severe iron deficiency

Hemoglobin

+ Main component of RBCs, which transport oxygen
+ Requires adequate supply of protein in the form of amino acids
+ Levels indicate blood's oxygen-carrying capacity
+ Diagnoses anemia, protein deficiency, and hydration status

Albumin

The serum albumin level test assesses protein levels in the body. Albumin makes up more than 50% of total proteins in blood and affects the cardiovascular system because it helps to maintain osmotic pressure. Keep in mind that albumin production requires functioning liver cells and an adequate supply of amino acids, the building blocks of proteins.

 ABNORMAL FINDINGS *When a patient's serum albumin level decreases this can be due to serious protein deficiency and loss of blood protein caused by burns, malnutrition, liver or renal disease, heart failure, major surgery, infections, or cancer.*

Decreased albumin levels correlate with poor clinical outcomes, increased length of hospitalization, and increased morbidity and mortality.

Creatinine height index

The creatinine height index involves a 24-hour urine collection to measure urinary excretion of creatinine. It helps define body protein mass and evaluate protein depletion. Test results are interpreted using a formula that compares results with ideal height standards.

The test is of limited value because results are greatly altered by age, amount of exercise, stress, menstruation, and the presence of severe illness. Increased values may indicate decreased protein stores.

 SPECIAL POINTS *Creatinine values decrease with age because of a normal decrease in lean muscle mass.*

Transferrin

Transferrin is a "carrier" protein that transports iron. The molecule is synthesized mainly in the liver. Transferrin levels decrease along with protein levels and indicate depletion of protein stores. Serum transferrin levels reflect the patient's current protein status more accurately than albumin levels because of their shorter half-life. A normal transferrin value is greater than 200 mg/dl.

 ABNORMAL FINDINGS *Decreased transferrin values may indicate inadequate protein production due to liver damage, protein loss from renal disease, acute or chronic infection, or cancer. Elevated levels may indicate severe iron deficiency.*

Hemoglobin

Hemoglobin (Hb) is the main component of red blood cells (RBCs), which transport oxygen. Its formation requires an adequate supply of protein in the form of amino acids. Hb levels help to assess the blood's oxygen-carrying capacity and are useful in diagnosing anemia, protein deficiency, and hydration status.

 ABNORMAL FINDINGS *Decreased Hb levels suggest iron deficiency anemia, protein deficiency, excessive blood loss, or overhydration. Increased Hb levels suggest dehydration or polycythemia.*

Normal Hb levels vary with the patient's age and type of blood sample tested. These values reflect normal Hb concentrations (in grams per deciliter):

+ neonates — 17 to 22 g/dl (SI, 170 to 220 g/L)
+ 1 week — 15 to 20 g/dl (SI, 150 to 200 g/L)
+ 1 month — 11 to 15 g/dl (SI, 110 to 150 g/L)
+ children — 11 to 13 g/dl (SI, 110 to 130 g/L)
+ adult males — 14 to 17.4 g/dl (SI, 140 to 174 g/L)
+ males after middle age — 12.4 to 14.9 g/dl (SI, 124 to 149/L)

✦ adult females — 12 to 16 g/dl (SI, 120 to 160 g/L)
✦ females after middle age — 11.7 to 13.8 g/dl (SI, 117 to 138 g/L).

Hematocrit

Hematocrit (HCT) reflects the proportion of blood occupied by the RBCs. This test helps diagnose anemia and dehydration.

 ABNORMAL FINDINGS *Decreased HCT suggests iron deficiency anemia or excessive fluid intake or blood loss. Increased HCT suggests severe dehydration or polycythemia.*

Normal HCT reflect age, gender, sample type, and the laboratory performing the test. These ranges represent normal HCT for different age-groups:
✦ neonates — 55% to 68% (SI, 0.55 to 0.68)
✦ 1 week — 47% to 65% (SI, 0.47 to 0.65)
✦ 1 month — 37% to 49% (SI, 0.37 to 0.49)
✦ 3 months — 30% to 36% (SI, 0.30 to 0.36)
✦ 1 year — 29% to 41% (SI, 0.29 to 0.41)
✦ 10 years — 36% to 40% (SI, 0.36 to 0.40)
✦ adult males — 42% to 52% (SI, 0.42 to 0.52)
✦ adult females — 36% to 48% (SI, 0.36 to 0.48).

Prealbumin

The prealbumin test is also more sensitive than the albumin test because of its shorter half-life (2 days). It isn't as affected by liver disease and hydration status as the albumin test is; however, it's more expensive to perform. A normal prealbumin value is 16 to 30 mg/dl.

Retinol binding protein

Retinol binding protein is a reliable measurement during acute response. It responds quickly to nutritional repletion due to a small body pool and short half-life (10 to 12 hours). A normal retinol binding protein value is 2.6 to 7.7 mg/dl.

Total lymphocyte count

A leukocyte is a white blood cell (WBC), which is the main cell responsible for fighting infection. Leukocytes are responsible for destroying organisms as well as for phagocytosis, which promotes cellular repair. Normal WBC counts range from 4,000 to 10,000/μl. This test is useful for diagnosing the severity of a disease.

There are five different types of leukocytes:
✦ neutrophils, which fight pyogenic infections
✦ eosinophils, which fight allergic disorders and parasitic infections
✦ basophils, which fight parasitic infections
✦ lymphocytes, which fight viral infections
✦ monocytes, which fight severe infections.

The WBC differential will provide specific information about which type of WBC is being affected and is a diagnostically useful test.

Malnutrition decreases the total number of lymphocytes, impairing the body's ability to fight infection. The total lymphocyte count is used in evaluating the health of the immune system and assists in evaluation of protein stores. The total lymphocyte count may also be affected by many medical conditions, so the value of this test is limited.

 ABNORMAL FINDINGS *Decreased total lymphocyte count may indicate malnutrition when no other cause is apparent. It may also point to infection, leukemia, or tissue necrosis.*

Cutaneous hypersensitivity reactions

+ Evaluate immunocompetence
+ Show positive reaction in 24 to 48 hours
+ Malnourished patients have delayed or no reaction

X-rays

+ Determine bone integrity to detect osteoporosis
+ Identify fractures, tumors, or inflammation
+ Evaluate GI tract for integrity
+ Diagnose disorders causing malnutrition

Nutritional disorders

+ Include protein-calorie malnutrition, obesity, anorexia nervosa, bulimia nervosa, or a vitamin deficiency

Facts about protein-calorie malnutrition

+ Caused by prolonged or chronic inadequate protein or caloric intake or by high metabolic protein and energy requirements
+ When protein or caloric intake is inadequate, the body breaks down stored proteins and fats to compensate

ASSESSING OTHER NUTRITIONAL DEFICIENCIES

Besides the patient's health history, physical findings, and laboratory data, you can use other criteria to measure poor nutrition.

Cutaneous hypersensitivity reactions

Immunocompetence may be evaluated by placing small quantities of recall antigens (Candida, mumps, or purified protein derivative of tuberculin) under the skin. Normally a positive reaction occurs in 24 to 48 hours with a red area of 5 mm or more. However, in the patient with malnutrition, a delayed reaction, reaction to only one antigen, or no reaction at all (anergy) may occur. (See *Delayed hypersensitivity reactions.*)

X-rays

X-rays may be used to determine bone integrity, especially in older women, to detect possible osteoporosis. A bone mineral density test is a specialized X-ray that detects the amount of change in a bone. The beam detects the intensity and shows the physician how dense the bones are. A bone scan, another type of X-ray, takes a picture of the bone and identifies fractures, tumors, or inflammation. It's also sensitive enough to recognize structural changes. X-rays may also be used to evaluate the GI tract for integrity and diagnose disorders that may cause malnutrition. The specific X-rays performed will be influenced by the patient's symptoms and diagnosis. Multiple tests may be necessary before a definitive diagnosis is made.

NUTRITIONAL DISORDERS

A patient with nutritional problems generally has one of these disorders: protein-calorie malnutrition, obesity, anorexia nervosa, bulimia nervosa, or a vitamin deficiency. Be aware that a patient hospitalized for more than 2 weeks is at risk for nutritional disorders.

PROTEIN-CALORIE MALNUTRITION

Protein-calorie, or protein-energy malnutrition is a term given to a spectrum of disorders caused by either prolonged or chronic inadequate protein or caloric intake or by high metabolic protein and energy requirements. When protein or caloric intake is inadequate, the body meets its energy needs by breaking down and using stored proteins and fats.

Three major disorders fall under the heading of protein-calorie malnutrition: marasmus, kwashiorkor, and marasmus-kwashiorkor mix.

KNOW-HOW

Detecting marasmus

In marasmus, the patient starves from prolonged lack of calories, protein, and nearly all other nutrients. This illness usually occurs in infants living in poverty but it may also occur in elderly or poor patients, or in young adults.

Diagnostic test results reveal vitamin and mineral deficiencies. With treatment, the patient has a fair prognosis.

SIGNS AND SYMPTOMS
Marasmus can lead to these signs and symptoms:
+ emaciated appearance
+ muscle wasting
+ loss of subcutaneous fat
+ subnormal body temperature
+ decreased resistance to infection
+ hair loss
+ dry, atrophic, loose skin, especially around the thighs and buttocks
+ mental and physical growth retardation in infants and children
+ failure to thrive in infants or elderly patients.

Marasmus

Marasmus, or protein-calorie malnutrition, occurs primarily in children ages 6 to 18 months and results from a chronic lack of nutrients. It impairs brain development and causes failure to thrive. It may also occur in patients with anorexia, starvation, bowel obstruction, and chronic illness. (See *Detecting marasmus*.)

Although blood and visceral protein levels may be normal, skeletal muscle wasting and loss of subcutaneous fat occurs. Skinfold and midarm muscle circumference measurements are smaller than normal, and the patient looks emaciated.

Kwashiorkor

Kwashiorkor, or protein malnutrition, occurs in young children, usually when they're weaned from breast-feeding to a diet consisting mainly of carbohydrates. Protein malnutrition can also occur in hospitalized adult patients who are receiving no protein. Anthropometric measurements may be normal. Children may even appear obese, but a loss of visceral protein occurs. (See *Detecting kwashiorkor*, page 86.)

Low-protein diets, fad diets, and the prolonged use of fluids without supplemental nutrition can all cause kwashiorkor. Edema, lack of pigmentation in the skin and hair, and depressed immune function may occur as well as decreased serum albumin and transferrin levels. Kwashiorkor develops much more quickly than marasmus.

Marasmus-kwashiorkor mix

Marasmus-kwashiorkor mix affects the chronically starved patient subjected to acute distress. It causes a loss of subcutaneous fat, immune system damage, and depletion of blood, visceral, and muscle protein. Of the three types of malnutrition, this type is the most serious and is associated with starvation, burns, and trauma. Usually, this mixed form of malnutrition is the result of a metabolic stressor superimposed on preexisting malnutrition.

Facts about marasmus
+ Occurs primarily in children ages 6 to 18 months
+ Results from chronic lack of nutrients and occurs with anorexia, starvation, bowel obstruction, and chronic illness
+ Impairs brain development
+ Causes failure to thrive

Facts about kwashiorkor
+ Occurs in young children, usually when they're weaned from breast-feeding to a diet high in carbohydrates
+ Results from low-protein diets, fad diets, and the prolonged use of fluids without supplemental nutrition
+ Causes edema, lack of pigmentation in the skin and hair, and depressed immune function
+ Decreases serum albumin and transferrin levels

Facts about marasmus-kwashiorkor mix
+ Affects chronically starved patients subjected to acute distress
+ Causes loss of subcutaneous fat, immune system damage, and blood, visceral, and muscle protein depletion
+ Occurs when a metabolic stressor combines with preexisting malnutrition

Facts about obesity

+ Weight more than 20% above ideal body weight
+ Caused by an imbalance of calorie intake and calorie use
+ Malnourishment caused by deficiencies in certain nutrients
+ Normal immune function
+ Increased anthropometric measurements

Facts about anorexia nervosa

+ Intentional loss of at least 25% of body weight
+ Causes muscle wasting; dry, inelastic skin; loss or change in hair; constipation; amenorrhea; hypotension; and bradycardia
+ Excessive vomiting causes loss of tooth enamel

Facts about bulimia nervosa

+ Normal or above-normal body weight or frequent fluctuations in weight
+ Excessive use of vomiting, emetics, laxatives, diuretics, and diet pills to control weight
+ Electrolyte imbalances, gum infections, and loss of tooth enamel occur

---

KNOW-HOW

Detecting kwashiorkor

A severe protein deficiency, kwashiorkor results from insufficient intake of quality protein. It's usually associated with adequate or even excessive calorie intake or with a high-carbohydrate diet, and it typically accompanies an acute illness. Diagnostic test results show vitamin and mineral deficiencies (especially vitamins A and B), anemia, and low serum albumin, potassium, lymphocyte, and transferrin levels.

Left untreated, kwashiorkor causes death in most instances. With treatment, however, the patient's prognosis is good.

SIGNS AND SYMPTOMS

Patients with kwashiorkor typically suffer from:

+ generalized illness, possibly involving fever
+ weight loss and muscle wasting, possibly masked by facial edema or edema in the lower body, producing a potbelly
+ sparse, thin, soft hair, possibly with parallel gray, red, or blond streaks
+ changes in the mucous membranes, including cracks at the corners of the mouth, mouth ulcerations and lesions, and tongue atrophy
+ scaly skin, dermatosis, and reddish skin and hair pigmentation
+ enlarged liver
+ apathy and irritability
+ poor appetite
+ anorexia
+ diarrhea
+ reduced resistance to infection
+ poor wound healing.

OBESITY

Obesity is defined as weight more than 20% above ideal body weight and is due to an imbalance of calorie intake and calorie use. Although an obese patient consumes more than adequate food quantities, he may still be malnourished and have deficiencies in certain nutrients as a result of eating an unbalanced diet. Causes of obesity are varied. Immune function is usually normal and anthropometric measurements are increased.

ANOREXIA NERVOSA

A psychosocial disorder, anorexia nervosa is an intentional loss of at least 25% of body weight. Signs and symptoms include muscle wasting; fat store depletion; dry, inelastic skin; loss or change in hair; constipation; amenorrhea; hypotension; and bradycardia. You may also find a loss of tooth enamel in the patient because of excessive vomiting.

BULIMIA NERVOSA

Bulimia nervosa, a binge-purge syndrome, is more deceptive than anorexia nervosa because the patient typically has normal or above-normal body weight or frequent fluctuations in weight. Weight is controlled though the use of excessive vomiting, emetics, laxatives, diuretics, and diet pills. Electrolyte imbalances, gum infections, and loss of tooth enamel may occur.

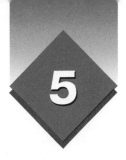

5

Cardiovascular system

Although people are living longer, they're increasingly living with chronic conditions or the sequelae of acute ones. No matter where you practice, you'll be dealing with cardiovascular patients more often. To provide effective care for these patients, you need a clear understanding of cardiovascular anatomy and physiology, assessment techniques, and how to interpret your findings.

A LOOK AT THE CARDIOVASCULAR SYSTEM

The cardiovascular system plays an important role in the body. It delivers oxygenated blood to tissues and removes waste products. The heart pumps blood to all organs and tissues of the body. The autonomic nervous system (ANS) controls how the heart pumps. The vascular network — the arteries and veins — carries blood throughout the body, keeps the heart filled with blood, and maintains blood pressure. Let's look at each part of this critical system.

HEART

The heart is a hollow, muscular organ about the size of a closed fist. It's approximately 5″ (12.5 cm) long and 3½″ (9 cm) in diameter at its widest point. It weighs 1 to 1¼ lb (250 to 300 g). The heart is located between the lungs in the mediastinum, behind and to the left of the sternum.

Anatomy of the heart
The heart spans the area from the second to the fifth intercostal space. The right border of the heart lines up with the right border of the sternum. The left border lines up with the left midclavicular line. The exact position of the heart may vary slightly with each patient. Leading into and out of the heart are the great vessels: the inferior vena cava, the superior vena cava, the aorta, the pulmonary artery, and four pulmonary veins.

The cardiovascular system
+ Heart pumps blood to all organs and tissues
+ Delivers oxygenated blood to tissues and removes waste products
+ ANS controls how heart pumps
+ Arteries and veins carry blood, keep heart filled with blood, and maintain blood pressure

Anatomy of the heart
+ Spans from the second to the fifth intercostal space
+ Right border lines up with the right border of the sternum
+ Left border lines up with the left midclavicular line

Facts about the heart wall

+ Formed by a thick myocardium with interlacing bundles of cardiac muscle fibers
+ A thin layer of endothelial tissue forms the inner endocardium
+ Makes up outside layer of the heart

Four chambers of the heart

+ Right atrium
+ Left atrium
+ Right ventricle
+ Left ventricle

Facts about blood flow

+ Deoxygenated venous blood returns to right atrium
+ Blood from upper body returns through the superior vena cava; lower body, the inferior vena cava
+ Empties into the right atrium then into the right ventricle and then ejects through the pulmonic valve into the pulmonary artery when the ventricle contacts
+ Enters the lungs to be oxygenated

Facts about valves

+ Keep blood flowing in one direction
+ Open and close passively as a result of pressure changes within the four heart chambers

The heart wall

The heart wall consists of three layers. A thick myocardium, composed of interlacing bundles of cardiac muscle fibers, forms most of the heart wall. A thin layer of endothelial tissue forms the inner endocardium. The epicardium makes up the outside layer.

The pericardium is a fibroserous sac that surrounds the heart and the roots of the great vessels. It consists of the serous pericardium and the fibrous pericardium. The serous pericardium consists of the parietal layer, which lines the inside of the fibrous pericardium, and the visceral layer, which adheres to the surface of the heart. The fibrous pericardium is a thicker layer that protects the heart. The space between the two layers, called the *pericardial space,* contains 10 to 30 ml of serous fluid, which prevents friction between the layers as the heart pumps. (See *Inside the heart.*)

Chambers

The heart contains four hollow chambers: two atria and two ventricles. The right atrium lies in front and to the right of the left atrium. It receives blood from the superior and inferior venae cavae. The left atrium, smaller but with thicker walls than the right atrium, forms the uppermost part of the heart's left border, extending to the left of and behind the right atrium. It receives blood from the pulmonary veins. The interatrial septum separates the left and right atria.

The right and left ventricles make up the two lower chambers. Both are large and thick-walled. The right ventricle lies behind the sternum and forms the largest part of the sternocostal surface and inferior border of the heart. The left ventricle is larger than the right because it must contract with enough force to eject blood into the aorta and the rest of the body. This ventricle forms the apex and most of the left border of the heart and its diaphragmatic surface.

Blood flow

Deoxygenated venous blood returns to the right atrium through three vessels: the superior vena cava, inferior vena cava, and coronary sinus. Blood from the upper body returns to the heart through the superior vena cava. Blood in the lower body returns through the inferior vena cava, and blood from the heart muscle itself returns through the coronary sinus. All of the blood from those vessels empties into the right atrium.

Blood in the right atrium empties into the right ventricle and is then ejected through the pulmonic valve into the pulmonary artery when the ventricle contracts. The blood then travels to the lungs to be oxygenated.

From the lungs, blood travels to the left atrium through the pulmonary veins. The left atrium empties the blood into the left ventricle, which then pumps the blood through the aortic valve into the aorta and throughout the body with each contraction. Because the left ventricle pumps blood against a much higher pressure than the right ventricle, its wall is three times thicker.

Valves

Valves in the heart keep blood flowing in only one direction through the heart. Think of the valves as traffic cops at the entrances to one-way streets, preventing blood from traveling the wrong way despite great pressure to do so. Healthy valves open and close passively as a result of pressure changes within the four heart chambers.

Valves between the atria and ventricles are called atrioventricular (AV) valves and include the tricuspid valve on the right side of the heart and the mitral valve on the left. The pulmonic valve (between the right ventricle and pulmonary artery)

Inside the heart

The heart's internal structure consists of the pericardium, three layers of the heart wall, four chambers, and four valves.

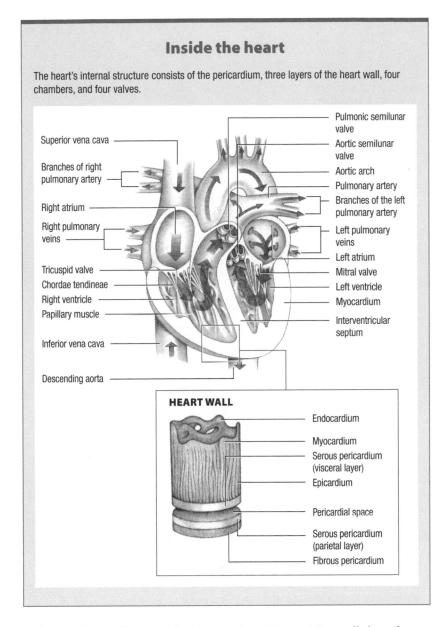

Superior vena cava

Branches of right pulmonary artery

Right atrium

Right pulmonary veins

Tricuspid valve

Chordae tendineae

Right ventricle

Papillary muscle

Inferior vena cava

Descending aorta

Pulmonic semilunar valve

Aortic semilunar valve

Aortic arch

Pulmonary artery

Branches of the left pulmonary artery

Left pulmonary veins

Left atrium

Mitral valve

Left ventricle

Myocardium

Interventricular septum

HEART WALL

Endocardium

Myocardium

Serous pericardium (visceral layer)

Epicardium

Pericardial space

Serous pericardium (parietal layer)

Fibrous pericardium

and the aortic valve (between the left ventricle and the aorta) are called *semilunar valves.*

Each valve's leaflets, or cusps, are anchored to the heart wall by cords of fibrous tissue. Those cords, called *chordae tendineae,* are controlled by papillary muscles. The cusps of the valves act to maintain tight closure. The tricuspid valve has three cusps. The mitral valve has two. The semilunar valves each have three cusps.

Physiology of the heart

An electrical conduction system regulates myocardial contraction. This system includes the nerve fibers of the autonomic nervous system (ANS) and specialized nerves and fibers in the heart. The ANS involuntarily increases or decreases heart action to meet the individual's metabolic needs. (See *Cardiac conduction,* page 90.)

Physiology of the heart
- ANS nerve fibers form the electrical conduction system that regulates myocardial contraction
- Causes involuntarily increased or decreased heart action to meet the individual's metabolic needs
- Allows both sympathetic and parasympathetic nerves to participate in the control of cardiac function
- Controls heart through branches of vagus nerve (cranial nerve X) through parasympathetic nervous system
- Stimulates heart's nerves and fibers to fire and contract during activity or stress

Elements of the cardiac conduction system

+ SA node
+ Interatrial tract (Bachmann's bundle)
+ Internodal tracts
+ AV node
+ AV bundle (bundle of His)
+ Right bundle branch
+ Left bundle branch
+ Purkinje fibers

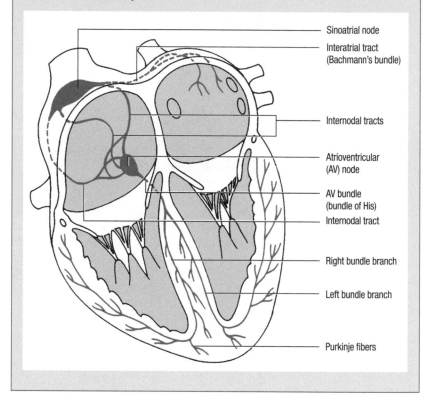

Cardiac conduction

In the heart's conduction system, specialized fibers spread an impulse quickly throughout the heart's muscle cell network, causing a generalized contraction. This illustration shows the elements of this conduction system.

Sinoatrial node
Interatrial tract (Bachmann's bundle)
Internodal tracts
Atrioventricular (AV) node
AV bundle (bundle of His)
Internodal tract
Right bundle branch
Left bundle branch
Purkinje fibers

Facts about pacemaker cells

+ Allow electrical impulse conduction
+ Control heart rate and rhythm and rate and rhythm of contractions
+ Stimulate SA node, which paces heart; and AV node, which takes up impulse conduction
+ Allow conduction to speed through the bundle of His

Both sympathetic and parasympathetic nerves participate in the control of cardiac function. With the body at rest, the parasympathetic nervous system controls the heart through branches of the vagus nerve (cranial nerve X). Heart rate and electrical impulse propagation are very slow.

In times of activity or stress, the sympathetic nervous system takes control. It stimulates the heart's nerves and fibers to fire and conduct more rapidly and the ventricles to contract more forcefully.

Pacemaker cells

Myocardial cells have specialized pacemaker cells that allow electrical impulse conduction. Pacemaker cells control heart rate and rhythm (a property known as *automaticity*). However, any myocardial muscle cell can control the rate and rhythm of contractions under certain circumstances.

Normally, the sinoatrial (SA) node (located on the endocardial surface of the right atrium, near the superior vena cava) paces the heart. SA node firing spreads an impulse throughout the right and left atria, by way of internodal pathways, resulting in atrial contraction.

The AV node (located low in the septal wall of the right atrium immediately above the coronary sinus opening) takes up impulse conduction. Normally, the AV node forms the only electrical connection between the atria and ventricles. It initially slows the impulse, delaying ventricular activity and allowing blood to fill from the atria. Then conduction speeds through the AV node and a network of fibers called the bundle of His.

The bundle of His arises in the AV node and continues along the right interventricular septum. It divides in the ventricular septum to form the right and left bundle branches. Its fibers rapidly spread the impulse throughout both ventricles.

Purkinje fibers, the distal portions of the left and right bundle branches, fan across the subendocardial surface of the ventricles from the endocardium through the myocardium. As the impulse spreads throughout the distal conduction system, it prompts ventricular contraction.

Cardiac cycle

The cardiac cycle describes the period from the beginning of one heartbeat to the beginning of the next. During this cycle, electrical and mechanical events must occur in the proper order and to the proper degree to provide adequate blood flow to all body parts. Basically, the cardiac cycle has two phases, systole and diastole.

Systole

At the beginning of systole, the ventricles contract, increasing pressure and forcing the mitral and tricuspid valves shut. This valvular closing prevents blood backflow into the atria and coincides with the first heart sound, known as S_1 or the "lub" of "lub-dub." As the ventricles contract, ventricular pressure builds until it exceeds that in the pulmonary artery and the aorta. Then the aortic and pulmonic semilunar valves open, and the ventricles eject blood into the aorta and the pulmonary artery.

Diastole

When the ventricles empty and relax, ventricular pressure falls below that in the pulmonary artery and the aorta. At the beginning of diastole, the semilunar valves close to prevent backflow into the ventricles. This coincides with the second heart sound, known as S_2 or the "dub" of "lub-dub."

As the ventricles relax the mitral and tricuspid valves open and blood begins to flow into the ventricles from the atria. When the ventricles become full, near the end of diastole, the atria contract to send the remaining blood to the ventricles. Then a new cardiac cycle begins as the heart enters systole again. (See *Phases of the cardiac cycle,* page 92.)

Cardiac output and stroke volume

Cardiac output refers to the amount of blood the heart pumps in 1 minute. Stroke volume, the amount of blood ejected with each beat multiplied by the number of beats per minute, determines cardiac output. Stroke volume depends on three major factors:

✦ preload—the stretching of heart muscle fibers caused by blood volume in the ventricles at the end of diastole
✦ afterload—the pressure that the ventricular muscles must generate to overcome the higher pressure in the aorta
✦ contractility—the myocardium's inherent ability to contract normally.

Understanding the cardiac cycle helps to assess the heart's hemodynamics. Many cardiac dysfunctions cause abnormal findings that correlate with specific events in the cardiac cycle. (See *Understanding preload and afterload,* page 93.)

The cardiac cycle

✦ Describes the period from the beginning of one heartbeat to the beginning of the next
✦ Electrical and mechanical events must occur in the proper order and to the proper degree to provide adequate blood flow to all body parts
✦ Has two phases: systole and diastole

Systole

✦ Ventricles contract increasing pressure
✦ Mitral and tricuspid valves are forced shut, preventing backflow into atria
✦ Coincides with S_1
✦ As ventricles contract, ventricular pressure builds
✦ Aortic and pulmonic semilunar valves open; ventricles eject blood into aorta and pulmonary artery

Diastole

✦ Ventricles empty and relax; pressure falls
✦ Semilunar valves close, preventing backflow into the ventricles
✦ Coincides with S_2
✦ Mitral and tricuspid valves open; blood flows into the ventricles from the atria
✦ When the ventricles become full, the atria contract, sending remaining blood to the ventricles

Cardiac output and stroke volume

Cardiac output

✦ Amount of blood the heart pumps in 1 minute

Stroke volume

✦ Amount of blood ejected with each beat multiplied by the number of beats per minute; determines cardiac output

Phases of the cardiac cycle

A coordinated sequence of events controls blood flow through the heart's chambers and valves. Called the cardiac cycle, it consists of two phases: systole and diastole.

In the upper illustration, which shows systolic events, the arrows indicate ventricular contraction, the opening of the aortic and pulmonic valves, and the ejection of blood into the aorta and pulmonary artery.

In the lower illustration, which shows diastolic events, the arrows indicate ventricular relaxation, the opening of the tricuspid and mitral valves, and the flow of blood into the ventricles.

Events on the heart's right side occur a fraction of a second after events on the left side because right-side pressure is lower.

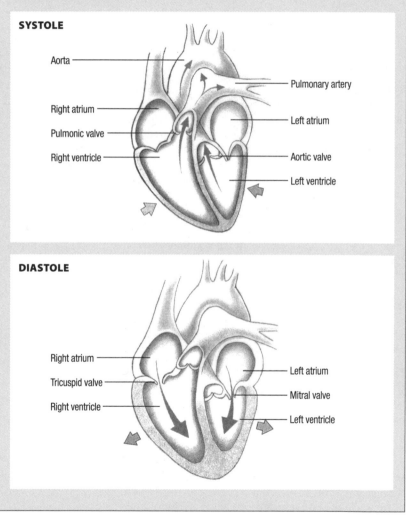

Understanding the vascular system

✦ Composed of arteries, arterioles, capillaries, venules, and veins

✦ Keeps blood circulating

✦ Has two branches: pulmonary and systemic circulation

VASCULAR SYSTEM

About 60,000 miles of arteries, arterioles, capillaries, venules, and veins keep blood circulating to and from every functioning cell in the body. This network has two branches: pulmonary circulation and systemic circulation. (See *Major blood vessels*, page 94.)

Understanding preload and afterload

Preload refers to a passive stretching force exerted on the ventricular muscle at end diastole by the amount of blood in the chamber. According to Starling's law, the more cardiac muscles are stretched in diastole, the more forcefully they contract in systole.

Afterload refers to the pressure the ventricular muscles must generate to overcome the higher pressure in the aorta. Normally, end-diastolic pressure in the left ventricle is 5 to 10 mm Hg; in the aorta, however, it's 70 to 80 mm Hg. This difference means that the ventricle must develop enough pressure to force open the aortic valve.

PRELOAD

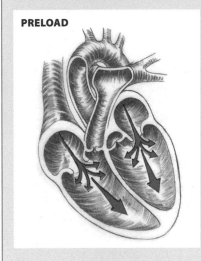

AFTERLOAD

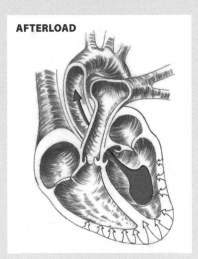

Preload and afterload

Preload
✦ Refers to a passive stretching force exerted on the ventricular muscle at end diastole by amount of blood in chamber

Afterload
✦ Refers to pressure the ventricular muscles generate to overcome the higher pressure in the aorta

Pulmonary circulation

Pulmonary circulation refers to blood that travels to the lungs to pick up oxygen and liberate carbon dioxide. It works as follows:
✦ Unoxygenated blood travels from the right ventricle through the pulmonic valve into the pulmonary arteries.
✦ Blood passes through progressively smaller arteries and arterioles into the capillaries of the lungs.
✦ Blood reaches the alveoli and exchanges carbon dioxide for oxygen.
✦ The oxygenated blood then returns via venules and veins to the pulmonary veins, which carry it back to the left atrium of the heart.

Systemic circulation

Through systemic circulation, blood carries oxygen and other nutrients to body cells and transports waste products for excretion. At specific sites, the pumping action of the heart that forces blood through the arteries becomes palpable. This regular expansion and contraction of the arteries is called the *pulse*.

The major artery—the aorta—branches into vessels that supply blood to specific organs and areas of the body. The left common carotid, left subclavian, and innominate arteries arise from the arch of the aorta and supply blood to the brain, arms, and upper chest. As the aorta descends through the thorax and abdomen, its branches supply blood to the GI and genitourinary organs, spinal column, and

Pulmonary circulation
✦ Blood travels to the lungs to pick up oxygen and liberate carbon dioxide
✦ Oxygenated blood returns to the pulmonary veins, which carry it back to heart's left atrium

Systemic circulation
✦ Blood carries oxygen and other nutrients to body cells and transports waste for excretion
✦ At specific sites, pumping action of heart forces blood through the arteries, becoming palpable—called the *pulse*

Five major blood vessels

+ Arteries
+ Arterioles
+ Capillaries
+ Venules
+ Veins

Major blood vessels

This illustration shows the body's major arteries and veins.

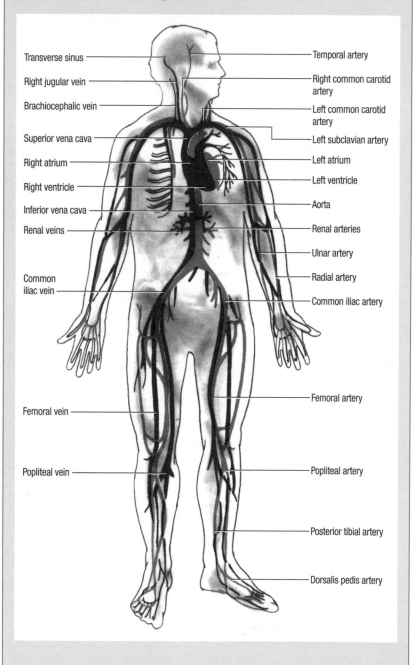

Transverse sinus

Right jugular vein

Brachiocephalic vein

Superior vena cava

Right atrium

Right ventricle

Inferior vena cava

Renal veins

Common iliac vein

Femoral vein

Popliteal vein

Temporal artery

Right common carotid artery

Left common carotid artery

Left subclavian artery

Left atrium

Left ventricle

Aorta

Renal arteries

Ulnar artery

Radial artery

Common iliac artery

Femoral artery

Popliteal artery

Posterior tibial artery

Dorsalis pedis artery

lower chest and abdominal muscles. Then the aorta divides into the iliac arteries, which further divide into femoral arteries.

As the arteries divide into smaller units, the number of vessels increases dramatically, thereby increasing the area of perfusion. Arteries are thick-walled because they transport blood under high pressure. Arterial walls contain a tough, elastic layer to help propel blood through the arterial system. At the end of the arterioles and the beginning of the capillaries, strong sphincters control blood flow into the tissues. These sphincters dilate to permit more flow when needed, close to shunt blood to other areas, or constrict to increase blood pressure.

Although the capillary bed contains the smallest vessels, it supplies blood to the largest area. Capillary pressure is extremely low to allow for the exchange of nutrients, oxygen, and carbon dioxide with body cells. From the capillaries, blood flows into venules and, eventually, into veins. Approximately 5% of the circulating blood volume at any given moment is contained within the capillary network.

Nearly all veins carry oxygen-depleted blood; the sole exception being the pulmonary vein, which carries oxygenated blood from the lungs to the left atrium. Veins serve as a large reservoir for circulating blood. Valves in the veins prevent blood backflow, and the pumping action of skeletal muscles assists venous return. The wall of a vein is thinner and more pliable than the wall of an artery. That pliability allows the vein to accommodate variations in blood volume. The veins merge until they form two main branches—the superior and inferior venae cavae—that return blood to the right atrium.

Coronary circulation

Blood flowing through the heart's chambers doesn't exchange oxygen and other nutrients with the myocardial cells. Instead, a specialized part of the systemic circulation, the coronary circulation, supplies blood to the heart. (See *The heart's blood supply,* page 96.)

Pulses

Arterial pulses are pressure waves of blood generated by the pumping action of the heart. All vessels in the arterial system have pulsations, but the pulsations can be felt only where an artery lies near the skin. You can palpate for these peripheral pulses: temporal, carotid, brachial, radial, ulnar, femoral, popliteal, posterior tibial, and dorsalis pedis.

 SPECIAL POINTS *Be aware that in older patients peripheral pulses may be diminished.*

OBTAINING A HEALTH HISTORY

To obtain a health history of a patient's cardiovascular system, begin by introducing yourself and explaining what will occur during the health history and physical examination. To take an effective history, you'll need to establish rapport with the patient. Ask open-ended questions and listen carefully to responses. Closely observe the patient's nonverbal behavior.

CHIEF COMPLAINT

You'll find that a patient with a cardiovascular problem typically cites specific complaints, such as:
+ chest pain
+ irregular heartbeat or palpitations

Facts about coronary circulation

+ Blood flowing through heart's chambers doesn't exchange oxygen and other nutrients with the myocardial cells
+ Coronary circulation, part of the systemic circulation, supplies blood to the heart

Facts about pulses

Arterial pulses
+ Pressure waves of blood generated by pumping action of heart felt only where an artery lies near the skin

Peripheral pulses
+ Include temporal, carotid, brachial, radial, ulnar, femoral, popliteal, posterior tibial, dorsalis pedis; in older patients, may be diminished

---

Obtaining a health history

+ Establish a rapport
+ Ask open-ended questions and listen to responses
+ Observe nonverbal behavior

Exploring the chief complaint

+ Chest pain
+ Irregular heartbeat or palpitations

Components of the heart's blood supply

✦ Coronary arteries and their branches—supply oxygenated blood
✦ Cardiac veins—remove oxygen-depleted blood
✦ Right coronary artery—supplies blood to the right atrium, part of the left atrium, most of the right ventricle, and the inferior part of the left ventricle
✦ Left coronary artery—supplies blood to the left atrium, most of the left ventricle, and most of the interventricular septum

Facts about cardiac veins

✦ Lie superficial to the arteries
✦ Coronary sinus—largest vein—lies in the posterior part of coronary sulcus, opening into the right atrium
✦ Most major cardiac veins empty into the coronary sinus
✦ Anterior cardiac vein empties into the right atrium

The heart's blood supply

The heart relies on the coronary arteries and their branches to supply itself with oxygenated blood, and on the cardiac veins to remove oxygen-depleted blood. During left ventricular systole, blood is ejected into the aorta. During diastole, blood flows into the coronary ostia and then through the coronary arteries to nourish the heart muscle.

The right coronary artery supplies blood to the right atrium (including the sinoatrial and atrioventricular nodes of the conduction system), part of the left atrium, most of the right ventricle, and the inferior part of the left ventricle.

The left coronary artery, which splits into the anterior descending and circumflex arteries, supplies blood to the left atrium, most of the left ventricle, and most of the interventricular septum. Many collateral arteries connect the branches of the right and left coronary arteries.

The cardiac veins lie superficial to the arteries. The largest vein, the coronary sinus, lies in the posterior part of the coronary sulcus and opens into the right atrium. Most of the major cardiac veins empty into the coronary sinus, except for the anterior cardiac veins, which empty into the right atrium.

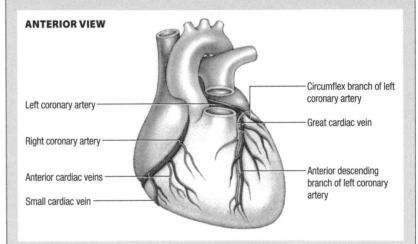

ANTERIOR VIEW

Left coronary artery

Right coronary artery

Anterior cardiac veins

Small cardiac vein

Circumflex branch of left coronary artery

Great cardiac vein

Anterior descending branch of left coronary artery

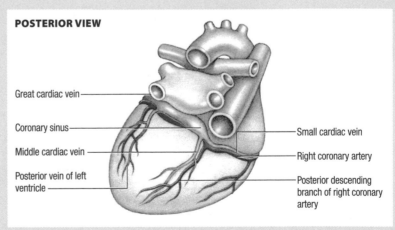

POSTERIOR VIEW

Great cardiac vein

Coronary sinus

Middle cardiac vein

Posterior vein of left ventricle

Small cardiac vein

Right coronary artery

Posterior descending branch of right coronary artery

+ shortness of breath on exertion, lying down, or at night
+ cough
+ cyanosis or pallor
+ weakness
+ fatigue
+ unexplained weight change
+ swelling of the extremities
+ dizziness
+ headache
+ high or low blood pressure
+ peripheral skin changes, such as decreased hair distribution, skin color changes, or a thin, shiny appearance to the skin
+ pain in the extremities, such as leg pain or cramps.

 SPECIAL POINTS *In pregnant patients in their third trimester, you might find 4+ pitting edema in the legs. Severe edema is common not just in the third trimester but also in pregnant women who stand for long periods of time. Varicose veins are another common finding in the third trimester.*

Ask the patient how long he has had the problem, how it affects his daily routine, and when it began. Find out about any associated signs and symptoms. Ask about the location, radiation, intensity, and duration of any pain and any precipitating, exacerbating, or relieving factors. Ask him to rate the pain on a scale of 1 to 10, in which 1 means negligible and 10 means the worst pain imaginable. (See *Understanding chest pain,* pages 98 and 99.)

Let the patient describe his problem in his own words. Avoid leading questions. Use familiar expressions rather than medical terms whenever possible. If the patient isn't in distress, ask questions that require more than a yes-or-no response. Try to obtain as accurate a description as possible of any chest pain.

 SPECIAL POINTS *Even a child old enough to talk may have difficulty describing chest pain, so be alert for nonverbal clues, such as restlessness, facial grimaces, or holding the painful area. Ask the child to point to the painful area and then to where the pain goes (to find out if it's radiating). Determine the pain's severity by asking the parents if the pain interferes with the child's normal activities and behavior.*

Because elderly patients have a higher risk of developing life-threatening conditions — such as a myocardial infarction (MI), angina, and aortic dissection — carefully evaluate chest pain in these patients.

CURRENT HEALTH HISTORY

Besides checking for pain, also ask the patient these questions:
+ Are you ever short of breath? If so, what activities cause you to be short of breath?

 ABNORMAL FINDINGS *Orthopnea or dyspnea that occurs when the patient is lying down and improves when he sits up, suggests left ventricular heart failure or mitral stenosis. It can also accompany obstructive lung disease.*
+ Do you feel dizzy or fatigued?

Exploring the chief complaint
(continued)

+ Shortness of breath or cough
+ Cyanosis or pallor
+ Weakness and fatigue
+ Unexplained weight change
+ Pain or swelling in extremities
+ Dizziness or headache
+ High or low blood pressure
+ Peripheral skin changes

Special points: Pregnant patients

+ Third trimester may reveal 4+ pitting edema in legs
+ Severe edema is also common in pregnant patients who stand for long periods of time
+ Varicose veins may also occur

Special points: Children and elderly patients

+ Be alert for nonverbal cues
+ Ask parents if pain interferes with the child's normal activities
+ Evaluate chest pain in elderly patients because they have a higher risk of developing life-threatening conditions

Current health history

+ Ask about shortness of breath
+ Ask if rings or shoes feel tight or if ankles swell
+ Ask about changes in color or sensation in the legs
+ Find out about sores or ulcers
+ Ask about standing or sitting for long periods
+ Find out how many pillows patient sleeps on at night
+ Ask about dizziness or fatigue

Abnormal findings

+ Orthopnea or dyspnea, occurring when lying down and improving when sitting up, suggests left ventricular failure or mitral stenosis

Types of chest pain

- Aching
- Tight with pressure
- Sharp and continuous
- Excruciating and tearing
- Sudden and severe
- Dull, pressurelike, and squeezing
- Burning
- Gripping, sharp
- Continuous or intermittent sharp
- Dull or stabbing

Locations of chest pain

- Substernal; radiating to jaw, neck, arms, and back
- Across chest
- Over lung area
- Lower chest or upper abdomen
- Right epigastric or abdominal areas; possibly radiating to shoulders

Understanding chest pain

This chart outlines the different types of chest pain including their location, exacerbating factors, causes, and alleviating factors. Use this chart to accurately assess chest pain in a patient.

DESCRIPTION	LOCATION
Aching, squeezing, pressure, heaviness, burning pain; usually subsides within 10 minutes	Substernal; may radiate to jaw, neck, arms, and back
Tightness or pressure; burning, aching pain; possibly accompanied by shortness of breath, diaphoresis, weakness, anxiety, or nausea; sudden onset; lasts ½ to 2 hours	Typically across chest but may radiate to jaw, neck, arms, or back
Sharp and continuous; may be accompanied by friction rub; sudden onset	Substernal; may radiate to neck or left arm
Excruciating, tearing pain; may be accompanied by blood pressure difference between right and left arm; sudden onset	Retrosternal, upper abdominal, or epigastric; may radiate to back, neck, or shoulders
Sudden, stabbing pain; may be accompanied by cyanosis, dyspnea, or cough with hemoptysis	Over lung area
Sudden and severe pain; sometimes accompanied by dyspnea, increased pulse rate, decreased breath sounds, or deviated trachea	Lateral thorax
Dull, pressurelike, squeezing pain	Substernal, epigastric areas
Sharp, severe pain	Lower chest or upper abdomen
Burning feeling after eating sometimes accompanied by hematemesis or tarry stools; sudden onset that generally subsides within 15 to 20 minutes	Epigastric
Gripping, sharp pain; possibly nausea and vomiting	Right epigastric or abdominal areas; possible radiation to shoulders
Continuous or intermittent sharp pain; possibly tender to touch; gradual or sudden onset	Anywhere in chest
Dull or stabbing pain usually accompanied by hyperventilation or breathlessness; sudden onset; lasting less than a minute or as long as several days	Anywhere in chest

 SPECIAL POINTS *When evaluating a child for fatigue, ask his parents if they have notice any change in his activity level. Fatigue without an organic cause occurs normally during accelerated growth phases in preschool-age and prepubescent children.*

EXACERBATING FACTORS	CAUSES	ALLEVIATING MEASURES
Eating, physical effort, smoking, cold weather, stress, anger, hunger, lying down	Angina pectoris	Rest, nitroglycerin (Note: Unstable angina appears even at rest.)
Exertion, anxiety	Acute myocardial infarction	Opioid analgesics such as morphine, nitroglycerin
Deep breathing, supine position	Pericarditis	Sitting up, leaning forward, anti-inflammatory drugs
Not applicable	Dissecting aortic aneurysm	Analgesics, surgery
Inspiration	Pulmonary embolus	Analgesics
Normal respiration	Pneumothorax	Analgesics, chest tube insertion
Food, cold liquids, exercise	Esophageal spasm	Nitroglycerin, calcium channel blockers
Eating a heavy meal, bending, lying down	Hiatal hernia	Antacids, walking, semi-Fowler's position
Lack of food or highly acidic foods	Peptic ulcer	Food, antacids
Eating fatty foods, lying down	Cholecystitis	Rest and analgesics, surgery
Movement, palpation	Chest-wall syndrome	Time, analgesics, heat applications
Increased respiratory rate, stress or anxiety	Acute anxiety	Slowing of respiratory rate, stress relief

Exacerbating factors of chest pain

✦ Physical effort, smoking, cold weather, hunger, lying down
✦ Exertion, anxiety
✦ Deep breathing, supine position
✦ Inspiration or normal respiration
✦ Cold liquids
✦ Lack of food or highly acidic foods
✦ Heavy meals and fatty foods
✦ Increased respiratory rate

Causes of chest pain

✦ Angina pectoris
✦ Acute myocardial infarction
✦ Pneumothorax
✦ Hiatal hernia
✦ Peptic ulcer
✦ Acute anxiety

Alleviating measures for chest pain

✦ Rest
✦ Nitroglycerin
✦ Analgesics
✦ Surgery
✦ Calcium channel blockers
✦ Food, antacids

Always ask the elderly patient about fatigue because this symptom may be insidious and mask a more serious underlying condition in this age-group.

✦ Do your rings or shoes feel tight?
✦ Do your ankles swell?

Past health history

✦ Reveals hypertension, rheumatic fever, scarlet fever, diabetes mellitus, hyperlipidemia, congenital heart defects, and syncope

Family history

✦ Hypertension
✦ MI
✦ Cardiomyopathy
✦ Diabetes mellitus
✦ CAD
✦ Vascular disease
✦ Hyperlipidemia
✦ Sudden death

Special points

✦ CAD affects more White men between ages 40 and 60
✦ Hypertension occurs most commonly in Blacks
✦ Heart disease affects more postmenopausal women and those with diabetes

---

Key questions for assessing cardiac function

These questions and statements will help you to assess the patient more accurately:

✦ Are you still in pain? Where's it located? Point to where you feel it.
✦ Describe what the pain feels like. (If the patient needs prompting, ask if he feels a burning, tightness, or squeezing sensation in his chest.)
✦ Does the pain radiate to any other part of your body? Your arm? Neck? Back? Jaw?
✦ When did the pain begin? What relieves it? What makes it feel worse?
✦ Tell me about any other feelings you're experiencing. (If the patient needs prompting, suggest nausea, dizziness, or sweating.)
✦ Tell me about any feelings of shortness of breath. Does a particular body position seem to bring this on? Which one? How long does any shortness of breath last? What relieves it?

✦ Has sudden breathing trouble ever awakened you from sleep? Tell me more about this.
✦ Do you ever wake up coughing? How often? Have you ever coughed up blood?
✦ Does your heart ever pound or skip a beat? If so, when does this happen?
✦ Do you ever feel dizzy or faint? What seems to bring this on?
✦ Tell me about any swelling in your ankles or feet. At what time of day?
✦ Does anything relieve the swelling?
✦ Do you urinate more frequently at night?
✦ Tell me how you feel while you're doing your daily activities. Have you had to limit your activities or rest more often while doing them?

✦ Have you noticed changes in color or sensation in your legs? If so, what are those changes?
✦ If you have sores or ulcers, how quickly do they heal?
✦ Do you stand or sit in one place for long periods at work?
✦ How many pillows do you sleep on at night? (See *Key questions for assessing cardiac function.*)

PAST HEALTH HISTORY

Ask the patient about any history of cardiac-related disorders, such as hypertension, rheumatic fever, scarlet fever, diabetes mellitus, hyperlipidemia, congenital heart defects, and syncope. Other questions to ask include:

✦ Have you ever had severe fatigue not caused by exertion?
✦ Are you taking any prescription, over-the-counter, or recreational drugs?
✦ Are you allergic to any drugs, foods, or other products? If yes, describe the reaction you experienced.

In addition, ask the female patient:

✦ Have you begun menopause?
✦ Do you use hormonal contraceptives or estrogen?
✦ Have you experienced any medical problems during pregnancy? Have you ever had pregnancy-induced hypertension?

FAMILY HISTORY

Information about the patient's blood relatives may suggest a specific cardiac problem. Ask him if anyone in his family has ever had hypertension, MI, cardiomyopathy, diabetes mellitus, coronary artery disease (CAD), vascular disease, hyperlipidemia, or sudden death.

 SPECIAL POINTS *As you analyze a patient's problems, remember that age, gender, and race are essential considerations in identifying the risk for cardiovascular disorders. For example, CAD most commonly affects White men between ages 40 and 60. Hypertension occurs most commonly in Blacks.*

Women are also vulnerable to heart disease, especially postmenopausal women and those with diabetes mellitus. Many elderly people often have increased systolic blood pressure because of an increase in the rigidity of their blood vessel walls with age. Overall, elderly people have a higher incidence of cardiovascular disease than do younger people.

PSYCHOSOCIAL HISTORY

Obtain information about your patient's occupation, educational background, living arrangements, daily activities, and family relationships.

Also, obtain information about:
+ stress levels and how he deals with them
+ current health habits, such as smoking, alcohol intake, caffeine intake, exercise, and dietary intake of fat and sodium
+ environmental or occupational considerations
+ activities of daily living (ADLs).

During the history-taking session, note the appropriateness of the patient's responses, his speech clarity, and his mood so that you can better identify changes later.

ASSESSING THE CARDIOVASCULAR SYSTEM

Cardiovascular disease affects people of all ages and can take many forms. Using a consistent, methodical approach to your assessment will help you identify abnormalities. The key to accurate assessment is regular practice, which will help improve technique and efficiency.

Before assessing the patient's cardiovascular system, you must assess the factors that reflect cardiovascular function. These include general appearance, body weight, vital signs, and related body structures.

PREPARING FOR THE ASSESSMENT

Wash your hands and gather the necessary equipment. Choose a private room. Adjust the thermostat, if necessary; cool temperatures may alter the patient's skin temperature and color, heart rate, and blood pressure. Make sure the room is quiet. If possible, close the door and windows and turn off radios and noisy equipment.

Combine parts of the assessment, as needed, to conserve time and the patient's energy. If the patient experiences cardiovascular difficulties, alter the order of your assessment as needed.

 CLINICAL ALERT If the patient develops chest pain and dyspnea, quickly check his vital signs and then auscultate the heart.

If a female patient feels embarrassed about exposing her chest, explain each assessment step beforehand, use drapes appropriately, and expose only the area being assessed.

ASSESSING VITAL SIGNS

Assessing vital signs includes measurement of temperature, blood pressure, pulse rate, and respiratory rate.

Psychosocial history
+ Reveals occupation, educational background, living arrangements, and family relationships
+ Uncovers stress levels, current health habits, environmental or occupational considerations, and ADLs

Assessing the cardiovascular system
+ Before beginning assessment, look at factors reflecting cardiovascular function: general appearance, body weight, vital signs, related body structures

Preparation
+ Wash your hands and gather equipment
+ Adjust room temperature; ensure quiet
+ Combine parts of assessment; if patient develops chest pain or dyspnea, promptly check vital signs and auscultate heart

Vital signs assessment
+ Temperature, blood pressure, pulse rate, respiratory rate

Measuring temperature

+ Measured in degrees Fahrenheit (°F) or degrees Celsius (°C)
+ Obtained by oral, tympanic, rectal, or axillary route
+ Route chosen based on patient's age and condition
+ Normal ranges — 98.6° F to 99.5° F (36° C to 37.5° C)

Abnormal findings

+ Fever may reveal cardiovascular inflammation or infection, heightened cardiac workload, MI or acute pericarditis, infections
+ Lower than normal body temperatures reveal poor perfusion and metabolic disorders

Measuring blood pressure

+ Palpate and auscultate blood pressure in an extremity
+ Between measurements, wait 3 to 5 minutes
+ Normal — less than 120/80 mm Hg in adult; 78/46 to 114/78 mm Hg in child
+ Rule out examination stress

Abnormal findings

+ A 10 mm Hg or more difference between arms may indicate thoracic outlet syndrome
+ High blood pressure in arms but low blood pressure in legs signals aortic coarctation

Determining pulse pressure

+ Subtract diastolic pressure from systolic pressure
+ Reflects arterial pressure during resting phase of cardiac cycle
+ Normal — 30 to 50 mm Hg

Abnormal findings

+ Rising or diminishing pulse pressure

Measuring temperature

Temperature is measured and documented in degrees Fahrenheit (°F) or degrees Celsius (°C). Choose the method of obtaining the patient's temperature (oral, tympanic, rectal, or axillary) based on the patient's age and condition. Normal body temperature ranges from 96.8° F to 99.5° F (36° C to 37.5° C).

 ABNORMAL FINDINGS In patients with fever, findings may indicate:
+ *cardiovascular inflammation or infection*
+ *heightened cardiac workload (assess a febrile patient with heart disease for signs of increased cardiac workload such as tachycardia)*
+ *MI or acute pericarditis (mild to moderate fever usually occurs 2 to 5 days after an MI when the healing infarct passes through the inflammatory stage)*
+ *infections, such as infective endocarditis, which cause fever spikes (high fever).*
In patients with lower than normal body temperatures, findings include poor perfusion and certain metabolic disorders.

Measuring blood pressure

First palpate and then auscultate the blood pressure in an arm or a leg. Wait 3 to 5 minutes between measurements. Normal blood pressure readings are less than 120/80 mm Hg in a resting adult and 78/46 to 114/78 mm Hg in a young child.

Emotional stress caused by physical examination may elevate blood pressure. If the patient's blood pressure is high, allow him to relax for several minutes and then measure again to rule out stress.

When assessing a patient's blood pressure for the first time, take measurements in both arms.

 ABNORMAL FINDINGS A difference of 10 mm Hg or more between the patient's arms may indicate thoracic outlet syndrome or other forms of arterial obstruction.

If blood pressure is elevated in both arms, measure the pressure in the thigh. Wrap a large cuff around the patient's upper leg at least 1″ (2.5 cm) above the knee. Place the stethoscope over the popliteal artery, located on the posterior surface slightly above the knee joint. Listen for sounds when the bladder of the cuff is deflated.

 ABNORMAL FINDINGS High blood pressure in the patient's arms with normal or low pressure in the legs suggests aortic coarctation.

Determining pulse pressure

To calculate the patient's pulse pressure, subtract the diastolic pressure from the systolic pressure. This reflects arterial pressure during the resting phase of the cardiac cycle and normally ranges from 30 to 50 mm Hg.

ABNORMAL FINDINGS Rising pulse pressure is seen with:
+ *increased stroke volume, which occurs with exercise, anxiety, and bradycardia*
+ *declined peripheral vascular resistance or aortic distention, which occurs with anemia, hyperthyroidism, fever, hypertension, aortic coarctation, and aging.*
    Diminishing pulse pressure occurs with:
+ *mitral or aortic stenosis, which occurs with mechanical obstruction*
+ *constricted peripheral vessels, which occurs with shock*
+ *declined stroke volume, which occurs with heart failure, hypovolemia, cardiac tamponade, or tachycardia.*

Checking radial pulse

If you suspect cardiac disease, palpate for 1 full minute to detect arrhythmias. Normally, an adult's pulse ranges from 60 to 100 beats/minute. Its rhythm should feel regular, except for a subtle slowing on expiration, caused by changes in intrathoracic pressure and vagal response. Note whether the pulse feels weak, normal, or bounding.

Evaluating respirations

Observe for eupnea—a regular, unlabored, and bilaterally equal breathing pattern.

ABNORMAL FINDINGS *In patients with irregular breathing, altered patterns may indicate:*
* *low cardiac output with tachypnea*
* *dyspnea, a possible indicator of heart failure (not evident at rest; however, pausing occurs after only a few words to take breaths)*
* *Cheyne-Stokes respirations may accompany severe heart failure (seen especially with coma)*
* *shallow breathing may be seen with acute pericarditis (shallow respirations occur in an attempt to reduce the pain associated with deep respirations).*

ASSESSING APPEARANCE

Begin by observing the patient's general appearance, particularly noting weight and muscle composition. Is he well-developed, well-nourished, alert, and energetic? Document any departures from normal. Does the patient appear older than his chronological age or seem unusually tired or slow-moving? Does the patient appear comfortable or does he seem to be anxious or in distress?

Measuring height and body weight

Accurately measure and record the patient's height and weight. These measurements will help determine risk factors, calculate hemodynamic indexes (such as cardiac index), guide treatment plans, determine medication dosages, assist with nutritional counseling, and detect fluid overload. Fluctuations in weight may prove significant, especially when extreme.

CLINICAL ALERT **An example of an extreme weight fluctuation would be the patient with developing heart failure gaining several pounds overnight.**

Next, assess for cachexia—weakness and muscle wasting. Observe the amount of muscle bulk in the upper arms, thighs, and chest wall. For a more precise measurement, calculate the percentage of body fat. For men, this should be 12%; for women, it should be 18%. Loss of the body's energy stores slows healing and impairs immune function. A patient with chronic cardiac disease may develop cachexia, losing body fat and muscle mass. However, be aware that edema may mask these effects.

Assessing the skin

Note the patient's skin color, temperature, turgor, and texture. Because normal skin color can vary widely among patients, ask him if his current skin tone is normal. Then inspect the skin color and note any cyanosis. Examine the underside of the tongue, buccal mucosa, and conjunctiva for signs of central cyanosis. Inspect the lips, tip of the nose, earlobes, and nail beds for signs of peripheral cyanosis.

SPECIAL POINTS *In a dark-skinned patient, inspect the oral mucous membranes, such as the lips and gingivae, which normally appear pink and moist but would appear ashen if cyanotic.*

Because the color range for normal mucous membranes is narrower than that for the skin, it provides a more accurate assessment.

Checking radial pulse
* Detect arrhythmias by palpating for 1 full minute
* Normal—60 to 100 beats/minute
* Subtle slowing on expiration

Evaluating respirations
* Normal: Eupnea

Abnormal findings
* Tachypnea
* Dyspnea
* Cheyne-Stokes respirations
* Shallow breathing

Assessing appearance
* Note weight and muscle tone
* Look for normal development, nourishment, alertness, and energy
* Observe for level of comfort or anxiety and distress

Height and body weight measurements
* Determines risk factors
* Used to calculate hemodynamic indexes
* Guides treatment plans and determines medication dosages
* Assists with nutritional counseling and detects fluid overload

Alert!
* Extreme overnight weight gain signals developing heart failure

Assessing the skin
* Note color, temperature, turgor, and texture
* Inspect the skin; note cyanosis.
* Examine tongue, buccal mucosa, and conjunctiva
* Inspect lips, tip of nose, earlobes, and nail beds

Assessing the skin
(continued)

Abnormal findings

- Central cyanosis — reduced oxygen intake or transport from lungs to bloodstream; occurs with heart failure
- Peripheral cyanosis — constriction of peripheral arterioles; results from hypovolemia, cardiogenic shock, or vasoconstrictive disease
- Flushing can result from medications, excess heat, anxiety, or fear
- Pallor can result from anemia or increased peripheral vascular resistance caused by atherosclerosis
- Dependent rubor may be a sign of chronic arterial insufficiency
- Foot showing marked pallor, delayed color return, delayed venous filling, or marked redness indicates arterial insufficiency
- Cool and clammy skin results from vasoconstriction
- Warm, moist skin results from vasodilation
- Taut and shiny skin may result from ascites or marked edema
- Tenting skin may be caused by dehydration, age, malnutrition, or adverse reactions to drugs
- Edema may be caused by varicosities or thrombophlebitis, ascites, or venous compression
- Edema may be caused by varicosities or thrombophlebitis, ascites, or venous compression
- Dry, open lesions on lower extremities, with pallor, cool skin, and lack of hair indicate arterial insufficiency; wet, open lesions, with red or purplish edges indicate venous stasis

 ABNORMAL FINDINGS *Two types of cyanosis can occur in patients:*
- *central cyanosis, suggesting reduced oxygen intake or transport from the lungs to the bloodstream, which may occur with heart failure*
- *peripheral cyanosis, suggesting constriction of peripheral arterioles, a natural response to cold or anxiety or a result of hypovolemia, cardiogenic shock, or a vasoconstrictive disease.*

When evaluating the patient's skin color, also observe for flushing, pallor, and rubor.

 ABNORMAL FINDINGS *Flushing of a patient's skin can result from medications, excess heat, anxiety, or fear. Pallor can result from anemia or increased peripheral vascular resistance caused by atherosclerosis. Dependent rubor may be a sign of chronic arterial insufficiency.*

Next, assess the patient's perfusion by evaluating the arterial flow adequacy. With the patient lying down, elevate one of the his legs 12″ (30.5 cm) above heart level for 60 seconds. Next, tell him to sit up and dangle both legs. Compare the color of both legs. The leg that was elevated should show mild pallor compared with the other leg. Color should return to the pale leg in about 10 seconds, and the veins should refill in about 15 seconds.

 ABNORMAL FINDINGS *Suspect arterial insufficiency if the patient's foot shows marked pallor, delayed color return that ends with a mottled appearance, delayed venous filling, or marked redness.*

Next, touch the patient's skin. It should feel warm and dry.

 ABNORMAL FINDINGS *If the patient's skin is cool and clammy, this results from vasoconstriction, which occurs when cardiac output is low such as during shock. Warm, moist skin results from vasodilation, which occurs when cardiac output is high — for example during exercise.*

Evaluate skin turgor by grasping and raising the skin between two fingers and then letting it go. Normally, the skin immediately returns to its original position.

ABNORMAL FINDINGS *If the patient's skin is taut and shiny and can't be grasped, this may result from ascites or the marked edema that accompanies heart failure. Skin that doesn't immediately return to the original position exhibits tenting, a sign of decreased skin turgor, which may result from dehydration, especially if the patient takes diuretics. It may also result from age, malnutrition, or an adverse reaction to corticosteroid treatment.*

Observe the skin for signs of edema. Inspect the patient's arms and legs for symmetrical swelling. Because edema usually affects lower or dependent areas of the body first, be especially alert when assessing the arms, hands, legs, feet, and ankles of an ambulatory patient or the buttocks and sacrum of a bedridden patient. Determine the type of edema (pitting or nonpitting), its location, its extent, and its symmetry (unilateral or symmetrical). If the patient has pitting edema, assess the degree of pitting.

ABNORMAL FINDINGS *Edema can result from heart failure or venous insufficiency caused by varicosities or thrombophlebitis. Chronic right-sided heart failure may even cause ascites, which leads to generalized edema and abdominal distention. Venous compression may result in localized edema along the path of the compressed vessel.*

While inspecting the patient's skin, note the location, size, number, and appearance of any lesions.

 ABNORMAL FINDINGS *Dry, open lesions on the patient's lower extremities accompanied by pallor, cool skin, and lack of hair growth signify arterial insufficiency, possibly caused by arterial peripheral vascular disease. Wet,*

open lesions with red or purplish edges that appear on the patient's legs may result from the venous stasis associated with venous peripheral vascular disease.

Assessing the arms and legs

Inspect the hair on the patient's arms and legs. Hair should be distributed symmetrically and should grow thicker on the anterior surface of the arms and legs. Note whether the length of the arms and legs is proportionate to the length of the trunk.

 ABNORMAL FINDINGS *If the patient's hair isn't thicker on the anterior of the surface of the arms and legs, this may indicate diminished arterial blood flow to these extremities.*

A patient with long, thin arms and legs may have Marfan syndrome, a congenital disorder that causes cardiovascular problems, such as aortic dissection, aortic valve incompetence, and cardiomyopathy.

Assessing the fingernails

Fingernails normally appear pinkish with no markings.

 ABNORMAL FINDINGS *A bluish color in the nail beds indicates peripheral cyanosis.*

To estimate the rate of peripheral blood flow, assess the capillary refill in the patient's fingernails (or toenails) by applying pressure to the nail for 5 seconds, then assessing the time it takes for color to return. In a patient with a good arterial supply, color should return in less than 3 seconds.

 ABNORMAL FINDINGS *Delayed capillary refill in the patient's fingernails suggests reduced circulation to that area, a sign of low cardiac output that may lead to arterial insufficiency.*

Assess the angle between the nail and the cuticle. An angle of 180 degrees or greater indicates finger clubbing. Check for enlarged fingertips with spongy, slightly swollen nail bases. Normally, the nail bases feel firm, but in early clubbing, they're spongy.

 ABNORMAL FINDINGS *Finger clubbing commonly indicates chronic tissue hypoxia.*

The shape of the patient's nails should be smooth and rounded.

ABNORMAL FINDINGS *A concave depression in the middle of a thin nail indicates koilonychia (spoon nail), a sign of iron deficiency anemia or Raynaud's disease, whereas thick, ridged nails can result from arterial insufficiency.*

Finally, check for splinter hemorrhages — small, thin, red or brown lines that run from the base to the tip of the nail, which may develop in patients with bacterial endocarditis.

Assessing the eyes

Inspect the eyelids for xanthelasma — small, slightly raised, yellowish plaques that usually appear around the inner canthus. The plaques that occur in xanthelasma result from lipid deposits and may signal severe hyperlipidemia, a risk factor of cardiovascular disease.

Next, observe the color of the patient's sclerae.

 ABNORMAL FINDINGS *Yellowish sclerae may be the first sign of jaundice, which occasionally results from liver congestion caused by right-sided heart failure.*

Next, check for arcus senilis — a thin grayish ring around the edge of the cornea.

Assessing the arms and legs

- Assess the hair on the patient's arms and legs
- Look for symmetry and thickness of hair on the anterior surface of the arms and legs
- Note whether the length of the extremities is proportionate to the length of the trunk

Abnormal findings

- Hair that isn't thicker on anterior surface may signal diminished arterial blood flow
- Long, thin arms and legs may indicate Marfan syndrome

Assessing the fingernails

- Assess for pinkish color with no markings
- Assess capillary refill by applying pressure to the nail for 5 seconds, then assess the time it takes for color to return (3 seconds)
- Look for clubbing, smoothness and roundness, and splinter hemorrhages

Abnormal findings

- Bluish color in nailbed
- Delayed capillary refill in fingernails
- Finger clubbing
- Concave depression in middle of a thin nail

Assessing the eyes

- Inspect the eyelids for xanthelasma
- Observe the color of the patient's sclerae
- Check for arcus senilis
- Examine the retinal vessels and background

Assessing the eyes
(continued)
Abnormal findings
+ Yellow sclerae may signal jaundice
+ Narrowing or blocking of a vein where an arteriole crosses over; soft exudates

Assessing head movement
+ Assess head at rest for abnormal position or movements
+ Check ROM and rotation

Abnormal findings
+ Slight, rhythmic bobbing may be caused by aortic insufficiency or aneurysm

Assessing the heart
+ Have patient lie on his back, with the head of the examination table at a 30- to 45-degree angle
+ Inspect, palpate, percuss, and auscultate the heart

Inspection
+ Expose anterior chest and observe appearance
+ Note deviations from typical chest shape
+ Identify cardiovascular landmarks
+ Look for pulsations, symmetry of movement, retractions, or heaves
+ Use a light source to cast a shadow on the chest
+ Note location of the apical pulse

Abnormal findings
+ Barrel chest
+ Pectus excavatum

 SPECIAL POINTS *A normal occurrence in older patients, arcus senilis can indicate hyperlipidemia in patients younger than age 65.*

Using an ophthalmoscope, examine the retinal structures, including the retinal vessels and background. The retina is normally light yellow to orange, and the background should be free from hemorrhages and exudates.

 ABNORMAL FINDINGS *Structural changes, such as narrowing or blocking of a vein where an arteriole crosses over, indicate hypertension. Soft exudates may suggest hypertension or subacute bacterial endocarditis.*

Assessing head movement
Assess the patient's head at rest and be alert for abnormal positioning or movements. Also check range of motion (ROM) and rotation of the neck.

 ABNORMAL FINDINGS *A slight, rhythmic bobbing of the patient's head in time with his heartbeat (Musset's sign) may accompany the high back-pressure caused by aortic insufficiency or aneurysm.*

ASSESSING THE HEART
Ask the patient to remove all clothing except his underwear and to put on an examination gown. Have the patient lie on his back, with the head of the examination table at a 30- to 45-degree angle. Stand on the patient's right side if you're right-handed or his left side if you're left-handed so you can auscultate more easily.

As with assessment of other body systems, you'll inspect, palpate, percuss, and auscultate in your assessment of the heart.

Inspection
First, inspect the patient's chest and thorax. Expose the anterior chest and observe its general appearance. Normally, the lateral diameter is twice the anteroposterior diameter. Note any deviations from typical chest shape.

Note landmarks you can use to describe your findings as well as structures underlying the chest wall. (See *Identifying cardiovascular landmarks.*)

Look for pulsations, symmetry of movement, retractions, or heaves. A heave is a strong outward thrust of the chest wall and occurs during systole.

Position a light source, such as a flashlight or gooseneck lamp, so that it casts a shadow on the patient's chest. Note the location of the apical impulse. This is also usually the point of maximal impulse and should be located in the fifth intercostal space medial to the left midclavicular line.

The apical impulse gives an indication of how well the left ventricle is working because it corresponds to the apex of the heart. The impulse can be seen in about 50% of adults.

 SPECIAL POINTS *You'll notice the apical impulse more easily in children and in patients with thin chest walls. To find the apical impulse in a woman with large breasts, displace the breasts during the examination. In thin adults and in children, you may see a slight sternal movement and pulsations over the pulmonary arteries or the aorta as well as visible pulsations in the epigastric area.*

 ABNORMAL FINDINGS *On inspection you may discover irregularities in the patient's thorax and spine, some of which can impair cardiac output by preventing chest expansion and inhibiting heart muscle movement, including:*
+ *barrel chest (rounded thoracic cage caused by chronic obstructive pulmonary disease)*
+ *pectus excavatum (depressed sternum)*

KNOW-HOW

Identifying cardiovascular landmarks

These views show where to find critical landmarks used in cardiovascular assessment.

ANTERIOR THORAX

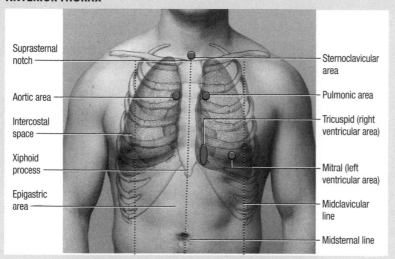

Suprasternal notch

Aortic area

Intercostal space

Xiphoid process

Epigastric area

Sternoclavicular area

Pulmonic area

Tricuspid (right ventricular area)

Mitral (left ventricular area)

Midclavicular line

Midsternal line

LATERAL THORAX

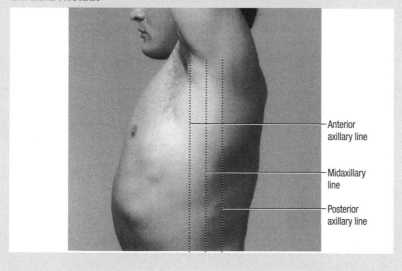

Anterior axillary line

Midaxillary line

Posterior axillary line

♦ *scoliosis (lateral curvature of the spine)*
♦ *pectus carinatum (protruding sternum)*
♦ *kyphosis (convex curvature of the thoracic spine)*
♦ *retractions (visible indentations of the soft tissue covering the chest wall) or the use of accessory muscles to breathe, which typically result from a respiratory disorder, but may also indicate congenital heart defect or heart failure*

Identifying cardiovascular landmarks

Anterior thorax
♦ Suprasternal notch, aortic area, intercostal space, xiphoid process, epigastric area, sternoclavicular area, pulmonic area, tricuspid (right ventricular area), mitral (left ventricular area), midclavicular line, midsternal line

Lateral thorax
♦ Anterior axillary line, midaxillary line, posterior axillary line

Inspection
(continued)

Abnormal findings
♦ Scoliosis
♦ Pectus carinatum
♦ Kyphosis
♦ Retractions

Assessing the apical impulse

The apical impulse is associated with the first heart sound and carotid pulsation. To ensure that you're feeling the apical impulse and not a muscle spasm or some other pulsation, use one hand to palpate the patient's carotid artery and the other to palpate the apical impulse. Then compare the timing and regularity of the impulses. The apical impulse should roughly coincide with the carotid pulsation.

Note the amplitude, size, intensity, location, and duration of the apical impulse. You should feel a gentle pulsation in an area about ½" to ¾" (1.5 to 2 cm) in diameter.

Inspection
(continued)

Abnormal findings
+ Visible pulsation to right of sternum
+ Pulsation in sternoclavicular epigastric area
+ Sustained, forceful apical impulse
+ Laterally displaced apical impulse

Palpation
+ Start at the sternoclavicular area, moving down to the epigastric area
+ Use the pads of the fingers to assess large pulse sites
+ Use the ball of your hand, then fingertips, to palpate over the precordium to find apical pulse, noting heaves or thrills
+ Have patient lie of left side or sit upright if palpation proves difficult lying on his back

Abnormal findings
+ Strong apical pulse, lasting longer than one-third of cycle
+ Displaced, diffuse pulse
+ Aortic, pulmonic, right ventricular area pulsation
+ Sternoclavicular, epigastric area pulsation
+ Palpable thrill

+ *visible pulsation to the right of the sternum, a possible indication of aortic aneurysm*
+ *pulsation in the sternoclavicular or epigastric area, a possible indication of aortic aneurysm*
+ *sustained, forceful apical impulse, a possible indication of left ventricular hypertrophy, which increases blood pressure and may cause cardiomyopathy and mitral insufficiency*
+ *laterally displaced apical impulse, a possible sign of left ventricular hypertrophy.*

Palpation

Maintain a gentle touch when you palpate so you won't obscure pulsations or similar findings. Follow a systematic palpation sequence covering the sternoclavicular, aortic, pulmonary right ventricular, left ventricular (apical), and epigastric areas. Use the pads of the fingers to effectively assess large pulse sites. Finger pads prove especially sensitive to vibrations.

Start at the sternoclavicular area and move methodically through the palpation sequence down to the epigastric area.

 SPECIAL POINTS *At the sternoclavicular area, you may feel pulsation of the aortic arch, especially in a thin or average-build patient. In a thin patient, you may palpate a pulsation in the abdominal aorta over the epigastric area.*

Using the ball of your hand, then your fingertips, palpate over the precordium to find the apical impulse. Note heaves or thrills, fine vibrations that feel like the purring of a cat. (See *Assessing the apical impulse.*)

 SPECIAL POINTS *Keep in mind that the apical impulse may be difficult to palpate in obese and pregnant patients and in patients with thick chest walls.*

If it's difficult to palpate with the patient lying on his back, have him lie on his left side or sit upright. It may also be helpful to have the patient exhale completely and hold his breath for a few seconds.

 ABNORMAL FINDINGS *Palpation of the patient's chest may reveal:*
+ *apical impulse that exerts unusual force and lasts longer than one-third of the cardiac cycle — a possible indication of increased cardiac output*
+ *displaced or diffuse impulse — a possible indication of left ventricular hypertrophy*
+ *pulsation in the aortic, pulmonic, or right ventricular area — a sign of chamber enlargement or valvular disease*
+ *pulsation in the sternoclavicular or epigastric area — a sign of aortic aneurysm*
+ *palpable thrill (fine vibration) — an indication of blood flow turbulence, usually*

related to valvular dysfunction (determine how far the thrill radiates and make a mental note to listen for a murmur at this site during auscultation)

✦ *heave (a strong outward thrust during systole) along the left sternal border—an indication of right ventricular hypertrophy*

✦ *heave over the left ventricular area—a sign of a ventricular aneurysm (a thin patient may experience a heave with exercise, fever, or anxiety because of increased cardiac output and more forceful contraction)*

✦ *displaced point of maximal impulse (PMI)—a possible indication of left ventricular hypertrophy caused by volume overload from mitral or aortic stenosis, septal defect, acute MI, or other disorder.*

Percussion

Although percussion isn't as useful as other methods of assessment, this technique may help you locate cardiac borders. Begin percussing at the anterior axillary line, and percuss toward the sternum along the fifth intercostal space.

The sound changes from resonance to dullness over the left border of the heart, normally at the midclavicular line.

 ABNORMAL FINDINGS *If the cardiac border extends to the left of the midclavicular line, the patient's heart—and especially the left ventricle—may be enlarged.*

The right border of the heart is usually aligned with the sternum and can't be percussed.

 SPECIAL POINTS *In patients who are obese, percussion may be difficult because of the fat overlying the chest or in female patients because of breast tissue. In these cases, a chest X-ray can be used to provide information about the heart border.*

Auscultating for heart sounds

You can learn a great deal about the heart by auscultating for heart sounds. Cardiac auscultation requires a methodical approach and lots of practice. Begin by warming the stethoscope in your hands, and then identify the sites where you'll auscultate: over the four cardiac valves and at Erb's point, the third intercostal space at the left sternal border. Use the bell to hear low-pitched sounds and the diaphragm to hear high-pitched sounds. (See *Auscultation sites*, page 110.)

Auscultate for heart sounds with the patient in three positions: lying on his back with the head of the bed raised 30 to 45 degrees, sitting up, and lying on his left side. You can start at the base and work downward or at the apex and work upward. Whichever approach you use, be consistent.

Use the diaphragm to listen as you go in one direction; use the bell as you come back in the other direction. Be sure to listen over the entire precordium, not just over the valves.

Note the heart rate and rhythm. Always identify the first heart sound (S_1) and the second heart sound (S_2), and then listen for adventitious sounds, such as third (S_3) and fourth heart sounds, (S_4), murmurs, and rubs.

Start auscultating at the aortic area where S_2, the second heart sound, is loudest. S_2 is best heard at the base of the heart at the end of ventricular systole. This sound corresponds to closure of the pulmonic and aortic valves and is generally described as sounding like "dub." It's a shorter, higher-pitched, louder sound than S_1. When the pulmonic valve closes later than the aortic valve during inspiration, you'll hear a split S_2.

From the base of the heart, move to the pulmonic area and then down to the tricuspid area. Then move to the mitral area, where S_1 is the loudest. S_1 is best heard at the apex of the heart. This sound corresponds to closure of the mitral and tricuspid valves and is generally described as sounding like "lub." It's low-pitched

Palpation
(continued)

Abnormal findings
✦ Heave along left sternal border
✦ Heave over left ventricular area
✦ Displaced PMI

Percussion
✦ Begin at the anterior axillary line, continuing toward sternum along fifth intercostal space
✦ Note sound changes from resonance to dullness over left border of heart, normally at midclavicular line

Abnormal findings
✦ If cardiac border extends to left of midclavicular line, heart may be enlarged

Auscultating for heart sounds
✦ Auscultate over the four cardiac valves, and at Erb's point, the third intercostal space at the left sternal border
✦ Auscultate with patient lying on his back with the head of the bed raised 30 to 45 degrees, sitting up, and lying on left side
✦ Use the bell to hear low-pitched sounds and the diaphragm to hear high-pitched sounds
✦ Always identify S_1 and S_2 first
✦ Start auscultating at aortic area where S_2 is loudest
✦ S_1 is described as a dull, low-pitched sound like "lub"
✦ S_2 is described as a short, high-pitched sound like "dub"
✦ When the pulmonic valve closes later than the aortic valve during inspiration, you'll hear a split S_2

KNOW-HOW

Auscultation sites

When auscultating for heart sounds, place the stethoscope over four different sites. Follow the same auscultation sequence during every cardiovascular assessment:

✦ Place the stethoscope in the second intercostal space along the right sternal border, as shown. In the aortic area, blood moves from the left ventricle during systole, crossing the aortic valve and flowing through the aortic arch.

✦ Move to the pulmonic area, located in the second intercostal space at the left sternal border. In the pulmonic area, blood ejected from the right ventricle during systole crosses the pulmonic valve and flows through the main pulmonary artery.

✦ In the third auscultation site, assess the tricuspid area, which lies in the fifth intercostal space along the left sternal border. In the tricuspid area, sounds reflect blood movement from the right atrium across the tricuspid valve, filling the right ventricle during diastole.

✦ Finally, listen in the mitral area, located in the fifth intercostal space near the midclavicular line. (If the patient's heart is enlarged, the mitral area may be closer to the anterior axillary line.) In the mitral (apical) area, sounds represent blood flow across the mitral valve and left ventricular filling during diastole.

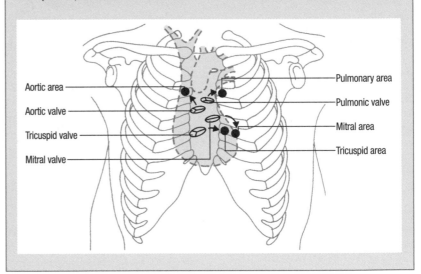

Auscultating for abnormal heart sounds

✦ S_1 and S_2 may be accentuated, diminished, or inaudible, which may result from pressure changes, valvular dysfunctions, and conduction defects

✦ A prolonged, persistent, or reversed spilt sound may result from a mechanical or electrical problem

✦ S_3 and S_4 may also occur as well as a click, an opening snap, and a summation gallop

Facts about S_3

✦ Also known as *ventricular gallop*

✦ Best heard with bell placed at the heart apex

✦ Rhythm resembles a horse galloping

✦ Cadence resembles the word "Ken-tuc-ky" ("lub-dub-by")

and dull. S_1 occurs at the beginning of ventricular systole. It may be split if the mitral valve closes just before the tricuspid.

Auscultating for abnormal heart sounds

Auscultation may detect S_1 and S_2 that are accentuated, diminished, or inaudible. These abnormalities may result from pressure changes, valvular dysfunctions, and conduction defects. A prolonged, persistent, or reversed split sound may result from a mechanical or electrical problem. Auscultation may also reveal an S_3, an S_4, or both. Other abnormal sounds include a click, an opening snap, and a summation gallop.

Third heart sound

Also known as a *ventricular gallop,* it's a low-pitched noise that's best heard by placing the bell of the stethoscope at the apex of the heart. Its rhythm resembles a horse galloping, and its cadence resembles the word "Ken-tuc-ky" ("lub-dub-by"). Listen for S_3 with the patient in a supine or left-lateral decubitus position.

S_3 usually occurs during early diastole to mid-diastole, at the end of the passive-filling phase of either ventricle.

Listen for this sound immediately after S_2. It may signify that the ventricle isn't compliant enough to accept the filling volume without additional force. If the right ventricle is noncompliant, the sound will occur in the tricuspid area; if the left ventricle is noncompliant, in the mitral area. A heave may be palpable when the sound occurs.

SPECIAL POINTS *An S_3 may occur normally in a child or young adult. It may also occur during the last trimester of pregnancy. In a patient over age 30, it usually indicates a disorder, such as right-sided heart failure, left-sided heart failure, pulmonary congestion, intracardiac shunting of blood, MI, anemia, or thyrotoxicosis.*

Fourth heart sound
The fourth heart sound is an abnormal heart sound that occurs late in diastole, just before the pulse upstroke. It immediately precedes the S_1 of the next cycle and is associated with acceleration and deceleration of blood entering a chamber that resists additional filling. Known as the *atrial* or *presystolic gallop*, it occurs during atrial contraction.

S_4 shares the same cadence as the word "Ten-nes-see" ("le-lub-dub"). Heard best with the bell of the stethoscope and with the patient in a supine position, S_4 may occur in the tricuspid or mitral area, depending on which ventricle is dysfunctional. Although rare, S_4 may occur normally in a young patient with a thin chest wall. More commonly, it indicates cardiovascular disease, such as acute MI, hypertension, CAD, cardiomyopathy, angina, anemia, elevated left ventricular pressure, or aortic stenosis. If the sound persists, it may indicate impaired ventricular compliance or volume overload.

SPECIAL POINTS *S_4 commonly appears in elderly patients with age-related systolic hypertension and aortic stenosis.*

Summation gallop
Occasionally, a patient may have both S_3 and S_4. Auscultation may reveal two separate abnormal heart sounds and two normal sounds. Usually, the patient has tachycardia and diastole is shortened. S_3 and S_4 occur so close together that they appear to be one sound—a summation gallop.

Clicks
Clicks are high-pitched abnormal heart sounds that result from tensing of the chordae tendineae structures and mitral valve cusps. Initially, the mitral valve closes securely, but a large cusp prolapses into the left atrium. The click usually precedes a late systolic murmur caused by regurgitation of a little blood from the left ventricle into the left atrium.

SPECIAL POINTS *Clicks occur in 5% to 10% of young adults and affect more women than men.*

To detect the high-pitched click of mitral valve prolapse in your patient, place the stethoscope diaphragm at the apex and listen during midsystole to late systole. To enhance the sound, change the patient's position to sitting or standing, and listen along the lower left sternal border.

Facts about S_3
(continued)
✦ Occurs during early diastole to mid-diastole, at the end of the passive-filling phase of either ventricle

Special points
✦ In a patient over age 30, may indicate right- or left-sided heart failure, pulmonary congestion, intracardiac shunting of blood, MI, anemia, or thyrotoxicosis

Facts about S_4
✦ Abnormal heart sound occurring late in diastole, immediately preceding S_1 of the next cycle
✦ Associated with acceleration and deceleration of blood entering a chamber that resists additional filling
✦ Also known as the *atrial* or *presystolic gallop*
✦ Shares the same cadence as the word "Ten-nes-see" ("le-lub-dub")
✦ Heard best with bell and patient in supine position
✦ Occurs in the tricuspid or mitral area

Facts about summation gallop
✦ S_3 and S_4 occur as two separate abnormal sounds and two normal sounds
✦ Patient experiences tachycardia and shortened diastole

Facts about clicks
✦ High-pitched abnormal sounds
✦ Result from tensing of the chordae tendineae structures and mitral valve cusps
✦ Precede a late systolic murmur caused by regurgitation of blood from left ventricle into left atrium

Facts about snaps

+ Occur immediately after S_2
+ Resemble normal S_1 and S_2 in quality
+ High pitch helps differentiate them from S_3
+ Usually precede mid-diastolic to late diastolic murmur

Facts about rubs

+ Harsh, scratchy, scraping, or squeaking sounds occurring through systole, diastole, or both
+ Sound enhanced by upright leaning forward position or exhalation
+ Usually indicate pericarditis

Facts about murmurs

+ Vibrating, blowing, or rumbling noises, produced by turbulent blood flow result from valvular stenosis, valvular insufficiency, or septal defect

Special points

+ Up to 25% of children experience innocent murmurs, usually disappearing by adolescence
+ Elderly patients experience nonpathologic murmurs as a short systolic murmur

KNOW-HOW

Grading murmurs

Use the system outlined here to describe the intensity of a murmur. When recording your findings, use Roman numerals as part of a fraction, always with VI as the denominator. For instance, a grade III murmur would be recorded as "grade III/VI."

+ Grade I is barely audible.
+ Grade II is audible but quiet and soft.
+ Grade III is moderately loud, without a thrust or thrill.
+ Grade IV is loud, with a thrill.
+ Grade V is very loud, with a thrust or a thrill.
+ Grade VI is loud enough to be heard before the stethoscope comes into contact with the chest.

Snaps

Upon placing the stethoscope diaphragm dial to the apex along the lower left sternal border, you may detect an opening snap immediately after S_2. The snap resembles the normal S_1 and S_2 in quality; its high pitch helps differentiate it from an S_3. Because the opening snap may accompany mitral or tricuspid stenosis, it usually precedes a middiastolic to late diastolic murmur—a classic sign of stenosis. It results from the stenotic valve attempting to open.

Rubs

To detect a pericardial friction rub, use the diaphragm of the stethoscope to auscultate in the third left intercostal space along the lower left sternal border. Listen for a harsh, scratchy, scraping, or squeaking sound that occurs throughout systole, diastole, or both. To enhance the sound, have the patient sit upright and lean forward or exhale. A rub usually indicates pericarditis.

Murmurs

Longer than a heart sound, a murmur occurs as a vibrating, blowing, or rumbling noise. Just as turbulent water in a stream babbles as it passes through a narrow point, turbulent blood flow produces a murmur. An innocent or functional murmur may appear in a patient without heart disease. Best heard in the pulmonic area, it occurs early in systole and seldom exceeds grade 2 in intensity. When the patient changes from a supine to a sitting position, the murmur may disappear. If fever, exercise, anemia, anxiety, pregnancy, or other factors increase cardiac output, the murmur may increase in intensity. (See *Grading murmurs*.)

 SPECIAL POINTS *Innocent murmurs affect up to 25% of all children but usually disappear by adolescence. Similarly, elderly patients who experience changes in the aortic valve structures and the aorta also experience a nonpathologic murmur—a short systolic murmur, best heard at the left sternal border.*

Pathologic murmurs in a patient may occur during systole or diastole and may affect any heart valve. These murmurs may result from valvular stenosis (inability of the heart valves to open properly), valvular insufficiency (inability of the heart valves to close properly, allowing regurgitation of blood), or a septal defect (a defect in the septal wall separating two heart chambers). The best way to hear murmurs is with the patient sitting up and leaning forward. You can also have him lie on his left side. (See *Positioning the patient for auscultation.* See also *Identifying heart murmurs,* page 114.)

KNOW-HOW

Positioning the patient for auscultation

FORWARD-LEANING POSITION
The forward-leaning position is best suited for hearing high-pitched sounds related to semilunar valve problems, such as aortic and pulmonic valve murmurs. To auscultate for these sounds, place the diaphragm of the stethoscope over the aortic and pulmonic areas in the right and left second intercostal spaces, as shown below.

LEFT LATERAL RECUMBENT POSITION
The left lateral recumbent position is best suited for hearing low-pitched sounds, such as mitral valve murmurs and extra heart sounds. To hear these sounds, place the bell of the stethoscope over the apical area, as shown below.

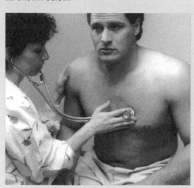
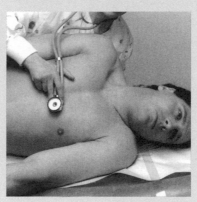

If you detect a murmur, identify where it's loudest, pinpoint the time it occurs during the cardiac cycle, and describe its pitch, pattern, quality, and intensity.

Location and timing
Murmurs may occur in any cardiac auscultatory site and may radiate from one site to another. To identify the radiation area, auscultate from the site where the murmur seems loudest to the farthest site it's still heard. Note the anatomic landmark of this farthest site.

Determine if the murmur occurs during systole (between S_1 and S_2) or diastole (between S_2 and the next S_1). Pinpoint when in the cardiac cycle the murmur occurs—for example, during middiastole or late systole. A murmur that is heard throughout systole is called *holosystolic* or *pansystolic*, while a murmur heard throughout diastole is called a *pandiastolic murmur*. Occasionally murmurs occur during both portions of the cycle (*continuous murmur*).

Pitch
Depending on rate and pressure of blood flow, pitch may be high, medium, or low. You can best hear a low-pitched murmur with the bell of the stethoscope, a high-pitched murmur with the diaphragm, and a medium-pitched murmur with both.

Pattern
Crescendo occurs when the velocity of blood flow increases and the murmur becomes louder. Decrescendo occurs when velocity decreases and the murmur be-

Facts about murmurs
(continued)

Location and timing
✦ Occur in any cardiac auscultatory site radiating from one side to the other

Pitch
✦ May be high, medium, or low

Pattern
✦ Loud murmur in crescendo, quiet murmur in decrescendo, and increasing loudness and softness in crescendo-decrescendo

Conditions associated with heart murmurs

+ Aortic stenosis
+ Pulmonic stenosis
+ Aortic insufficiency
+ Pulmonic insufficiency
+ Mitral stenosis
+ Mitral insufficiency
+ Tricuspid stenosis
+ Tricuspid insufficiency

Facts about murmurs
(continued)

Quality
+ Described as musical, blowing, harsh, rasping, rumbling, or machinelike

Intensity
+ Graded by a six-level scale

Identifying heart murmurs

Heart murmurs can occur as a result of various conditions and have wide-ranging characteristics. Here's a list of some conditions and their associated murmurs.

AORTIC STENOSIS
In a patient with aortic stenosis, the aortic valve has calcified and restricts blood flow, causing a midsystolic, low-pitched, harsh murmur that radiates from the valve to the carotid artery. The murmur shifts from crescendo to decrescendo and back.

The crescendo-decrescendo murmur of aortic stenosis results from the turbulent, highly pressured flow of blood across stiffened leaflets and through a narrowed opening.

PULMONIC STENOSIS
During auscultation, listen for a murmur near the pulmonic valve. In a patient with this type of murmur it might indicate pulmonic stenosis, a condition in which the pulmonic valve has calcified and interferes with the flow of blood out of the right ventricle. The murmur is medium-pitched, systolic, and harsh and shifts from crescendo to decrescendo and back. The murmur is caused by turbulent blood flow across a stiffened, narrowed valve.

AORTIC INSUFFICIENCY
In a patient with aortic insufficiency, the blood flows backward through the aortic valve and causes a high-pitched, blowing, decrescendo, diastolic murmur. The murmur radiates from the aortic valve area to the left sternal border.

PULMONIC INSUFFICIENCY
In a patient with pulmonic insufficiency, the blood flows backward through the pulmonic valve, causing a blowing, diastolic, decrescendo murmur at Erb's point (at the left sternal border of the third intercostal space). If the patient has a higher-than-normal pulmonary

pressure, the murmur is high-pitched. If not, it will be low-pitched.

MITRAL STENOSIS
In a patient with mitral stenosis, the mitral valve has calcified and is blocking blood flow out of the left atrium. Listen for a low-pitched, rumbling, crescendo-decrescendo murmur in the mitral valve area. This murmur results from turbulent blood flow across the stiffened, narrowed valve.

MITRAL INSUFFICIENCY
In a patient with mitral insufficiency, blood regurgitates into the left atrium. The regurgitation produces a high-pitched, blowing murmur throughout systole (pansystolic or holosystolic). The murmur may radiate from the mitral area to the left axillary line. You can hear it best at the apex.

TRICUSPID STENOSIS
In a patient with tricuspid stenosis, the tricuspid valve has calcified and is blocking blood flow through the valve from the right atrium. Listen for a low, rumbling, crescendo-decrescendo murmur in the tricuspid area. The murmur results from turbulent blood flow across the stiffened, narrowed valvular leaflets.

TRICUSPID INSUFFICIENCY
In a patient with tricuspid insufficiency, blood regurgitates into the right atrium. This backflow of blood through the valve causes a high-pitched, blowing murmur throughout systole in the tricuspid area. The murmur becomes louder when the patient inhales.

---

comes quieter. A crescendo-decrescendo pattern describes a murmur with increasing loudness followed by increasing softness.

Quality
The volume of blood flow, the force of the contraction, and the degree of valve compromise all contribute to murmur quality. Terms used to describe quality include musical, blowing, harsh, rasping, rumbling, or machinelike.

Intensity

Use a standard, six-level grading scale to describe the intensity of the murmur.

ASSESSING THE VASCULAR SYSTEM

Assessment of the vascular system is an important part of a full cardiovascular assessment. Examination of the patient's arms and legs can reveal arterial or venous disorders. Examine the patient's arms when you take his vital signs. Check the legs later during the physical examination, when the patient is lying on his back. Remember to evaluate leg veins when the patient is standing.

Inspection

Start your assessment of the vascular system the same way you start an assessment of the cardiac system — by making general observations. Are the patient's arms equal in size? Are the legs symmetrical?

Inspect the patient's skin color. Note how body hair is distributed. Note lesions, scars, clubbing, and edema of the extremities. If the patient is bedridden, be sure to check the sacrum for swelling. Examine the fingernails and toenails for abnormalities.

ABNORMAL FINDINGS *Upon inspection of the patient's vascular system you may uncover irregularities, including:*
- *cyanosis, pallor, or cool or cold skin, indicating poor cardiac output and tissue perfusion*
- *warm skin caused by fever or increased cardiac output*
- *absence of body hair on the patient's arms or legs, indicating diminished arterial blood flow to those areas (see Findings in arterial and venous insufficiency, page 116)*
- *swelling or edema, indicating heart failure or venous insufficiency, or varicosities or thrombophlebitis*
- *ascites and generalized edema, indicating chronic right-sided heart failure*
- *localized swelling, indicating compressed veins*
- *swelling in the lower legs, indicating right-sided heart failure.*

Start your inspection by observing vessels in the patient's neck. The carotid artery should show a brisk, localized pulsation. The internal jugular vein has a softer, undulating pulsation. The carotid pulsation doesn't decrease when the patient is upright, when he inhales, or when you palpate the carotid. The internal jugular pulsation, on the other hand, changes in response to position, breathing, and palpation.

Check carotid artery pulsations. Are they weak or bounding? Inspect the jugular veins. Inspection of these vessels can provide information about blood volume and pressure in the right side of the heart.

To check the jugular venous pulse, have the patient lie on his back. Elevate the head of the bed 30 to 45 degrees, and turn the patient's head slightly away from you. Normally, the highest pulsation occurs no more than 1½" (4 cm) above the sternal notch.

ABNORMAL FINDINGS *If the patient's pulsations appear higher, this indicates elevation in central venous pressure and jugular vein distention. Characterize this distention as mild, moderate, or severe. Determine the level of distention in fingerbreadths above the clavicle or in relation to the jaw or clavicle. Also, note the amount of distention in relation to head elevation.*

Assessing the vascular system

- ✦ Examine patient's arms and legs for arterial or venous disorders
- ✦ Observe his arms when you take his vital signs
- ✦ Check his legs later during the physical examination, when he's lying on his back
- ✦ Evaluate his leg veins while he's standing

Inspection

- ✦ Assess arms and legs for equality and symmetry
- ✦ Inspect skin color and body hair distribution
- ✦ Note lesions, scars, clubbing, and edema
- ✦ If the patient is bedridden, check sacrum for swelling
- ✦ Examine fingernails and toenails for abnormalities
- ✦ Observe the carotid artery and internal jugular vein pulsations

Abnormal findings

- ✦ Cyanosis, pallor, cool skin
- ✦ Warm skin
- ✦ Absence of arm or leg hair
- ✦ Swelling, edema, ascites, generalized edema
- ✦ Localized swelling
- ✦ Swelling in lower legs
- ✦ Jugular venous pulsations appearing higher than 1½" above sternal notch

Findings in arterial and venous insufficiency

Assessment findings differ in patients with arterial insufficiency and those with chronic venous insufficiency. These illustrations show those differences.

ARTERIAL INSUFFICIENCY

In a patient with arterial insufficiency, pulses may be decreased or absent. His skin will be cool, pale, and shiny, and he may have pain in his legs and feet. Ulcerations typically occur in the area around the toes, and the foot usually turns deep red when dependent. Nails may be thick and ridged.

CHRONIC VENOUS INSUFFICIENCY

In a patient with chronic venous insufficiency, check for ulcerations around the ankle. Pulses are present but may be difficult to find because of edema. The foot may become cyanotic when dependent.

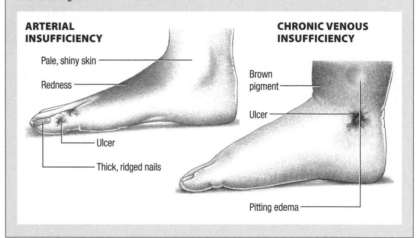

ARTERIAL INSUFFICIENCY — Pale, shiny skin — Redness — Ulcer — Thick, ridged nails

CHRONIC VENOUS INSUFFICIENCY — Brown pigment — Ulcer — Pitting edema

Palpation

- ✦ Assess skin temperature, texture, and turgor
- ✦ Check capillary refill time in nail beds on fingers and toes
- ✦ Palpate arms and legs for temperature and edema
- ✦ Palpate for arterial pulses
- ✦ Check carotid, brachial, radial, femoral, popliteal, posterior tibial, and dorsalis pedis pulses

Alert!

- ✦ Don't palpate both carotid arteries at the same time or press too firmly; patient may faint or become bradycardic

Palpation

The first step in palpating the vascular system is to assess skin temperature, texture, and turgor. Then check capillary refill time by assessing the nail beds on the fingers and toes. Refill time should be no more than 3 seconds, or long enough to say "capillary refill."

Palpate the patient's arms and legs for temperature and edema. Edema is graded on a four-point scale. If your finger leaves a slight imprint, the edema is recorded as +1. If your finger leaves a deep imprint that only slowly returns to normal, the edema is recorded as +4.

Palpate for arterial pulses by gently pressing with the pads of your index and middle fingers. Start at the top of the patient's body at the temporal artery, and work your way down. Check the carotid, brachial, radial, femoral, popliteal, posterior tibial, and dorsalis pedis pulses.

Palpate for the pulse on each side, comparing pulse volume and symmetry.

 CLINICAL ALERT **Don't palpate both carotid arteries at the same time or press too firmly. If you do, the patient may faint or become bradycardic.**

If you haven't put on gloves for the examination, do so when you palpate the femoral arteries.

KNOW-HOW

Assessing arterial pulses

To assess arterial pulses, apply pressure with your index and middle fingers. The following illustrations show where to position your fingers when palpating for various pulses.

CAROTID PULSE
Lightly place your fingers just medial to the trachea and below the jaw angle. Never palpate both carotid arteries at the same time.

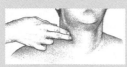

BRACHIAL PULSE
Position your fingers medial to the biceps tendon.

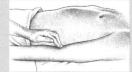

RADIAL PULSE
Apply gentle pressure to the medial and ventral side of the wrist, just below the base of the thumb.

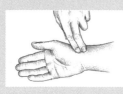

FEMORAL PULSE
Press relatively hard at a point inferior to the inguinal ligament. For an obese patient, palpate in the crease of the groin, halfway between the pubic bone and the hip bone.

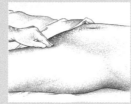

POPLITEAL PULSE
Press firmly in the popliteal fossa at the back of the knee.

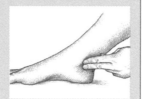

POSTERIOR TIBIAL PULSE
Apply pressure behind and slightly below the malleolus of the ankle.

DORSALIS PEDIS PULSE
Place your fingers on the medial dorsum of the foot while the patient points his toes down. (*Note:* The pulse is difficult to detect here and may be nonpalpable in healthy patients.)

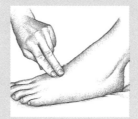

All pulses should be regular in rhythm and equal in strength. Pulses are graded on the following scale: 4+ is bounding, 3+ is increased, 2+ is normal, 1+ is weak, and 0 is absent. (See *Assessing arterial pulses.*)

 ABNORMAL FINDINGS *A weak arterial pulse may indicate decreased cardiac output or increased peripheral vascular resistance, both pointing to arterial atherosclerotic disease.*

 SPECIAL POINTS *Elderly patients often have weak pedal pulses.*

Assessing arterial pulses
+ Carotid pulse — medial to trachea and below jaw angle
+ Brachial pulse — medial to biceps tendon
+ Radial pulse — medial and ventral side of wrist below thumb base
+ Femoral pulse — point inferior to inguinal ligament
+ Popliteal pulse — popliteal fossa at back of knee
+ Posterior tibial pulse — behind and slightly below malleolus of ankle
+ Dorsalis pedis pulse — medial dorsum of foot while patient points toes down

Pulse gradings
+ Pulses are graded on a four-point scale: 4+ (bounding), 3+ (increased), 2+ (normal), 1+ (weak) 0 (absent)

Abnormal findings
+ Weak arterial pulse
+ Strong or bounding pulsations

Characteristics of pulse waveforms

+ Weak—decreased amplitude with slower upstroke and downstroke
+ Bounding—sharp upstroke and downstroke with pointed peak
+ Pulsus alternans — regular, alternating pattern of a weak and strong pulse
+ Pulsus bigeminus—occurs at irregular intervals caused by premature atrial or ventricular beats
+ Pulsus paradoxus—increases and decreases in amplitude associated with respiratory cycle
+ Pulsus biferiens—initial upstroke, a subsequent downstroke, then another upstroke during systole

Pulse waveforms

To identify abnormal arterial pulses, check the waveforms below and see which one matches the patient's peripheral pulse.

WEAK PULSE

A weak pulse has a decreased amplitude with a slower upstroke and downstroke. Possible causes of a weak pulse include increased peripheral vascular resistance, such as happens in cold weather or severe heart failure, and decreased stroke volume, as with hypovolemia or aortic stenosis.

BOUNDING PULSE

A bounding pulse has a sharp upstroke and downstroke with a pointed peak. The amplitude is elevated. Possible causes of a bounding pulse include increased stroke volume, as with aortic regurgitation, or stiffness of arterial walls, as with aging.

PULSUS ALTERNANS

Pulsus alternans has a regular, alternating pattern of a weak and a strong pulse. This pulse is associated with left-sided heart failure.

PULSUS BIGEMINUS

Pulsus bigeminus is similar to alternating pulse but occurs at irregular intervals. This pulse is caused by premature atrial or ventricular beats.

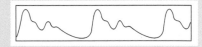

PULSUS PARADOXUS

Pulsus paradoxus has increases and decreases in amplitude associated with the respiratory cycle. Marked decreases occur when the patient inhales. Pulsus paradoxus is associated with pericardial tamponade, advanced heart failure, and constrictive pericarditis.

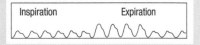

Inspiration   Expiration

PULSUS BIFERIENS

Pulsus biferiens shows an initial upstroke, a subsequent downstroke, and then another upstroke during systole. Pulsus biferiens is caused by aortic stenosis and aortic insufficiency.

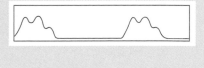

Auscultation

+ Follow palpation sequence; listen over each artery
+ Assess upper abdomen for abnormal pulsations
+ Auscultate femoral and popliteal pulses; check for a bruit or other abnormal sounds

 ABNORMAL FINDINGS *Strong or bounding pulsations usually occur in a patient with a condition that causes increased cardiac output, such as hypertension, hypoxia, anemia, exercise, or anxiety. (See* Pulse waveforms.*)*

Auscultation

After you palpate, use the bell of the stethoscope to begin auscultating the vascular system; then follow the palpation sequence and listen over each artery. You shouldn't hear sounds over the carotid arteries. A hum, or bruit, sounds like buzzing or blowing and could indicate arteriosclerotic plaque formation.

Assess the upper abdomen for abnormal pulsations, which could indicate the presence of an abdominal aortic aneurysm. Finally, auscultate for the femoral and popliteal pulses, checking for a bruit or other abnormal sounds.

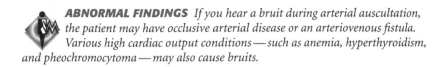

ABNORMAL FINDINGS *If you hear a bruit during arterial auscultation, the patient may have occlusive arterial disease or an arteriovenous fistula. Various high cardiac output conditions—such as anemia, hyperthyroidism, and pheochromocytoma—may also cause bruits.*

INTERPRETING YOUR FINDINGS

Your assessment will reveal a group of findings that may lead you to suspect a particular disorder. (See *The cardiovascular system: Interpreting your findings,* pages 120 to 122.)

CARDIOVASCULAR SYSTEM DISORDERS

CONGENITAL HEART DEFECTS

Congenital heart defects are typed as either acyanotic or cyanotic. Acyanotic defects have a left-to-right shunt, delivering richly oxygenated blood from the left side of the heart to the right side. Examples of acyanotic defects include ventricular and atrial septal defects, coarctation of the aorta, and patent ductus arteriosus. Cyanotic defects have a right-to-left shunt, delivering deoxygenated blood to the systemic circulation, causing hypoxia and cyanosis. Cyanotic defects include tetralogy of Fallot and transposition of the great arteries.

Atrial septal defect

In atrial septal defect (ASD), an opening between the left and right atria allows shunting of blood between the chambers. Because left atrial pressure is normally slightly higher than right atrial pressure, blood shunts from left to right. The pressure difference forces large amounts of blood through the defect and leads to volume overload in the right side of the heart affecting the right atrium, right ventricle, and pulmonary arteries. Eventually, the right atrium enlarges, and the right ventricle dilates to accommodate the increased blood volume.

 SPECIAL POINTS *Although ASD is usually a benign defect during infancy and childhood, delayed development of symptoms and complications make it one of the most common congenital heart defects diagnosed in adults. Asymptomatic patients have an excellent chance of recovery; the outlook is less hopeful for patients with cyanosis caused by large, untreated defects.*

The young patient is commonly asymptomatic, especially if he's a preschooler. He may only complain of feeling tired after extreme exertion. If large amounts of shunting occur, his growth may be retarded.

Auscultation at the second or third left intercostal space may reveal a superficial, early to midsystolic murmur. You may hear a fixed, widely split second heart sound (S_2) and a systolic click or late systolic murmur at the apex. In a patient with a large shunt, auscultation at the lower left sternal border may reveal a low-pitched diastolic murmur that becomes more pronounced on inspiration. Note that this murmur may be difficult to hear.

Older patients may develop pronounced fatigability, clubbing, and cyanosis as increased pulmonary vascular resistance (PVR) leads to reverse shunting. Dyspnea on exertion may severely limit the patient's activity, especially after age 40.

In older patients with large, uncorrected defects and fixed pulmonary hypertension, auscultation may reveal an accentuated S_2, a pulmonary ejection click, an audible S_4, and atrial arrhythmias. *(Text continues on page 122.)*

Cardiovascular system disorders

Congenital heart defects

+ Typed as acyanotic or cyanotic
+ Acyanotic—ventricular and atrial septal defects, coarctation of the aorta, and patent ductus arteriosus
+ Cyanotic—tetralogy of Fallot, transposition of the great arteries

Facts about ASD

+ Opening between left and right atria allows shunting of blood between chambers
+ Pressure difference forces large amounts of blood through the defect and leads to volume overload
+ The right atrium enlarges and the right ventricle dilates to accommodate the increased blood volume
+ Auscultation reveals a widely split S_2 and a systolic click or late systolic murmur at the apex

Special points
+ Delayed onset of symptoms and complications make ASD one of the most common congenital heart defects

The cardiovascular system: Interpreting your findings

This chart shows some common groups of findings for signs and symptoms of cardiovascular system disorders, along with their probable causes.

SIGN OR SYMPTOM AND FINDINGS	PROBABLE CAUSE
Chest pain	
✦ A feeling of tightness or pressure in the chest described as pain or a sensation of indigestion or expansion ✦ Pain may radiate to the neck, jaw, and arms; classically to the inner aspect of the left arm ✦ Pain begins gradually, reaches a maximum, then slowly subsides ✦ Pain is provoked by exertion, emotional stress, or a heavy meal ✦ Pain typically lasts 2 to 10 minutes (usually no more than 20 minutes) ✦ Dyspnea ✦ Nausea and vomiting ✦ Tachycardia ✦ Dizziness ✦ Diaphoresis	Angina
✦ Crushing substernal pain, unrelieved by rest or nitroglycerin ✦ Pain that may radiate to the left arm, jaw, neck, or shoulder blades ✦ Pain that lasts from 15 minutes to hours ✦ Pallor ✦ Clammy skin ✦ Dyspnea ✦ Diaphoresis ✦ Feeling of impending doom	Myocardial infarction
✦ Sharp, severe pain aggravated by inspiration, coughing, or pressure ✦ Shallow, splinted breaths ✦ Dyspnea ✦ Cough ✦ Local tenderness and edema	Rib fracture
Fatigue	
✦ Fatigue following mild activity ✦ Pallor ✦ Tachycardia ✦ Dyspnea	Anemia
✦ Persistent fatigue unrelated to exertion ✦ Headache ✦ Anorexia ✦ Constipation ✦ Sexual dysfunction ✦ Loss of concentration ✦ Irritability	Depression

The cardiovascular system:
Interpreting your findings *(continued)*

SIGN OR SYMPTOM AND FINDINGS	PROBABLE CAUSE
***Chest pain** (continued)*	
✦ Progressive fatigue ✦ Cardiac murmur ✦ Exertional dyspnea ✦ Cough ✦ Hemoptysis	Valvular heart disease
Palpitations	
✦ Paroxysmal palpitations ✦ Diaphoresis ✦ Facial flushing ✦ Trembling ✦ Impending sense of doom ✦ Hyperventilation ✦ Dizziness	Acute anxiety attack
✦ Paroxysmal or sustained palpitations ✦ Dizziness ✦ Weakness ✦ Fatigue ✦ Irregular, rapid, or slow pulse rate ✦ Decreased blood pressure ✦ Confusion ✦ Diaphoresis	Arrhythmias
✦ Sustained palpitations ✦ Fatigue ✦ Irritability ✦ Hunger ✦ Cold sweats ✦ Tremors ✦ Anxiety	Hypoglycemia
Peripheral edema	
✦ Headache ✦ Bilateral leg edema with pitting ankle edema ✦ Weight gain despite anorexia ✦ Nausea ✦ Chest tightness ✦ Hypotension ✦ Pallor ✦ Palpitations ✦ Inspiratory crackles	Heart failure

(continued)

The cardiovascular system: Interpreting your findings (continued)

SIGN OR SYMPTOM AND FINDINGS	PROBABLE CAUSE
Peripheral edema (continued)	
✦ Bilateral arm edema accompanied by facial and neck edema ✦ Edematous areas marked by dilated veins ✦ Headache ✦ Vertigo ✦ Vision disturbances	Superior vena cava syndrome
✦ Moderate to severe, unilateral or bilateral leg edema ✦ Darkened skin ✦ Stasis ulcers around the ankle	Venous insufficiency

Facts about coarctation of the aorta

✦ Aorta narrows below left subclavian artery, causing hypertension and diminishing pressure in vessels below constriction
✦ Cardinal signs include resting systolic hypertension, absent or diminished femoral pulses, and widened pulse pressure

Special points

✦ Infants — look for tachypnea, dyspnea, pallor, tachycardia, failure to thrive, and cardiomegaly and hepatomegaly
✦ Adolescents — look for dyspnea, claudication, headache, and epistaxis

Facts about PDA

✦ Abnormal opening between pulmonary artery and aorta
✦ Allows left-to-right shunting of blood from aorta to pulmonary artery, resulting in recirculation of arterial blood through lungs
✦ Effects precipitate pulmonary vascular disease
✦ Can be fatal if it advances to intractable heart failure
✦ Associated with other congenital defects

Syncope or hemoptysis may occur in adults with severe pulmonary vascular complications.

Coarctation of the aorta

Coarctation of the aorta is the narrowing of the aorta that usually occurs just below the left subclavian artery, near the site where the ligamentum arteriosum (the remnant of the ductus arteriosus, a fetal blood vessel) joins the pulmonary artery to the aorta. The obstructive process causes hypertension in the aortic branches above the constriction (arteries that supply the arms, neck, and head) and diminished pressure in the vessels below the constriction.

Usually, prognosis depends on the severity of associated cardiac anomalies. Prognosis for isolated coarctation is good if the patient undergoes corrective surgery before his condition induces severe systemic hypertension or degenerative changes in the aorta.

Cardinal signs include resting systolic hypertension, absent or diminished femoral pulses, and widened pulse pressure.

 SPECIAL POINTS When assessing an infant for coarctation of the aorta, look for tachypnea, dyspnea, pallor, tachycardia, failure to thrive, and cardiomegaly and hepatomegaly. In an adolescent patient, look for signs and symptoms that may include dyspnea, claudication, headache, and epistaxis. Inspection and palpation may reveal a visible aortic pulsation in the suprasternal notch. Auscultation may reveal a continuous systolic murmur with an accentuated S_2 and S_3.

Patent ductus arteriosus

Patent ductus arteriosus (PDA) is an abnormal opening between the pulmonary artery and the aorta. It allows left-to-right shunting of blood from the aorta to the pulmonary artery. This results in recirculation of arterial blood through the lungs.

Initially, PDA may produce no clinical effects, but in time it can precipitate pulmonary vascular disease, causing symptoms to appear by age 40. Patients with a small shunt or those who undergo effective surgical repair have a good chance of recovery. Otherwise, PDA may advance to intractable heart failure, which may be fatal.

Most prevalent in premature neonates, PDA commonly accompanies rubella syndrome. It may be associated with other congenital defects, such as coarctation of the aorta, ventricular septal defect, and pulmonary and aortic stenoses.

 SPECIAL POINTS *Neonates, especially premature ones, with a large PDA usually develop respiratory distress with signs of heart failure. Other findings may include frequent respiratory infections, slow motor development, and failure to thrive. Most children with PDA have only cardiac symptoms. Others may exhibit signs of heart disease, such as physical underdevelopment and fatigability. By age 40, adults with untreated PDA may develop fatigability and dyspnea on exertion with cyanosis appearing in the final stages of the illness.*

Auscultation reveals the classic machinery murmur (Gibson murmur). This continuous murmur is best heard at the base of the heart, at the second left intercostal space under the left clavicle in 85% of children with PDA. The murmur may obscure S_2. With a right-to-left shunt, however, the murmur may not occur. You may also palpate a thrill at the left sternal border and a prominent left ventricular impulse. Palpation will reveal bounding peripheral arterial pulses (Corrigan's pulse). Look for widened pulse pressure.

Other clinical findings include cardiomegaly, especially of the left atrium and left ventricle; dilated ascending aorta; and tachycardia.

Tetralogy of Fallot

Tetralogy of Fallot is a complex of four cardiac defects: ventricular septal defect (VSD), right ventricular outflow tract obstruction (pulmonary stenosis), right ventricular hypertrophy, and dextroposition of the aorta, with overriding of the VSD. Blood shunts right to left through the VSD, permitting unoxygenated blood to mix with oxygenated blood, resulting in cyanosis. (See *Tetralogy of Fallot: Four defects in one,* page 124.)

Tetralogy of Fallot sometimes coexists with other congenital heart defects, such as patent ductus arteriosus or atrial septal defect. It accounts for about 10% of all congenital heart disease and occurs equally in boys and girls. Before surgical advances made correction possible, approximately one-third of these children died in infancy.

The degree of pulmonary stenosis, interacting with VSD size and location, determines the clinical effects of this complex condition.

 SPECIAL POINTS *In infants, the hallmark sign of tetralogy of Fallot is cyanosis but it can also produce dyspnea; deep, sighing respirations; bradycardia; fainting; seizures; and loss of consciousness.*

In toddlers, tetralogy of Fallot produces clubbing, diminished exercise tolerance, increasing dyspnea on exertion, growth retardation, and eating difficulties. The child may squat when short of breath.

Transposition of the great arteries

In transposition of the great arteries, the great arteries are reversed. The aorta arises from the right ventricle and the pulmonary artery from the left ventricle, producing two noncommunicating circulatory systems (pulmonary and systemic). Transposition accounts for up to 5% of all congenital heart defects and commonly coexists with other congenital heart defects, such as VSD, VSD with pulmonary stenosis, ASD, and PDA.

Facts about PDA
(continued)

Special points
+ Neonates, especially premature ones, develop respiratory distress with signs of heart failure
+ Other findings include frequent respiratory infections, slow motor development, and failure to thrive
+ By age 40, adults with untreated PDA may develop fatigue and dyspnea on exertion with cyanosis

Facts about tetralogy of Fallot
+ Complex of four cardiac defects
+ Blood shunts from right-to-left through VSD, permitting unoxygenated blood to mix with oxygenated blood (cyanosis)
+ Accounts for 10% of all congenital heart disease, coexisting with other congenital heart defects
+ Degree of pulmonary stenosis, interacting with VSD size and location, determines clinical effects

Special points
+ Infants—cyanosis; dyspnea; deep, sighing respirations; bradycardia; fainting; seizures; and loss of consciousness
+ Toddlers—clubbing, diminished exercise tolerance, increasing dyspnea on exertion, growth retardation, and eating difficulties

Facts about transposition of the great arteries
+ Produces two noncommunicating circulatory systems: pulmonary and systemic
+ Accounts for up to 5% of all congenital heart defects, commonly coexisting with other congenital heart defects

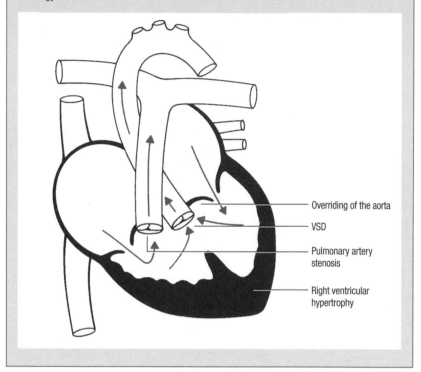

Tetralogy of Fallot: Four defects in one

This illustration shows a heart with ventricular septal detect (VSD), overriding the aorta, pulmonary artery stenosis, and right ventricular hypertrophy. All of these defects occur in tetralogy of Fallot.

Overriding of the aorta

VSD

Pulmonary artery stenosis

Right ventricular hypertrophy

Facts about transposition of the great arteries

Special points

✦ Affects males two to three times more commonly than females
✦ In neonates, cyanosis and tachypnea worsens with crying and heart failure
✦ In older children, diminished exercise tolerance, fatigability, coughing, and clubbing may occur

Facts about VSD

✦ Opening in the septum between ventricles
✦ Blood shunts between the left and right ventricles
✦ Most common congenital heart disorder, accounting for up to 30% of all congenital heart defects
✦ Auscultating may reveal loud S_2, possible murmurs, and other associated signs

 SPECIAL POINTS *Transposition of the great arteries affects males two to three times more commonly than females.*

In neonates, cyanosis and tachypnea occur that worsens with crying and signs of heart failure (typically gallop rhythm, tachycardia, dyspnea, hepatomegaly, and cardiomegaly).

If the patient also has ASD, VSD, PDA, or pulmonary stenosis, auscultation may reveal a loud S_2, possible murmurs, and other associated signs.

SPECIAL POINTS *Older children with transposition of the great arteries may show diminished exercise tolerance, fatigability, coughing, and clubbing.*

Ventricular septal defect

In VSD, an opening in the septum between the ventricles allows blood to shunt between the left and right ventricles. The most common congenital heart disorder, VSD accounts for up to 30% of all congenital heart defects. Some defects close spontaneously and others are surgically correctable.

Clinical features vary with the size of the defect, the effect of shunting on the pulmonary vasculature, and the infant's age.

A small VSD produces a functional murmur or a loud, harsh systolic murmur. A moderate-sized VSD produces a murmur (typically at least a grade III, pansystolic, loudest at the fourth intercostal space) and, possibly, a thrill. In addition, the pulmonary component of S_2 sounds loud and S_2 is widely-split. Palpation indicates that the PMI is displaced to the left.

 SPECIAL POINTS *An infant with a large VSD appears thin and small and gains weight slowly. He may have heart failure, with dusky skin; liver, heart, and spleen enlargement; diaphoresis; feeding difficulties; rapid, grunting respirations; and increased heart rate.*

On auscultation and palpation, the murmur produced by a large VSD can't be distinguished from that produced by a moderate-sized VSD. Because the patient may develop pulmonary hypertension, you may hear a diastolic murmur on auscultation that becomes quieter during systole and a greatly accentuated S_2.

INFLAMMATORY HEART DISEASE

Although inflammation is normally a protective mechanism, its effects on the heart are potentially devastating. For instance, in endocarditis, myocarditis, pericarditis, and rheumatic heart disease, scar formation and other healing processes cause debilitating structural damage, especially in the valves.

Endocarditis

Endocarditis, infection of the endocardium, heart valves, or cardiac prosthesis, results from bacterial invasion. In I.V. drug abusers, it may also result from fungal invasion. This invasion produces vegetative growths on the heart valves, endocardial lining of a heart chamber, or the endothelium of a blood vessel that may embolize to the spleen, kidneys, central nervous system, extremities, and lungs.

Acute infective endocarditis usually results from bacteremia that follows septic thrombophlebitis, open-heart surgery involving prosthetic valves, or skin, bone, and pulmonary infections. This form of endocarditis also occurs in I.V. drug abusers.

Subacute infective endocarditis typically occurs in patients with acquired valvular or congenital cardiac lesions. It can also follow dental, genitourinary, gynecologic, and GI procedures.

Rheumatic endocarditis commonly affects the mitral valve; less frequently, the aortic or tricuspid valve; and rarely, the pulmonic valve. Preexisting rheumatic endocardial lesions are a common predisposing factor.

Untreated endocarditis usually proves fatal, but with proper treatment, 70% of patients recover. Prognosis becomes much worse when endocarditis causes severe valvular damage (leading to insufficiency and heart failure) or when it involves a prosthetic valve.

Early clinical features are usually nonspecific and include weakness, fatigue, weight loss, anorexia, arthralgia, night sweats, intermittent fever (may recur for weeks), and a loud, regurgitant murmur. This murmur is typical of the underlying rheumatic or congenital heart disease. A suddenly-changing murmur or the discovery of a new murmur along with fever is a classic sign of endocarditis.

Other signs include petechiae on the skin (especially common on the upper anterior trunk); the buccal, pharyngeal, or conjunctival mucosa; and the nails (splinter hemorrhages). Osler's nodes, Roth's spots, and Janeway lesions occur rarely.

In subacute endocarditis, embolization from vegetating lesions or diseased valve tissue may produce these features:
+ splenic infarction (pain in the left upper quadrant, radiating to the left shoulder; abdominal rigidity)
+ renal infarction (hematuria, pyuria, flank pain, decreased urine output)

Facts about VSD

Special points
+ An infant with a large VSD appears thin and small and gains weight slowly
+ Infant may have heart failure; liver, heart, and spleen enlargement; diaphoresis; feeding difficulties; rapid, grunting respirations; and increased heart rate

Types of inflammatory heart disease
+ Endocarditis
+ Myocarditis
+ Pericarditis
+ Rheumatic fever and rheumatic heart disease

Facts about endocarditis
+ Infection of the endocardium, heart valves, or cardiac prosthesis, resulting from bacterial invasion
+ Can produce vegetative growths on the heart valves, endocardial lining of a heart chamber, or endothelium of a blood vessel, which may embolize to the spleen, kidneys, central nervous system, extremities, and lungs
+ Types include acute infective endocarditis, subacute infective endocarditis, and rheumatic endocarditis
+ May prove fatal if left untreated; with treatment, 70% of patients recover
+ Produces fatigue, weight loss, arthralgia, night sweats, fever, murmur, petechiae on the skin, the buccal, pharyngeal, or conjunctival mucosa, and the nails

✦ cerebral infarction (hemiparesis, aphasia, or other neurologic deficits)
✦ pulmonary infarction (most common in right-sided endocarditis, which commonly occurs among I.V. drug abusers and after cardiac surgery; cough, pleuritic pain, pleural friction rub, dyspnea, and hemoptysis)
✦ peripheral vascular occlusion (numbness and tingling in an arm, leg, finger, or toe, or signs of impending peripheral gangrene).

Myocarditis

Facts about myocarditis

✦ Focal or diffuse inflammation of the cardiac muscle
✦ Acute or chronic, striking at any age
✦ Fails to produce specific symptoms or ECG abnormalities
✦ Occasionally complicated by heart failure
✦ Produces fatigue, dyspnea, palpitations, fever

Myocarditis, a focal or diffuse inflammation of the cardiac muscle (myocardium), may be acute or chronic and can strike at any age. In many cases, myocarditis fails to produce specific cardiovascular symptoms or electrocardiogram (ECG) abnormalities. The patient will usually experience spontaneous recovery, without residual defects. Occasionally, myocarditis is complicated by heart failure and, rarely, leads to cardiomyopathy.

Look for fatigue, dyspnea, palpitations, fever, and occasionally, mild continuous pressure or soreness in the chest.

On auscultation, be alert for supraventricular and ventricular arrhythmias, S_3 and S_4 gallops, a faint S_1, possibly a murmur of mitral insufficiency (from papillary muscle dysfunction), and, if pericarditis is present, a pericardial friction rub.

With more advanced disease, signs and symptoms of heart failure may be present, including pulmonary edema, diaphoresis, and distended jugular veins.

Pericarditis

Facts about pericarditis

✦ Acute or chronic inflammation affects pericardium, fibrous sac that envelops, supports, and protects heart
✦ Causes sharp, sudden pain over sternum radiating to neck, shoulders, back, and arms
✦ Pain increases with deep inspiration and decreases with sitting up and leaning forward
✦ Causes pericardial friction rub
✦ Indicated by gradual increases in systemic venous pressure
✦ Causes fluid retention, ascites, and hepatomegaly

Pericarditis is an acute or chronic inflammation that affects the pericardium, the fibroserous sac that envelops, supports, and protects the heart. Acute pericarditis can be fibrinous or effusive, with purulent serous or hemorrhagic exudate. Chronic constrictive pericarditis characteristically leads to dense fibrous pericardial thickening. Because pericarditis commonly coexists with other conditions, diagnosis of acute pericarditis depends on typical clinical features and the elimination of other possible causes. Prognosis depends on the underlying cause. Most patients recover from acute pericarditis, unless constriction occurs.

The patient frequently experiences sharp, typically sudden pain that usually starts over the sternum and radiates to the neck, shoulders, back, and arms. Unlike the pain of MI, pericardial pain is commonly pleuritic, increasing with deep inspiration and decreasing when the patient sits up and leans forward.

You may hear a pericardial friction rub. A classic sign, this grating sound occurs as the heart moves. You will usually hear the friction rub best during forced expiration while the patient leans forward or is on his hands and knees in bed. It may have up to three components, corresponding to the timing of atrial systole, ventricular systole, and the rapid-filling phase of ventricular diastole. Occasionally, friction rub is heard only briefly or not at all.

When assessing for chronic constrictive pericarditis, look for a gradual increase in systemic venous pressure and signs similar to those of chronic right-sided heart failure including fluid retention, ascites, and hepatomegaly.

Rheumatic fever and rheumatic heart disease

Facts about rheumatic fever and rheumatic heart disease

✦ Rheumatic fever — systemic inflammatory disease of childhood following a group A beta-hemolytic streptococcal infection
✦ Rheumatic heart disease — includes pancarditis (myocarditis, pericarditis, and endocarditis) during early acute phase and chronic valvular disease in later phases

Commonly recurrent, rheumatic fever is a systemic inflammatory disease of childhood that follows a group A beta-hemolytic streptococcal infection. Rheumatic heart disease refers to the cardiac manifestations of rheumatic fever. It includes pancarditis (myocarditis, pericarditis, and endocarditis) during the early acute phase and chronic valvular disease in the later phases. Long-term antibiotic therapy can minimize recurrence of rheumatic fever, reducing the risk of permanent cardiac damage and eventual valvular deformity. However, severe pancarditis occasionally produces fatal heart failure during the acute phase.

Signs and symptoms may include fever; migratory joint pain; skin lesions; firm, movable, nontender subcutaneous nodules near tendons or bony prominences of joints; chorea (later symptom); or pleural friction rub and pain.

The patient may also have a heart murmur. This may be a systolic murmur of mitral insufficiency (high-pitched, blowing, holosystolic, loudest at apex, possibly radiating to the anterior axillary line). Alternatively, the patient may have a midsystolic murmur (caused by stiffening and swelling of the mitral leaflet) or, occasionally, a diastolic murmur of aortic insufficiency (low-pitched, rumbling, almost inaudible).

CORONARY ARTERY DISEASE

Coronary artery disease (CAD) refers to any narrowing or obstruction of arterial lumina that interferes with cardiac perfusion. Deprived of sufficient blood, the myocardium can develop various ischemic diseases, including angina pectoris, MI, heart failure, sudden death, and cardiac arrhythmias.

 SPECIAL POINTS *CAD affects more Whites than Blacks, and more men than women. However, after menopause, women with CAD are increasing in numbers to equal that of men. This disease occurs more commonly in industrial than in underdeveloped countries and affects more affluent than poor people.*

Angina, the classic symptom of CAD, occurs as a burning, squeezing, or crushing tightness in the substernal or precordial chest. It may radiate to the left arm, neck, jaw, or shoulder blade.

 SPECIAL POINTS *Women with CAD commonly experience atypical chest pain, vague chest pain, or a lack of chest pain. However, they may also experience classic chest pain, which may occur without any relationship to activity or stress. While men tend to complain of crushing pain in the center of the chest, women are more likely to experience arm or shoulder pain; jaw, neck, or throat pain; toothache; back pain; or pain under the breastbone or in the stomach. Other signs and symptoms include nausea or dizziness; shortness of breath; unexplained anxiety, weakness, or fatigue; and palpitations, cold sweat or paleness.*

Angina most frequently follows physical exertion but may also follow emotional excitement, exposure to cold, or a large meal. Less severe and shorter than the pain associated with acute MI, angina is commonly relieved by nitroglycerin. Other possible signs and symptoms include nausea, vomiting, weakness, diaphoresis, and cool extremities.

Angina has four major forms: stable (predictable pain, in frequency and duration, which can be relieved with nitrates and rest), unstable (increased pain which is easily induced), Prinzmetal's or variant (from unpredictable coronary artery spasm), and microvascular (in which impairment of vasodilator reserve causes angina-like chest pain in a patient with normal coronary arteries).

HEART FAILURE

A syndrome rather than a disease, heart failure occurs when the heart no longer provides enough blood to meet the body's metabolic needs. Pump failure usually occurs in a damaged left ventricle (left-sided heart failure), but may happen in the right ventricle, either as primary failure or secondary to left-sided heart failure. Sometimes, left- and right-sided heart failure develop simultaneously. Heart failure may also be classified according to the phase of the cardiac cycle in which the dysfunction occurs; systolic and diastolic heart failure may occur alone or together.

Facts about CAD
+ Refers to any narrowing or obstruction of arterial lumina that interferes with cardiac perfusion
+ Due to blood insufficiency, myocardium at risk for developing angina pectoris, myocardial infarction, heart failure, cardiac arrhythmias, and sudden death

Special points
+ Affects more Whites than Blacks
+ Affects more men than women
+ Number of postmenopausal women with CAD increasing to equal that of men
+ Occurs more commonly in industrial than in underdeveloped countries
+ Affects more affluent than poor people
+ Women commonly experience atypical chest pain
+ Men commonly experience crushing pain

Facts about heart failure
+ Occurs when heart no longer provides enough blood to meet body's metabolic needs
+ Pump failure occurs in damaged left ventricle (left-sided heart failure), but may happen in right ventricle
+ Also classified according to phase of cardiac cycle

Reviewing acute heart failure

+ Results from MI
+ Associated with renal retention of sodium and water
+ Left-sided heart failure — dyspnea, paroxysmal nocturnal dyspnea, Cheyne-Stokes respirations, cough, and orthopnea
+ Right-sided heart failure — edema; distended and rigid jugular veins; hepatomegaly leading to anorexia, nausea, and vague abdominal pain; ascites or a ventricular heave

Facts about MI

+ Occlusion of a coronary artery leading to oxygen deprivation, myocardial ischemia, and eventual necrosis; leading cause of death in United States

---

Comparing signs and symptoms of left- and right-sided heart failure

Below are signs and symptoms of left-sided heart failure, both early and later, and right-sided heart failure.

LEFT-SIDED
Early
+ Dyspnea on exertion
+ Paroxysmal nocturnal dyspnea
+ Orthopnea
+ Fatigue
+ Nonproductive cough
+ Increased blood pressure

Later
+ Decreased functional capacity
+ Cognitive impairment
+ Third or fourth heart sound
+ Tachypnea
+ Increased heart rate
+ Low arterial oxygen saturation
+ Anxiety
+ Pulsus alternans
+ Pleural effusion
+ Arrhythmias
+ Severe respiratory distress
+ Pale or cyanotic appearance

+ Diaphoresis
+ Crackles
+ Cough that produces pink, frothy sputum
+ Tachycardia

RIGHT-SIDED
+ Respiratory distress
+ Peripheral edema
+ Nausea, anorexia
+ GI bloating
+ Dyspnea
+ Dependent edema
+ Right upper quadrant discomfort or pain
+ Fatigue
+ Hepatojugular reflux
+ Hepatomegaly
+ Ascites
+ Weight gain
+ Heart murmurs
+ Pleural effusion
+ Jugular vein distention
+ Nocturia

Acute heart failure may result from MI, but most patients experience a chronic form of the disorder associated with renal retention of sodium and water. Advances in diagnostic and therapeutic techniques have greatly improved the outlook for patients with heart failure, but prognosis still depends on the underlying cause and its response to treatment.

Clinical signs of left-sided heart failure include dyspnea, initially upon exertion. The patient also develops paroxysmal nocturnal dyspnea, Cheyne-Stokes respirations, cough, and orthopnea. Check also for tachycardia, fatigue, muscle weakness, edema and weight gain, irritability, restlessness, and a shortened attention span. Auscultate for a ventricular gallop (heard over the apex) and bibasilar crackles. (See *Comparing signs and symptoms of left- and right-sided heart failure.*)

The patient with right-sided heart failure may develop edema. Initially dependent, edema may progress. The patient's jugular veins may become distended and rigid. Hepatomegaly may eventually lead to anorexia, nausea, and vague abdominal pain. Also, observe the patient for ascites or a ventricular heave.

MYOCARDIAL INFARCTION

Myocardial infarction (MI) is an occlusion of a coronary artery that leads to oxygen deprivation, myocardial ischemia, and eventual necrosis. The extent of functional impairment and the patient's prognosis depend on the size and location of the infarct, the condition of the uninvolved myocardium, the potential for collateral circulation, and the effectiveness of compensatory mechanisms. In the United States, MI is the leading cause of death.

The patient experiences severe, persistent chest pain that is unrelieved by rest or nitroglycerin. He may describe pain as crushing or squeezing. Usually substernal, pain may radiate to left arm, jaw, neck, or shoulder blades. Other signs and symptoms include a feeling of impending doom, fatigue, nausea and vomiting, shortness of breath, cool extremities, perspiration, anxiety, hypotension or hypertension, palpable precordial pulse and possibly, muffled heart sounds.

ABDOMINAL AORTIC ANEURYSM

Abdominal aortic aneurysm, an abnormal dilation in the arterial wall, most commonly occurs in the aorta between the renal arteries and the iliac branches. More than 50% of all patients with untreated abdominal aortic aneurysms die, primarily from aneurysm rupture, within 2 years of diagnosis. More than 85% die within 5 years.

When aneurysmal rupture isn't imminent, you may be able to see an asymptomatic pulsating mass in the patient's periumbilical area. Auscultation may reveal a systolic bruit over the aorta, and tenderness may be present on deep palpation.

When aneurysmal rupture is imminent, pressure on lumbar nerves may lead to lumbar pain that radiates to the flank and groin.

If the aneurysm ruptures into the peritoneal cavity, it causes severe, persistent abdominal and back pain, mimicking renal or ureteral colic. The patient may hemorrhage; however, retroperitoneal bleeding may make such signs and symptoms as weakness, sweating, tachycardia, and hypotension appear rather subtle.

 CLINICAL ALERT Abdominal bleeding due to an aneurysmal rupture is life-threatening and produces such signs and symptoms of shock as pallor, tachycardia, hypotension, diaphoresis, and oliguria.

ARTERIAL OCCLUSIVE DISEASE

In arterial occlusive disease, obstruction or narrowing of the lumen of the aorta and its major branches causes an interruption of blood flow, usually to the legs and feet. A frequent complication of atherosclerosis, arterial occlusive disease may affect the carotid, vertebral, innominate, subclavian, mesenteric, and celiac arteries. Occlusions may be acute or chronic.

 SPECIAL POINTS *Men suffer from arterial occlusive disease more commonly than women.*

Prognosis depends on the location of the occlusion, the development of collateral circulation to counteract reduced blood flow and, in acute disease, the time elapsed between occlusion and its removal.

Signs and symptoms depend on the severity and site of the arterial occlusion. For example, a single mild stenosis in the superficial femoral segment may have no obvious effect on the legs. However, a multiple-segment occlusion typically causes severe ischemia, leading to intermittent claudication, severe burning pain in the toes (aggravated by elevating the extremity and sometimes relieved by keeping the extremity in a dependent position), ulcers, and gangrene.

Other signs include dependent rubor, pallor on elevation, delayed capillary filling or hair loss, and trophic nail changes. Progressive arterial disease can cause diminished or absent pedal pulses.

Facts about arterial occlusive disease
(continued)

+ Acute arterial occlusion producing the five classic P's: paralysis, pain, paresthesia, pallor, and pulselessness

Special points
+ Affects more men than women

Facts about thrombophlebitis

+ Involves inflammation and thrombus formation
+ Occurs in deep (intermuscular or intramuscular) or superficial (subcutaneous) veins
+ Deep vein thrombophlebitis — affects small or large veins; leading to pulmonary embolism; producing severe pain, fever, chills, malaise, and swelling and cyanosis of affected arm or leg
+ Complications include chronic venous insufficiency and varicose veins
+ Superficial thrombophlebitis — causes heat, pain, swelling, rubor, tenderness, and induration along length of the vein

Progressive narrowing of the arterial lumen stimulates the development of collateral circulation in surrounding blood vessels. With insufficient collateral development, thrombosis or total occlusion may occur, severely jeopardizing the limb.

Acute arterial occlusion may produce the five classic P's: paralysis, pain, paresthesia, pallor, and pulselessness. Impaired circulation produces varying degrees of neurologic dysfunction.

THROMBOPHLEBITIS

An acute condition characterized by inflammation and thrombus formation, thrombophlebitis may occur in deep (intermuscular or intramuscular) or superficial (subcutaneous) veins.

Deep vein thrombophlebitis affects small veins, such as the soleal venous sinuses, or large veins, such as the vena cava, and the femoral, iliac, and subclavian veins. Usually progressive, this disorder may lead to pulmonary embolism, a potentially fatal condition.

Superficial thrombophlebitis is usually self-limiting and rarely leads to pulmonary embolism.

Clinical features vary with the site and length of the affected vein. Deep vein thrombophlebitis may produce severe pain, fever, chills, malaise, and swelling and cyanosis of the affected arm or leg. The affected area may feel warm to the touch. Some patients may have a positive Homans' sign (pain on dorsiflexion of the foot); however, false-positives are common. Complications of this disorder include chronic venous insufficiency and varicose veins.

Superficial thrombophlebitis leads to heat, pain, swelling, rubor, tenderness, and induration along the length of the affected vein. Extensive vein involvement may cause lymphadenitis.

Respiratory system

A LOOK AT THE RESPIRATORY SYSTEM

The respiratory system includes the airways, lungs, bony thorax, respiratory muscles, and central nervous system (CNS). They all work together to deliver oxygen to the bloodstream and remove excess carbon dioxide from the body. Knowing the basic structures and functions of the respiratory system will help you perform a comprehensive respiratory assessment and recognize any abnormalities. (See *The respiratory system*, page 132.)

ANATOMY

Airways and lungs

The airways are divided into the upper and lower airways. The upper airways include the nasopharynx (nose), oropharynx (mouth), laryngopharynx, and larynx. Their purpose is to warm, filter, and humidify inhaled air. They also help to make sound and send air to the lower airways.

The epiglottis is a flap of tissue that closes over the top of the larynx when the patient swallows. The epiglottis protects the patient from aspirating food or fluid into the lower airways.

The larynx is located at the top of the trachea and houses the vocal cords. It's the transition point between the upper and lower airways.

The lower airways begin with the trachea, which then divides into the right and left mainstem bronchial tubes. The bronchial tubes divide into bronchi, which are lined with mucus-producing ciliated epithelium, one of the lungs' major defense systems.

The bronchi then divide into secondary bronchi, tertiary bronchi, terminal bronchioles, respiratory bronchioles, alveolar ducts and, finally, into the alveoli, the gas-exchange units of the lungs. The lungs in an adult typically contain about 300 million alveoli.

The respiratory system

+ Airways
+ Lungs
+ Bony thorax
+ Respiratory muscles
+ CNS

Anatomy

Upper airways

+ Nasopharynx, oropharynx, laryngopharynx, and larynx
+ Warm, filter, and humidify inhaled air
+ Help make sound and send air into lower airways
+ Larynx is the transition point between upper and lower airways; contains vocal cords
+ Epiglottis protects from aspiration of food or fluid into lower airways

Lower airways

+ Trachea, bronchial tubes, bronchi, bronchioles, alveolar ducts, alveoli
+ Mucus-producing ciliated epithelium of bronchi is a major defense system of lungs

The respiratory system

The major structures of the upper and lower airways are illustrated below.

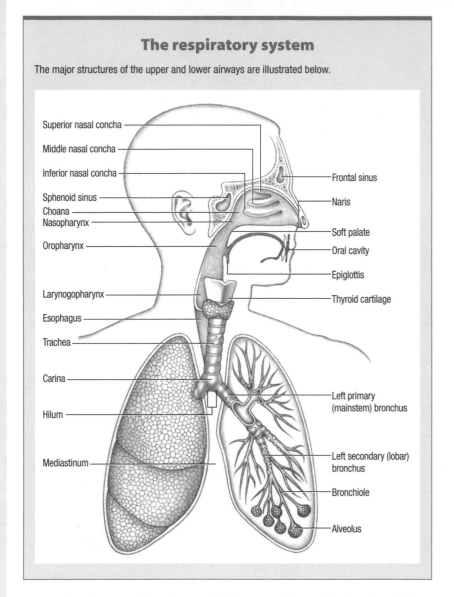

Superior nasal concha
Middle nasal concha
Inferior nasal concha
Sphenoid sinus
Choana
Nasopharynx
Oropharynx
Larynogopharynx
Esophagus
Trachea
Carina
Hilum
Mediastinum

Frontal sinus
Naris
Soft palate
Oral cavity
Epiglottis
Thyroid cartilage
Left primary (mainstem) bronchus
Left secondary (lobar) bronchus
Bronchiole
Alveolus

Anatomy
(continued)

Lungs

✦ Adult lungs contain about 300 million alveoli
✦ Are wrapped in a lining called the *visceral pleura*
✦ Larger right lung contains upper, middle, and lower lobes
✦ Smaller left lung contains an upper and a lower lobe
✦ Share space with heart and great vessels, trachea, esophagus, and bronchi
✦ Parietal pleura lines thoracic cavity around lungs; emits pain signals when inflammation occurs
✦ Pleural fluid fills the area between parietal and visceral pleurae, allowing for chest expansion and contractions

Each lung is wrapped in a lining called the *visceral pleura*. The right lung is larger and has three lobes: upper, middle, and lower. The left lung is smaller and has only an upper and a lower lobe.

The lungs share space in the thoracic cavity with the heart and great vessels, the trachea, the esophagus, and the bronchi. All areas of the thoracic cavity that come in contact with the lungs are lined with parietal pleura.

A small amount of fluid fills the area between the two layers of the pleura. That fluid, called pleural fluid, allows the layers of the pleura to slide smoothly over one another as the chest expands and contracts. The parietal pleura also contains nerve endings that emit pain signals when inflammation occurs.

Thorax

Composed of bone and cartilage, the thoracic cage supports and protects the lungs. The vertebral column and 12 pairs of ribs form the posterior portion of the thoracic cage. The ribs, the major portion of the thoracic cage, extend from the thoracic vertebrae toward the anterior thorax. Along with the vertebrae, they support and protect the thorax, permitting the lungs to expand and contract. Both are numbered from top to bottom. Posteriorly, certain landmarks are used as well to help identify specific vertebrae. In 90% of people , the seventh cervical vertebra (C7) is the most prominent vertebra on a flexed neck; for the remaining 10%, it's the first thoracic vertebra (T1). Thus, to locate a specific vertebra, count down along the vertebrae from C7 or T1.

The manubrium, sternum, xiphoid process, and ribs form the anterior thoracic cage, which has the additional duty of protecting the mediastinal organs that lie between the right and left pleural cavities. Ribs 1 through 7 attach directly to the sternum; ribs 8 through 10 attach to the cartilage of the preceding rib. The other two pairs of ribs are "free-floating"; they don't attach to any part of the anterior thoracic cage. Rib 11 ends anterolaterally, and rib 12 ends laterally. The lower parts of the rib cage (the costal margins) near the xiphoid process form the borders of the costal angle — an angle of about 90 degrees in a normal person.

Above the anterior thorax is a depression called the *suprasternal notch.* Because this notch isn't covered by the rib cage like the rest of the thorax, it allows you to palpate the trachea and check aortic pulsation. (See *Respiratory assessment landmarks,* page 134.)

Respiratory muscles

The diaphragm and the external intercostal muscles are the primary muscles used in breathing. They contract when the patient inhales and relax when the patient exhales.

The respiratory center in the medulla initiates each breath by sending messages to the primary respiratory muscles over the phrenic nerve. Impulses from the phrenic nerve adjust the rate and depth of breathing, depending on the carbon dioxide and pH levels in the cerebrospinal fluid (CSF). (See *The mechanics of breathing,* page 135.)

Other muscles assist in breathing. Accessory inspiratory muscles include the trapezius, the sternocleidomastoid, and the scalenes, which combine to elevate the scapula, clavicle, sternum, and upper ribs. That elevation expands the front-to-back diameter of the chest when use of the diaphragm and intercostal muscles isn't effective.

Expiration occurs when the diaphragm and external intercostal muscles relax. If the patient has an airway obstruction, he may also use the abdominal muscles and internal intercostal muscles to exhale.

PHYSIOLOGY

Pulmonary circulation

Oxygen-depleted blood enters the lungs from the pulmonary artery of the right ventricle, then flows through the main pulmonary arteries into the pleural cavities and the main bronchi, where it continues to flow through progressively smaller vessels until it reaches the single-celled endothelial capillaries serving the alveoli. Here, oxygen and carbon dioxide diffusion takes place. After passing through the pulmonary capillaries, blood flows through progressively larger vessels, enters the main pulmonary veins, finally flowing into the left atrium.

Anatomy
(continued)

Thorax
- Composed of bone and cartilage; supports and protects lungs
- Vertebral column and 12 pairs of ribs form posterior thoracic cage
- Ribs permit lungs to expand and contract
- Manubrium, sternum, xiphoid process, and ribs form anterior thoracic cage
- Suprasternal notch not covered by the rib cage, allowing palpation of the trachea and assessment of aortic pulsation

Respiratory muscles
- Include diaphragm and external intercostal muscles, the primary muscles of breathing
- Contract on inhalation and relax on exhalation
- Respiratory center in the medulla initiates each breath via phrenic nerve, which adjusts breath rate and depth
- Include trapezius, sternocleidomastoid, and scalenes, elevating the scapula, clavicle, sternum, and upper ribs

Facts about pulmonary circulation
- Oxygen-depleted blood enters lungs from pulmonary artery of the right ventricle
- Blood flows through main pulmonary arteries into pleural cavities, main bronchi, progressively smaller vessels to alveolar capillaries where oxygen and carbon dioxide diffusion occurs
- Oxygenated blood flows through progressively larger vessels to main pulmonary veins, and atrium

Respiratory assessment landmarks

This illustration shows common landmarks used in respiratory assessment.

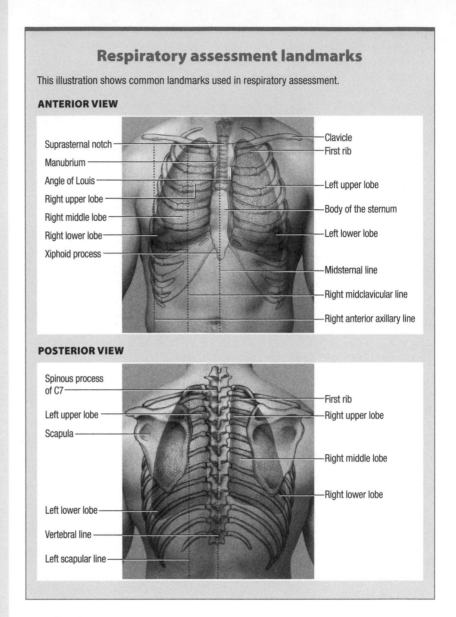

ANTERIOR VIEW

- Suprasternal notch
- Manubrium
- Angle of Louis
- Right upper lobe
- Right middle lobe
- Right lower lobe
- Xiphoid process
- Clavicle
- First rib
- Left upper lobe
- Body of the sternum
- Left lower lobe
- Midsternal line
- Right midclavicular line
- Right anterior axillary line

POSTERIOR VIEW

- Spinous process of C7
- Left upper lobe
- Scapula
- Left lower lobe
- Vertebral line
- Left scapular line
- First rib
- Right upper lobe
- Right middle lobe
- Right lower lobe

Facts about respiration

+ Requires gas exchange in lungs (external respiration) and tissues (internal respiration)
+ External respiration includes ventilation, pulmonary perfusion, and diffusion
+ Internal respiration occurs only through diffusion
+ Maintains adequate oxygenation and acid-base balance

Respiration

Effective respiration requires gas exchange in the lungs (external respiration) and in the tissues (internal respiration). Three processes contribute to external respiration: ventilation (gas distribution into and out of the pulmonary airways), pulmonary perfusion (blood flow from the right side of the heart, through the pulmonary circulation, and into the left side of the heart), and diffusion (gas movement from an area of greater to lesser concentration through a semipermeable membrane). Internal respiration occurs only through diffusion. These processes are vital to maintain adequate oxygenation and acid-base balance.

The mechanics of breathing

These illustrations show how mechanical forces, such as the movement of the diaphragm and intercostal muscles, produce a breath. A plus sign (+) indicates positive pressure, and a minus sign (−) indicates negative pressure.

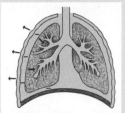 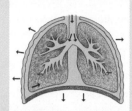 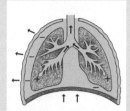

AT REST
+ Inspiratory muscles relax.
+ Atmospheric pressure is maintained in the tracheobronchial tree.
+ No air movement occurs.

INSPIRATION
+ Inspiratory muscles contract.
+ The diaphragm descends and flattens.
+ Negative alveolar pressure is maintained.
+ Air moves into the lungs.

EXPIRATION
+ Inspiratory muscles relax, causing lungs to recoil to their resting size and position.
+ The diaphragm ascends to its resting position.
+ Positive alveolar pressure is maintained.
+ Air moves out of the lungs.

Ventilation

Adequate ventilation depends on the nervous, musculoskeletal, and pulmonary systems for the requisite lung pressure changes. Any dysfunction in these systems increases the work of breathing, diminishing its effectiveness.

Nervous system effects

Although ventilation is largely involuntary, individuals can control its rate and depth. Involuntary breathing results from neurogenic stimulation of the respiratory center in the medulla and the pons of the brain stem. The medulla regulates the rate and depth of respiration; the pons moderates the rhythm of the switch from inspiration to expiration. Specialized neurovascular tissue alters these phases of the breathing process automatically and instantaneously.

When carbon dioxide in the blood diffuses into the CSF, specialized tissue in the respiratory center of the brain stem responds. At the same time, peripheral chemoreceptors in the aortic arch and the bifurcation of the carotid arteries respond to reduced oxygen levels in the blood. When the carbon dioxide level rises or the oxygen level falls noticeably, the respiratory center of the medulla initiates respiration.

Musculoskeletal effects

The adult thorax is a flexible structure — its shape can be altered by contracting the chest muscles. The medulla controls ventilation primarily by stimulating contraction of the diaphragm and the external intercostals, the major muscles of breathing. The diaphragm descends to expand the length of the chest cavity, while the external intercostals contract to expand the anteroposterior and lateral chest diameter. These actions produce changes in intrapulmonary pressure that cause inspiration.

Facts about ventilation
+ Gas distribution into and out of the pulmonary airways
+ Dysfunction increases work of breathing

Nervous system effects
+ Involuntary breathing is controlled in medulla and pons of the brain stem
+ Medulla regulates rate and depth of respiration; pons moderates switch from inspiration to expiration
+ When carbon dioxide level rises or oxygen level falls, respiratory center of the medulla initiates respiration

Musculoskeletal effects
+ Medulla controls ventilation by stimulating contraction of the diaphragm and the external intercostals
+ Diaphragm descends, expanding the chest cavity length
+ External intercostals contract to expand the chest diameter
+ Resulting changes in intrapulmonary pressure cause inspiration

Facts about ventilation
(continued)
Pulmonary effects
+ Inspiration causes airflow into lungs
+ Factors altering airflow distribution include air flow pattern, volume and location of the functional reserve capacity, amount of intrapulmonary resistance, and presence of lung disease
+ Normal breathing: active inspiration and passive expiration
+ Forced breathing: active inspiration and expiration

Facts about pulmonary perfusion
+ Aids external respiration and promotes efficient alveolar gas exchange
+ Less efficient gas transport results from reduced cardiac output, elevated pulmonary and systemic vascular resistance, abnormal or insufficient Hb, or gravity

Facts about diffusion
+ Oxygen and carbon dioxide moves between the alveoli and capillaries
+ Partial pressure dictating direction of movement
+ Oxygen crosses the alveolar and capillary membranes, dissolves in the plasma, and passes into RBCs; carbon dioxide moves in the opposite direction
+ RBCs carry oxygen to cells, where oxygen in RBCs and carbon dioxide switch places
+ Most transported oxygen binds with Hb to form oxyhemoglobin; remainder in plasma is measurable as Pao_2

Pulmonary effects

During inspiration, air flows through the right and left mainstem bronchi into increasingly smaller bronchi, then into bronchioles, alveolar ducts, and alveolar sacs, finally reaching the alveolar membrane. Many factors can alter airflow distribution, including air flow pattern, volume and location of the functional reserve capacity (air retained in the alveoli that prevents their collapse during respiration), amount of intrapulmonary resistance, and presence of lung disease. If disrupted, airflow distribution will follow the path of least resistance. For example, an intrapulmonary obstruction or forced inspiration will cause an uneven distribution of air.

Normal breathing requires active inspiration and passive expiration. Forced breathing, as in cases of emphysema, demands both active inspiration and expiration. It activates accessory muscles of respiration, which requires additional oxygen to work, resulting in less efficient ventilation with an increased workload.

Other alterations in airflow, such as changes in compliance (distensibility of the lungs and thorax) and resistance (interference with airflow in the tracheobronchial tree), can also increase oxygen and energy demands and lead to respiratory muscle fatigue.

Pulmonary perfusion

Optimal pulmonary perfusion aids external respiration and promotes efficient alveolar gas exchange. However, factors that reduce blood flow, such as a cardiac output that is less than average (5 L/minute) and elevated pulmonary and systemic vascular resistance, can interfere with gas transport to the alveoli. Also, abnormal or insufficient hemoglobin (Hb) picks up less oxygen than is needed for efficient gas exchange.

Gravity can affect oxygen and carbon dioxide transport by influencing pulmonary circulation. Gravity pulls more unoxygenated blood to the lower and middle lung lobes relative to the upper lobes, where most of the tidal volume also flows. As a result, neither ventilation nor perfusion is uniform throughout the lung. Areas of the lung where perfusion and ventilation are similar have good ventilation-perfusion matching. In such areas, gas exchange is most efficient. Areas of the lung that demonstrate ventilation-perfusion inequality result in less efficient gas exchange. (See *What happens in ventilation-perfusion mismatch.*)

Diffusion

In diffusion, molecules of oxygen and carbon dioxide move between the alveoli and the capillaries. Partial pressure — the pressure exerted by one gas in a mixture of gases — dictates the direction of movement, which is always from an area of greater concentration to one of lesser concentration. During diffusion, oxygen moves across the alveolar and capillary membranes, then dissolves in the plasma, and passes through the red blood cell (RBC) membrane. Carbon dioxide moves in the opposite direction.

Successful diffusion requires an intact alveolocapillary membrane. Both the alveolar epithelium and the capillary endothelium are composed of a single layer of cells. Between these layers are minute interstitial spaces filled with elastin and collagen. Normally, oxygen and carbon dioxide move easily through all of these layers. Oxygen moves from the alveoli into the bloodstream, where it's taken up by Hb in the RBCs. When there, it displaces carbon dioxide (the by-product of metabolism), which diffuses from the RBCs into the blood and then to the alveoli. Most transported oxygen binds with Hb to form oxyhemoglobin, while a small portion dissolves in the plasma (measurable as the partial pressure of oxygen in arterial blood [Pao_2]).

What happens in ventilation-perfusion mismatch

Effective gas exchange depends on the relationship between ventilation and perfusion ($\dot{V}/\dot{Q}$). The diagrams below show what happens when the $\dot{V}/\dot{Q}$ ratio is normal and abnormal.

NORMAL VENTILATION AND PERFUSION

When $\dot{V}/\dot{Q}$ are matched, unoxygenated blood from the venous system returns to the right ventricle through the pulmonary artery to the lungs, carrying carbon dioxide. The arteries branch into the alveolar capillaries. Gas exchange takes place in the alveolar capillaries.

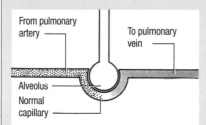

INADEQUATE PERFUSION (DEAD-SPACE VENTILATION)

When the $\dot{V}/\dot{Q}$ ratio is high, as shown here, ventilation is normal, but alveolar perfusion is reduced or absent. Note the narrowed capillary, indicating poor perfusion. This commonly results from a perfusion defect such as pulmonary embolism or a disorder that decreases cardiac output.

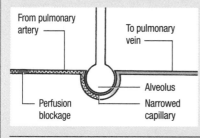

INADEQUATE VENTILATION (SHUNT)

When the $\dot{V}/\dot{Q}$ ratio is low, pulmonary circulation is adequate, but not enough oxygen is available to the alveoli for normal diffusion. A portion of the blood flowing through the pulmonary vessels doesn't become oxygenated.

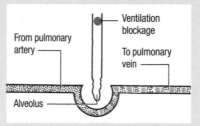

INADEQUATE VENTILATION AND PERFUSION (SILENT UNIT)

The silent unit indicates an absence of ventilation and perfusion to the lung area. The silent unit may help compensate for a $\dot{V}/\dot{Q}$ imbalance by delivering blood flow to better-ventilated areas.

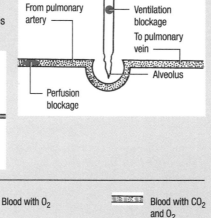

Blood with CO_2 — Blood with O_2 — Blood with CO_2 and O_2

What happens in $\dot{V}/\dot{Q}$ mismatch

+ Inadequate perfusion (dead-space ventilation) — occurs when $\dot{V}/\dot{Q}$ ratio is high, ventilation is normal, but alveolar perfusion is reduced or absent; results from perfusion defect or disorder that decreases cardiac output

+ Inadequate ventilation (shunt) — occurs when $\dot{V}/\dot{Q}$ ratio is low, pulmonary circulation is adequate, but not enough oxygen is available to the alveoli for normal diffusion

+ Inadequate ventilation and perfusion (silent unit) — occurs with the absence of ventilation and perfusion to the lung area; silent unit may be helping to compensate for a $\dot{V}/\dot{Q}$ imbalance by delivering blood flow to better-ventilated areas

After oxygen binds to Hb, the RBCs travel to the tissues. At this point, the blood cells contain more oxygen, and the tissue cells contain more carbon dioxide. Internal respiration occurs during cellular diffusion, as RBCs release oxygen and absorb carbon dioxide. The RBCs then transport carbon dioxide back to the lungs for removal during expiration.

Facts about acid-base balance

+ Lungs help maintain acid-base balance through external and internal respiration
+ Carbon dioxide dissolves in the blood forming bicarbonate (base) and carbonic acid (acid)
+ Medulla changes rate and depth of ventilation to maintain acid-base balance by adjusting the amount of carbon dioxide lost

Abnormal findings

+ Hypoventilation results in carbon dioxide retention, causing respiratory acidosis
+ Hyperventilation leads to increased exhalation of carbon dioxide, resulting in respiratory alkalosis

Obtaining a health history

+ Ask open-ended questions
+ Conduct interview in several short sessions
+ Establish a rapport with the patient
+ Gain trust by being sensitive to concerns and feelings
+ Be alert to nonverbal responses

Exploring the chief complaint

+ When did patient first notice the problem?
+ What's similar about this and previous episodes?
+ What relief measures were helpful or unhelpful?

Acid-base balance

The lungs help maintain acid-base balance in the body by maintaining external and internal respiration. Oxygen collected in the lungs is transported to the tissues by the circulatory system, which exchanges it for the carbon dioxide produced by cellular metabolism. Because carbon dioxide is 20 times more soluble than oxygen, it dissolves in the blood, where most of it forms bicarbonate (base) and smaller amounts form carbonic acid (acid).

The lungs control bicarbonate levels by converting bicarbonate to carbon dioxide and water for excretion. In response to signals from the medulla, the lungs can change the rate and depth of ventilation. Such changes maintain acid-base balance by adjusting the amount of carbon dioxide that is lost. For example, in metabolic alkalosis, which results from excess bicarbonate retention, the rate and depth of ventilation decrease so that carbon dioxide is retained. This increases carbonic acid levels. In metabolic acidosis (a condition resulting from excess acid retention or excess bicarbonate loss), the lungs increase the rate and depth of ventilation to exhale excess carbon dioxide, thereby reducing carbonic acid levels.

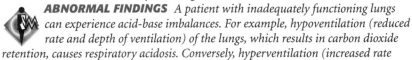 *ABNORMAL FINDINGS A patient with inadequately functioning lungs can experience acid-base imbalances. For example, hypoventilation (reduced rate and depth of ventilation) of the lungs, which results in carbon dioxide retention, causes respiratory acidosis. Conversely, hyperventilation (increased rate and depth of ventilation) of the lungs, leads to increased exhalation of carbon dioxide and will result in respiratory alkalosis.*

OBTAINING A HEALTH HISTORY

Build the patient's history by asking him open-ended questions. If possible, ask these questions systematically to avoid overlooking important information.

You may have to conduct the interview in several short sessions, depending on the severity of your patient's condition, and his expectations as well as staffing constraints.

During the interview, establish a rapport with the patient by explaining who you are and what you'll be doing. The quantity and quality of the information you gather depends on your relationship with the patient. Try to gain his trust by being sensitive to his concerns and feelings. Be alert to nonverbal responses that support or contradict his verbal responses. He may, for example, deny chest pain verbally but reveal it through his facial expression. If the patient's verbal and nonverbal responses contradict each other, explore this with him to clarify your assessment.

CHIEF COMPLAINT

Ask your patient to tell you about his chief complaint. Use such questions as "When did you first notice you weren't feeling well?" and "What's happened since then that brings you here today?" Because many respiratory disorders are chronic, be sure to ask him how the latest episode compared with the previous episode, and what relief measures were helpful or unhelpful.

CURRENT HEALTH HISTORY

The current health history includes the patient's biographic data and an analysis of his symptoms. Determine the patient's age, gender, marital status, occupation, education, religion, and ethnic background. These factors provide clues to potential risks and to the patient's interpretation of his respiratory condition. Advanced age, for example, suggests physiologic changes such as decreased vital capacity. Alternatively, the patient's occupation may alert you to problems related to hazardous materials. Don't forget to ask him for the name, address, and phone number of a relative who can be contacted in an emergency.

After you've obtained biographic data, ask the patient to describe his symptoms chronologically. Concentrate on the symptoms':

✦ onset — When did the symptom first occur? Did it appear suddenly or gradually?

✦ incidence — How often does the symptom occur? For example, would he describe pain as constant, intermittent, steadily worsening, or crescendo-decrescendo?

✦ duration — How long does the symptom last? Use precise terms to describe his answers, such as 30 minutes after meals, twice a day, or for 3 hours.

✦ manner — How does the symptom change over time?

Next, ask the patient to characterize his symptoms. Have him describe:

✦ aggravating factors — What increases the symptom's intensity? For example, if he has dyspnea, ask him how many blocks he can walk before he feels short of breath.

✦ alleviating factors — What relieves the symptom? Determine if he's tried any home remedies, such as over-the-counter (OTC) medications, alternative therapies, and a change in sleeping position.

✦ associated factors — Do other symptoms occur at the same time as the primary symptom?

✦ location — Where does he experience the symptom? Can he pinpoint it? Does it radiate to other areas?

✦ quality — Can he describe the feeling that accompanies the symptom? Has he experienced anything similar before? Ask him to characterize the symptom in his own words. Document his description, including the words he chooses to describe pain — for example, sharp, stabbing, or throbbing.

✦ setting — Where was he when the symptom occurred? What was he doing? Who was with him? Be sure to document your findings.

A patient with a respiratory disorder may complain of shortness of breath, cough, sputum production, wheezing, and chest pain.

Here are some helpful assessment techniques to gain information about each of those signs and symptoms.

Shortness of breath

Dyspnea, or shortness of breath, occurs when breathing is inappropriately difficult for the activity that the patient is performing.

You can gain a history of shortness of breath by using several scales. Ask the patient to rate his usual level of dyspnea on a scale of 0 to 10, in which 0 means no dyspnea and 10 means the worst he has experienced. Then ask him to rate the level that day. Another method to assess dyspnea is to count the number of words the patient speaks between breaths. A normal individual can speak 10 to 12 words. A severely dyspneic patient may speak only 1 to 2 words per breath.

Other scales grade dyspnea as it relates to activity. You might also ask these questions: What do you do to relieve the dyspnea? How well does it work? (See *Grading dyspnea*, page 140.) Dyspnea occurs when ventilation is disturbed. When ventilatory demands exceed the actual or perceived capacity of the lungs to respond, the patient becomes short of breath. In addition, dyspnea is caused by decreased lung compliance, disturbances in the chest bellows system, airway obstruction, or exogenous factors (such as obesity).

Current health history

Biographic data
✦ Age and gender
✦ Marital status
✦ Education and occupation
✦ Religious and ethnic background

Symptom analysis
✦ Onset
✦ Incidence
✦ Duration
✦ Change over time
✦ Aggravating, alleviating, and associated factors
✦ Location
✦ Quality
✦ Setting when occurred

Questions about shortness of breath

✦ Ask the patient to rate his usual level of dyspnea, then today's level, on a scale of 0 to 10
✦ Count the number of words he speaks between breaths (normal 10 to 12; dyspneic 1 to 2)
✦ Ask him to relate dyspnea to activity, what he does to relieve it, and how well that measure works

Causes
✦ Decreased lung compliance
✦ Disturbances in chest bellows system
✦ Airway obstruction
✦ Obesity

Grading dyspnea

To assess dyspnea as objectively as possible, ask your patient to briefly describe how various activities affect his breathing. Then document his response using the grading system.

◆ *Grade 0*—not troubled by breathlessness except with strenuous exercise

◆ *Grade 1*—troubled by shortness of breath when hurrying on a level path or walking up a slight hill

◆ *Grade 2*—walks more slowly on a level path because of breathlessness than people of the same age do or has to stop to breathe when walking on a level path at his own pace

◆ *Grade 3*—stops to breathe after walking about 100 yards (91 m) on a level path

◆ *Grade 4*—too breathless to leave the house or breathless when dressing or undressing

---

Questions about shortness of breath
(continued)

Special points

◆ Suspect dyspnea in an infant who breathes costally; in an older child who breathes abdominally; or in any child who uses neck and shoulder muscles to help in breathing

Facts about orthopnea

◆ Increases in supine position

◆ Measured by degree of elevation or by number of pillows needed to prop patient before dyspnea resolves

◆ Possible causes: pulmonary hypertension, left-sided heart failure, obesity, diaphragmatic paralysis, asthma, or COPD

Questions about cough

◆ Is the cough productive?

◆ If it's chronic, has it changed recently?

◆ What makes it better or worse?

◆ Is it severe and disruptive, dry, hacking, congested, or mucoid?

◆ What time of day does it occur?

To find out if the dyspnea stems from pulmonary disease, ask your patient about its onset and severity:

◆ A sudden onset may indicate an acute problem, such as pneumothorax or pulmonary embolus, or may also result from anxiety caused by hyperventilation.

◆ A gradual onset suggests a slow, progressive disorder, such as emphysema, whereas acute intermittent attacks may indicate asthma.

 SPECIAL POINTS *Normally, an infant's respirations are abdominal, gradually changing to costal by age 7. Suspect dyspnea in an infant who breathes costally, in an older child who breathes abdominally, or in any child who uses neck or shoulder muscles to help in breathing.*

Orthopnea

Orthopnea is increased dyspnea when the patient is in a supine position. It's traditionally measured in "pillows"—as in the number (usually 1 to 3) of pillows needed to prop the patient before dyspnea resolves. A better method is to record the degree of head elevation at which dyspnea is relieved. For example, a goniometer—a device used by physical therapists to determine range of motion—may be used to measure that a patient's "orthopnea is relieved at 35 degrees." Orthopnea in patients may be caused by:

◆ pulmonary hypertension

◆ left-sided heart failure

◆ obesity

◆ diaphragmatic paralysis

◆ asthma

◆ chronic obstructive pulmonary disease (COPD).

Cough

Ask the patient with a cough these questions: Is the cough productive? If the cough is a chronic problem, has it changed recently? If so, how? What makes the cough better? What makes it worse?

If your patient experiences coughing, investigate its characteristics:

◆ severe, disrupting daily activities and causing chest pain or acute respiratory distress

+ dry, signaling a cardiac condition
+ hacking, signaling pneumonia
+ congested, signaling a cold, pneumonia, or bronchitis
+ increased amounts of mucoid sputum, suggesting acute tracheobronchitis or acute asthma
+ chronic productive with mucoid sputum, signaling asthma or chronic bronchitis
+ changing sputum, from white to yellow or green, suggesting a bacterial infection
+ occurring in the early morning , indicating chronic airway inflammation, possibly from cigarette smoke
+ occurring in late afternoon, indicating exposure to irritants
+ occurring in the evening, suggesting chronic postnasal drip or sinusitis.

> *SPECIAL POINTS In children, evaluate a cough for these characteristics:*
> + *a barking cough indicates croup.*
> + *a nonproductive cough may indicate obstruction with a foreign body, asthma, pneumonia, or acute otitis media, or it may be an early indicator of cystic fibrosis.*
> + *a productive cough, which is accompanied by thick or excessive secretions, can quickly develop and occlude the child's narrow airway, causing respiratory distress, asthma, bronchiectasis, bronchitis, cystic fibrosis, and pertussis.*

Sputum

When a patient produces sputum, ask him to estimate the amount produced in teaspoons or some other common measurement. At what time of day does he usually cough? What is the color and consistency of his sputum? If his sputum is a chronic problem, has it changed recently? If so, how? Does he cough up blood? If so, how much and how often?

> *ABNORMAL FINDINGS If a patient is experiencing hemoptysis (coughing up blood), this may result from violent coughing or from serious disorders, such as pneumonia, lung cancer, lung abscess, tuberculosis, pulmonary embolism, bronchiectasis, and left-sided heart failure. If the hemoptysis is mild (sputum streaked with blood), reassure the patient and report this finding to the physician, making sure to ask the patient when he first noticed it and how often it occurs.*

> *SPECIAL POINTS Hemoptysis in children may stem from Goodpasture's syndrome, cystic fibrosis or, in rare cases, idiopathic primary pulmonary hemosiderosis. Sometimes no cause can be found for pulmonary hemorrhage occurring within the first 2 weeks of life; in such cases, the prognosis is poor. If an elderly patient with hemoptysis is receiving anticoagulants, determine changes that need to be made in diet or medications (including OTC and herbal supplements) because these factors may affect clotting.*

> *CLINICAL ALERT If hemoptysis is severe (frank bleeding), place the patient in a semirecumbent position, call the physician immediately, and note the patient's pulse rate, blood pressure, and general condition. When his condition stabilizes, ask whether he has ever experienced similar bleeding. (See Hemoptysis or hematemesis? page 142.)*

Wheezing

If a patient wheezes, ask him these questions: When does wheezing occur? What makes you wheeze? Do you wheeze loudly enough for others to hear it? What helps stop your wheezing?

Questions about cough
(continued)

Special points: Children
+ Barking cough indicates croup
+ Nonproductive cough may indicate obstruction, asthma, or pneumonia
+ Productive cough may indicate asthma or cystic fibrosis

Questions about sputum

+ What's the amount of sputum produced in teaspoons or other common measurement?
+ What's the color and consistency of the sputum?
+ If sputum is a chronic problem, has it changed recently?

Abnormal findings
+ Hemoptysis (coughing up blood)

Special points
+ Hemoptysis in children may stem from Goodpasture's syndrome, cystic fibrosis or, rarely, from idiopathic primary pulmonary hemosiderosis
+ In the elderly patient (with hemoptysis) taking anticoagulants, changes in diet or medications must be determined because they affect clotting

Alert!
+ If hemoptysis is severe, place patient in semirecumbent position; call physician immediately
+ Note pulse rate, blood pressure, and general condition
+ Ask about similar bleeding experiences

Questions about wheezing
+ When does the wheezing occur?
+ What instigates it?
+ Is it so loud that others hear it?
+ What does the patient do to stop it?

Hemoptysis or hematemesis?

If your patient begins bleeding from his mouth, determine if he's experiencing hemoptysis (coughing blood from the lungs), hematemesis (vomiting blood from the stomach), or bleeding from a site in the upper respiratory tract. Here's how the conditions compare.

HEMOPTYSIS
+ Bright red or pink, frothy blood
+ Blood mixed with sputum
+ Negative litmus paper test of blood (paper remains blue)

HEMATEMESIS
+ Dark red blood, possibly with coffee-ground appearance
+ Blood mixed with food
+ Positive litmus paper test of blood (paper turns pink)

BLEEDING FROM THE UPPER RESPIRATORY TRACT
Oral sources
+ Blood mixed with saliva
+ Evidence of mouth or tongue laceration
+ Negative litmus paper test of blood (paper remains blue)

Nasal or sinus source
+ Tickling sensation in nasal passages
+ Sniffing behavior

Questions about wheezing
(continued)

Special points
+ Children are more susceptible because their smaller airways allow for rapid obstruction

Alert!
+ Assess ABCs
+ Assess chest excursion, accessory muscle use, and body position during breathing
+ Assess LOC
+ Assess skin color and feel

Questions about chest pain
+ Where's the chest pain located?
+ Is the pain sharp, stabbing, burning, or aching?
+ Is it referred to another area of the body?
+ How long does it last, what causes it, and what makes it better?

 CLINICAL ALERT If the patient is in distress, immediately assess the patient's ABCs — airway, breathing, and circulation. Does he have an open airway? Is he breathing? Does he have a pulse? If these are absent, call for help and start cardiopulmonary resuscitation.

Next, quickly check for these signs of impending crisis:
+ Is the patient having difficulty breathing?
+ Is he using accessory muscles to breathe? If chest excursion is less than the normal 1⅛" to 2" (3 to 5 cm), he'll use accessory muscles when he breathes. Look for shoulder elevation, intercostal muscle retraction, and use of scalene and sternocleidomastoid muscles.
+ Has his level of consciousness diminished?
+ Is he confused, anxious, or agitated?
+ Does he change his body position to ease breathing?
+ Does his skin look pale, diaphoretic, or cyanotic?

 SPECIAL POINTS *Children are especially susceptible to wheezing because their small airways allow for rapid obstruction.*

Chest pain

If the patient has chest pain, ask him these questions: Where is the pain located? What does it feel like? Is it sharp, stabbing, burning, or aching? Does it move to another area in your body? If so, where? How long does it last? What causes it to occur? What makes it better?

Your patient may describe different types of chest pain, such as:
+ substernal pain, which is sharp, stabbing pain in the middle of his chest, indicating spontaneous pneumothorax
+ tracheal pain, which is a burning sensation that intensifies with deep breathing or coughing, suggesting oxygen toxicity or aspiration
+ esophageal pain, which is a burning sensation that intensifies with swallowing, indicating local inflammation
+ pleural pain, associated with pulmonary infarction, pneumothorax, or pleurisy, which is a stabbing, knifelike pain that increases with deep breathing or coughing

✦ chest wall pain, which is localized and tender, indicating an infection or inflammation of the chest wall, intercostal nerves, or intercostal muscles, or possibly, blunt chest trauma.

No matter what type of pain he describes, remember to assess associated factors, such as breathing, body position, and ease or difficulty of movement.

PAST HEALTH HISTORY

The information you gain from the patient's past health history helps you understand his current symptoms. It also helps to identify patients at risk for developing respiratory difficulty.

First, focus on identifying previous respiratory problems, such as asthma and emphysema. A history of these provides instant clues to the patient's current condition. Then ask about childhood illnesses. Infantile eczema, atopic dermatitis, or allergic rhinitis, for example, may precipitate current respiratory problems such as asthma.

Obtain an immunization history (especially of influenza and pneumococcal vaccination), which may provide clues about the potential for respiratory disease. A travel history may be useful and should include dates, destinations, and lengths of stay.

Next, ask what problems caused the patient to see a physician or required hospitalization in the past. Again, pay particular attention to respiratory problems. For example, chronic sinus infection or postnasal discharge may lead to recurrent bronchitis, and repeated episodes of pneumonia involving the same lung lobe may accompany bronchogenic carcinoma.

Ask the patient to describe the prescribed treatment, whether he followed the treatment plan, and whether the treatment helped. Determine whether he has suffered any traumatic injuries. If he has, note when they occurred and how they were treated.

The history should also include brief personal details. Ask the patient if he smokes; if he does, ask when he started and how many cigarettes he smokes per day. By calculating his smoking in pack-years, you can assess his risk of respiratory disease. To estimate pack-years, use this simple formula: number of packs smoked per day multiplied by the number of years the patient has smoked. For example, a patient who has smoked 2 packs of cigarettes per day for 42 years has accumulated 84 pack-years.

Remember to ask about alcohol use and about his diet, because nutritional status commonly influences a patient's risk of respiratory infection.

FAMILY HISTORY

Obtaining a family history helps determine whether a patient is at risk for hereditary or infectious respiratory diseases. First, ask if any of his immediate blood relatives (parents, siblings, and children) have had cancer, sickle cell anemia, heart disease, or a chronic illness, such as asthma or emphysema. Remember that diabetes can lead to cardiac, and possibly respiratory problems. If an immediate relative has one or more of these, ask for more information about the patient's maternal and paternal grandparents, aunts, and uncles.

Be sure to determine whether the patient lives with anyone who has an infectious disease, such as influenza or tuberculosis.

Past health history
✦ Reveals information about current health and symptoms
✦ Identifies patients at risk for developing respiratory difficulty
✦ Reveals previous respiratory problems, childhood illnesses, and travel history
✦ Uncovers immunization history
✦ Shows whether previous treatment plan helped
✦ Reveals smoking history, alcohol use, and diet

Family history
✦ Helps determine risk for hereditary or infectious respiratory diseases
✦ Suspect diseases: cancer, sickle cell anemia, heart disease, asthma or emphysema, diabetes, influenza, tuberculosis

Psychosocial history
+ Reveals lifestyle
+ Detects exposure to environmental irritants
+ Uncovers interpersonal relationships, mental status, stress management, and coping style

Assessing the respiratory system
+ Use inspection, palpation, percussion, and auscultation
+ Observe patient for alertness, comfort, anxiety, and general appearance
+ Seat patient in a position that allows access to the anterior and posterior thorax
+ If the patient can't sit up, use semi-Fowler's position to examine the anterior chest wall; side-lying position to assess posterior thorax

Inspecting the chest
+ Determine the rate, rhythm, and quality of respirations
+ Inspect chest configuration, tracheal position, chest symmetry, skin condition, nostrils, and accessory muscle use
+ Observe breathing and inspect his anterior and posterior thorax

PSYCHOSOCIAL HISTORY

Ask your patient about his psychosocial history to assess his lifestyle. Be sure to cover his home, community, and other environmental factors that might influence how he deals with his respiratory problems. People who work in mining, construction, or chemical manufacturing are commonly exposed to environmental irritants. Also ask about interpersonal relationships, mental status, stress management, and coping style. Keep in mind that a patient's sexual habits or drug use may be connected with acquired immunodeficiency syndrome-related pulmonary disorders.

ASSESSING THE RESPIRATORY SYSTEM

Any patient can develop a respiratory disorder. By using a systematic assessment, you'll be able to detect subtle or obvious respiratory changes. The depth of your assessment will depend on several factors, including the patient's primary health problem and his risk of developing respiratory complications.

A physical examination of the respiratory system follows four steps: inspection, palpation, percussion, and auscultation. Before you begin, make sure the room is well-lit and warm.

Make a few observations about the patient as soon as you enter the room. Note how the patient is seated, which will most likely be the position most comfortable for him. Take note of his level of awareness and general appearance. Does he appear relaxed? Anxious? Uncomfortable? Is he having trouble breathing? You'll include those observations in your final assessment.

When you're ready to begin, seat the patient in a position that allows access to the anterior and posterior thorax. Provide a gown that offers easy access to the chest and back without requiring unnecessary exposure. Make sure the patient isn't cold because shivering may alter breathing patterns.

If the patient can't sit up, use the semi-Fowler position to assess the anterior chest wall and the side-lying position to assess the posterior thorax. Keep in mind that these positions may cause some distortion of findings.

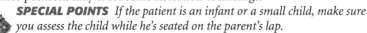 **SPECIAL POINTS** *If the patient is an infant or a small child, make sure you assess the child while he's seated on the parent's lap.*

When performing the assessment, you may find it easier to inspect, palpate, percuss, and auscultate the anterior chest before the posterior. However, this section covers inspection of the entire chest, then palpation, percussion, and auscultation of the entire chest.

INSPECTING THE CHEST

To assess respiratory function, determine the rate, rhythm, and quality of the patient's respirations and inspect his chest configuration, tracheal position, chest symmetry, skin condition, nostrils (for flaring), and accessory muscle use. Accomplish this by observing the patient's breathing and inspecting his anterior and posterior thorax. Note all abnormal findings.

Respiration
To find the patient's respiratory rate, count for a full minute—longer if you note abnormalities. Don't tell him what you're doing, or he might alter his natural breathing pattern.

SPECIAL POINTS *Adults normally breathe at a rate of 12 to 20 breaths/ minute. An infant's breathing rate may reach about 40 breaths/minute.*

      The respiratory pattern should be even, coordinated, and regular, with occasional sighs. The ratio of inspiration to expiration (I:E) is about 1:2.

 SPECIAL POINTS *Men, children, and infants usually use abdominal, or diaphragmatic, breathing. Athletes and singers do as well. Most women, however, usually use chest, or intercostal breathing.*

 ABNORMAL FINDINGS *Paradoxical, or uneven, movement of the chest wall may appear as an abnormal collapse of part of the chest wall when the patient inhales or an abnormal expansion when the patient exhales. In either case, this uneven movement indicates a loss of normal chest-wall function.*

    When the patient inhales, his diaphragm should descend and the intercostal muscles should contract. This dual motion causes the abdomen to push out and the lower ribs to expand laterally.

    When the patient exhales, his abdomen and ribs return to their resting position. The upper chest shouldn't move much. Accessory muscles may hypertrophy, indicating frequent use.

ABNORMAL FINDINGS *Identifying abnormal respiratory patterns can help you assess more completely a patient's respiratory status and his overall condition. (See* Spotting abnormal respiratory patterns, *page 146.)*
Upon examining your patient, you may find these respiratory abnormalities:
✦ *Frequent use of accessory muscles indicates a respiratory problem, particularly when the patient purses his lips and flares his nostrils when breathing.*
✦ *Tachypnea is a respiratory rate greater than 20 breaths/minute with shallow breathing. It's commonly seen in patients with restrictive lung disease, pain, sepsis, obesity, or anxiety. Fever may be another cause. The respiratory rate may increase by 4 breaths/minute for every 1° F (0.6° C) rise in body temperature.*
✦ *Bradypnea is a respiratory rate below 10 breaths/minute and is commonly noted just before a period of apnea or full respiratory arrest. Patients with bradypnea might have CNS depression as a result of excessive sedation, tissue damage, or diabetic coma, which all depress the brain's respiratory control center. (The respiratory rate normally decreases during sleep.)*
✦ *Apnea is the absence of breathing. Periods of apnea may be short and occur sporadically during Cheyne-Stokes respirations, Biot's respirations, or other abnormal respiratory patterns.*

 CLINICAL ALERT Apnea in patients may be life-threatening if the periods of apnea last long enough.
    ✦ Characterized by deep breathing, hyperpnea occurs in patients who exercise or who have anxiety, pain, or metabolic acidosis. In a comatose patient, hyperpnea may indicate hypoxia or hypoglycemia.
✦ Kussmaul's respirations are rapid, deep, sighing breaths that occur in patients with metabolic acidosis, especially when associated with diabetic ketoacidosis.
✦ Cheyne-Stokes respirations have a regular pattern of variations in the rate and depth of breathing. Deep breaths alternate with short periods of apnea. This respiratory pattern is seen in patients with heart failure, kidney failure, or CNS damage. Biot's respirations involve rapid deep breaths that alternate with abrupt periods of apnea. Biot's respirations are an ominous sign of severe CNS damage.

SPECIAL POINTS *Cheyne-Stokes respirations may be normal in children and elderly patients during sleep.*

Inspecting the chest

Special points
✦ Normal adult breath rate: 12 to 20 breaths/minute
✦ Normal infant rate: up to 40 breaths/minute
✦ Men, children, and infants usually use abdominal (diaphragmatic) breathing
✦ Women usually use chest (intercostal) breathing
✦ During sleep in children and elderly patients, Cheyne-Stokes respirations may be normal

Abnormal findings
✦ Paradoxical, uneven chest movement
✦ Frequent accessory muscle use, pursed lips, flared nostrils
✦ Tachypnea — more than 20 breaths/minute with shallow breathing
✦ Bradypnea — fewer than 10 breaths/minute; commonly occurs just before apnea or full respiratory arrest
✦ Hyperpnea — deep breathing at a normal rate
✦ Apnea — absence of breathing; occurs sporadically during Cheyne-Stokes respirations, Biot's respirations, or other abnormal respiratory patterns

Alert!
✦ Hyperpnea occurs in patients who exercise or who have had anxiety, pain, or metabolic acidosis
✦ Kussmaul's respirations occur in patients with metabolic acidosis
✦ Cheyne-Stokes respirations occur in patients with heart failure, kidney failure, or CNS damage
✦ Biot's respirations are an ominous sign of severe CNS damage

Spotting abnormal respiratory patterns

Here are typical characteristics of the more common abnormal respiratory patterns.

TACHYPNEA
Shallow breathing with increased respiratory rate

KUSSMAUL'S RESPIRATIONS
Rapid, deep breathing without pauses; in adults, more than 20 breaths/minute; breathing usually sounds labored with deep breaths that resemble sighs

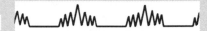

BRADYPNEA
Decreased rate but regular breathing

CHEYNE-STOKES RESPIRATIONS
Breaths that gradually become faster and deeper than normal, then slower, during a 30- to 170-second period; alternates with 20-to 60-second periods of apnea

APNEA
Absence of breathing; may be periodic

HYPERPNEA
Deep breathing at a normal rate

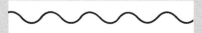

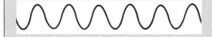

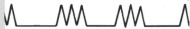

BIOT'S RESPIRATIONS
Rapid, deep breathing with abrupt pauses between each breath; equal depth to each breath

Inspecting the anterior thorax

✦ Abnormalities include concave or convex curvature of the anterior chest wall over the sternum and retractions (sinking of soft tissues between and around ribs)
✦ Respiratory pattern and chest expansion should be symmetric
✦ Thorax should have a greater diameter laterally than anteroposteriorly
✦ Sternocostal angle (between ribs and sternum at point immediately above the xiphoid process) should be less than 90 degrees in adults
✦ Skin on anterior chest should have normal color, and be free from lumps or lesions

Anterior thorax

After assessing respiration, inspect the thorax for structural deformities such as a concave or convex curvature of the anterior chest wall over the sternum. Inspect between and around the ribs for visible sinking of soft tissues (retractions). Assess the patient's respiratory pattern for symmetry. Look for abnormalities in skin color or alterations in muscle tone. For future documentation, note the location of abnormalities according to regions delineated by imaginary lines on the thorax.

Initially inspect the chest wall to identify the shape of the thoracic cage. In an adult, the thorax should have a greater diameter laterally (from side to side) than anteroposteriorly (from front to back).

Note the angle between the ribs and the sternum at the point immediately above the xiphoid process. This angle, called the *sternocostal angle,* should be less than 90 degrees in an adult; it widens if the chest wall is chronically expanded, as in cases of increased anteroposterior diameter, or barrel chest.

To inspect the anterior chest for symmetry of movement, have the patient lie in a supine position. Stand at the foot of the bed and carefully observe the patient's quiet and deep breathing for equal expansion of the chest wall.

ABNORMAL FINDINGS *Watch for abnormal collapse of part of the chest wall during inspiration, along with abnormal expansion of the same area during expiration (paradoxical movement). Paradoxical movement indicates a loss of normal chest wall function. Also check whether one portion of the chest wall lags behind the others as the chest moves. This may indicate an obstructive component to the patient's lung disease.*

Next, check for use of accessory muscles for respiration by observing the sternocleidomastoid, scalene, and trapezius muscles in the shoulders and neck. During normal inspiration and expiration, the diaphragm and external intercostal muscles should easily maintain the breathing process.

 ABNORMAL FINDINGS *Hypertrophy of any of the accessory muscles may indicate frequent abnormal use, especially if found in an elderly patient— although hypertrophy may be normal in a well-conditioned athlete.*

Also note the position the patient assumes to breathe.

ABNORMAL FINDINGS *A patient who depends on accessory muscles may assume a "tripod position," where he rests his arms on his knees or on the sides of a chair and supports his head.*

Observe the patient's skin on the anterior chest for any unusual color, lumps, or lesions, and note the location of any abnormality. Unless the patient has been exposed to significant sun or heat, the skin color of the chest should match the rest of the patient's complexion. A skin abnormality may reflect problems in the underlying structure, so note the location of underlying ribs and other bones, cartilage, and lung lobes. Also check for any chest wall scars from surgery. If the patient didn't mention surgery during the health history, ask about it now.

Posterior thorax

To inspect the posterior thorax, observe the patient's breathing again. If he can't sit in a backless chair or lean forward against a supporting structure, direct him to lie in a lateral position. Be aware that this may distort your findings in some situations.

 ABNORMAL FINDINGS *Your findings in an obese patient may be distorted because he may be unable to fully expand the lower lung from the lateral position, leaving breath sounds on that side diminished.*

Assess the posterior chest wall for the same characteristics as the anterior: chest structure, respiratory pattern, symmetry of expansion, skin color and muscle tone, and accessory muscle use. As you examine a patient for chest wall abnormalities, keep in mind he might have completely normal lungs and that the lungs might be cramped within the chest. The patient might have a smaller-than-normal lung capacity and limited exercise tolerance, and he may more easily develop respiratory failure from a respiratory tract infection.(See *Identifying chest deformities*, page 148.)

 ABNORMAL FINDINGS *Chest wall abnormalities include the following:*
✦ A barrel chest, which looks like its name implies: The chest is abnormally round and bulging, with a greater-than-normal front-to-back diameter. It occurs as a result of chronic obstructive pulmonary disease, indicating that the lungs have lost their elasticity and that the diaphragm is flattened. The patient typically uses accessory muscles when he inhales and easily becomes breathless. You'll also note kyphosis of the thoracic spine, ribs that run horizontally rather than tangentially, and a prominent sternal angle. Barrel chest may be normal in an infant or in an elderly patient.

Inspecting the anterior thorax
(continued)

Abnormal findings
✦ Paradoxical movement (abnormal collapse of part of chest wall during inspiration) may indicate a loss of normal chest wall function
✦ Delayed movement of part of chest wall may indicate obstruction
✦ Hypertrophy of accessory muscles and tripod position during breathing may signal abnormal accessory muscle use (hypertrophy may be normal in athletes)

Inspecting the posterior thorax

✦ If patient can't sit or lean forward against a support, have him lie in a lateral position
✦ Assess chest structure, respiratory pattern, symmetry of expansion, skin color, muscle tone, and accessory muscle

Abnormal findings
✦ Obesity may prevent full inspiration
✦ Chest deformities include barrel chest (may be normal in infant or elderly person), pigeon chest, funnel chest, and thoracic kyphoscoliosis

Identifying chest deformities

As you inspect the patient's chest, note deviations in size and shape. These illustrations show a normal adult chest and four common chest deformities.

NORMAL ADULT CHEST

BARREL CHEST
Increased anteroposterior diameter

FUNNEL CHEST
Depressed lower sternum

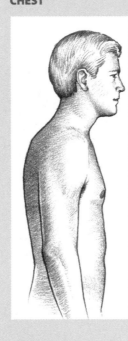

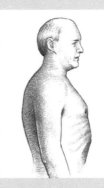

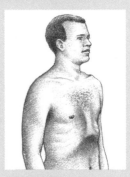

PIGEON CHEST
Anteriorly displaced sternum

THORACIC KYPHOSCOLIOSIS
Raised shoulder and scapula, thoracic convexity, and flared interspaces

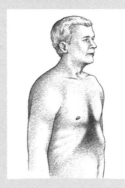

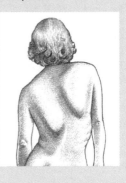

✦ *Pigeon chest, or pectus carinatum, is characterized by a chest with a sternum that protrudes beyond the front of the abdomen. The displaced sternum increases the front-to-back diameter of the chest.*
✦ *Funnel chest, or pectus excavatum, is characterized by a funnel-shaped depression on all or part of the sternum. The shape of the chest may interfere with respiratory and cardiac function. If cardiac compression occurs, you may hear a murmur.*
✦ *Thoracic kyphoscoliosis occurs when the patient's spine curves to one side and the vertebrae are rotated. Because the rotation distorts lung tissues, you may have a more difficult time assessing respiratory status.*

KNOW-HOW

Checking for clubbed fingers

To assess the patient for chronic tissue hypoxia, check his fingers for clubbing. Normally, the angle between the fingernail and the point where the nail enters the skin is about 160 degrees, as shown below left. Clubbing occurs when that angle increases to 180 degrees or more, as shown below right.

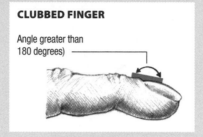

NORMAL FINGER

Normal angle (160 degrees)

CLUBBED FINGER

Angle greater than 180 degrees

Inspecting related structures

Inspecting the patient's skin and nails will give you an overview of the patient's clinical status along with an assessment of his peripheral oxygenation.

ABNORMAL FINDINGS A dusky or bluish tint (cyanosis) to the patient's skin may indicate decreased hemoglobin oxygen saturation. Distinguishing central from peripheral cyanosis is important:

✦ *Central cyanosis results from hypoxemia and may appear in patients with right-to-left cardiac shunting or a pulmonary disease that causes hypoxemia, such as chronic bronchitis. It appears on the skin; the mucous membranes of the mouth, lips, and conjunctivae; or in other highly vascular areas, such as the earlobes, tip of the nose, and nail beds.*

✦ *Peripheral cyanosis, commonly seen in patients exposed to the cold, results from vasoconstriction, vascular occlusion, or reduced cardiac output and appears in the nail beds, nose, ears, and fingers. Note that unlike central cyanosis, it doesn't affect the mucous membranes. Peripheral cyanosis indicates oxygen depletion in non-perfused areas of the body because oxyhemoglobin reduced by metabolism isn't replaced by fresh blood.*

SPECIAL POINTS A dark-skinned patient may be more difficult to assess for central cyanosis. In this patient, inspect the oral mucous membranes and lips, which will appear ashen-gray rather than bluish. Facial skin may appear pale gray or ashen in a cyanotic black-skinned patient and yellowish brown in a cyanotic brown-skinned patient.

Next, assess the patient's nail beds and toes for abnormal enlargement.

ABNORMAL FINDINGS Abnormal enlargement of the patient's nail beds and toes is called clubbing, *which results from chronic tissue hypoxia. Nail thinning accompanied by an abnormal alteration of the angle of the finger and toe bases distinguishes clubbing. (See* Checking for clubbed fingers.*)*

Inspecting related structures

✦ Skin and nails reveal peripheral oxygenation

Abnormal findings
✦ Cyanosis
✦ Clubbing of nails

Special points
✦ In dark-skinned patients, assess for central cyanosis by inspecting the oral mucous membranes and lips (ashen-gray rather than bluish)
✦ Facial skin may appear pale gray or ashen in a cyanotic black-skinned patient and yellowish brown in a cyanotic brown-skinned patient

KNOW-HOW

Palpating the trachea

To palpate the trachea, stand in front of the patient and place one thumb on either side of the trachea above the suprasternal notch. Gently slide both thumbs, at equal speed, along the upper edge of the patient's clavicle until you reach the sternocleidomastoid muscle. Each thumb should cover an equal distance, indicating a midline trachea.

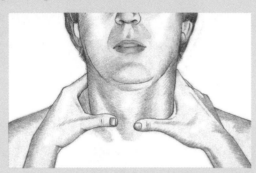

Palpating the chest

✦ Palpate the trachea and anterior and posterior thorax to detect structural and skin abnormalities, areas of pain, and chest asymmetry

Palpating the trachea

✦ Palpate the trachea for position
✦ Palpate the suprasternal notch for strength and regularity of aortic pulsations

Abnormal findings

✦ Trachea isn't midline

Palpating the anterior thorax

✦ Palpate to assess skin and underlying tissues for density
✦ Palpate areas that looked abnormal on inspection
✦ The chest wall should feel smooth, warm, and dry
✦ If patient complains of pain, assess for localization, radiation, and severity
✦ Palpate the costal angle
✦ Palpate for symmetrical movement during inspiration

PALPATING THE CHEST

By carefully palpating the trachea and the anterior and posterior thorax, you can detect structural and skin abnormalities, areas of pain, and chest asymmetry.

Trachea and anterior thorax

First, palpate the trachea for position. (See *Palpating the trachea.*)

 ABNORMAL FINDINGS *Palpation of the patient's trachea may show that the trachea isn't midline (possibly resulting from collapsed lung tissue [at-electasis], thyroid enlargement, or fluid accumulation in the air spaces of the lungs [pleural effusion]). A tumor or collapsed lung (pneumothorax) may have also displaced the trachea to one side.*

Observe the patient to determine whether he uses accessory neck muscles to breathe.

Next, palpate the suprasternal notch. In most patients, the arch of the aorta lies close to the surface just behind the suprasternal notch. Use your fingertips to gently evaluate the strength and regularity of the patient's aortic pulsations in this area.

Then palpate the thorax to assess the skin and underlying tissues for density. (See *Palpating the thorax.*)

Gentle palpation shouldn't be painful, so assess any complaints of pain for localization, radiation, and severity. Be especially careful to palpate any areas that looked abnormal during inspection. If necessary, support the patient during the procedure with one hand while using your other hand to palpate one side at a time, continuing to compare sides. Note any unusual findings, such as masses, crepitus, skin irregularities, and painful areas.

The chest wall should feel smooth, warm, and dry.

ABNORMAL FINDINGS *If the patient has subcutaneous air in the chest, this indicates crepitus, an abnormal condition that feels like puffed-rice cereal crackling under the skin and indicates that air is leaking from the airways or lungs. If a patient has a chest tube, you may find a small amount of subcutaneous air around the insertion site.*

Identifying cardiovascular landmarks and sites for heart sounds

This illustration shows where to find critical landmarks used in cardiovascular assessment. When auscultating for heart sounds, place the stethoscope over the four different sites shown below. Auscultation sites are identified by the names of the heart valves but aren't located directly over the valves. Rather, these sites are located along the pathway blood takes as it flows through the heart's chambers and valves.

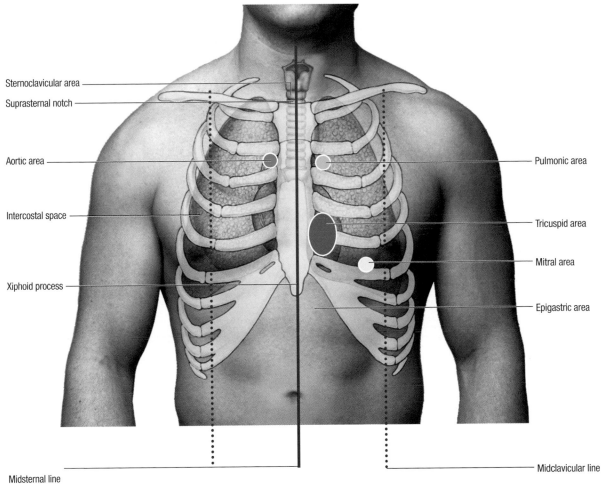

Cycle of heart sounds

When you auscultate a patient's chest and hear that familiar "lub-dub," you're hearing the first and second heart sounds, S_1 and S_2. At times, two other sounds may occur, S_3 and S_4.

Heart sounds are generated by events in the cardiac cycle. When valves close or blood fills the ventricles, vibrations of the heart muscle can be heard through the chest wall.

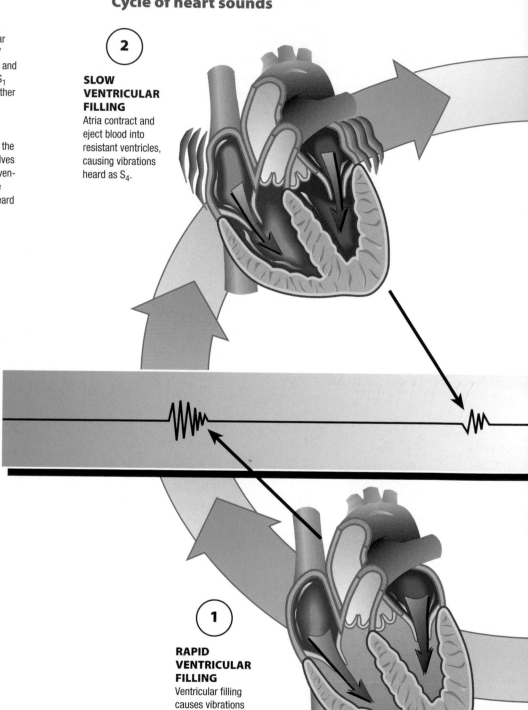

2

SLOW VENTRICULAR FILLING
Atria contract and eject blood into resistant ventricles, causing vibrations heard as S_4.

1

RAPID VENTRICULAR FILLING
Ventricular filling causes vibrations heard as S_3.

KEY

 Diastole

Systole

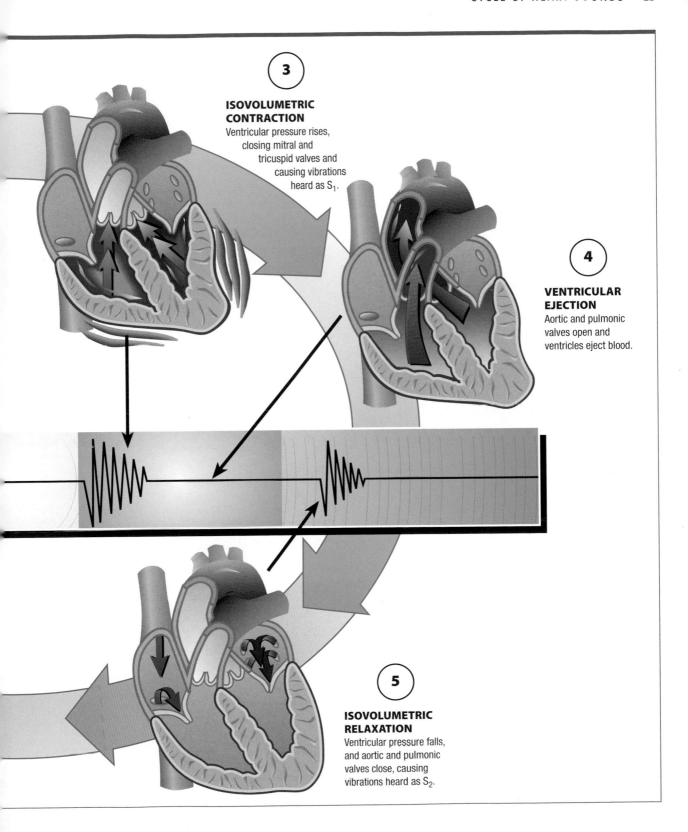

3

ISOVOLUMETRIC CONTRACTION
Ventricular pressure rises, closing mitral and tricuspid valves and causing vibrations heard as S_1.

4

VENTRICULAR EJECTION
Aortic and pulmonic valves open and ventricles eject blood.

5

ISOVOLUMETRIC RELAXATION
Ventricular pressure falls, and aortic and pulmonic valves close, causing vibrations heard as S_2.

Understanding murmurs

Normally, heart valves close tightly and then open completely to let blood flow through. However, various conditions may alter blood flow through the valves, causing murmurs and, in many cases, increasing the workload of the heart.

The first two illustrations show a normal valve open and closed. The other illustrations portray three common reasons for the development of murmurs.

NORMAL VALVE OPEN

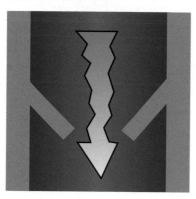

NORMAL VALVE CLOSED

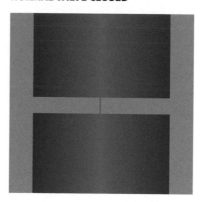

HIGH BLOOD FLOW

High blood flow through a normal valve may cause a murmur. For example, an aortic systolic murmur, which can be caused by anemia, causes a subsequent compensatory increase in cardiac output.

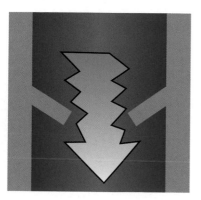

DECREASED BLOOD FLOW

Low blood flow through a stenotic valve can cause a murmur. The valves can't open or close properly because they're thickened, fibrotic, or calcified. Common examples include aortic and mitral stenosis.

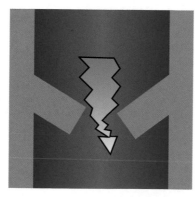

BACKFLOW OF BLOOD

A backflow of blood through an insufficient or incompetent valve can cause a murmur. Because the valve can't close properly, blood can leak back or regurgitate into the heart chamber from which it came. Common examples include aortic and mitral insufficiency.

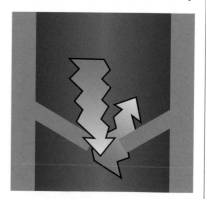

Expected percussion notes

When you're percussing the thorax and upper abdomen, certain areas will produce expected areas of dullness, flatness, resonance, and tympany. These illustrations show the areas of expected percussion notes in the anterior and posterior thorax.

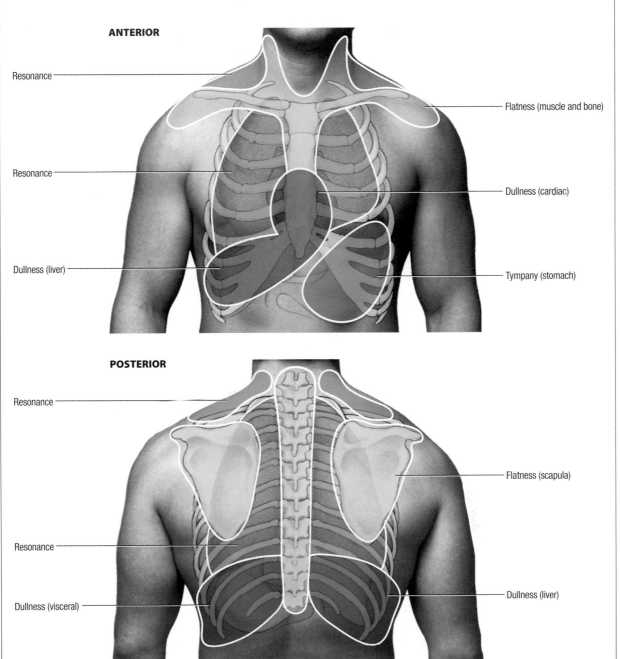

ANTERIOR

Resonance

Resonance

Dullness (liver)

Flatness (muscle and bone)

Dullness (cardiac)

Tympany (stomach)

POSTERIOR

Resonance

Resonance

Dullness (visceral)

Flatness (scapula)

Dullness (liver)

Respiratory assessment landmarks

By recognizing respiratory landmarks, you can perform your assessment more proficiently. Use these illustrations to familiarize yourself with these anterior and posterior landmarks of the respiratory system.

ANTERIOR VIEW

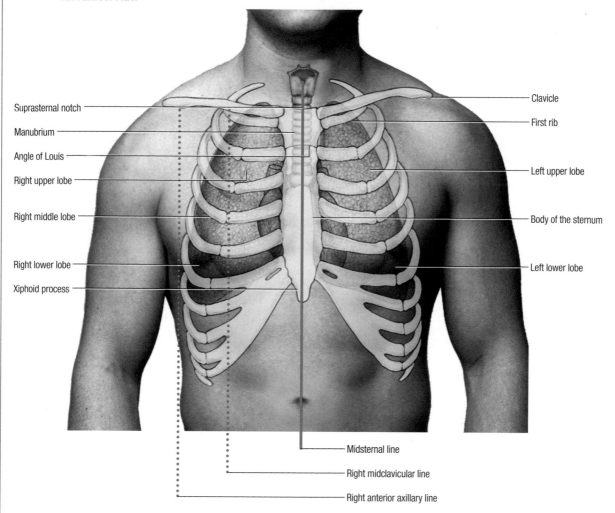

POSTERIOR VIEW

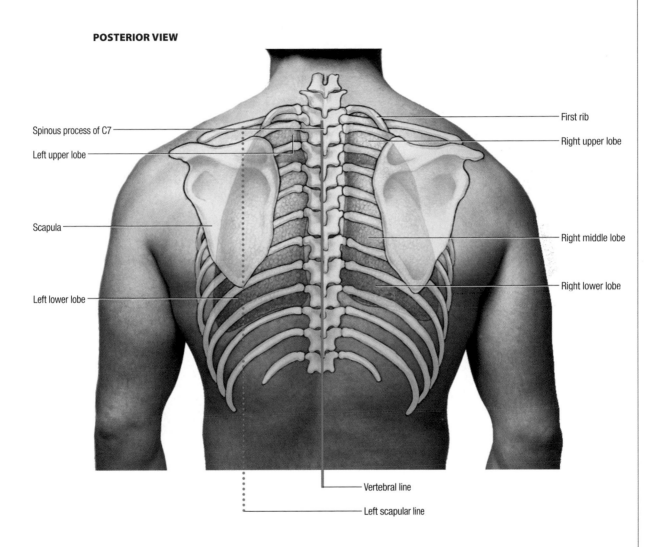

Spinous process of C7

Left upper lobe

Scapula

Left lower lobe

First rib

Right upper lobe

Right middle lobe

Right lower lobe

Vertebral line

Left scapular line

Abdominal quadrants

To perform a systematic GI assessment, try to visualize the abdominal structures by dividing the abdomen into four quadrants, as shown here.

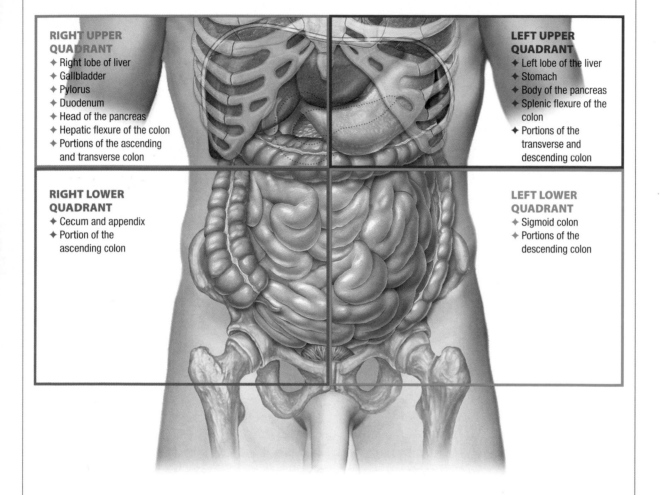

RIGHT UPPER QUADRANT
- Right lobe of liver
- Gallbladder
- Pylorus
- Duodenum
- Head of the pancreas
- Hepatic flexure of the colon
- Portions of the ascending and transverse colon

LEFT UPPER QUADRANT
- Left lobe of the liver
- Stomach
- Body of the pancreas
- Splenic flexure of the colon
- Portions of the transverse and descending colon

RIGHT LOWER QUADRANT
- Cecum and appendix
- Portion of the ascending colon

LEFT LOWER QUADRANT
- Sigmoid colon
- Portions of the descending colon

KNOW-HOW

Palpating the thorax

To palpate the thorax, place the palm of your hand (or hands) lightly over the thorax, as shown. Palpate for tenderness, alignment, bulging, or retractions of the chest and intercostal spaces. Assess the patient for crepitus, especially around drainage sites. Repeat this procedure on the patient's back.

Next, use the pads of your lingers, as shown, to palpate the front and back of the thorax. Pass your fingers over the ribs and any scars, lumps, lesions, or ulcerations. Note the skin temperature, turgor, and moisture. Also note tenderness or bony or subcutaneous crepitus. The muscles should feel firm and smooth.

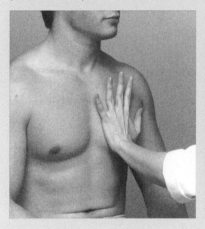
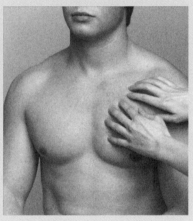

 CLINICAL ALERT If the patient has no chest tube or the area of crepitus is getting larger, alert the physician immediately.

If the patient complains of chest pain, attempt to determine the cause by palpating the anterior chest.

ABNORMAL FINDINGS *Increased pain during palpation may be caused by certain conditions—such as musculoskeletal pain, an irritation of the nerves covering the xiphoid process, and an inflammation of the cartilage connecting the bony ribs to the sternum (costochondritis). These conditions may also produce pain during inspiration, causing the patient to breathe shallowly to decrease his discomfort. Keep in mind that palpation doesn't worsen pain caused by cardiac or pulmonary disorders, such as angina and pleurisy.*

Next, palpate the costal angle. The area around the xiphoid process contains many nerve endings, so be gentle to avoid causing pain.

ABNORMAL FINDINGS *If a patient frequently uses the internal intercostal muscles to breathe, these muscles will eventually pull the chest cavity upward and outward. If this has occurred, the costal angle will be greater than the normal 90 degrees.*

To evaluate how symmetrical the patient's chest wall is and how much it expands, place your hands on the front of the chest wall, with your thumbs touching each other at the second intercostal space. As the patient inhales deeply, watch your

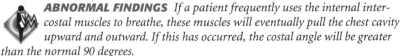

Alert!
✦ If the patient has no chest tube or the area of crepitus is getting larger, alert physician immediately

Palpating the anterior thorax
(continued)

Abnormal findings
✦ Subcutaneous air in the chest (crepitus)
✦ Skin irregularities
✦ Pain during palpation or inspiration (musculoskeletal pain, irritation of nerves or xiphoid process, costochondritis)
✦ Costal angle greater than 90 degrees (frequent use of internal intercostal muscles to breathe)

KNOW-HOW

Palpating the thorax for tactile fremitus

When you check the back of the thorax for tactile fremitus, ask the patient to fold his arms across his chest. This movement shifts the scapulae out of the way.

WHAT TO DO
Check for tactile fremitus by lightly placing your open palms on both sides of the patient's back, as shown, without touching his back with your fingers. Ask the patient to repeat the phrase "ninety-nine" loud enough to produce palpable vibrations. Then palpate the front of the chest using the same hand positions.

INTERPRETING THE RESULTS
Vibrations that feel more intense on one side than the other indicate tissue consolidation on that side. Less intense vibrations may indicate emphysema, pneumothorax, or pleural effusion. Faint or no vibrations in the upper posterior thorax may indicate bronchial obstruction or a fluid-filled pleural space.

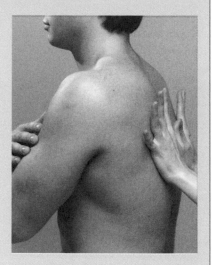

Palpating the anterior thorax
(continued)

Abnormal findings

+ Asymmetrical expansion
+ Decreased expansion at the level of the diaphragm
+ Absent or delayed chest movement during respiratory excursion

Palpating the posterior thorax

+ Use palmar surface of fingertips of one or both hands
+ Identify first thoracic vertebra and count the number of spinous processes from this landmark to the abnormal finding
+ Identify the inferior scapular tips and medial borders of both bones to define the margins of the upper and lower lung lobes posteriorly
+ Palpate for symmetrical movement during inspiration
+ Evaluate abnormalities such as use of accessory muscles and complaints of pain

thumbs. They should separate simultaneously and equally, to a distance several centimeters away from the sternum.

Repeat the measurement at the fifth intercostal space. The same measurement may be made on the back of the chest near the tenth rib.

 ABNORMAL FINDINGS *During chest palpation you may find these abnormal signs in the patient's chest:*

+ it expands asymmetrically if he has pleural effusion, atelectasis, pneumonia, or pneumothorax
+ it has decreased expansion at the level of the diaphragm if he has emphysema, respiratory depression, diaphragm paralysis, atelectasis, obesity, or ascites
+ it has absent or delayed chest movement during respiratory excursion, indicating previous surgical removal of the lung, complete or partial obstruction of the airway or underlying lung, or diaphragmatic dysfunction on the affected side.

Posterior thorax
Palpate the posterior thorax in a similar manner, using the palmar surface of the fingertips of one or both hands. During the process, identify bony structures, such as the vertebrae and the scapulae.

To determine the location of abnormalities, identify the first thoracic vertebra (with the patient's head tipped forward) and count the number of spinous processes from this landmark to the abnormal finding. Use this reference point for documentation. Also, identify the inferior scapular tips and medial borders of both bones to define the margins of the upper and lower lung lobes posteriorly. Locate and describe all abnormalities in relation to these landmarks. Remember to evaluate abnormalities, such as use of accessory muscles and complaints of pain.

KNOW-HOW

Percussing the chest

To percuss the chest, hyperextend the middle finger of your left hand if you're right-handed and the middle finger of your right hand if you're left-handed. Place your hand firmly on the patient's chest. Use the tip of the middle finger of your dominant hand — your right hand if you're right-handed, left hand if you're left-handed — to tap on the middle finger of your other hand just below the distal joint (as shown).

The movement should come from the wrist of your dominant hand, not your elbow or upper arm. Keep the fingernail you use for tapping short so you won't hurt yourself. Follow the standard percussion sequence over the front and back chest walls.

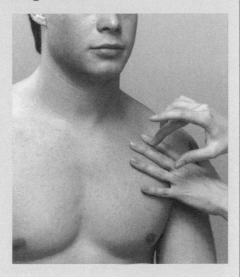

Tactile fremitus

Because sound travels more easily through solid structures than through air, checking for tactile fremitus (the palpation of vocalizations) helps you learn about the contents of the lungs. (See *Palpating the thorax for tactile fremitus*.)

The patient's vocalization should produce vibrations of equal intensity on both sides of the chest. Normally, vibrations should occur in the upper chest, close to the bronchi, and then decrease and finally disappear toward the periphery of the lungs.

Conditions that restrict air movement, such as pneumonia, pleural effusion, and chronic obstructive pulmonary disease with overinflated lungs, cause decreased tactile fremitus. Conditions that consolidate tissue or fluid in a portion of the pleural area, such as a lung tumor, pneumonia, and pulmonary fibrosis, increase tactile fremitus.

 ABNORMAL FINDINGS *A grating feeling when palpating the patient's chest may signify a pleural friction rub.*

PERCUSSING THE CHEST

You'll percuss the patient's chest to find the boundaries of the lungs; to determine whether the lungs are filled with air, fluid, or solid material; and to evaluate the distance the diaphragm travels between the patient's inhalation and exhalation. (See *Percussing the chest*.)

Percussion allows you to assess structures as deep as 3″ (7.6 cm). You'll hear different percussion sounds in different areas of the chest. (See *Percussion sounds*, page 154.)

Facts about tactile fremitus

✦ Gives information about lung contents
✦ Patient's vocalization should produce palpable vibrations of equal intensity on both sides of upper chest
✦ Decreases with conditions that restrict air movement
✦ Increases with conditions that consolidate tissue or fluid

Abnormal findings

✦ Grating feeling may signal pleural friction rub

Percussing the chest

✦ Locates lung boundaries
✦ Determines lung contents: air, fluid, or solid material
✦ Evaluates diaphragmatic excursion between inhalation and exhalation

Facts about percussion sounds

✦ Resonant sounds heard over normal lung tissue
✦ Dull sounds heard in the left front chest over the heart
✦ Sequence heard in the posterior thorax is slightly different

Percussing the chest
(continued)

Abnormal findings

✦ Hyperresonance indicates pneumothorax, acute asthma, bullous emphysema, and gastric distention
✦ Abnormal dullness indicates pleural fluid, consolidation, atelectasis, or tumor

Percussing the diaphragm

✦ Descends 2″ to 2½″ on inhalation
✦ Restricted in emphysema, respiratory depression, diaphragm paralysis, atelectasis, obesity, or ascites

---

Percussion sounds

This chart describes percussion sounds in various parts of the body and their clinical significance.

SOUND	DESCRIPTION	CLINICAL SIGNIFICANCE
Flat	Short, soft, high-pitched, extremely dull, found over the thigh	Consolidation as in atelectasis and extensive pleural effusion
Dull	Medium in intensity and pitch, moderate length, thudlike, found over the liver	Solid area as in pleural effusion, mass, or lobar pneumonia
Resonant	Long, loud, low-pitched, hollow	Normal lung tissue, bronchitis
Hyperresonancy	Very loud, lower-pitched, found over the stomach	Hyperinflated lung as in emphysema or pneumothorax
Tympanic	Loud, high-pitched, moderate length, musical, drumlike, found over a puffed-out cheek	Air collection as in a gastric air bubble or air in the intestines, large pneumothorax

---

You may also hear different sounds after certain treatments. For instance, if your patient has atelectasis and you percuss his chest before chest physiotherapy, you'll hear a high-pitched, dull, soft sound. After physiotherapy, you should hear a low-pitched, hollow sound. In all cases, make sure you use other assessment techniques to confirm percussion findings.

You'll hear resonant sounds over normal lung tissue, which you should find over most of the chest. In the left front chest, from the third or fourth intercostal space at the sternum to the third or fourth intercostal space at the midclavicular line, you should hear a dull sound. Percussion is dull here because that's the space occupied by the heart. Resonance resumes at the sixth intercostal space. The sequence of sounds in the back is slightly different. (See *Percussion sequences.*)

 ABNORMAL FINDINGS *Hyperresonance during percussion indicates an area of increased air in the lung or pleural space that's associated with pneumothorax, acute asthma, bullous emphysema (large holes in the lungs from alveolar destruction), and gastric distention that pushes up on the diaphragm. Abnormal dullness during percussion indicates areas of decreased air in the lungs that's associated with pleural fluid, consolidation, atelectasis, or a tumor.*

Movement of the diaphragm

Percussion also allows you to assess how much the diaphragm moves during inspiration and expiration. The normal diaphragm descends 2″ to 2½″ (5 to 6 cm) when the patient inhales.

 ABNORMAL FINDINGS *The diaphragm doesn't move as far in a patient with emphysema, respiratory depression, diaphragm paralysis, atelectasis, obesity, or ascites. (See Measuring diaphragmatic movement, page 156.)*

AUSCULTATING THE CHEST

As air moves through the bronchial tubes, it creates sound waves that travel to the chest wall. The sounds produced by breathing change as air moves from larger air-

KNOW-HOW

Percussion sequences

Follow these percussion sequences to distinguish between normal and abnormal sounds in the patient's lungs. Remember to compare sound variations from one side to the other as you proceed. Carefully describe abnormal sounds you hear and include their locations. You'll follow the same sequences for auscultation.

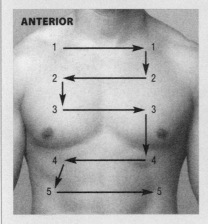

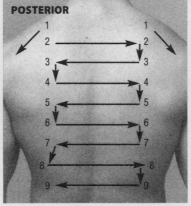

ways to smaller airways. Sounds also change if they pass through fluid, mucus, or narrowed airways.

Auscultation helps you to determine the condition of the alveoli and surrounding pleura.

Preparing to auscultate

Auscultation sites are the same as percussion sites. Listen to a full inspiration and a full expiration at each site, using the diaphragm of the stethoscope. Ask the patient to breathe through his mouth; nose-breathing alters the pitch of breath sounds.

If the patient has abundant chest hair, mat it down with a damp washcloth so the hair doesn't make sounds like crackles.

To auscultate for breath sounds, you'll press the stethoscope firmly against the skin. Remember that if you listen through clothing or dry chest hair, you may hear unusual and deceptive sounds.

Normal breath sounds

You'll hear four types of breath sounds over normal lungs. The type of sound you hear depends on where you listen. (See *Qualities of normal breath sounds*, page 157, and *Locations of normal breath sounds*, page 158.)

✦ Tracheal breath sounds are harsh, high-pitched, and discontinuous sounds heard over the trachea. They occur when a patient inhales or exhales.

✦ Bronchial breath sounds are loud, high-pitched sounds normally heard over the manubrium. They're discontinuous, and they're loudest when the patient exhales.

Auscultating the chest

✦ Helps to determine the condition of the alveoli and surrounding pleura

✦ Detects sound changes as air moves through fluid, mucus, or narrowed airways

Preparing to auscultate

✦ Use same sites as percussion sites

✦ Ask patient to breathe through his mouth

✦ Mat down chest hair so sounds don't resemble crackles

✦ Listen to full inspiration and full expiration at each site

Normal breath sounds

✦ Tracheal — harsh, high-pitched

✦ Bronchial — loud, high-pitched

Measuring diaphragmatic movement

You can measure how much the diaphragm moves by first asking the patient to exhale. Percuss the back on one side to locate the upper edge of the diaphragm, the point at which normal lung resonance changes to dullness. Use a pen to mark the spot indicating the position of the diaphragm at full expiration on that side of the back.

Then ask the patient to inhale as deeply as possible. Percuss the back when the patient has breathed in fully until you locate the diaphragm. Use the pen to mark this spot as well. Repeat on the opposite side of the back.

Use a ruler or tape measure to determine the distance between the marks. The distance, normally 1¼" to 2" (3 to 5 cm) long, should be equal on both the right and left sides.

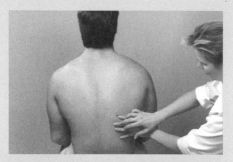

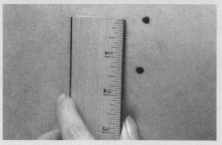

Normal breath sounds
(continued)
✦ Bronchovesicular — medium in loudness and pitch
✦ Vesicular — soft, low-pitched

Abnormal findings
✦ Specific type of breath sound heard in an area where it isn't normally heard
✦ Diminished
✦ Absent
✦ Crackles
✦ Wheezes
✦ Rhonchi
✦ Stridor
✦ Pleural friction rub

✦ Bronchovesicular sounds are medium-pitched, continuous sounds. They're heard when the patient inhales or exhales and are best heard over the upper third of the sternum and between the scapulae.
✦ Vesicular sounds are soft, low-pitched sounds heard over the remainder of the lungs. They're prolonged when the patient inhales and shortened during exhalation in about a 3:1 ratio.

 ABNORMAL FINDINGS If you hear diminished but normal breath sounds in both lungs, the patient may have emphysema, atelectasis, severe bronchospasm, or shallow breathing. If breath sounds are heard in one lung only, the patient may have pleural effusion, pneumothorax, a tumor, or mucus plugs in the airways.

Classify each sound according to its intensity, location, pitch, duration, and characteristic. Note whether the sound occurs when the patient inhales, exhales, or both.

 ABNORMAL FINDINGS If you hear a sound in an area other than where you would expect to hear it, consider the sound abnormal. For instance, bronchial or bronchovesicular breath sounds found in an area where vesicular breath sounds would normally be heard indicates that the alveoli and small bronchioles in that area might be filled with fluid or exudate, as happens in pneumonia and atelectasis. You won't hear vesicular sounds in those areas because no air is moving through the small airways.

A patient with abnormal findings during a respiratory assessment may be further evaluated using such diagnostic tests as arterial blood gas analysis or pulmonary function tests.

Qualities of normal breath sounds

BREATH SOUND	QUALITY	INSPIRATION-EXPIRATION RATIO	LOCATION
Tracheal	Harsh, high-pitched	I about = E	Over trachea
Bronchial	Loud, high-pitched	I < E	Over the manubrium
Bronchovesicular	Medium in loudness and pitch	I = E	Next to sternum, between scapula
Vesicular	Soft, low-pitched	I > E	Over most of both lungs

ABNORMAL FINDINGS *Upon examining your patient, you may hear abnormal breath sounds, including:*
✦ diminished or absent, if a foreign body, pus, fluid, or secretions obstruct a bronchus, over lung tissue located distal to the obstruction
✦ crackles, which are caused by collapsed or fluid-filled alveoli popping open when the patient inhales; classified as either fine or coarse and usually don't clear with coughing (See Types of crackles, page 158.)
✦ wheezes, which are high-pitched sounds heard on exhalation when airflow is blocked (As severity of the block increases, wheezes may also be heard when the patient inhales. The sound of a wheeze doesn't change with coughing. Patients may wheeze as a result of asthma, infection, heart failure, or airway obstruction from a tumor or foreign body.)
✦ rhonchi, which are low-pitched, snoring, rattling sounds heard on exhalation, though they may also be heard on inhalation, change in sound or disappear with coughing when fluid partially blocks the large airways
✦ stridor, which is a loud, high-pitched crowing sound heard (usually without a stethoscope) during inspiration (louder in the neck than over the chest wall) and is caused by an obstruction in the upper airway warrants immediate medical attention
✦ pleural friction rub, which is a low-pitched, grating, rubbing sound heard when the patient inhales and exhales, caused by pleural inflammation of the two layers of pleura rubbing together. (The patient may complain of pain in areas where the rub is heard.)

CLINICAL ALERT Keep in mind these important interventions when assessing your patient's respiratory system:
✦ If your patient is having an acute asthma attack, the absence of wheezing sounds may not mean that the attack is over. When bronchospasm and mucosal swelling become severe, little air can move through the patient's airways. As a result, you won't hear wheezing.
✦ If all other assessment criteria — labored breathing, prolonged expiratory time, accessory muscle use — point to acute bronchial obstruction, maintain the pa-

Alert!
✦ Absence of wheezes may not signal end to acute asthma attack
✦ Wheezing may resume when obstruction begins to resolve

Locations of normal breath sounds

These photographs show the normal locations of different types of breath sounds.

ANTERIOR THORAX

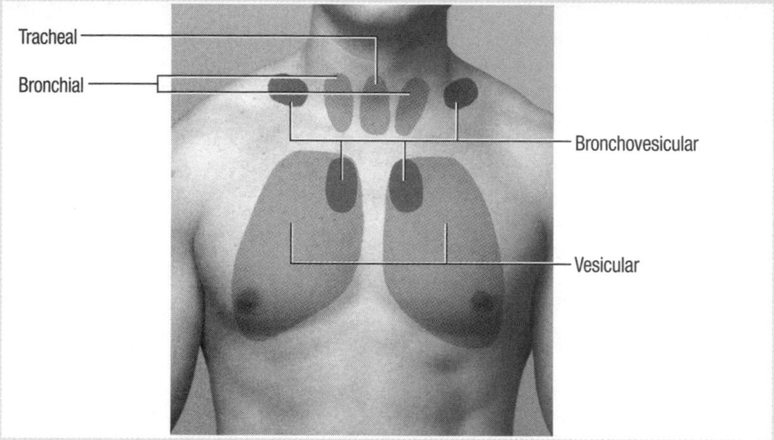

Tracheal
Bronchial
Bronchovesicular
Vesicular

POSTERIOR THORAX

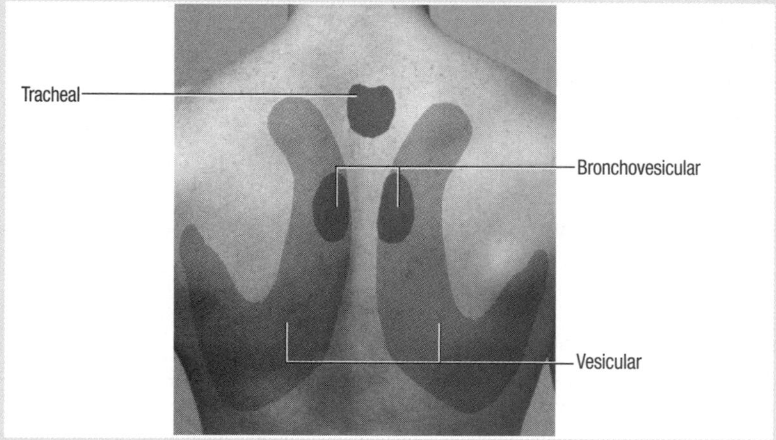

Tracheal
Bronchovesicular
Vesicular

Signs and symptoms of airway obstruction

+ Anxiety, dyspnea, stridor, or wheezes
+ Decreased or absent breath sounds
+ Use of accessory muscles
+ Seesaw movement between chest and abdomen
+ Inability to speak
+ Cyanosis

tient's airway and give oxygen, as ordered. The patient may begin wheezing again when the airways open more.

+ If your patient can't maintain a patent airway, he may end up in respiratory arrest. Refer to this list of potential signs and symptoms when assessing a patient for partial or complete airway obstruction:

+ anxiety
+ dyspnea
+ stridor
+ wheezes
+ decreased or absent breath sounds
+ use of accessory muscles
+ seesaw movement between chest and abdomen

KNOW-HOW

Types of crackles

When assessing the patient's lungs, it's critical to differentiate fine from coarse crackles.

FINE CRACKLES
These characteristics distinguish fine crackles:
+ Occur when the patient stops inhaling and alveoli "pop" open
+ Are usually heard in lung bases
+ Sound like a piece of hair being rubbed between the fingers or like Velcro being pulled apart
+ Occur in restrictive diseases, such as pulmonary fibrosis, asbestosis, silicosis, atelectasis, congestive heart failure, and pneumonia
+ Are soft, high-pitched, and very brief sounds unaffected by coughing

COARSE CRACKLES
These characteristics distinguish coarse crackles:
+ Are somewhat louder, lower in pitch, and not as brief as fine crackles
+ Are heard primarily in the trachea and bronchi
+ Are usually clear or diminish after coughing
+ Occur when the patient starts to inhale; may be present when the patient exhales
+ May be heard through the lungs and even at the mouth
+ Sound more like bubbling or gurgling, as air moves through secretions in larger airways
+ Occur in chronic obstructive pulmonary disease, bronchiectasis, pulmonary edema, and with severely ill patients who can't cough; also called the "death rattle"

+ inability to speak (complete obstruction)
+ cyanosis.

Vocal fremitus
Vocal fremitus is the sound that chest vibrations produce as the patient speaks. Abnormal voice sounds—the most common of which are bronchophony, egophony, and whispered pectoriloquy—may occur over areas that are consolidated. Ask the patient to repeat the words listed beside each abnormal sound, while you listen. Auscultate over an area where you hear vesicular sounds and then again over an area where you hear bronchial breath sounds.

Bronchophony
Ask the patient to say "ninety-nine" or "blue moon". Over normal lung tissue, the words sound muffled. Over consolidated areas, the words sound unusually loud.

Egophony
Ask the patient to say "E". Over normal lung tissue, the sound is muffled. Over consolidated lung tissue, it will sound like the letter a.

Whispered pectoriloquy
Ask the patient to whisper "1, 2, 3". Over normal lung tissue, the numbers will be almost indistinguishable. Over consolidated lung tissue, the numbers will be loud and clear.

Facts about vocal fremitus
+ Sounds that chest vibrations produce as patient speaks
+ Auscultation area includes areas where you hear vesicular sounds and areas where you hear bronchial breath sounds
+ Abnormal sounds include bronchophony, egophony, and whispered pectoriloquy

Bronchophony
+ Ask the patient to say "ninety-nine" or "blue moon"
+ Sound is normally muffled; loud over consolidated tissue

Egophony
+ Ask the patient to say "E"
+ Sound is normally muffled; sounds like "A" over consolidated tissue

Whispered pectoriloquy
+ Ask the patient to whisper "1, 2, 3"
+ Numbers are normally almost indistinguishable; loud and clear over consolidated tissue

INTERPRETING YOUR FINDINGS

Your assessment will reveal a group of findings that may lead you to suspect a particular disorder. (See *The respiratory system: Interpreting your findings.*)

RESPIRATORY SYSTEM DISORDERS

ASTHMA

Asthma is a chronic disorder in which the airways are hyperreactive. The patient will have acute episodes of airway obstruction resulting from bronchospasm, increased mucus secretion, and mucosal edema.

Expect dyspnea, cough, and wheezing with increasing respiratory distress. You'll notice wheezing, exhalation that takes longer and is more strenuous than normal, and accessory muscle use. Intercostal and supraclavicular retraction in inspiration is noticeable. The patient may be anxious, become cyanotic, and complain of chest tightness. You may hear rhonchi if mucus is present. Tactile fremitus is decreased. Percussion is usually hyperresonant. You may detect vocal fremitus, diminished or distant breath sounds, and hyperresonance in the lungs.

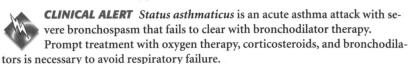 ***CLINICAL ALERT*** *Status asthmaticus* is an acute asthma attack with severe bronchospasm that fails to clear with bronchodilator therapy. Prompt treatment with oxygen therapy, corticosteroids, and bronchodilators is necessary to avoid respiratory failure.

ATELECTASIS

A patient with atelectasis has a section of alveoli or an entire lung that has collapsed from airway obstruction, lack of surfactant (liquid in the alveoli), or compression of the chest wall. Hypoxemia occurs when collapsed tissue can't perform gas exchange, allowing unoxygenated blood to pass through without obtaining oxygen. This is referred to as a *shunt*. Atelectasis may be chronic or acute and commonly occurs to some degree in patients undergoing abdominal or thoracic surgery. The prognosis depends on prompt removal of airway obstruction, relief of hypoxia, and reexpansion of the collapsed lobules or lungs.

Your assessment findings will vary with the cause and degree of hypoxia. You may see decreased chest expansion on the affected side, an increased respiratory rate, dyspnea, cyanosis and, in severe cases, a shift of the trachea toward the affected side. You'll also note a lack of tactile fremitus over the area, dullness in percussion, and decreased or absent breath sounds. Tachycardia and fever are commonly present.

Respiratory system disorders

Facts about asthma

- ✦ Acute episodes of airway obstruction
- ✦ Dyspnea, cough, wheezing, and labored exhalation
- ✦ Anxiety, cyanosis, and chest tightness
- ✦ Rhonchi, decreased tactile fremitus, or hyperresonant percussion
- ✦ Possible vocal fremitus, diminished or distant breath sounds, and hyperresonance in lungs

Alert!

- ✦ Status asthmaticus involves severe bronchospasm
- ✦ Requires prompt treatment with oxygen, corticosteroids, and bronchodilators

Facts about atelectasis

- ✦ Collapse of alveoli or entire lung causing shunting and hypoxemia
- ✦ May cause decreased chest expansion, increased respiratory rate, dyspnea, cyanosis, and tracheal shift
- ✦ Causes lack of tactile fremitus, dullness in percussion, decreased or absent breath sounds, tachycardia, and fever

The respiratory system:
Interpreting your findings

The chart below shows some common groups of findings for signs and symptoms of the respiratory system, along with their probable causes.

SIGN OR SYMPTOM AND FINDINGS	PROBABLE CAUSE
Cough	
◆ Nonproductive cough ◆ Pleuritic chest pain ◆ Dyspnea ◆ Tachypnea ◆ Anxiety ◆ Decreased vocal fremitus ◆ Tracheal deviation toward the affected side	Atelectasis
◆ Productive cough with small amounts of purulent (or mucopurulent), blood-streaked sputum or large amounts of frothy sputum ◆ Dyspnea ◆ Anorexia ◆ Fatigue ◆ Weight loss ◆ Wheezing ◆ Clubbing	Lung cancer
◆ Nonproductive cough ◆ Dyspnea ◆ Pleuritic chest pain ◆ Decreased chest motion ◆ Pleural friction rub ◆ Tachypnea ◆ Tachycardia ◆ Flatness on percussion ◆ Egophony	Pleural effusion
Dyspnea	
◆ Acute dyspnea ◆ Tachypnea ◆ Crackles and rhonchi in both lung fields ◆ Intercostal and suprasternal retractions ◆ Restlessness ◆ Anxiety ◆ Tachycardia	Acute respiratory distress syndrome
◆ Progressive exertional dyspnea ◆ History of smoking ◆ Barrel chest ◆ Accessory muscle hypertrophy ◆ Diminished breath sounds ◆ Pursed-lip breathing ◆ Prolonged expiration ◆ Anorexia ◆ Weight loss	Emphysema

(continued)

The respiratory system:
Interpreting your findings *(continued)*

SIGN OR SYMPTOM AND FINDINGS	PROBABLE CAUSE
Dyspnea (continued)	
◆ Acute dyspnea ◆ Pleuritic chest pain ◆ Tachycardia ◆ Decreased breath sounds ◆ Low-grade fever ◆ Dullness on percussion ◆ Cool, clammy skin	Pulmonary embolism
Hemoptysis	
◆ Sputum ranging in color from pink to dark brown ◆ Productive cough ◆ Dyspnea ◆ Chest pain ◆ Crackles on auscultation ◆ Chills ◆ Fever	Pneumonia
◆ Frothy, blood-tinged pink sputum ◆ Severe dyspnea ◆ Orthopnea ◆ Gasping ◆ Diffuse crackles ◆ Cold, clammy skin ◆ Anxiety	Pulmonary edema
◆ Blood-streaked or blood-tinged sputum ◆ Chronic productive cough ◆ Fine crackles after coughing ◆ Dyspnea ◆ Dullness to percussion ◆ Increased tactile fremitus	Pulmonary tuberculosis
Wheezing	
◆ Sudden onset of wheezing ◆ Stridor ◆ Dry, paroxysmal cough ◆ Gagging ◆ Hoarseness ◆ Decreased breath sounds ◆ Dyspnea ◆ Cyanosis	Aspiration of a foreign body

The respiratory system: Interpreting your findings *(continued)*

SIGN OR SYMPTOM AND FINDINGS	PROBABLE CAUSE
Wheezing (continued)	
✦ Audible wheezing on expiration ✦ Prolonged expiration ✦ Apprehension ✦ Intercostal and supraclavicular retractions ✦ Rhonchi ✦ Nasal flaring ✦ Tachypnea	Asthma
✦ Wheezing ✦ Coarse crackles ✦ Hacking cough that later becomes productive ✦ Dyspnea ✦ Barrel chest ✦ Clubbing ✦ Edema ✦ Weight gain	Chronic bronchitis

CHRONIC BRONCHITIS

In chronic bronchitis, changes in the tracheobronchial tree lead to inflammation, increased mucus production, ciliary damage, and blocked airways. Expect to see dyspnea, chronic cough with sputum production and tachypnea, and accessory muscle use. The lungs will be resonant, and you'll detect normal tactile fremitus. The patient may wheeze.

EMPHYSEMA

In a patient with emphysema, recurrent inflammation of the lungs destroys alveolar walls. Destruction of the alveoli creates large air spaces, decreases the elastic recoil of the lungs, and leads to trapped air and hyperinflated lungs.

Expect shortness of breath, a chronic cough, and possibly a barrel chest. The patient may breathe through pursed lips and use accessory muscles. His fingernails may be clubbed. Tactile fremitus and breath sounds will be decreased. Adventitious breath sounds, including wheezing, may vary. Percussion will be resonant to diffusely hyperresonant. Vocal fremitus will be normal or decreased.

PNEUMONIA

In a patient with pneumonia, an infection in the lungs causes fluid and cell debris to build up in the alveoli, which interferes with gas exchange. Prognosis is usually good for patients who have normal lungs and adequate host defenses before the onset of pneumonia; however bacterial pneumonia is the fifth leading cause of death in debilitated patients.

The patient will be tachypneic and will possibly have pleuritic-type chest pain with guarding and less motion on the affected side, sputum production, fever, and chills. Tactile fremitus is usually increased over the affected areas.

Facts about chronic bronchitis

✦ Inflammation, increased mucus, ciliary damage, and blocked airways
✦ Dyspnea, chronic cough with sputum production and tachypnea, and accessory muscle use
✦ Resonant lungs, tactile fremitus, possible wheezing

Facts about emphysema

✦ Alveolar walls destroyed by recurrent lung inflammation
✦ Shortness of breath, decreased tactile fremitus and breath sounds, chronic cough, barrel chest, and possible pursed-lip breathing, accessory muscle use, and clubbed fingers
✦ Resonant to diffusely hyperresonant percussion
✦ Normal or decreased vocal fremitus

Facts about pneumonia

✦ Lung infection causes fluid and cell debris to build up in alveoli
✦ Prognosis usually good for patients with normal lungs and adequate host defenses before its onset
✦ Tachypnea, pleuritic-type chest pain, increased tactile fremitus

Facts about
pneumonia
(continued)

- Dullness, bronchial breath sounds, and crackles over affected area; increased vocal fremitus

Facts about pleural effusion

- Transudative pleural effusion — increased capillary permeability due to pressure changes
- Exudative pleural effusion — increased capillary permeability with or without pressure changes
- Causes dyspnea, pleural friction rub, pleuritic pain, dry cough, dullness on percussion, tachycardia, tachypnea, and decreased chest motion and breath sounds

Facts about pneumothorax

- Air movement into pleural space causes full or partial lung collapse

Tension pneumothorax

- Air in pleural space under higher pressure than air in adjacent lung and vascular structures
- Fatal without prompt treatment

Spontaneous pneumothorax

- May produce no symptoms in mild cases; profound respiratory distress in moderate to severe cases — weak, rapid pulse; pallor; jugular vein distention; anxiety
- Causes decreased or absent tactile fremitus, vocal fremitus, and breath sounds
- Hyperresonance or tympanic percussion

You may find dullness over the airless area and increased vocal fremitus. Also, expect bronchial breath sounds and crackles over the affected area.

PLEURAL EFFUSION

Pleural effusion results from an excess of fluid in the pleural space. In transudative pleural effusion, excessive hydrostatic pressure or decreased osmotic pressure allows excessive fluid to pass across intact capillaries. In exudative pleural effusion, capillaries exhibit increased permeability, with or without changes in hydrostatic and colloid osmotic pressures, allowing protein-rich fluid to leak into the pleural space.

Assess your patient for these signs and symptoms:

- dyspnea
- pleural friction rub
- possible pleuritic pain that worsens with coughing or deep breathing
- dry cough
- dullness on percussion
- tachycardia
- tachypnea
- decreased chest motion and breath sounds.

PNEUMOTHORAX

In a patient with pneumothorax, air moves into the pleural space and causes collapse of part or all of the lung. The severity of the patient's distress varies with the size of the pneumothorax. With tension pneumothorax, air in the pleural space is under higher pressure than air in the adjacent lung and vascular structures.

 CLINICAL ALERT Unless treated quickly, tension or large-volume pneumothorax results in fatal pulmonary and circulatory impairment.

Spontaneous pneumothorax may produce no symptoms in mild cases, but profound respiratory distress occurs in moderate to severe cases. Weak and rapid pulse, pallor, jugular vein distention, and anxiety indicate tension pneumothorax. In most cases, expect tachypnea, shortness of breath, pleuritic chest pain, cyanosis, decreased chest-wall expansion on the affected side, and possibly tracheal deviation away from the affected side. Tactile fremitus, vocal fremitus, and breath sounds will be decreased or absent over the area. Percussion will reveal hyperresonance or tympanic percussion.

Gastrointestinal system

A LOOK AT THE GI SYSTEM

As the site of the body's digestive processes, the GI system has the critical task of supplying essential nutrients to fuel the brain, heart, and lungs. GI function also profoundly affects the quality of life through its impact on a person's overall health.

The GI system consists of two major components: the alimentary canal and the accessory GI organs. The alimentary canal, or GI tract, consists essentially of a hollow muscular tube that begins in the mouth and extends to the anus. It includes the pharynx, esophagus, stomach, small intestine, and large intestine. Accessory organs aiding GI function include the salivary glands, liver, biliary duct system (gallbladder and bile ducts), and pancreas.

Together, the GI tract and accessory organs serve two major functions: digestion, the breaking down of food and fluid into simple chemicals that can be absorbed into the bloodstream and transported throughout the body, and the elimination of waste products from the body through excretion of stool. (See *Anatomic structures of the GI system*, page 166.)

ANATOMY

The GI tract is a hollow tube that begins at the mouth and ends at the anus. About 25′ (7.5 m) long, the GI tract consists of smooth muscle alternating with blood vessels and nerve tissue. Specialized circular and longitudinal fibers contract, causing peristalsis, which aids in propelling food through the GI tract. The GI tract includes the pharynx, esophagus, stomach, small intestine, and large intestine.

Mouth

Digestive processes begin in the mouth with chewing (mastication), salivating (the beginning of starch digestion), and swallowing (deglutition). The tongue provides the sense of taste. Saliva is produced by three pairs of glands: the parotid, submandibular, and sublingual.

A look at the GI system

+ Supplies essential nutrients to fuel the brain, heart, and lungs
+ Consists of alimentary canal and accessory organs
+ Serves as digestion and elimination

Anatomy

+ Hollow tube begins at mouth and ends at anus, consisting of smooth muscle, alternating with blood vessels and nerve tissue
+ Circular and longitudinal fibers
+ Pharynx, esophagus, stomach, small intestine, large intestine

Facts about the mouth

+ Digestive process begins with chewing, salivating, and swallowing
+ Tongue provides sense of taste
+ Parotid, submandibular, and sublingual glands produce saliva

Anatomic structures of the GI system

This illustration shows the GI system's major anatomic structures. Knowing these structures will help you conduct an accurate physical assessment.

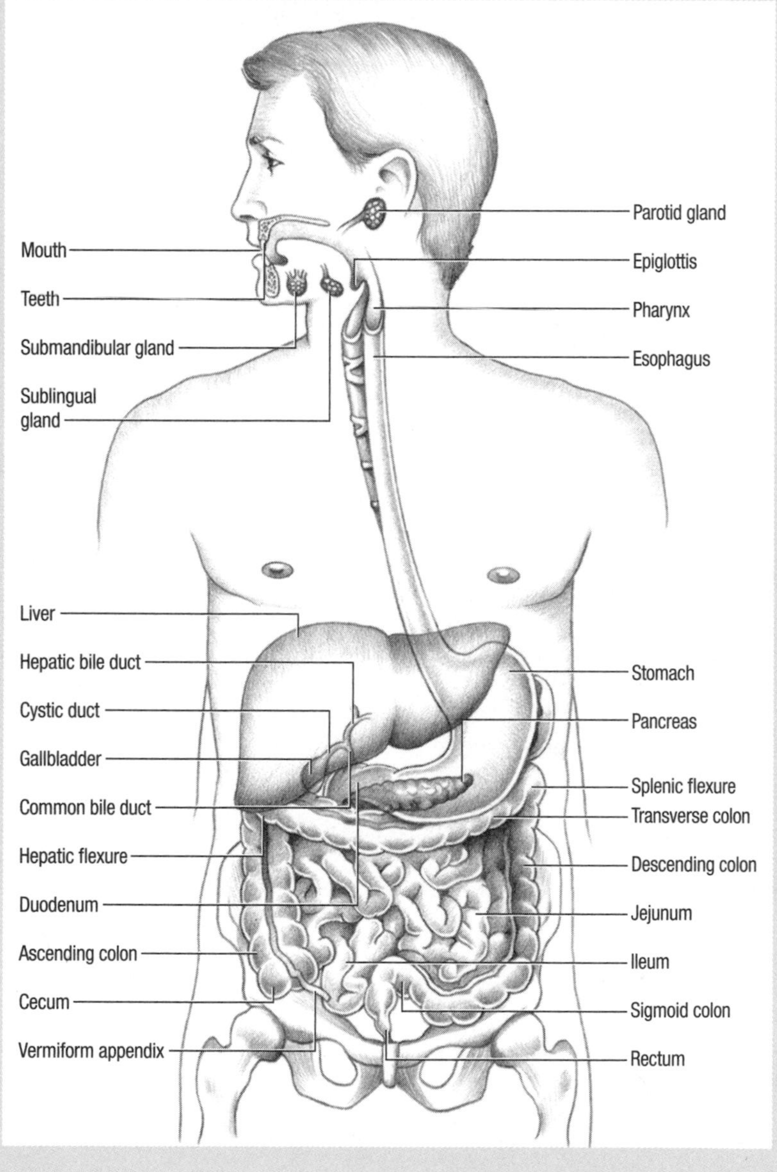

Labels (left side): Mouth, Teeth, Submandibular gland, Sublingual gland, Liver, Hepatic bile duct, Cystic duct, Gallbladder, Common bile duct, Hepatic flexure, Duodenum, Ascending colon, Cecum, Vermiform appendix

Labels (right side): Parotid gland, Epiglottis, Pharynx, Esophagus, Stomach, Pancreas, Splenic flexure, Transverse colon, Descending colon, Jejunum, Ileum, Sigmoid colon, Rectum

Facts about the pharynx

+ Allows passage of food from mouth to esophagus
+ Secretes mucus that aids in digestion
+ Includes epiglottis, which keeps food and fluid from being aspirated into the airway

Pharynx

The pharynx, or throat, allows the passage of food from the mouth to the esophagus. The pharynx assists in the swallowing process and secretes mucus that aids in digestion. The epiglottis — a thin, leaf-shaped structure made of fibrocartilage — is located directly behind the root of the tongue. When food is swallowed, the epiglottis closes over the larynx, and the soft palate lifts to block the nasal cavity. These actions keep food and fluid from being aspirated into the airway.

Esophagus

The esophagus is a muscular, hollow tube about 10″ (25.5 cm) long that moves food from the pharynx to the stomach. When food is swallowed, the upper esophageal sphincter relaxes, and the food moves into the esophagus. Peristalsis then propels the food toward the stomach. The gastroesophageal sphincter at the lower end of the esophagus normally remains closed to prevent reflux of gastric contents. The sphincter opens during swallowing, belching, and vomiting. As food moves through the esophagus, glands in the esophageal mucosal layer secrete mucus, which lubricates the bolus and protects the esophageal mucosal layer from being damaged by poorly chewed foods.

Stomach

The stomach, a reservoir for food, is a dilated, saclike structure that lies obliquely in the left upper quadrant below the esophagus and diaphragm, to the right of the spleen, and partly under the liver. The stomach contains two important sphincters: the cardiac sphincter, which protects the entrance to the stomach, and the pyloric sphincter, which guards the exit.

The stomach has three major functions. It:
+ stores food
+ mixes food with gastric juices (hydrochloride acid)
+ parcels food into the small intestine for further digestion and absorption.

Except for alcohol, little food absorption normally occurs in the stomach. Peristaltic contractions churn the food into tiny particles and mix it with gastric juices, forming a thick, almost liquid food bolus known as *chyme*. After mixing, stronger peristaltic waves move the chyme into the antrum, where it's backed up against the pyloric sphincter before being released into the duodenum, triggering the intestinal phase of digestion.

The rate of stomach emptying depends on a complex interplay of factors, including gastrin release and neural signals caused by stomach wall distention and the enterogastric reflex. In this reaction, the duodenum releases secretin and gastric-inhibiting peptide, and the jejunum secretes cholecystokinin—all of which act to decrease gastric motility.

An average meal can remain in the stomach for 3 to 4 hours. Rugae, accordion-like folds in the stomach lining, allow the stomach to expand when large amounts of food and fluid are ingested.

Small intestine

The small intestine performs most of the work of digestion and absorption. It's about 20′ (6.1 m) long and is named for its diameter, not its length. It has three sections: the duodenum, the jejunum, and the ileum. As chyme passes into the small intestine, the end products of digestion are absorbed through its thin mucous membrane lining into the bloodstream.

Carbohydrates, fats, and proteins are broken down in the small intestine. Enzymes from the pancreas, bile from the liver, and hormones from glands of the small intestine all aid digestion. These secretions mix with the chyme as it moves through the intestines. Chyme passes through the small intestine by peristalsis.

Large intestine

The large intestine, or colon, is about 5′ (1.5 m) long and is responsible for:
+ absorbing excess water and electrolytes
+ storing food residue

Facts about the esophagus

+ Muscular, hollow tube; moves food from pharynx to stomach
+ Upper esophageal sphincter relaxes when food is swallowed
+ Peristalsis propels food toward stomach
+ Gastroesophageal sphincter opens during swallowing, belching, and vomiting
+ Glands secrete mucus, which lubricate bolus, preventing damage from poorly chewed foods

Facts about the stomach

+ Dilated, saclike structure serves as a reservoir for food
+ Contains cardiac sphincter and pyloric sphincter
+ Mixes food with gastric juices to form chyme, which then moves into antrum, then the duodenum for further digestion
+ Rugae, accordion-like folds in the lining, allow expansion

Facts about the small intestine

+ Performs most of the work of digestion and absorption
+ Includes duodenum, jejunum, and ileum
+ Absorbs end products of food digestion
+ Breaks down carbohydrates, fats, and proteins using enzymes, bile, and hormones
+ Peristalsis moves chyme through

Facts about the large intestine

+ Absorbs excess water and electrolytes
+ Stores food residue

Facts about the large intestine
(continued)

+ Eliminates waste products in the form of feces
+ Chyme has been reduced to indigestible substances by the time it enters large intestine
+ The bolus travels through the large intestine, eventually arriving at the anal canal
+ Through blood and lymph vessels, the intestine absorbs water as well as sodium and chloride
+ Bacteria synthesizes vitamin K and breaks down cellulose into useable carbohydrate, producing flatus
+ Alkaline mucus lubricates intestinal walls as food pushes through to lower colon for elimination

Physiology

+ Accessory organs include the liver, bile ducts, gallbladder, and pancreas

Facts about the liver

+ Metabolizes carbohydrates, fats, and proteins
+ Detoxifies blood
+ Converts ammonia to urea

+ eliminating waste products in the form of feces.

By the time chyme passes through the small intestine and enters the ascending colon of the large intestine, it has been reduced to mostly indigestible substances.

The bolus begins its journey through the large intestine at the juncture of the ileum and cecum with the ileocecal pouch. Then the bolus moves up the ascending colon past the right abdominal cavity to the liver's lower border, crosses horizontally below the liver and stomach via the transverse colon, and descends the left abdominal cavity to the iliac fossa through the descending colon.

From there, the bolus travels through the sigmoid colon to the lower midline of the abdominal cavity, then to the rectum, and finally to the anal canal. The anus opens to the exterior through two sphincters. The internal anal sphincter contains thick, circular smooth muscle under autonomic control. The external sphincter contains skeletal muscle under voluntary control.

Circular and longitudinal fibers of the tunica muscularis move and mix intestinal contents, and the longitudinal muscle gives the large intestine its familiar shape. These fibers gather into three narrow bands (teniae coli) down the middle of the colon and pucker the intestine into characteristic pouches (haustra coli).

The ascending and descending colons attach directly to the posterior abdominal wall for support. The transverse and sigmoid colons attach indirectly through sheets of connective tissue (mesocolon).

Although the large intestine produces no hormones or digestive enzymes, it continues the absorptive process. Through blood and lymph vessels in the submucosa, the proximal half of the intestine absorbs all but about 100 ml of the remaining water in the colon plus large amounts of sodium and chloride. The large intestine also harbors the bacteria *Escherichia coli, Enterobacter aerogenes, Clostridium welchii,* and *Lactobacillus bifidus,* which help synthesize vitamin K and break down cellulose into usable carbohydrate. Bacterial action also produces flatus, which helps propel stool toward the rectum. In addition, the mucosa produces alkaline secretions from tubular glands composed of goblet cells. This alkaline mucus lubricates the intestinal walls as food pushes through and protects the mucosa from acidic bacterial action.

In the lower colon, long and relatively sluggish contractions cause propulsive waves known as *mass movements.* These movements, which normally occur several times a day, propel intestinal contents into the rectum and produce the urge to defecate. Defecation normally results from the defecation reflex, a sensory and parasympathetic nerve-mediated response, along with the person's relaxation of the external anal sphincter.

PHYSIOLOGY

Accessory organs

Accessory GI organs include the liver, bile ducts, gallbladder, and pancreas. The abdominal aorta and the gastric and splenic veins also aid the GI system.

Liver

The liver is located in the right upper quadrant under the diaphragm. It has two major lobes, divided by the falciform ligament. The liver is the heaviest organ in the body, weighing about 3 lbs (1.5 kg) in the adult.

The liver's functions include:

+ metabolizing carbohydrates, fats, and proteins
+ detoxifying blood
+ converting ammonia to urea for excretion

✦ synthesizing plasma proteins, nonessential amino acids, vitamin A, and essential nutrients, such as iron and vitamins D, K, and B$_{12}$.

The liver metabolizes digestive end products by regulating blood glucose levels. When glucose is being absorbed through the intestine (anabolic state), the liver stores glucose as glycogen. When glucose isn't being absorbed or when blood glucose levels fall (catabolic state), the liver mobilizes glucose to restore blood levels necessary for brain function.

The liver also secretes bile, a greenish fluid that helps digest fats and absorb fatty acids, cholesterol, and other lipids. Bile also gives stool its color.

The bile ducts provide a passageway for bile to travel from the liver to the intestines. Two hepatic ducts drain the liver and the cystic duct drains the gallbladder. These ducts converge into the common bile duct, which then empties into the duodenum.

Function of bile

A greenish liquid composed of water, cholesterol, bile salts, electrolytes, and phospholipids, bile is important in fat emulsification (breakdown) and intestinal absorption of fatty acids, cholesterol, and other lipids. When bile salts are absent from the intestinal tract, lipids are excreted and fat-soluble vitamins are absorbed poorly. Bile also aids in excretion of conjugated bilirubin (an end product of hemoglobin degradation) from the liver and thereby prevents jaundice.

The liver recycles about 80% of bile salts into bile, combining them with bile pigments (biliverdin and bilirubin — the breakdown products of red blood cells [RBCs]) and cholesterol. The liver produces about 500 ml of this alkaline bile in continuous secretion. Enhanced bile production can result from vagal stimulation, release of the hormone secretin, increased liver blood flow, and the presence of fat in the intestine.

Function of the lobule

The liver's functional unit, the lobule, consists of a plate of hepatic cells (hepatocytes) that encircle a central vein and radiate outward. The plates of hepatocytes are separated from one another by sinusoids, the liver's capillary system. Lining the sinusoids are reticuloendothelial macrophages (Kupffer's cells), which remove bacteria and toxins that have entered the blood through the intestinal capillaries.

The sinusoids carry oxygenated blood from the hepatic artery and nutrient-rich blood from the portal vein. Unoxygenated blood leaves through the central vein and flows through hepatic veins to the inferior vena cava. Bile, recycled from bile salts in the blood, leaves through bile ducts (canaliculi) that merge into the right and left hepatic ducts to form the common hepatic duct. This common duct joins the cystic duct from the gallbladder to form the common bile duct to the duodenum.

Gallbladder

The gallbladder, a 3″ to 4″ (7.5- to 10-cm) long, pear-shaped organ, is joined to the liver's ventral surface by the cystic duct. It stores and concentrates bile produced by the liver. Its 30- to 50-ml storage load increases up to tenfold in potency. Secretion of the hormone cholecystokinin causes gallbladder contraction and relaxation of the sphincter of Oddi, releasing bile into the common bile duct for delivery to the duodenum. When the sphincter closes, bile shunts to the gallbladder for storage.

Pancreas

The pancreas, which measures 6″ to 8″ (15 to 20.5 cm) in length, lies horizontally in the abdomen, behind the stomach. It consists of a head, tail, and body. The head of

---

Facts about the liver
(continued)

✦ Synthesizes plasma proteins, nonessential amino acids, vitamin A, and essential nutrients
✦ Metabolizes digestive end products by regulating blood glucose levels
✦ Secretes bile

Function of bile

✦ Emulsifies fat and aids intestinal absorption of fatty acids, cholesterol, and other lipids
✦ Aids in excretion of conjugated bilirubin from liver

Function of the lobule

✦ Consists of a plate of hepatic cells that encircle a central vein and radiate outward
✦ Kupffer's cells lining the sinusoids remove bacteria and toxins that have entered the blood through the intestinal capillaries
✦ Sinusoids carry oxygenated blood from hepatic artery and nutrient-rich blood from portal vein; unoxygenated blood leaves via central vein to inferior vena cava

Facts about the gallbladder

✦ Joins liver's ventral surface by cystic duct
✦ Stores and concentrates bile produced by liver
✦ Releases bile for delivery to duodenum

Facts about the pancreas

✦ Consists of head, tail, and body

Facts about the pancreas
(continued)

+ Performs both exocrine and endocrine functions
+ Secretes over 1,000 ml of digestive enzymes daily
+ Islets of Langerhans secrete glucagon and insulin

Facts about the vascular structures

+ Abdominal aorta — supplies blood to GI tract
+ Gastric and splenic veins — drain absorbed nutrients into portal vein of the liver

Obtaining a health history

+ Tracks the development of relevant signs and symptoms over time
+ Includes chief complaint, current and past health, body system review, and family and psychosocial history

Exploring the chief complaint

+ Ask about onset, duration, location, quality, frequency, and severity
+ Pain, heartburn, nausea, vomiting, and altered bowel habits

the pancreas is located in the right upper quadrant; the tail, in the left upper quadrant, is attached to the duodenum and touches the spleen.

The pancreas performs both exocrine and endocrine functions. Its exocrine function involves scattered cells that secrete more than 1,000 ml of digestive enzymes daily. Lobules and lobes of the clusters (acini) of enzyme-producing cells release their secretions into ducts that merge into the pancreatic duct. The pancreatic duct runs the length of the pancreas and joins the bile duct from the gallbladder before entering the duodenum. Vagal stimulation and release of the hormones secretin and cholecystokinin control the rate and amount of pancreatic secretion.

The endocrine function of the pancreas involves the islets of Langerhans, which are located between the acinar cells. Over one million of these islets house two cell types: Alpha cells secrete glucagon, which stimulates glycogenolysis in the liver; beta cells secrete insulin to promote carbohydrate metabolism. Both hormones flow directly into the blood; their release is stimulated by blood glucose levels.

Vascular structures

The abdominal aorta supplies blood to the GI tract. It enters the abdomen, separates into the common iliac arteries, and then branches into many arteries extending the length of the GI tract.

The gastric and splenic veins drain absorbed nutrients into the portal vein of the liver. After entering the liver, the venous blood circulates and then exits the liver through the hepatic vein, emptying into the inferior vena cava.

OBTAINING A HEALTH HISTORY

GI signs and symptoms can have many baffling causes. For instance, if your patient is vomiting, what does this sign mean? The patient could be pregnant, could have a viral infection or, possibly, could have a severe metabolic disorder such as hyperkalemia. Maybe the patient merely has indigestion — or maybe a cardiac crisis is building.

To help track the development of relevant signs and symptoms over time, you'll need to develop a detailed patient history. The history includes the patient's chief complaint, present and previous illnesses, a review of all body systems, and family and social history. For best results, establish rapport with the patient by using your best communication skills. Conduct this part of the assessment as privately as possible; many patients feel embarrassed to talk about GI functions. Speak softly so that others won't overhear the discussion.

If your patient has a hearing problem, perform the assessment in a private area or at a time when his roommate is out of the room. If the patient is in pain, help him into a comfortable position before asking questions.

CHIEF COMPLAINT

If your patient has a GI problem, he'll usually complain about pain, heartburn, nausea, vomiting, or altered bowel habits. To investigate these and other signs and symptoms, ask him about the onset, duration, location, quality, frequency, and severity of each.

Ask the patient why he's seeking care and record his words verbatim. Ask when he first noticed symptoms, keeping in mind that his answer may indicate only how long the symptoms have been intolerable, not necessarily their true duration. Clarify this point with the patient.

Assessing abdominal pain

If your patient complains of abdominal pain, ask him to describe the type of pain he's experiencing and how and when it started. This table will help you assess the patient's pain and determine the possible causes.

TYPE OF PAIN	PROBABLE CAUSE
Burning	Peptic ulcer, gastroesophageal reflux disease
Cramping	Biliary colic, irritable bowel syndrome, diarrhea, constipation, flatulence
Severe cramping	Appendicitis, Crohn's disease, diverticulitis
Stabbing	Pancreatitis, cholecystitis

Knowing what precipitates and relieves the patient's symptoms will help you perform a more accurate physical assessment and better plan your care. (See *Assessing abdominal pain*.) Abdominal pain arises from the abdominopelvic viscera, the parietal peritoneum, or the capsules of the liver, kidney, or spleen, and may be acute or chronic, diffuse, or localized.

Types of abdominal pain

Several types of abdominal pain exist, including:

✦ visceral — pain that develops slowly into a deep, dull, aching pain that's poorly localized in the epigastric, periumbilical, or hypogastric region.

✦ somatic (parietal or peritoneal) — pain that produces sharp, more intense, and well-localized discomfort that rapidly follows the attack. Movement or coughing aggravates this pain.

✦ referred — pain that occurs from another site with the same or similar nerve supply. This sharp, well-localized, pain is felt in skin or deeper tissues and may coexist with skin hyperesthesia and muscle hyperalgesia.

✦ inflammatory — pain that's associated with such disorders as ulcers, intestinal obstruction, appendicitis, cholecystitis, or peritonitis. (For example, a duodenal ulcer can cause gnawing abdominal pain in the midepigastrium 1½ to 3 hours after eating and may even awaken the patient; antacids or food may relieve it.)

✦ other — pain that occurs from stretching or tension of the gut wall, traction on the peritoneum or mesentery, vigorous intestinal contraction, ischemia, and sensory nerve irritation.

 SPECIAL POINTS *Because many children have difficulty describing abdominal pain, pay close attention to such nonverbal cues as wincing, lethargy, or unusual positioning (for example, a side-lying position with knees flexed to the abdomen). Observing the child while he coughs, walks, or climbs may offer some diagnostic clues. Also, remember that a parent's description of the child's complaints is a subjective interpretation of what the parent believes is wrong.*

In children, abdominal pain can signal a disorder with greater severity or different associated signs than in adults. For example:

✦ *Appendicitis has a higher rupture rate and mortality in children, and vomiting may be the only other sign.*

✦ *Acute pyelonephritis may cause abdominal pain, vomiting, and diarrhea, but not*

Types of abdominal pain

✦ Visceral — deep, dull, aching; poorly localized
✦ Somatic (parietal or peritoneal) — sharp, intense, and well-localized discomfort
✦ Referred — from another site with same or similar nerve supply
✦ Inflammatory — associated with ulcers, intestinal obstruction, appendicitis, cholecystitis, or peritonitis
✦ Other — occurs from stretching or tension of gut wall, traction on peritoneum or mesentery, intestinal contraction, ischemia, and sensory nerve irritation

Special points: Abdominal pain in children

✦ Disclosed by wincing, fatigue, or unusual positions
✦ Diagnostic clues revealed by observing coughing, walking, or climbing
✦ Know that parent's description is subjective
✦ May signal disorders with greater severity or different associated signs than in adults

the classic urologic signs found in adults.

✦ *Peptic ulcer, which is becoming increasingly common in teenagers, causes nocturnal pain and colic that, unlike peptic ulcer in adults, may not be relieved by food.*

  Abdominal pain in children can also result from:

✦ *lactose intolerance*

✦ *allergic-tension-fatigue syndrome*

✦ *volvulus*

✦ *Meckel's diverticulum*

✦ *intussusception*

✦ *mesenteric adenitis*

✦ *diabetes mellitus*

✦ *juvenile rheumatoid arthritis*

✦ *heavy metal poisoning (uncommon)*

✦ *an emotional need, such as a wish to avoid school or to gain adult attention.*

CURRENT HEALTH HISTORY

The current health history describes information relevant to the chief complaint.
To establish a baseline for comparison, ask the patient about his present state of
health. Concentrate on the:

✦ onset — How did the problem start? Was it gradual or sudden, with or without
previous symptoms? What was the patient doing when he first noticed it?

✦ duration — When did the problem start? Has the patient had the problem before? If he's in pain, find out when the problem began. Is the pain continuous, intermittent, or colicky (cramplike)?

✦ quality — Ask the patient to describe the problem. Has he had it before? Was it
diagnosed? If he's in pain, find out whether the pain feels sharp, dull, aching, or
burning.

✦ severity — Ask the patient to describe how badly the problem bothers him, for
example, have him rate it on a scale of 1 to 10. Does it keep him from his normal
activities? Has it improved or worsened since he first noticed it? Does it wake him
at night? If he's in pain, does he double over from it?

✦ location — Where does the patient feel the problem? Does it spread, radiate, or
shift? Ask him to point to where he feels it most. Does he feel any pain in his shoulder, back, flank, or groin? Keep in mind pain may be referred near or far from its
origin. (See *Identifying areas of referred pain.*)

  Next, ask the patient to characterize his symptoms. Have him describe:

✦ precipitating factors — Does anything seem to bring on the problem? What
makes it worse? Does it occur at the same time each day or with certain positions?
Does the patient notice it after eating or drinking certain foods or after certain activities?

✦ alleviating factors — Does anything relieve the problem? Does the patient take
any prescribed or over-the-counter (OTC) medications for relief? Has he tried anything else for relief?

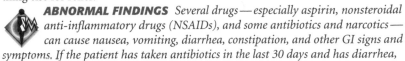 ***ABNORMAL FINDINGS*** *Several drugs — especially aspirin, nonsteroidal
anti-inflammatory drugs (NSAIDs), and some antibiotics and narcotics —
can cause nausea, vomiting, diarrhea, constipation, and other GI signs and
symptoms. If the patient has taken antibiotics in the last 30 days and has diarrhea,
suspect* Clostridium difficile *infection.*

✦ associated symptoms — What else bothers the patient when he has the problem?
Has he had nausea, vomiting, dry heaves? Has he seen blood in his vomitus? (If so,
this could indicate duodenal or peptic ulcer, esophageal or gastric varices, or gastri-
tis.)

Current health history

✦ Onset — how did the problem
start?

✦ Duration — when did it start?

✦ Quality — how would he describe it

✦ Severity — how would he describe its severity?

✦ Location — where does the patient feel it?

✦ Precipitating factors — what
seems to bring it on?

✦ Alleviating factors — what alleviates it?

✦ Associated symptoms — what
else bothers it?

Abnormal findings

✦ Aspirin, NSAIDs, antibiotics, and
narcotics can cause nausea,
vomiting, diarrhea, and constipation

✦ *Clostridium difficile* infection
may be causing diarrhea

KNOW-HOW

Identifying areas of referred pain

Pain may occur relatively near its source or distant from it. These illustrations will help you identify the areas and causes of referred pain.

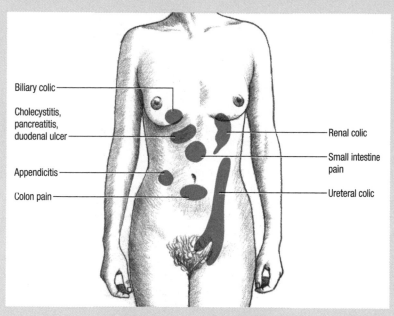

Biliary colic

Cholecystitis, pancreatitis, duodenal ulcer

Appendicitis

Colon pain

Renal colic

Small intestine pain

Ureteral colic

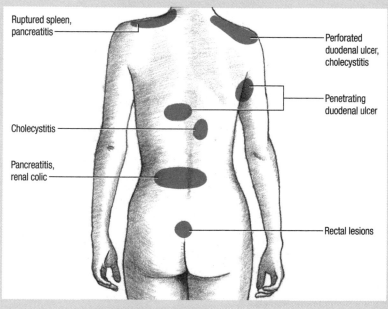

Ruptured spleen, pancreatitis

Cholecystitis

Pancreatitis, renal colic

Perforated duodenal ulcer, cholecystitis

Penetrating duodenal ulcer

Rectal lesions

Current health history
(continued)

Abnormal findings: Nausea and vomiting

+ Occur with fluid and electrolyte imbalance; infection; metabolic, endocrine, labyrinthine, and cardiac disorders; certain drugs; and surgery or radiation therapy
+ May arise from severe pain, anxiety, alcohol intoxication, overeating, or ingestion of distasteful food or liquid

Special points: Nausea

+ Often described as stomachache in children
+ Pyloric obstruction may cause projectile vomiting in neonates
+ Intussusception may lead to bile and fecal vomiting in infants or toddlers
+ Intestinal ischemia common in elderly patients

Abnormal findings: Diarrhea

+ May result from ingestion of contaminated food or water
+ Acute infection, stress, fecal impaction, and certain drugs are possible causes
+ Chronic infection, obstructive or inflammatory bowel disease, malabsorption syndrome, endocrine disorders, or GI surgery also may be causes

Special points: Diarrhea

+ In children, commonly results from infection
+ In elderly patients, consider ischemia before Crohn's disease

Abnormal findings: Constipation

+ Caused by immobility, sedentary lifestyle, habitual laxative use, medications, or IBS
+ Complete intestinal obstruction signaled by absence of flatus, stool, or bowel sounds

 ABNORMAL FINDINGS *Nausea and vomiting, common indications of a GI disorder, also occur with fluid and electrolyte imbalance; infection; metabolic, endocrine, labyrinthine, and cardiac disorders; use of certain drugs; surgery; and radiation. Nausea and vomiting can be caused by existing illnesses, such as myocardial infarction, gastric and peritoneal irritation, appendicitis, bowel obstruction, cholecystitis, acute pancreatitis, and neurologic disturbances.*

Commonly present during the first trimester of pregnancy, nausea and vomiting may also arise from severe pain, anxiety, alcohol intoxication, overeating, or ingestion of distasteful food or liquid.

 SPECIAL POINTS *In children, nausea—often described as stomachache—is one of the most common complaints. It can result from overeating or from any of several diverse disorders, ranging from an acute infection to a conversion reaction caused by fear.*

In neonates, pyloric obstruction may cause projectile vomiting, whereas Hirschsprung's disease may cause fecal vomiting. Intussusception may lead to vomiting of bile and fecal matter in an infant or toddler. Because a neonate may aspirate vomitus as a result of immature cough and gag reflexes, position him on his side or abdomen, and clear any vomitus immediately.

Elderly patients have increased dental caries; tooth loss; decreased salivary gland function, which causes mouth dryness; decreased gastric acid output and motility; and decreased sense of taste and smell. All of these can contribute to nonpathologic nausea. However, intestinal ischemia, which is common in this age-group, should always be ruled out as a potential cause for nausea and vomiting.

+ If the patient's chief complaint is diarrhea, find out if he recently traveled abroad.

 ABNORMAL FINDINGS *Diarrhea as well as hepatitis and parasitic infections can result from ingesting contaminated food or water. Acute diarrhea may also result from acute infection, stress, fecal impaction, or use of certain drugs. Chronic diarrhea may result from chronic infection, obstructive or inflammatory bowel disease, malabsorption syndrome, an endocrine disorder, or GI surgery. Periodic diarrhea may result from food intolerance or from ingestion of spicy or high-fiber foods or caffeine.*

Toxins, medications, or a GI disorder, such as Crohn's disease, can cause diarrhea. Cramping, abdominal tenderness, anorexia, and hyperactive bowel sounds may accompany diarrhea. If fever occurs, the diarrhea may be caused by a toxin. One or more pathophysiologic mechanisms may contribute to diarrhea, and the fluid and electrolyte imbalances it produces may precipitate life-threatening arrhythmias or hypovolemic shock.

 SPECIAL POINTS *Diarrhea in children commonly results from infection, although chronic diarrhea may be a sign of malabsorption syndrome, an anatomic defect, or allergies. Because dehydration and electrolyte imbalance occur rapidly in children, diarrhea can be life-threatening. Diligently monitor all episodes of diarrhea in this patient-group, and replace fluids immediately. In the elderly patient with new-onset segmental colitis, always consider ischemia before labeling the patient as having Crohn's disease.*

+ Is the patient complaining of constipation?

ABNORMAL FINDINGS *Constipation can be caused by immobility, a sedentary lifestyle, habitual laxative use, and certain medications, especially in older patients. The patient may complain of a dull ache in the abdomen, a full feeling, and hyperactive bowel sounds, which may be caused by irritable bowel syndrome (IBS). A patient with complete intestinal obstruction won't pass flatus or stool and won't have bowel sounds below the obstruction.*

✦ Ask about changes in bowel habits. When was the patient's last bowel movement? Was it unusual? Has the patient's stool changed in size or color or included mucus? Has he ever seen blood in his stool?

 ABNORMAL FINDINGS *Although hematochezia (blood in the stool) is commonly associated with GI disorders, it may also result from a coagulation disorder, exposure to toxins, or a diagnostic test. Always a significant sign, hematochezia may precipitate life-threatening hypovolemia.*

 SPECIAL POINTS *Hematochezia is much less common in children than in adults; however, when it does occur in children, it may result from a structural disorder, such as intussusception or Meckel's diverticulum, or from inflammatory disorders, such as peptic ulcer disease or ulcerative colitis. In children, ulcerative colitis typically produces chronic, rather than acute, signs and symptoms and may also cause slow growth and maturation related to malnutrition. Suspect sexual abuse in all cases of rectal bleeding in children.*

Because elderly patients are at increased risk for colon cancer, hematochezia should be evaluated with a colonoscopy after perirectal lesions have been ruled out as the cause of bleeding.

✦ Has the patient lost his appetite or lost any weight? Does he have excessive belching or passing of gas? Has he been drinking excessively? Can he eat normally and hold down foods and liquids, or does he have difficulty chewing or swallowing?

 ABNORMAL FINDINGS *Dysphagia, or difficulty in swallowing, may be accompanied by weight loss. It can be caused by an obstruction, achalasia of the lower esophagogastric junction, or a neurologic disease, such as stroke or Parkinson's disease. Dysphagia can lead to aspiration and pneumonia.*

PAST HEALTH HISTORY

Ask the patient whether he has had similar symptoms before. If so, did he seek medical attention? What was the medical diagnosis and treatment, if any? Has he had any major acute or chronic illnesses requiring hospitalization? Note the course of the illness, treatment, and any consequences. Record surgeries in chronological order and briefly describe them. Also ask about allergies, chronic diseases, possible genetic or environmental causes, GI disorders, lifestyle, and medications.

Allergies
Ask the patient whether he's allergic to any drugs, foods, or other agents. If so, have him describe his reaction.

Chronic diseases
Has the patient had cardiac or renal disease, diabetes mellitus, or cancer?

Genetic or environmental factors
Have the patient's family, friends, or coworkers had symptoms similar to his?

GI disorders
Ask about past GI illnesses, such as an ulcer; liver, pancreas, or gallbladder disease; inflammatory bowel disease; hiatal hernia; IBS; diverticulosis or diverticulitis; gastroesophageal reflux disease (GERD); hemorrhoids; cancer; or GI bleeding. Also, ask if he has had rectal or abdominal surgery or trauma.

Lifestyle
Ask whether the patient exercises. Also ask whether he drinks coffee, tea, or other caffeinated beverages such as colas. Does he smoke? If he does, how much each day? For how many years?

Ask the patient what he has had to eat and drink in the last 24 hours and explore his usual eating habits. Some GI problems can result from certain diets or eating patterns. Ask about any late-night eating or habitually large meals. Because lack of dietary fiber (roughage) may contribute to colorectal cancer and diverticular disease, find out about the patient's fiber intake.

Medications

Record all prescribed and OTC medications the patient has taken and note their dosages and amounts, if known. *Important:* Many patients won't mention OTC preparations unless you specifically ask. However, some OTC medications, such as ibuprofen or aspirin (or those containing aspirin), herbal remedies, and vitamins, can have GI effects. For instance, vitamins with iron may turn stool black.

Ask about illicit drug use and alcohol consumption. Remain tactful and nonjudgmental so the patient doesn't become defensive and give inaccurate answers.

FAMILY HISTORY

Questioning the patient about his family may reveal environmental, genetic, or familial illnesses that may influence his current health problems and needs. Ask about the general health of his immediate relatives and spouse. If the patient's diagnoses or suspected illness has possible familial or genetic tendencies, find out whether family members have had similar problems.

Disorders with a familial link include:
+ ulcerative colitis
+ colorectal cancer
+ peptic ulcers
+ gastric cancer
+ alcoholism.
+ Crohn's disease.

 SPECIAL POINTS *When taking a health history, consider your patient's ethnic background. For instance, patients from Japan, Iceland, Chile, and Austria die more of gastric cancer than patients from other countries. Also, Crohn's disease is more common in Jewish patients.*

PSYCHOSOCIAL HISTORY

Psychological and sociologic factors as well as physical environment can profoundly affect health. To find out whether such factors have contributed to your patient's problem, ask about his occupation, family size, cohabitants, and home environment. Has the patient been exposed to occupational or environmental hazards? Does he dislike his job? Duodenal ulcers arise more commonly in individuals with marked stress or job responsibility; gastric ulcers, in laborers. Inquire about the patient's history of blood transfusions and tattoos.

Assess the patient's financial status. Inadequate resources can add to the stress of being ill and exacerbate the underlying problem.

When talking to the patient, assess his cognition and comprehension levels to help determine his health education needs. Does he understand the importance of appropriate treatment?

Past health history
(continued)

Medications
+ Record all prescribed and OTC medications
+ Ask about herbal remedies, vitamins, illicit drug use, and alcohol consumption

Family history
+ Ulcerative colitis
+ Colorectal and gastric cancer
+ Peptic ulcer
+ Alcoholism
+ Crohn's disease

Special points
+ Consider ethnic background
+ Know that patients from Japan, Iceland, Chile, and Austria die more of gastric cancer
+ Crohn's disease more common in Jewish patients

Psychosocial history
+ Identifies occupation and exposure to hazard
+ Finds out about family, cohabitants, and home environment
+ Reveals history of blood transfusions and tattoos
+ Elicits financial status
+ Establishes comprehension levels in determining health education needs

ASSESSING THE GI SYSTEM

A physical assessment of the GI system should include a thorough examination of the mouth, abdomen, and rectum. To perform an abdominal assessment, use this sequence: inspection, auscultation, percussion, and palpation. Palpating or percussing the abdomen before you auscultate can change the character of the patient's bowel sounds and lead to an inaccurate assessment.

Before beginning your examination, explain the techniques you'll be using, and warn the patient that some procedures might be uncomfortable. Perform the examination in a private, quiet, warm, and well-lighted room.

ASSESSING THE ORAL CAVITY

To examine your patient's GI system, start by assessing the oral structures. Structural problems or disorders here may affect GI functioning. Use these guidelines when inspecting and palpating oral structures.

First, inspect the patient's mouth and jaw for asymmetry and swelling. Check his bite, noting malocclusion from an overbite or underbite. Inspect the inner and outer lips, teeth, gums, and oral mucosa with a penlight. Note bleeding; ulcerations; carious, loose, missing, or broken teeth; and color changes, including rashes. Palpate the gums, inner lips, and cheeks for tenderness, lumps, and lesions.

Assess the sides and undersurface of the tongue checking for coating, swelling, white or reddened areas, nodules, and ulcerations. Note unusual breath odors. Finally, examine the pharynx by pressing a tongue blade firmly down on the middle of the tongue and asking the patient to say "ah." Look for uvular deviation, tonsillar abnormalities, lesions, plaques, and exudate.

ASSESSING THE ABDOMEN

Use inspection, auscultation, percussion, and palpation to examine the abdomen. To ensure an accurate assessment, take these actions before the examination:
+ Ask the patient to empty his bladder.
+ Drape the genitalia and the breasts of a female patient.
+ Place a small pillow under the patient's knees to help relax the abdominal muscles.
+ Ask the patient to keep his arms at his sides.
+ Keep the room warm. Chilling can cause abdominal muscles to become tense.
+ Warm your hands and the stethoscope.
+ Approach the patient slowly and avoid quick, unexpected movements.
+ Speak softly, and encourage the patient to perform breathing exercises or use imagery during uncomfortable procedures. Distract the patient with conversation or questions.
+ Ask the patient to point to any areas of pain.
+ Assess painful areas last to help prevent the patient from becoming tense.
+ Watch the patient's face for signs of pain such as grimacing.

Inspection

Begin by mentally dividing the abdomen into four quadrants and then imagining the organs in each quadrant. (See *Abdominal quadrants,* page 178.) You can more accurately pinpoint your physical findings by knowing these three terms:
+ epigastric — above the umbilicus and between the costal margins
+ umbilical — around the navel
+ suprapubic — above the symphysis pubis.
   Observe the abdomen for symmetry, checking for bumps, bulges, or masses.

Assessing the GI system
+ Includes examination of mouth, abdomen, and rectum
+ Involves inspection, auscultation, percussion, and palpation

Assessing the oral cavity
+ Mouth and jaw — asymmetry and swelling, note bite
+ Lips, teeth, gums, and oral mucosa — note bleeding; ulcerations; carious, loose, missing, or broken teeth; and color changes
+ Tongue — coating, swelling, white or reddened areas, nodules, and ulcerations; note unusual breath odors
+ Pharynx — uvular deviation
+ Tonsils — lesions, plaques, and exudate

Assessing the abdomen
+ Ask patient to empty his bladder.
+ Help patient to relax and keep his arms at his sides
+ Ask patient to point to any areas of pain, assessing these areas last
+ Watch patient's face for signs of pain such as wincing

Facts about inspection
+ Mentally divide abdomen into four quadrants
+ Epigastric — above umbilicus and between costal margins
+ Umbilical — around navel
+ Suprapubic — above symphysis pubis
+ Observe for symmetry, bumps, bulges, or masses

Abdominal quadrants

To perform a systematic GI assessment, try to visualize the abdominal structures by dividing the abdomen into four quadrants, as shown here.

RIGHT UPPER QUADRANT
+ Right lobe of liver
+ Gallbladder
+ Pylorus
+ Duodenum
+ Head of the pancreas
+ Hepatic flexure of the colon
+ Portions of the ascending and transverse colon

LEFT UPPER QUADRANT
+ Left lobe of liver
+ Stomach
+ Tail of the pancreas
+ Splenic flexure of the colon
+ Portions of the transverse and descending colon

RIGHT LOWER QUADRANT
+ Cecum and appendix
+ Portion of the ascending colon

LEFT LOWER QUADRANT
+ Sigmoid colon
+ Portion of the descending colon

Facts about inspection
(continued)

Abnormal findings: Abdominal area

+ Bulging abdomen (bladder distention or hernia)
+ Protruding abdomen (obesity, pregnancy, ascites, abdominal distention, gas, tumor, or colon filled with feces)
+ Protruding umbilicus (pregnancy, ascites, or an underlying mass)
+ Striae (pregnancy, excessive weight gain, or ascites)
+ Redness (inflammation); bruising on the flank, or Turner's sign, (retroperitoneal hemorrhage)
+ Dilated, tortuous, visible veins (inferior vena cava obstruction)
+ Cutaneous angiomas (liver disease)

Also, note the patient's abdominal shape and contour. The abdomen should be flat to rounded in people of average weight. A slender person may have a slightly concave abdomen. Assess the umbilicus, which should be located midline in the abdomen and inverted.

 ABNORMAL FINDINGS *A bulge in the abdominal area may indicate bladder distention or hernia. A protruding abdomen may be caused by obesity, pregnancy, ascites, or abdominal distention. Gas, a tumor, or a colon filled with feces can all cause abdominal distention.*

Such conditions as pregnancy, ascites, or an underlying mass can cause the umbilicus to protrude. Have the patient raise his head and shoulders. If his umbilicus protrudes, he may have an umbilical hernia. A bluish umbilicus, called Cullen's sign, indicates intra-abdominal hemorrhage.

The skin of the abdomen should be smooth and uniform in color. Note dilated veins. Record the length of surgical scars on the abdomen.

 ABNORMAL FINDINGS *Striae, or stretch marks, can be caused by pregnancy, excessive weight gain, or ascites. New striae are pink or blue; old striae are silvery white (in patients with darker skin striae may be dark brown). Areas of abdominal redness may indicate inflammation. Bruising on the flank, or Turner's sign, indicates retroperitoneal hemorrhage. Dilated, tortuous, visible abdominal veins may indicate inferior vena cava obstruction. Cutaneous angiomas may signal liver disease.*

Note abdominal movements and pulsations. Usually, waves of peristalsis can't be seen; if they're visible, they look like slight, wavelike motions.

 ABNORMAL FINDINGS *Visible rippling waves in the abdomen may indicate bowel obstruction and should be reported immediately. In thin patients, pulsation of the aorta is visible in the epigastric area. Marked pulsations may occur with hypertension, aortic insufficiency, aortic aneurysm, and other conditions causing widening pulse pressure.*

Auscultation

Lightly place the stethoscope diaphragm in the right lower quadrant, slightly below and to the right of the umbilicus. Auscultate in a clockwise fashion in each of the four quadrants. Note the character and quality of bowel sounds in each quadrant. In some cases, you may need to auscultate for 5 minutes before you hear sounds. Make sure you allow enough time for listening in each quadrant before you decide that bowel sounds are absent.

Before auscultating the abdomen of a patient with a nasogastric tube or another abdominal tube connected to suction, briefly clamp the tube or turn off the suction. Suction noises can obscure or mimic actual bowel sounds.

Normal bowel sounds are high-pitched, gurgling noises caused by air mixing with fluid during peristalsis. The noises vary in frequency, pitch, and intensity and occur irregularly from 5 to 34 times per minute. They're loudest before mealtimes. Borborygmus, or stomach growling, is the loud, gurgling, splashing bowel sound heard over the large intestine as gas passes through it.

Bowel sounds are classified as normal, hypoactive, or hyperactive.

 ABNORMAL FINDINGS *Hyperactive bowel sounds—loud, high-pitched, tinkling sounds that occur frequently—indicate increased intestinal motility and have many causes, such as diarrhea, constipation, gastroenteritis, laxative use, and life-threatening intestinal obstruction.*

Hypoactive bowel sounds are heard infrequently. They're associated with ileus, bowel obstruction, or peritonitis and indicate diminished peristalsis. Recent bowel surgery or a full colon can all cause hypoactive bowel sounds. Paralytic ileus, torsion of the bowel, and the use of narcotics and other medications can decrease peristalsis. (See Interpreting abnormal abdominal sounds, *page 180.)*

Auscultate for vascular sounds with the bell of the stethoscope. Using firm pressure, listen over the aorta and renal, iliac, and femoral arteries for bruits, venous hums, and friction rubs.

 ABNORMAL FINDINGS *Friction rubs over the liver and spleen in the epigastric region may indicate splenic infarction or hepatic tumor. Abdominal bruits may be caused by aortic aneurysms or partial arterial obstruction. (See* Auscultating for vascular sounds, *page 181.)*

Percussion

Direct or indirect percussion is used to detect the size and location of abdominal organs and to detect air or fluid in the abdomen, stomach, or bowel.

In direct percussion, you strike your hand or finger directly against the patient's abdomen. With indirect percussion, you use the middle finger of your dominant hand or a percussion hammer to strike a finger resting on the patient's abdomen. Begin percussion in the right lower quadrant and proceed clockwise, covering all four quadrants.

Facts about inspection
(continued)

Abnormal findings: Abdominal area
- Visible rippling waves (bowel obstruction)
- Marked pulsations (hypertension, aortic insufficiency, and aortic aneurysm)

Facts about auscultation
- Performed in a clockwise fashion in each quadrant
- Reveals character and quality of bowel sounds
- Uncovers absent bowel signs
- Detects bruits, venous hums, and friction rubs over renal, iliac, and femoral arteries

Abnormal findings
- Hyperactive bowel sounds — frequently loud, high-pitched, tinkling sounds, indicating increased intestinal motility
- Hypoactive bowel sounds — infrequent; associated with ileus, bowel obstruction, or peritonitis, indicating diminished peristalsis
- Friction rubs over liver and spleen
- Abdominal bruits

Facts about percussion
- Direct or indirect — detects size and location of abdominal organs and presence of air or fluid
- Follows clockwise direction, covering all four quadrants

Interpreting abnormal abdominal sounds

✦ Abnormal bowel sounds — possible causes include diarrhea, laxative use, early intestinal obstruction, paralytic ileus, peritonitis, intestinal fluid, or intestinal obstruction

✦ Systolic bruits — possible causes include partial arterial obstruction or turbulent blood flow, renal artery stenosis, hepatomegaly, or arterial insufficiency in the legs

✦ Venous hum — a possible cause is increased collateral circulation between portal and systemic venous systems, such as with cirrhosis

✦ Friction rub — possible causes include inflammation of peritoneal surface of liver from a tumor or splenic infarct

Alert!

✦ Abdominal percussion or palpation contraindicated in patients with suspected appendicitis or abdominal aortic aneurysm, abdominal organ transplants, and children with suspected Wilms' tumor

KNOW-HOW

Interpreting abnormal abdominal sounds

SOUND AND DESCRIPTION	LOCATION	POSSIBLE CAUSE
Abnormal bowel sounds Hyperactive sounds (unrelated to hunger)	Any quadrant	Diarrhea, laxative use, or early intestinal obstruction
Hypoactive, then absent sounds	Any quadrant	Paralytic ileus or peritonitis
High-pitched tinkling sounds	Any quadrant	Intestinal fluid and air under tension in a dilated bowel
High-pitched rushing sounds coinciding with abdominal cramps	Any quadrant	Intestinal obstruction
Systolic bruits Vascular blowing sounds resembling cardiac murmurs	Over abdominal aorta	Partial arterial obstruction or turbulent blood flow
	Over renal artery	Renal artery stenosis
	Over iliac artery	Hepatomegaly
	Over femoral artery	Arterial insufficiency in the legs
Venous hum (rare) Continuous, medium-pitched tone with both systolic and diastolic components, created by blood flow in a large engorged vascular organ such as the liver	Epigastric and umbilical regions	Increased collateral circulation between portal and systemic venous systems such as with cirrhosis
Friction rub (rare) Harsh, grating sound like two pieces of sandpaper rubbing together	Over liver and spleen	Inflammation of the peritoneal surface of liver, such as from a tumor or splenic infarct (When a systolic bruit is also present, suspect liver cancer.)

CLINICAL ALERT Keep in mind that abdominal percussion or palpation is contraindicated in patients with suspected abdominal aortic aneurysm, those who have received abdominal organ transplants, and in children with suspected Wilms' tumor. If performing abdominal percussion or palpation in patients with suspected appendicitis, use extreme caution so as not to precipitate a rupture.

You normally hear two sounds during percussion of the abdomen: tympany and dullness. When you percuss over hollow organs, such as an empty stomach or bow-

Auscultating for vascular sounds

Use the bell of your stethoscope to auscultate for vascular sounds at the sites shown in the illustration.

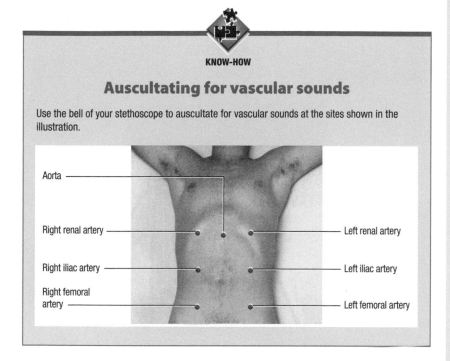

Aorta

Right renal artery — — Left renal artery

Right iliac artery — — Left iliac artery

Right femoral artery — — Left femoral artery

el, you hear a clear, hollow sound like a drum beating. This sound, tympany, predominates because air is normally present in the stomach and bowel. The degree of tympany depends on the amount of air and gastric dilation.

When you percuss over solid organs—such as the liver, kidney, urine-filled bladder, or feces-filled intestines—the sound changes to dullness. Note where percussed sounds change from tympany to dullness. (See *Sites of tympany and dullness,* page 182.)

Liver

Percussion of the liver can help you estimate its size. (See *Percussing and measuring the liver,* page 183.)

 ABNORMAL FINDINGS *Hepatomegaly is commonly associated with patients who have hepatitis and other liver diseases. Liver borders may be obscured and difficult to assess due to effusion, fluid, or infection in the lung, or gas in the colon.*

Spleen

The spleen is located at about the level of the 10th rib, in the left midaxillary line. Percussion may produce a small area of dullness, generally 7″ (18 cm) or less in adults. However, the spleen usually can't be percussed because tympany from the colon masks the dullness of the spleen. It's difficult to distinguish between the dullness of the posterior flank and the dullness of the spleen.

 ABNORMAL FINDINGS *Conditions that cause splenomegaly include mononucleosis, trauma, and illnesses that destroy RBCs, such as sickle cell anemia and some cancers. To assess a patient for splenic enlargement, ask him to breathe deeply and then percuss along the 9th to 11th intercostal spaces on the left, listening for a change from tympany to dullness. Measure the area of dullness, which is called a* positive splenic percussion sign.

Facts about liver percussion
+ Helps estimate size

Abnormal findings
+ Hepatomegaly (hepatitis and other liver diseases)
+ Obscured liver borders (effusion, fluid, infection in lungs, or gas in colon)

Facts about spleen percussion
+ Produces area of dullness, generally 7″ or less in adults
+ Usually can't be percussed due to tympany from the colon

Abnormal findings
+ Splenomegaly (mononucleosis, trauma, sickle cell anemia, or cancer)

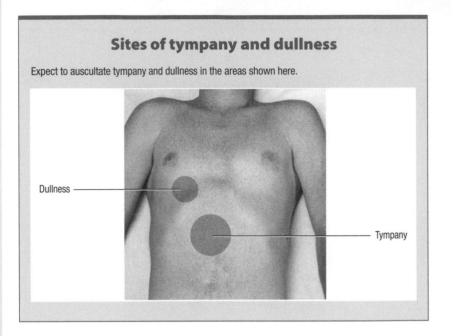

Sites of tympany and dullness

Expect to auscultate tympany and dullness in the areas shown here.

Dullness

Tympany

Facts about palpation

✦ Involves light and deep touch to determine size, shape, position, and tenderness of major abdominal organs and to detect masses and fluid accumulation

Facts about light palpation

✦ Requires use of fingers of one hand with gentle rotating movements

✦ Helps identify muscle resistance and tenderness

✦ Locates superficial organs, masses, and areas of tenderness or increased resistance

Facts about deep palpation

✦ Involves pushing abdomen down 2″ to 3″

✦ Reveals tenderness, pulsations, organ enlargement, and masses

✦ Detects mass location, size, shape, consistency, type of border, tenderness, pulsations, and degree of mobility

Palpation

Abdominal palpation includes light and deep touch to help determine the size, shape, position, and tenderness of major abdominal organs, and to detect masses and fluid accumulation. Palpate all four quadrants, leaving painful and tender areas for last. (See *Recognizing types of abdominal pain,* page 184.)

Light palpation

Light palpation helps identify muscle resistance and tenderness as well as the location of some superficial organs. To palpate, put the fingers of one hand close together, depress the skin about ½″ (1.5 cm) with your fingertips, and make gentle, rotating movements. Avoid short, quick jabs.

The abdomen should be soft and nontender. As you palpate the four quadrants, note organs, masses, and areas of tenderness or increased resistance. Determine whether resistance is due to the patient's being cold, tense, or ticklish, or whether it's due to involuntary guarding or rigidity from muscle spasms or peritoneal inflammation.

Help the ticklish patient relax by putting his hand over yours as you palpate. This usually decreases involuntary muscle contractions in response to touch. If he complains of abdominal tenderness even before you touch him, palpate by placing your stethoscope lightly on his abdomen.

Deep palpation

To perform deep palpation, push the abdomen down about 2″ to 3″ (5 to 7.5 cm). In an obese patient, put one hand on top of the other and push. Palpate the entire abdomen in a clockwise direction, checking for tenderness, pulsations, organ enlargement, and masses. If you detect a mass on light or deep palpation, note its location, size, shape, consistency, type of border, degree of tenderness, presence of pulsations, and degree of mobility (fixed or mobile).

KNOW-HOW

Percussing and measuring the liver

To percuss and measure the liver, follow these steps:

✦ Identify the upper border of liver dullness. Start in the right midclavicular line in an area of lung resonance, and percuss downward toward the liver. Use a pen to mark the spot where the sound changes to dullness.

✦ Start in the right midclavicular line at a level below the umbilicus, and lightly percuss upward toward the liver. Mark the spot where the sound changes from tympany to dullness.

✦ Use a ruler to measure the vertical span between the two marked spots, as shown. In an adult, a normal liver span ranges from 2½″ to 4¾″ (6.5 to 12 cm).

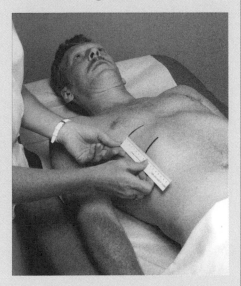

 CLINICAL ALERT If the patient's abdomen is rigid, don't palpate it. He could have peritoneal inflammation, and palpation could cause pain or could rupture an inflamed organ.

If the patient's abdomen is distended, assess its progression by taking serial measurements of abdominal girth. To do so, wrap a tape measure around the patient's abdomen at the level of the umbilicus and record the measurement. Be sure to mark the point of measurement with a felt-tip pen to ensure that subsequent readings are taken at the same point.

 CLINICAL ALERT Don't palpate a pulsating midline mass; it may be a dissecting aneurysm, which can rupture under the pressure of palpation. Report such a mass to the physician immediately.

Liver palpation
Palpate the patient's liver to check for enlargement and tenderness. (See *Palpating the liver,* page 185.)

Spleen palpation
Unless the spleen is enlarged, it isn't palpable. If you do feel the spleen, stop palpating immediately because compression can cause rupture. (See *Palpating the spleen,* page 186.)

 ABNORMAL FINDINGS *A markedly enlarged spleen descends into the left lower quadrant of the abdomen. A notch felt along its medial border distinguishes an enlarged spleen from an enlarged kidney.*

Alerts!
✦ Don't palpate a rigid abdomen; it could indicate peritoneal inflammation and palpation could cause rupture
✦ Don't palpate a pulsating midline mass; it could indicate dissecting aneurysm and palpation could cause rupture

Facts about liver palpation
✦ Helps check for enlargement and tenderness

Facts about spleen palpation
✦ The spleen usually can't be palpated, unless it's enlarged

Abnormal findings
✦ An enlarged spleen descends into left lower quadrant of abdomen, indicated by a notch felt along its medial border

KNOW-HOW

Recognizing types of abdominal pain

When assessing a patient with abdominal pain, use this chart to get a quick idea of the affected organ and the most likely source of the pain.

AFFECTED ORGAN	VISCERAL PAIN	PARIETAL PAIN	REFERRED PAIN
Stomach	Midepigastrium	Midepigastrium and left upper quadrant	Shoulders
Small intestine	Periumbilical area	Over affected site	Midback (rare)
Appendix	Periumbilical area	Right lower quadrant	Right lower quadrant
Proximal colon	Periumbilical area and right flank for ascending colon	Over affected site	Right lower quadrant and back (rare)
Distal colon	Hypogastrium and left flank for descending colon	Over affected site	Left lower quadrant and back (rare)
Gallbladder	Midepigastrium	Right upper quadrant	Right subscapular area
Ureters	Costovertebral angle	Over affected site	Groin; scrotum in men, labia in women (rare)
Pancreas	Midepigastrium and left upper quadrant	Midepigastrium and left upper quadrant	Back and left shoulder
Ovaries, fallopian tubes, and uterus	Hypogastrium and groin	Over affected site	Inner thighs

Special assessment procedures
+ May require checking for rebound tenderness or ascites

Facts about rebound tenderness
+ Detects suspected peritoneal inflammation
+ Requires pushing down slowly and deeply into the abdomen, withdrawing quickly, and noting rebound and any sharp pain
+ Can't be repeated, may rupture an inflamed appendix

Special assessment procedures
In your assessment you may encounter the need to perform special procedures to check for rebound tenderness or ascites. Use the following procedures.

Rebound tenderness
Perform the test for rebound tenderness when you suspect peritoneal inflammation. Check for rebound tenderness at the end of your examination.

Choosing a site away from the painful area, position your hand at a 90-degree angle to the abdomen. Push down slowly and deeply into the abdomen, then withdraw your hand quickly. Rapid withdrawal causes the underlying structures to rebound suddenly and results in a sharp, stabbing pain on the inflamed side. Don't repeat this maneuver or you may rupture an inflamed appendix.

KNOW-HOW

Palpating the liver

PALPATING THE LIVER
◆ Place the patient in the supine position. Standing at his right side, place your left hand under his back at the approximate location of the liver.
◆ Place your right hand slightly below the mark you made earlier at the liver's upper border. Point the fingers of your right hand toward the patient's head just under the right costal margin.
◆ As the patient inhales deeply, gently press in and up on the abdomen until the liver brushes under your right hand. The edge should be smooth, firm, and somewhat round. Note any tenderness.

HOOKING THE LIVER
◆ Hooking is an alternate way of palpating the liver. To hook the liver, stand next to the patient's right shoulder, facing his feet. Place your hands side by side, and hook your fingertips over the right costal margin, below the lower mark of dullness.
◆ Ask the patient to take a deep breath as you push your fingertips in and up. If the liver is palpable, you may feel its edge as it slides down in the abdomen as he inhales.

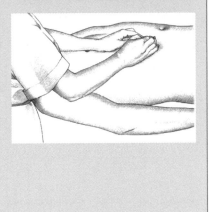

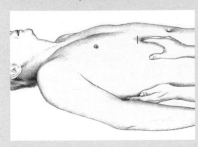

Facts about rebound tenderness
(continued)
◆ May be caused by appendicitis
◆ Increased abdominal wall resistance and guarding
◆ Older adults have less rigidity

Facts about ascites
◆ Large accumulation of fluid in peritoneal cavity
◆ Caused by advanced liver disease, heart failure, pancreatitis, or cancer
◆ Checked for by assessing for a fluid wave and shifting dullness

Characteristics of a fluid wave
◆ Elicited by giving the right abdomen a firm tap with your left hand
◆ If ascites is present, you may see and feel a "fluid wave" ripple across abdomen

Peritonitis or appendicitis can cause rebound tenderness. Appendicitis may be accompanied by increased abdominal wall resistance and guarding. Not all patients have the classic right lower quadrant pain. Some older adults with appendicitis have less abdominal rigidity than younger patients.

Ascites
Ascites, a large accumulation of fluid in the peritoneal cavity, can be caused by advanced liver disease, heart failure, pancreatitis, or cancer.

If ascites is present, use a tape measure to measure the fullest part of the abdomen. Mark this point on the patient's abdomen with indelible ink so you'll be sure to measure it consistently. This measurement is important, especially if fluid removal or paracentesis is performed.

Two maneuvers are useful in checking for ascites: assessing for a fluid wave and assessing for shifting dullness.

Fluid wave
Have an assistant place the ulnar edge of her hand firmly on the patient's abdomen at its midline. Then, as you stand facing the patient's head, place the palm of your right hand against the patient's left flank. Give the right abdomen a firm tap with

Palpating the spleen

Although a normal spleen isn't palpable, an enlarged spleen is. To palpate the spleen, stand on the patient's right side. Use your left hand to support his posterior left lower rib cage. Ask him to take a deep breath. Then, with your right hand on his abdomen, press up and in toward the spleen.

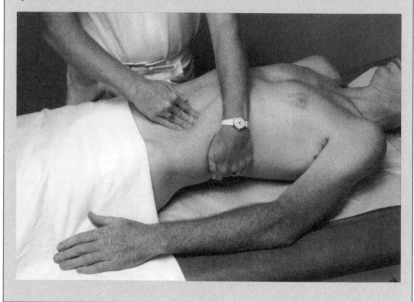

Characteristics of shifting dullness

+ Dependent areas of abdomen reveal dullness and a gas-filled bowel displaying tympany
+ If ascites is present, dullness shifts to more dependent side and tympany shifts to top

Facts about ballottement

+ Involves tapping or bouncing fingertips against abdominal wall
+ Helps to elicit abdominal muscle resistance or guarding, or the movement or bounce of a freely movable mass

your left hand. If ascites is present, you may see and feel a "fluid wave" ripple across the abdomen.

Shifting dullness

A protuberant abdomen with bulging flanks suggests ascites. Percuss the abdomen outward from the umbilicus in several directions. Fluid sinks with gravity so if ascites is present, dependent areas of the abdomen will be dull and gas-filled bowel that floats to the top will be tympanic.

Now ask the patient to turn on his side. Percuss again. In a patient without ascites the borders between tympany and dullness will remain about the same. If ascites is present, the dullness shifts to the more dependent side and the tympany shifts to the top.

Ballottement

Ballottement involves lightly tapping or bouncing your fingertips against the abdominal wall. This technique helps elicit abdominal muscle resistance or guarding that can be missed with deep palpation, or it may detect the movement or bounce of a freely movable mass. Your fingers should also bounce at the underlying dense liver tissue in the right upper quadrant. If the patient has ascites, you may need to use deep ballottement. To do so, push your fingertips deeply inward in a rapid motion; then quickly release the pressure, maintaining fingertip contact with the abdominal wall. You should feel the movement of an underlying organ or a movable mass toward your fingertips.

EXAMINING THE RECTUM AND ANUS

If your patient is age 40 or older, perform a rectal examination as part of your GI assessment. Make sure you explain the procedure to the patient.

Inspection

First, inspect the perianal area. Put on gloves and spread the buttocks to expose the anus and surrounding tissue, checking for fissures, lesions, scars, inflammation, discharge, rectal prolapse, and external hemorrhoids. Ask the patient to strain as if he's having a bowel movement; this may reveal internal hemorrhoids, polyps, or fissures. The skin in the perianal area is normally somewhat darker than that of the surrounding area.

Palpation

Next palpate the rectum. Apply a water-soluble lubricant to your gloved index finger. Warn the patient that he'll feel some pressure. Ask the patient to strain down. As the sphincter relaxes, gently insert your finger into the rectum, toward the umbilicus. If you feel the sphincter tighten, pause and reassure the patient. Continue the examination when the sphincter relaxes again. Rotate your finger clockwise and counterclockwise to palpate all aspects of the rectal wall for nodules, tenderness, irregularities, and fecal impaction. The rectal wall should feel smooth and soft. In a female patient, try to feel the posterior side of the uterus through the anterior rectal wall. In a male patient, assess the prostate gland when palpating the anterior rectal wall; the prostate should feel firm and smooth.

With your finger fully inserted, ask the patient to bear down again; this may cause any lesions higher in the rectum to move down to a palpable level. To assess anal sphincter competence, ask the patient to tighten the anal muscles around your finger. Finally, withdraw your finger and examine it for blood, mucus, or stool. Test fecal matter adhering to the glove for occult blood using a guaiac test.

ONGOING ASSESSMENT

Whenever a patient reports a GI complaint, he'll need reassessment. You can't assume, for instance, that a previously assessed dysfunction is causing the patient's present abdominal pain. The pain's nature and location may have changed, indicating more extensive involvement or perhaps a new disorder. To avoid unduly alarming your patient, reassure him that ongoing assessment doesn't necessarily mean he has a significant health problem. Tell him that repeated evaluations aid diagnosis and treatment.

INTERPRETING YOUR FINDINGS

Your assessment will reveal a group of findings that may lead you to suspect a particular disorder. (See *The GI system: Interpreting your findings,* pages 188 and 189.)

Examining the rectum and anus
+ Performed in patients age 40 and older

Facts about anus inspection
+ Detects fissures, lesions, rectal prolapse, and hemorrhoids
+ Reveals internal hemorrhoids, polyps, or fissures

Facts about rectum palpation
+ Reveals nodules, tenderness, irregularities, and fecal impaction
+ Assesses sphincter competence
+ Helps to test for occult blood, using guaiac test

Ongoing assessment
+ Reassess any patient who reports GI complaints
+ Reassure patient that repeated evaluations aid diagnosis and treatment

The GI system: Interpreting your findings

This chart shows some common groups of findings for signs and symptoms of the GI system, along with their probable causes.

SIGN OR SYMPTOM AND FINDINGS	PROBABLE CAUSE
Abdominal pain	
✦ Localized abdominal pain, described as steady, gnawing, burning, aching, or hungerlike, high in the midepigastrium, slightly off center, usually on the right ✦ Pain begins 2 to 4 hours after a meal ✦ Ingestion of food or antacids brings relief ✦ Changes in bowel habits ✦ Heartburn or retrosternal burning	Duodenal ulcer
✦ Pain and tenderness in the right or left lower abdominal quadrant, may become sharp and severe on standing or stooping ✦ Abdominal distention ✦ Mild nausea and vomiting ✦ Occasional menstrual irregularities ✦ Slight fever	Ovarian cyst
✦ Referred, severe upper abdominal pain, tenderness, and rigidity that diminish with inspiration ✦ Fever, shaking chills, achiness ✦ Blood-tinged or rusty sputum ✦ Dry, hacking cough ✦ Dyspnea	Pneumonia
Diarrhea	
✦ Soft, unformed stools or watery diarrhea that may be foul-smelling or grossly bloody ✦ Abdominal pain, cramping, and tenderness ✦ Fever	*Clostridium difficile* infection
✦ Diarrhea occurs within several hours of ingesting milk or milk products ✦ Abdominal pain, cramping, and bloating ✦ Borborygmi ✦ Flatus	Lactose intolerance
✦ Recurrent bloody diarrhea with pus or mucus ✦ Hyperactive bowel sounds ✦ Cramping lower abdominal pain ✦ Occasional nausea and vomiting	Ulcerative colitis
Hematochezia	
✦ Moderate to severe rectal bleeding ✦ Epistaxis ✦ Purpura	Coagulation disorders

The GI system: Interpreting your findings *(continued)*

SIGN OR SYMPTOM AND FINDINGS	PROBABLE CAUSE
Hematochezia (continued)	
✦ Bright-red rectal bleeding with or without pain ✦ Diarrhea or ribbon-shaped stools ✦ Stools may be grossly bloody ✦ Weakness and fatigue ✦ Abdominal aching and dull cramps	Colon cancer
✦ Chronic bleeding with defecation ✦ Painful defecation	Hemorrhoids
Nausea and vomiting	
✦ Nausea and vomiting follow or accompany abdominal pain ✦ Pain progresses rapidly to severe, stabbing pain in the right lower quadrant (McBurney's sign) ✦ Abdominal rigidity and tenderness ✦ Constipation or diarrhea ✦ Tachycardia	Appendicitis
✦ Nausea and vomiting of undigested food ✦ Diarrhea ✦ Abdominal cramping ✦ Hyperactive bowel sounds ✦ Fever	Gastroenteritis
✦ Nausea and vomiting ✦ Headache with severe, constant, throbbing pain ✦ Fatigue ✦ Photophobia ✦ Light flashes ✦ Increased noise sensitivity	Migraine headache

GI SYSTEM DISORDERS

APPENDICITIS

Appendicitis occurs when the appendix becomes inflamed. It's the most common major surgical emergency. Distention and contractions of the appendix cause pain that's initially generalized and then localized in the right lower abdomen. Other signs and symptoms include anorexia, nausea or vomiting, and low-grade fever. Symptoms of rupture include pain, tenderness, and spasm followed by brief cessation of abdominal pain.

CHOLECYSTITIS

In patients with cholecystitis, the gallbladder becomes inflamed, usually by a gallstone that has become lodged in the cystic duct, causing painful gallbladder distention.

GI system disorders

Facts about appendicitis
✦ Inflamed appendix
✦ Signs and symptoms include pain in right lower abdomen, anorexia, nausea or vomiting, and low-grade fever
✦ Symptoms of rupture include pain, tenderness, and spasm

Facts about cholecystitis
✦ Inflamed gallbladder

Signs and symptoms of acute cholecystitis often may include acute abdominal pain in the right upper quadrant that may radiate to the back, between the shoulders, or to the front of the chest and tenderness over the gallbladder that increases on inspiration (Murphy's sign). These signs and symptoms generally strike after meals that are rich in fats. The patient may also experience belching, flatulence, indigestion, nausea, vomiting, chills, low-grade fever, pallor, and diaphoresis.

CROHN'S DISEASE

Slow, progressive inflammation of the bowel with gradual onset of signs and symptoms, marked by periods of remission and exacerbation, is called *Crohn's disease.* Complications may include edema, mucosal ulceration, fissures, abscesses, intestinal obstruction or perforation, and nutritional deficiencies. The patient may report fatigue, weakness, fever, flatulence, nausea, weight loss, and steady, colicky, or cramping abdominal pain that usually occurs in the right lower abdominal quadrant. He may also report diarrhea that worsens after emotional upset or eating poorly tolerated foods, such as milk, fatty foods, or spices.

DIVERTICULAR DISEASE

Diverticula are bulging pouches in the intestinal wall, most commonly found in the sigmoid colon. When retained food mixed with bacteria accumulates in the diverticulum, inflammation follows, causing diverticulitis. The patient may complain of nausea, gas, diarrhea, or intermittent constipation. Sometimes rectal bleeding, low-grade fever, and muscle spasms may occur. He may also complain of dull or steady pain in the left lower abdominal quadrant, which is aggravated by straining, lifting, or coughing.

GASTROESOPHAGEAL REFLUX DISEASE

GERD occurs when gastric or duodenal contents backflow into the esophagus due to pyloric surgery, hiatal hernia, or other condition that increases abdominal pressure. The patient may have minimal or no symptoms or may report heartburn that occurs $\frac{1}{2}$ to 2 hours after eating and worsens with vigorous exercise, bending, lying down, wearing tight clothing, coughing, constipation, and obesity that's relieved by using antacids or sitting upright. Other symptoms include regurgitation; fluid in the back of the throat; pain radiating to the neck, jaws, and arms that mimics angina; nocturnal hypersalivation and wheezing; chronic cough; laryngitis; and morning hoarseness.

IRRITABLE BOWEL SYNDROME

IBS is a common condition marked by chronic or periodic diarrhea alternating with constipation. IBS is also known as *spastic colon* or *functional bowel disease.* The cause is unknown but anxiety, stress, and dietary factors (such as raw fruits; coffee; alcohol; cold, highly seasoned, or laxative-type foods; and lack of fiber) are felt to contribute to the development of IBS. Signs and symptoms include dyspepsia, heartburn, abdominal bloating and pain, mucusy stools, faintness, weakness, and fatigue.

PANCREATITIS

Pancreatitis occurs when pancreatic enzymes that are normally excreted into the duodenum digest pancreatic tissue and cause inflammation. The patient may experience hypotension, fever, dyspnea, orthopnea, jaundice, nausea, vomiting, weight loss, and intense epigastric pain around the umbilicus and radiating to the back. Pain may be aggravated by fatty foods, alcohol consumption, or recumbent position.

PEPTIC ULCER

A peptic ulcer is a circumscribed lesion in the mucosal membrane. Peptic ulcers can develop in the lower esophagus, stomach, duodenum, or jejunum. Symptoms include left epigastric pain, heartburn, indigestion, and feeling of fullness or distention. In addition, the patient with a gastric ulcer may report recent loss of weight or appetite, nausea or vomiting, and pain triggered or aggravated by eating. The patient with a duodenal ulcer may report weight gain, pain that wakens the patient from sleep, pain relieved by eating or pain that occurs 1½ to 3 hours after eating.

VIRAL HEPATITIS

Viral hepatitis is a common infection of the liver. In most patients, damaged liver cells eventually regenerate with little or no permanent damage. However, old age and serious underlying disorders make complications more likely. In the prodromal stage, the patient may complain of fatigue, anorexia, mild weight loss, general malaise, depression, headache, weakness, joint pain, muscle pain, photophobia, nausea, vomiting, fever, dark-colored urine, and clay-colored stools. In the clinical stage, the patient may report indigestion, pruritus, rashes, right upper quadrant tenderness, and jaundice of the sclerae and skin.

Facts about peptic ulcer

+ Circumscribed lesion in the mucosal membrane
+ Develop in lower esophagus, stomach, duodenum, or jejunum
+ Left epigastric pain, heartburn, indigestion, and distention

Facts about viral hepatitis

+ Infection of the liver
+ Prodromal stage causing fatigue, anorexia, mild weight loss, headache, weakness, joint pain, photophobia, nausea, vomiting, fever, dark-colored urine, and clay-colored stools
+ Clinical stage causing indigestion, pruritus, rashes, tenderness, and jaundice

8

Neurologic system

A look at the neurologic system

+ Controls body function and relates to all body systems
+ Consists of CNS, peripheral nervous system, and ANS, which integrates all physical, intellectual, and emotional activities

Facts about the CNS

+ Includes the brain and the spinal cord
+ Collects and interprets voluntary and involuntary motor and sensory stimuli

A LOOK AT THE NEUROLOGIC SYSTEM

The neurologic system controls body function and is related to every other body system. Consequently, patients who suffer from diseases of other body systems can develop neurologic impairments related to the disease. One example of this is a patient who has heart surgery and then suffers a stroke.

Because the neurologic system is so complex, evaluating it can seem overwhelming at first. Although tests for neurologic status are extensive, they're also basic and straightforward. In fact, you may routinely include some of these tests in your practice.

Just talking with a patient helps you assess his orientation, level of consciousness (LOC), and ability to formulate and produce speech. Having him perform a simple task, such as walking, allows you to evaluate motor ability. Your knowledge of neurologic anatomy, physiology, and assessment will enhance your patient care and may save some patients from irreversible neurologic damage.

The neurologic system is divided into the central nervous system (CNS), the peripheral nervous system, and the autonomic nervous system (ANS). Through complex and coordinated interactions, these three parts integrate all physical, intellectual, and emotional activities. Understanding how each part works is essential to conducting an accurate neurologic assessment.

CENTRAL NERVOUS SYSTEM

The CNS includes the brain and the spinal cord. These two structures collect and interpret voluntary and involuntary motor and sensory stimuli. (See *The CNS.*)

The CNS

This illustration shows a cross section of the brain and spinal cord, which together make up the central nervous system (CNS). The brain joins the spinal cord at the base of the skull and ends between the first and second lumbar vertebrae. Note the H-shaped mass of gray matter in the spinal cord.

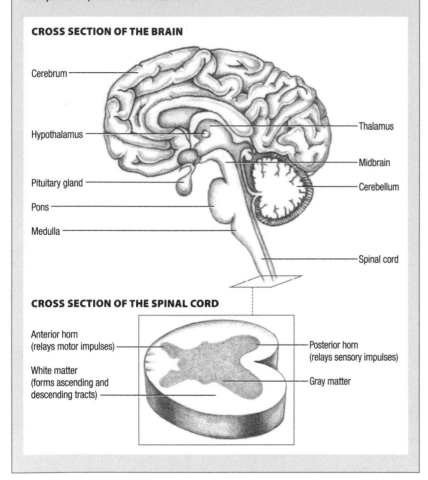

CROSS SECTION OF THE BRAIN

- Cerebrum
- Hypothalamus
- Pituitary gland
- Pons
- Medulla
- Thalamus
- Midbrain
- Cerebellum
- Spinal cord

CROSS SECTION OF THE SPINAL CORD

- Anterior horn (relays motor impulses)
- White matter (forms ascending and descending tracts)
- Posterior horn (relays sensory impulses)
- Gray matter

Brain

The brain consists of the cerebrum or cerebral cortex, the brain stem, and the cerebellum. It collects, integrates, and interprets all stimuli and initiates and monitors voluntary and involuntary motor activity.

Cerebrum

The cerebrum gives us the ability to think and reason. It's encased by the skull and enclosed by three membrane layers called *meninges*. If blood or fluid accumulates between these layers, pressure builds inside the skull and compromises brain function.

The cerebrum consists of a left and a right hemisphere joined by the corpus callosum, a mass of nerve fibers that allows communication between corresponding centers in the right and left hemispheres. Each hemisphere is divided into four

Facts about the brain

- ✦ Consists of cerebrum, brain stem, and cerebellum
- ✦ Collects, integrates, and interprets all stimuli
- ✦ Initiates and monitors voluntary and involuntary motor activity

Facts about the cerebrum

- ✦ Provides ability to think and reason
- ✦ Encased by skull and enclosed by meninges
- ✦ Blood or fluid may accumulate between meninges, which compromises brain function
- ✦ Consists of left and right hemispheres joined by corpus callosum

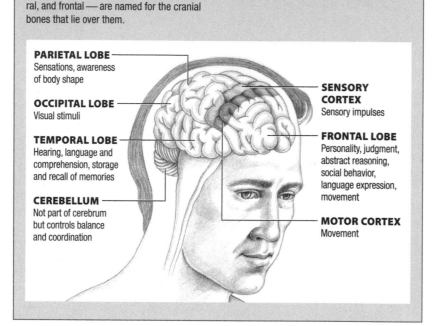

The cerebrum and its functions

The cerebrum is divided into four lobes, based on anatomic landmarks and functional differences. The lobes — parietal, occipital, temporal, and frontal — are named for the cranial bones that lie over them.

This illustration shows the locations of the cerebral lobes and explains their functions. It also shows the location of the cerebellum.

PARIETAL LOBE
Sensations, awareness of body shape

OCCIPITAL LOBE
Visual stimuli

TEMPORAL LOBE
Hearing, language and comprehension, storage and recall of memories

CEREBELLUM
Not part of cerebrum but controls balance and coordination

SENSORY CORTEX
Sensory impulses

FRONTAL LOBE
Personality, judgment, abstract reasoning, social behavior, language expression, movement

MOTOR CORTEX
Movement

Four lobes of the cerebrum

✦ Frontal — influences personality, judgment, abstract reasoning, social behavior, language expression, and movement
✦ Temporal — controls hearing, language comprehension, and storage and recall of memories
✦ Parietal — interprets and integrates sensations, including pain, temperature, and touch; also interprets size, shape, distance, and texture
✦ Occipital — interprets visual stimuli

Facts about the brain stem

✦ Lies below diencephalon; divides into midbrain, pons, and medulla
✦ Cranial nerves III and IV and corticospinal tract originate in midbrain

lobes, based on anatomic landmarks and functional differences. The lobes are named for the cranial bones that lie over them (frontal, temporal, parietal, and occipital). The cerebral cortex, the surface layer of the cerebrum, is composed of gray matter (unmyelinated cell bodies). The cerebrum has a rolling surface made up of convolutions (gyri) and creases or fissures (sulci).

The frontal lobe influences personality, judgment, abstract reasoning, social behavior, language expression, and movement. The temporal lobe controls hearing, language comprehension, and the storage and recall of memories (although some memories are stored throughout the brain). The parietal lobe interprets and integrates sensations, including pain, temperature, and touch. It also interprets size, shape, distance, and texture. The parietal lobe of the nondominant hemisphere, usually the right, is especially important for awareness of body schema (shape). The occipital lobe functions primarily in interpreting visual stimuli.

In addition, cranial nerves I and II originate in the cerebrum. The cerebrum is considered the area involving upper motor neuron function. (See *The cerebrum and its functions*.)

The diencephalon, a division of the cerebrum, contains the thalamus and hypothalamus. The thalamus is a relay station for sensory impulses. The hypothalamus has many regulatory functions, including temperature control, pituitary hormone production, and water balance.

Brain stem

The brain stem lies below the diencephalon and is divided into the midbrain, pons, and medulla. The midbrain is the origination site for cranial nerves III and IV and the corticospinal tract, which is the main motor pathway from the cerebrum. The midbrain mediates the auditory and visual reflexes. The pons is the origination area for cranial nerves V, VI, and VII and it contains one of the respiratory centers. The pons connects the cerebellum to the cerebrum and the midbrain to the medulla. The medulla is the origination area for cranial nerves VIII to XII. The medulla regulates respiratory, vasomotor, and cardiac function. Areas below the cerebrum are considered the areas involving lower motor neuron function.

Cerebellum

The cerebellum, the most posterior part of the brain, contains the major motor and sensory pathways. It facilitates smooth, coordinated muscle movement and helps to maintain equilibrium.

Spinal cord

The spinal cord is the primary pathway for messages traveling between the peripheral areas of the body and the brain. It also mediates the sensory-to-motor transmission path known as the *reflex arc.* Because the reflex arc enters and exits the spinal cord at the same level, reflex pathways don't need to travel up and down the way other stimuli do. Reflex responses occur automatically, without brain involvement, to protect the body. For example, if the brain can't send a message to a patient's leg after a severe spinal cord injury, a stimulus can still cause a knee jerk (patellar) reflex as long as the spinal cord remains intact at the level of the reflex. (See *How the reflex arc functions,* page 196.)

The spinal cord extends from the upper border of the first cervical vertebrae to the lower border of the first lumbar vertebrae. The spinal cord is encased in the spinal column by the uninterrupted meningeal linings and spinal fluid that protect the brain. Further protection of the spinal cord is provided by the bony vertebrae and the intervertebral disks.

A cross section of the spinal cord reveals a central H-shaped mass of gray matter divided into dorsal (posterior) and ventral (anterior) horns. Gray matter in the dorsal horns relays sensory (afferent) impulses; in the ventral horns, motor (efferent) impulses. White matter (myelinated axons of sensory and motor nerves) surrounds these horns and forms the ascending and descending tracts.

For the purpose of documenting sensory function, the body is divided into dermatomes. Each dermatome represents an area supplied with afferent, or sensory, nerve fibers from an individual spinal root — cervical, thoracic, lumbar, or sacral. This body "map" is used when testing sensation and trying to identify the source of a lesion. (See *Dermatomes,* page 197.)

Bone, meninges, and cerebrospinal fluid

Bone, meninges, and cerebrospinal fluid (CSF) protect the brain and the spinal cord from shock and infection. Formed of cranial bones, the skull completely surrounds the brain and opens at the base (the foramen magnum), where the spinal cord exits.

The vertebral column protects the spinal cord. It consists of 30 vertebrae, each separated by an intervertebral disk that allows flexibility.

The meninges cover and protect the cerebral cortex and spinal column. They consist of three layers of connective tissue: the dura mater, the arachnoid membrane, and the pia mater. (See *Protecting the CNS,* page 198.)

CSF nourishes cells, transports metabolic waste, and cushions the brain. This colorless fluid circulates through the ventricular system, into the subarachnoid space of the brain and spinal cord, and back to the venous sinuses on top of the brain where it's reabsorbed. The ependymal cells that cover the surface of the

---

Facts about the brain stem *(continued)*

- ✦ Cranial nerves V, VI, and VII originate in pons
- ✦ Cranial nerves VII to XII originate in medulla

Facts about the cerebellum

- ✦ Most posterior portion of the brain
- ✦ Contains major motor and sensory pathways
- ✦ Helps maintain equilibrium

Facts about the spinal cord

- ✦ Functions as main pathway for messages
- ✦ Encased by meningeal linings and spinal fluid; protected by vertebrae and intervertebral disks
- ✦ Contains dorsal horns, relaying sensory impulses; and ventral horns, relaying motor impulses

Functions of the bones, meninges, and CSF

- ✦ Protect brain and spinal cord from shock and infection

Bones
- ✦ Protect spinal cord with vertebral spinal column

Meninges
- ✦ Cover and protect cerebral cortex and spinal column

CSF
- ✦ Nourishes cells, transports metabolic waste, and cushions brain

How the reflex arc functions

Spinal nerves, which have sensory and motor portions, control deep tendon and superficial reflexes. A simple reflex arc requires a sensory (afferent) neuron and a motor (efferent) neuron. The knee jerk (patellar) reflex illustrates the sequence of events in a normal reflex arc.

First, a sensory receptor detects the mechanical stimulus produced by the reflex hammer striking the patellar tendon. Then the sensory neuron carries the impulse along its

axon by way of the spinal nerve to the dorsal root, where it enters the posterior horn of the spinal cord.

Next, in the anterior horn of the spinal cord, shown here, the sensory neuron joins with a motor neuron, which carries the impulse along its axon by way of spinal nerve to the muscle. The motor neuron transmits the impulse to the muscle fibers through stimulation of the motor end plate. This triggers the muscle to contract and the leg to extend.

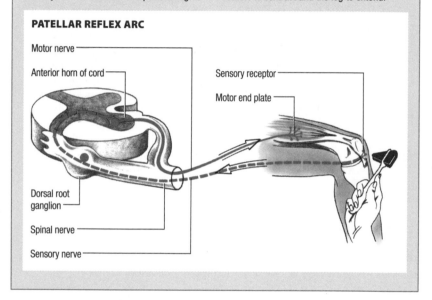

PATELLAR REFLEX ARC

Motor nerve

Anterior horn of cord

Sensory receptor

Motor end plate

Dorsal root ganglion

Spinal nerve

Sensory nerve

Facts about nervous system cells

+ Neurons — detect and transmit stimuli by electromechanical messages
+ Neuroglial cells — serve as supportive cells of CNS

Four types of neuroglial cells

+ Astroglia — form part of blood-brain barrier; supply nutrients to neurons and help maintain their electrical potential
+ Ependymal cells — line brain's four ventricles and choroid plexus and help produce CSF
+ Microglia — phagocytize waste products from injured neurons
+ Oligodendroglia — support and electrically insulate CNS axons

---

choroid plexus (a tangled mass of tiny blood vessels lining the ventricles) constantly produce CSF at a rate of about 150 ml/day.

Nervous system cells

Two major cell types, neurons and neuroglia, compose the nervous system. The conducting cells of the CNS, neurons (nerve cells) detect and transmit stimuli by electromechanical messages. These specialized cells don't reproduce themselves.

Neuroglial cells, or glial cells (derived from the Greek word for glue because they hold the neurons together), serve as the supportive cells of the CNS and form roughly 40% of the brain's bulk. Four types of neuroglial cells exist.

+ Astroglia, or astrocytes, exist throughout the nervous system and form part of the blood-brain barrier. They supply nutrients to the neurons and help maintain their electrical potential.

+ Ependymal cells line the brain's four ventricles and the choroid plexus and help produce CSF.

+ Microglia phagocytize waste products from injured neurons and are deployed throughout the nervous system.

+ Oligodendroglia support and electrically insulate CNS axons by forming protective myelin sheaths.

Dermatomes

Knowledge of dermatomes is useful to localize neurologic lesions. The following two illustrations demonstrate the patterns of dermatomes on the body.

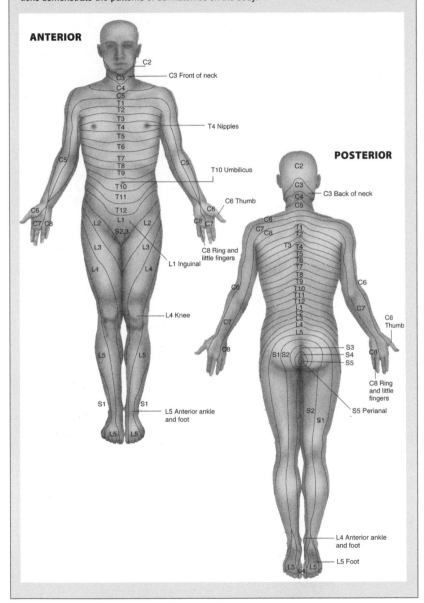

ANTERIOR

POSTERIOR

Understanding dermatomes

♦ Divide body into areas supplied with afferent, or sensory, nerve fibers from an individual spinal root
♦ Include cervical, thoracic, lumbar, or sacral roots
♦ Used to test sensation and identify sources of lesions

Facts about the peripheral nervous system

♦ Includes peripheral and cranial nerves
♦ Transmits stimuli to dorsal horn of spinal cord from sensory receptors in skin, muscles, sensory organs, and viscera

PERIPHERAL NERVOUS SYSTEM

The peripheral nervous system includes the peripheral and cranial nerves. Peripheral sensory nerves transmit stimuli to the dorsal horn of the spinal cord from sensory receptors located in the skin, muscles, sensory organs, and viscera. The upper

Protecting the CNS

- ◆ Dura mater — fibrous membrane that lines and provides stability
- ◆ Arachnoid membrane — fragile, fibrous layer that lies between the dura and pia mater
- ◆ Pia mater — thin, highly vascular membrane covering brain's surface and forms the choroid plexuses of the brain
- ◆ Additional layers — epidural, subdural, and subarachnoid spaces

Protecting the CNS

Three primary membranes, or meninges, help protect the central nervous system (CNS): the dura mater, the arachnoid membrane, and the pia mater.

DURA MATER

The dura mater, a fibrous membrane, lines the skull and forms folds (reflections) that descend into the brain's fissures and provide stability. The dural folds include the falx cerebri (which lies in the longitudinal fissure and separates the hemispheres of the cerebrum), the tentorium cerebelli (which separates the cerebrum from the cerebellum), and the falx cerebelli (which separates the two cerebellar lobes). The arachnoid villi, projections of the dura mater into the superior sagittal and transverse sinuses, serve as the exit points for cerebrospinal fluid (CSF) drainage into venous circulation.

ARACHNOID MEMBRANE

A fragile, fibrous layer with moderate vascularity, the arachnoid membrane lies between the dura and pia mater. Injury to its blood vessels during head trauma, lumbar puncture, or cisternal puncture may cause hemorrhage.

PIA MATER

An extremely thin and highly vascular membrane, the pia mater closely covers the brain's surface and extends into its fissures. Its intimate invaginations help form the choroid plexuses of the brain's ventricular system.

ADDITIONAL LAYERS

Three layers of space further cushion the brain and spinal cord against injury. The epidural space (a potential space) lies over the dura mater. The subdural space lies between the dura mater and the arachnoid membrane and is commonly the site of hemorrhage after head trauma. The subarachnoid space, which is filled with CSF, lies between the arachnoid membrane and the pia mater.

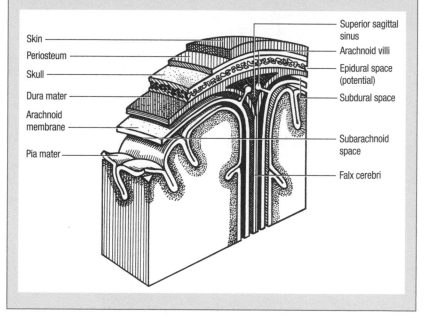

motor neurons of the brain and the lower motor neurons of the cell bodies in the ventral horn of the spinal cord carry impulses that affect movement.

The 12 pairs of cranial nerves are the primary motor and sensory pathways between the brain, head, neck, trunk, and abdomen. (See *Cranial nerves.*)

Cranial nerves

The 12 pairs of cranial nerves (CNs) transmit motor or sensory messages, or both, primarily between the brain or brain stem and the head and neck. All cranial nerves, except for the olfactory and optic nerves, exit from the midbrain, pons, or medulla of the brain stem.

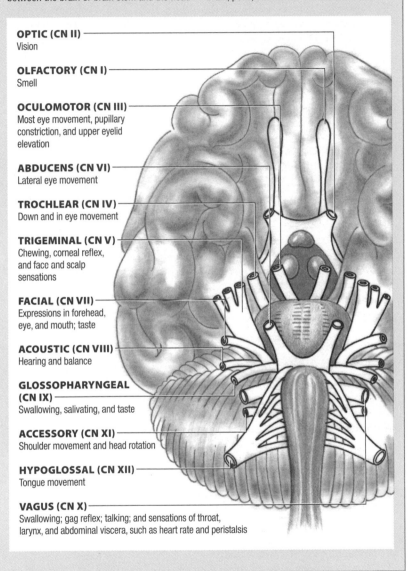

OPTIC (CN II)
Vision

OLFACTORY (CN I)
Smell

OCULOMOTOR (CN III)
Most eye movement, pupillary constriction, and upper eyelid elevation

ABDUCENS (CN VI)
Lateral eye movement

TROCHLEAR (CN IV)
Down and in eye movement

TRIGEMINAL (CN V)
Chewing, corneal reflex, and face and scalp sensations

FACIAL (CN VII)
Expressions in forehead, eye, and mouth; taste

ACOUSTIC (CN VIII)
Hearing and balance

GLOSSOPHARYNGEAL (CN IX)
Swallowing, salivating, and taste

ACCESSORY (CN XI)
Shoulder movement and head rotation

HYPOGLOSSAL (CN XII)
Tongue movement

VAGUS (CN X)
Swallowing; gag reflex; talking; and sensations of throat, larynx, and abdominal viscera, such as heart rate and peristalsis

AUTONOMIC NERVOUS SYSTEM

The vast ANS enervates all internal organs. Sometimes known as the *visceral efferent nerves*, the nerves of the ANS carry messages to the viscera from the brain stem and neuroendocrine system. The ANS has two major divisions: the sympathetic nervous system and the parasympathetic nervous system.

Facts about the ANS

+ Enervates all internal organs
+ Visceral efferent nerves carry messages to viscera from brain stem and neuroendocrine system
+ Two major divisions: sympathetic nervous system and parasympathetic nervous system

Facts about the sympathetic nervous system

+ Involves sympathetic nerves exiting spinal cord between first thoracic and second lumbar vertebrae, then entering small relay stations (ganglia) near cord
+ Disseminates impulses reaching organs and glands and producing widespread responses

Facts about the parasympathetic nervous system

+ Involves fibers leaving CNS by way of cranial nerves from midbrain and medulla and also from spinal nerves
+ Creates a more specific response involving only one organ or gland
+ Effects of activity range from reduced heart rate to increased GI tract tone and peristalsis

Obtaining a health history

+ Tracks relevant signs and symptoms over time
+ Includes chief complaint, current and past health, body system review, and family and psychosocial history
+ May include accounts from family members or friends

Exploring the chief complaint

+ Ask about onset and frequency, what precipitates or exacerbates it, what alleviates it, and if other symptoms accompany it
+ Headache, dizziness, or faintness; confusion or impaired mental status; balance and gait disturbances; LOC changes

Sympathetic nervous system

Sympathetic nerves, called *preganglionic neurons,* exit the spinal cord between the first thoracic and second lumbar vertebrae. After these nerves leave the spinal cord, they enter small relay stations (ganglia) near the cord. The ganglia form a chain that disseminates the impulse to postganglionic neurons. These neurons reach many organs and glands and can produce widespread, generalized responses.

The physiologic effects of sympathetic activity include vasoconstriction; elevated blood pressure; enhanced blood flow to skeletal muscles; increased heart rate and contractility; heightened respiratory rate; smooth-muscle relaxation of the bronchioles, GI tract, and urinary tract; sphincter contraction; pupillary dilation and ciliary muscle relaxation; increased sweat gland secretion; and reduced pancreatic secretion.

Parasympathetic nervous system

The fibers of the parasympathetic nervous system leave the CNS by way of the cranial nerves from the midbrain and medulla and also from the spinal nerves between the second and fourth sacral vertebrae (S2 to S4).

After leaving the CNS, the long preganglionic fiber of each parasympathetic nerve travels to a ganglion near a particular organ or gland; the short postganglionic fiber enters the organ or gland. This creates a more specific response involving only one organ or gland.

The physiologic effects of parasympathetic system activity include reduced heart rate, contractility, and conduction velocity; bronchial smooth-muscle constriction; increased GI tract tone and peristalsis with sphincter relaxation; urinary system sphincter relaxation and increased bladder tone; vasodilation of external genitalia, causing erection; pupillary constriction; and increased pancreatic, salivary, and lacrimal secretions. The parasympathetic system has little effect on mental or metabolic activity.

OBTAINING A HEALTH HISTORY

Begin by asking about the patient's chief complaint. Then gather details about his current illness, past illnesses, family history, and social history. Also perform a systems review.

If possible, include the patient's family members or close friends when taking the history. Don't assume that the patient remembers accurately; corroborate the details with others to get a better picture.

CHIEF COMPLAINT

The most common complaints about the neurologic system include headache, dizziness, faintness, confusion, impaired mental status, disturbances in balance and gait, and changes in LOC. When documenting the chief complaint, record the information in the patient's own words.

When you learn the patient's chief complaint, ask him about the onset and frequency of the problem, what precipitates or exacerbates it, and what alleviates it. Ask whether other symptoms accompany the problem and whether he has had adverse effects from treatments.

Also ask about other aspects of his current health and about his health and family history. Help him describe problems by asking pertinent questions.

CURRENT HEALTH HISTORY

Ask the patient whether he has headaches. If so, how often, and what seems to bring them on? Does light bother his eyes during a headache? What other symptoms occur with the headache?

 SPECIAL POINTS *If a patient is too young to describe his symptoms, suspect a headache if you see him banging or holding his head. In an infant, a shrill cry or bulging fontanels may indicate increased intracranial pressure (ICP) and headache. In children older than age 3, headache is the most common symptom of a brain tumor. In a school-aged child, ask the parents about the child's recent scholastic performance and about problems at home that may produce a tension headache. (Twice as many young boys have migraine headaches than girls.)*

Does the patient have dizziness, numbness, tingling, seizures, tremors, weakness, or paralysis? Does he have problems with his senses or with walking, keeping his balance, swallowing, or urinating?

How does he rate his memory and ability to concentrate? Does he ever have trouble speaking or understanding people? Does he have difficulty reading or writing? If he has these problems, how much do they interfere with his daily activities?

Keep in mind that some neurologic changes, such as decreased reflexes, hearing, and vision, are a normal part of aging.

 SPECIAL POINTS *Because neurons undergo various degenerative changes, aging can lead to:*
   ✦ *diminished reflexes*
✦ *decreased hearing, vision, taste, and smell*
✦ *slowed reaction time*
✦ *decreased agility*
✦ *decreased vibratory sense in the ankles*
✦ *development of muscle tremors, such as in the head and hands.*
Remember that not all neurologic changes in elderly patients are caused by aging and that certain drugs can cause changes as well. Find out if the changes are symmetric, indicating a pathologic condition, or if other abnormalities need further investigation.

PAST HEALTH HISTORY

Explore all of the patient's previous major illnesses, recurrent minor illnesses, accidents or injuries, surgical procedures, and allergies. Also explore his health and dietary habits. Does he exercise daily? Does he smoke, drink alcohol, or use illicit drugs?

Ask the patient if he's taking prescription or over-the-counter drugs or herbal preparations. If so, document the name and dosage of each drug or preparation, the duration of therapy, and the reason for it. If the patient can't remember which medications or herbal preparations he's taking, find out if he has brought them with him. If he has, examine the labels and contents yourself.

FAMILY HISTORY

Information about the patient's family may help uncover hereditary disorders. Ask him if anyone in his family has had diabetes, cardiac or renal disease, high blood pressure, cancer, bleeding disorders, mental disorders, or a stroke.

Some genetic diseases are degenerative; others cause muscle weakness. For example, seizures are more common in patients whose family history shows idiopathic epilepsy, and more than 50% of patients with migraine headaches have a family history of the disorder.

Current health history
✦ Reveals headaches, dizziness, numbness, tingling, seizures, tremors, weakness, or paralysis
✦ Detects impairment of memory and concentration
✦ Evaluates speech, comprehension, reading or writing skills
✦ Identifies interference with ADLs

Special points: Children and headace
✦ Suspect headache in child who bangs or holds his head
✦ In an infant, a shrill cry or bulging fontanels may indicate increased ICP and headache
✦ In children older than age 3, headache is the most common symptom of brain tumor

Special points: Neurologic changes with aging
✦ Note that not all neurologic changes in elderly patients are caused by aging, and that certain drugs can also cause changes

Past health history
✦ Previous major illnesses, recurrent minor illnesses, accidents or injuries, surgical procedures, and allergies
✦ Health and dietary habits and drug use

Family history
✦ Diabetes
✦ Cardiac or renal disease
✦ High blood pressure or stroke
✦ Cancer
✦ Bleeding or mental disorders

Facts about psychosocial history

+ Reveals occupation, home environment, religion, and hobbies
+ Assesses patient's self-image

Assessing the neurologic system

Facts about vital signs

+ Controlled by CNS
+ Involves body temperature, heart rate and rhythm, blood pressure, and respiratory rate

Facts about temperature

+ Normal range — 96.7° F to 100.5° F

Abnormal findings

+ Ability to maintain a constant temperature can be impaired due to hypothalamus or upper brain stem damage

Facts about heart rate

+ Controlled by ANS
+ Slows due to pressure on brain stem and cranial nerves

Abnormal findings

+ Bradycardia
+ Tachycardia

Facts about blood pressure

+ Continuously monitored by pressor receptors in the medulla

Abnormal findings

+ Rising systolic blood pressure in a patient with no history of hypertension may signal rising ICP

PSYCHOSOCIAL HISTORY

Always consider the patient's cultural and social background when planning his care. For example, what's his religion? Does he actively practice his beliefs? Also note the patient's education level and occupation: Does he have a stable or erratic employment history? Does he live alone or with someone? Does he have hobbies? How does he view his illness? Assess the patient's self-image as you gather this information.

ASSESSING THE NEUROLOGIC SYSTEM

A complete neurologic examination is so long and detailed that you probably won't ever perform one in its entirety. However, if your initial screening examination suggests a neurologic problem, you may want to perform a more detailed assessment.

Always examine the patient's neurologic system in an orderly fashion.

VITAL SIGNS

The CNS, primarily by way of the brain stem and the ANS, controls the body's vital functions: body temperature; heart rate and rhythm; blood pressure; and respiratory rate, depth, and pattern. However, because these vital control centers lie deep within the cerebral hemispheres and in the brain stem, changes in vital signs — temperature, heart rate, blood pressure, and respiration — aren't usually early indicators of CNS deterioration. When evaluating the significance of vital sign changes, consider each sign individually as well as in relation to the others.

Temperature

Normal body temperature ranges from 96.7° F to 100.5° F (35.9° C to 38.1° C), depending upon the route used for measurement.

ABNORMAL FINDINGS Damage to the hypothalamus or upper brain stem can impair the body's ability to maintain a constant temperature, resulting in profound hypothermia (temperature below 94° F [34.4° C]) or hyperthermia (temperature above 106° F [41.1° C]). Such damage can result from petechial hemorrhages in the hypothalamus or brain stem, trauma (causing pressure, twisting, or traction), or destructive lesions.

Heart rate

Because the ANS controls heart rate and rhythm, pressure on the brain stem and cranial nerves slows the heart rate by stimulating the vagus nerve.

ABNORMAL FINDINGS Bradycardia occurs in patients in the later stages of increasing ICP and with cervical spinal cord injuries; it's usually accompanied by rising systolic blood pressure, widening pulse pressure, and bounding pulse. Tachycardia occurs in patients with acutely increased ICP or a brain injury; it signals decompensation (a condition in which the body has exhausted its compensatory measures for managing ICP), which rapidly leads to death.

Blood pressure

Pressor receptors in the medulla continually monitor blood pressure.

ABNORMAL FINDINGS Keep in mind that in a patient with no history of hypertension, rising systolic blood pressure may signal rising ICP. If ICP continues to rise, the patient's pulse pressure widens as his systolic pressure climbs and diastolic pressure remains stable or falls. In the late stages of acutely elevated ICP, blood pressure plummets as cerebral perfusion fails, resulting in the patient's death.

Hypotension accompanying a brain injury is also an ominous sign. In addition, cervical spinal cord injuries may interrupt sympathetic nervous system pathways, causing peripheral vasodilation and hypotension.

Respiration

Respiratory centers in the medulla and pons control the rate, depth, and pattern of respiration. Neurologic dysfunction, particularly when it involves the brain stem or both cerebral hemispheres, commonly alters respirations. Assessment of respiration provides valuable information about a CNS lesion's site and severity.

ABNORMAL FINDINGS *Several conditions that display impaired respiration include:*

✦ *Cheyne-Stokes respiration—a waxing and waning period of hyperpnea that alternates with a shorter period of apnea, which usually indicates increased ICP from a deep cerebral or brain stem lesion, or a metabolic disturbance in the brain*

✦ *Central neurogenic hyperventilation—a type of hyperpnea that indicates damage to the lower midbrain or upper pons, which may occur as a result of severe head injury*

✦ *Apneustic respiration—an irregular breathing pattern characterized by prolonged, gasping inspiration, with a pause at full inspiration followed by expiration (there can also be a pause after expiration) that's an important localizing sign of severe brain stem damage*

✦ *Biot's respiration—late signs of neurologic deterioration, which are rare and may appear abruptly; characterized by irregular and unpredictable rate, rhythm, and depth of respiration; they may reflect increased pressure on the medulla coinciding with brain stem compression*

✦ *Respiration impairment—varying degrees can occur due to spinal cord damage above C7, which could weaken or paralyze the respiratory muscles.*

ASSESSING MENTAL STATUS AND SPEECH

Your mental status assessment actually begins when you talk to the patient during the health history. How he responds to your questions gives clues to his orientation and memory and guides you during your physical assessment.

Ask the patient questions that require more than yes or no answers. Otherwise, confusion or disorientation might not be immediately apparent. If you have doubts about a patient's mental status, perform a screening examination. (See *Checking mental status,* page 204.)

Another guide during the physical assessment is the patient's history and chief complaint. For example, if he complains about confusion or memory problems, you'll want to concentrate on the mental status part of the examination.

The mental status examination consists of checking LOC, appearance, behavior, communication, cognitive function, and constructional ability.

Level of consciousness

In performing an initial assessment, first evaluate the LOC of the patient. If the patient's behavior is threatening while doing this initial assessment, the patient may not be in immediate danger, but as the health care provider, you may be at risk. Therefore, you may need to change the order of the assessment. Always consider the environment and physical condition. For example, an elderly patient admitted to the hospital for several days may not be oriented to time, especially if he's bedridden. Also, consider the patients vital signs and need for immediate lifesaving care.

Facts about respiration

✦ Respiratory centers in medulla and pons regulate rate, depth, and pattern of respiration
✦ Neurologic dysfunction alters respirations
✦ Uncovers a CNS lesion's site and severity

Abnormal findings

✦ Cheyne-Stokes respiration
✦ Central neurogenic hyperventilation
✦ Apneustic and Biot's respirations
✦ Impaired respiration

Assessing mental status and speech

✦ Begins during health history
✦ Gives clues to orientation and memory, guides physical assessment
✦ Assesses LOC, appearance, behavior, communication, cognitive function, constructional ability

Facts about LOC

✦ Can change assessment order, depending on patient's state
✦ Tactile stimulus can be used if no response
✦ Painful stimuli can be used to assess unconscious patient or patient with markedly decreased LOC who doesn't respond to other stimuli

KNOW-HOW

Checking mental status

To screen patients for disordered thought processes, ask these questions. An incorrect answer to any question may indicate the need for a complete mental status examination.

QUESTION	FUNCTION SCREENED
What's your name?	Orientation to person
What's your mother's name?	Orientation to other people
What year is it?	Orientation to time
Where are you now?	Orientation to place
How old are you?	Memory
Where were you born?	Remote memory
What did you have for breakfast?	Recent memory
Who is the U.S. president?	General knowledge
Can you count backward from 20 to 1?	Attention span and calculation skills

A change in the patient's LOC is the earliest and most sensitive indicator that his neurologic status has changed.

A fully awake patient is alert, open-eyed, and attentive to environmental stimuli. A less awake patient appears drowsy, has reduced motor activity, and seems less attentive to environmental stimuli. Decreased arousal often precedes disorientation.

Speak the patient's name in a normal tone of voice and note the response to an auditory stimulus. If he doesn't respond, use a tactile stimulus, such as touching him gently, squeezing his hand, or shaking his shoulder.

Use painful stimuli only to assess a patient who's unconscious or who has a markedly decreased LOC and doesn't respond to other stimuli. To test response to pain, you can apply firm pressure over a nail bed with a blunt hard object such as a pen. Other acceptable methods include:

✦ squeezing the trapezius muscle
✦ applying supraorbital pressure
✦ applying mandibular pressure
✦ performing a sternal rub
✦ applying nailbed pressure.

Next, note the type and intensity of stimulus required to elicit a response. Is the response an appropriate verbal one, unintelligible mumbling, body movement, eye opening, or nothing at all? After you remove the stimulus, how alert is the patient? Wide awake? Drowsy? Drifting to sleep?

Other methods to assess LOC
✦ Squeeze trapezius muscle
✦ Apply supraorbital pressure
✦ Apply mandibular pressure
✦ Perform a sternal rub
✦ Apply nailbed pressure

After assessing the patient's level of arousal, compare the findings with results of previous assessments. Note trends. For example, is the patient lethargic more often than usual? Consider factors that could affect patient responsiveness. For example, a normally alert patient may become drowsy after administration of such CNS depressant medications as sedatives and opioids.

Learn to describe a patient's responsiveness objectively. For example, describe a lethargic patient's responses this way: "awakened when called loudly, then immediately fell asleep."

Many terms are used to describe LOC, but their definitions may differ slightly among practitioners. To avoid confusion, clearly describe the patient's response to various stimuli using these guidelines:

✦ alert—follows commands and responds completely and appropriately to stimuli
✦ lethargic—is drowsy; has delayed responses to verbal stimuli; may drift off to sleep during examination
✦ stuporous—requires vigorous stimulation for a response
✦ comatose—doesn't respond appropriately to verbal or painful stimuli; can't follow commands or communicate verbally.

 CLINICAL ALERT If the patient has sustained a skull fracture, but appears lucid, and later has a decreased LOC, this could indicate arterial epidural bleeding that requires immediate surgery.

To minimize the subjectivity of LOC assessment and to establish a greater degree of reliability, you may use the Glasgow Coma Scale. This scale evaluates the patient's LOC according to three objective behaviors: eye opening, verbal responsiveness (which includes orientation), and motor response. (See *Using the Glasgow Coma Scale*, page 206.) A patient's orientation to time is usually disrupted first and his orientation to person is disrupted last.

Several disorders can affect the cerebral hemisphere of the brain stem—and consciousness can be impaired by any one of them. Consciousness is the most sensitive indicator of neurologic dysfunction and may be a valuable adjunct to other findings. When assessing LOC, make sure you provide a stimulus that's strong enough to get a true picture of the patient's baseline. (See *Detecting increased ICP,* page 207.)

 CLINICAL ALERT A change in the patient's LOC commonly serves as the earliest indication of a brain disorder. Rapid deterioration of LOC (minutes to hours) usually indicates an acute neurologic disorder requiring immediate intervention. A gradually decreasing LOC (weeks to months) may reflect a progressive or degenerative neurologic disorder.

Disorders that affect LOC include:
✦ toxic encephalopathy
✦ hemorrhage
✦ extensive, generalized cortical atrophy
✦ tumor or intracranial hemorrhage.

Orientation
The orientation portion of the assessment measures the ability of the cerebral cortex to receive and accurately interpret sensory stimuli. It includes three aspects: orientation to person, place, and time. Always ask questions that require the patient to provide information, rather than a yes-or-no answer:
✦ person—Is the patient aware of his identity? Ask him his name, and note the response.

KNOW-HOW

Using the Glasgow Coma Scale

The Glasgow Coma Scale describes a patient's baseline mental status and helps to detect and interpret changes from baseline findings. When using the Glasgow Coma Scale, test the patient's ability to respond to verbal, motor, and sensory stimulation, and grade your findings according to the scale. A score of 15 indicates that the patient is alert, can follow simple commands, and is oriented to person, place, and time. A decreased score in one or more categories may signal an impending neurologic crisis. A score of 7 or less indicates severe neurologic damage.

Glasgow Coma Scale

+ Minimizes LOC subjectivity
+ Establishes greater degree of reliability
+ Describes patient's baseline mental status
+ Detects and interprets changes from baseline findings
+ Evaluates patient's LOC according to eye opening, verbal, and motor responsiveness

TEST	SCORE	PATIENT RESPONSE
Eye opening response		
Spontaneously	4	Opens eyes spontaneously
To speech	3	Opens eyes when told to
To pain	2	Opens eyes only to painful stimulus
None	1	Doesn't open eyes in response to stimuli
Motor response		
Obeys	6	Shows two fingers when asked
Localizes	5	Reaches toward painful stimulus and tries to remove it
Withdraws	4	Moves away from painful stimulus
Abnormal flexion	3	Assumes a decorticate posture (shown below)
Abnormal extension	2	Assumes a decerebrate posture (shown below)
None	1	No response; just lies flaccid (an ominous sign)
Verbal response (to question, "What year is this?")		
Oriented	5	Tells correct date
Confused	4	Tells incorrect year
Inappropriate words	3	Replies randomly with incorrect words
Incomprehensible	2	Moans or screams
No response	1	No response
Total score		

Detecting increased ICP

The earlier you can recognize the signs of increased intracranial pressure (ICP), the more quickly you can intervene and improve the patient's chance of recovery. By the time late signs appear, interventions may be useless.

	EARLY SIGNS	LATE SIGNS
Level of consciousness	✦ Requires increased stimulation ✦ Subtle orientation loss ✦ Restlessness and anxiety ✦ Sudden quietness	✦ Unarousable
Pupils	✦ Pupil changes on side of lesion ✦ One pupil constricts but then dilates (unilateral hippus) ✦ Sluggish reaction of both pupils ✦ Unequal pupils	✦ Pupils fixed and dilated or "blown"
Motor response	✦ Sudden weakness ✦ Motor changes on side opposite the lesion ✦ Positive pronator drift; with palms up, one hand pronates	✦ Profound weakness
Vital signs	✦ Intermittent increases in blood pressure	✦ Increased systolic pressure, profound bradycardia, abnormal respirations (Cushing's syndrome)

ABNORMAL FINDINGS *A patient disoriented to person may not be able to tell his name. When asked, he may look baffled or may stammer and finally produce an unintelligible or inaccurate answer. Self-identity usually remains intact until late in decreasing LOC, making disorientation to person an ominous sign.*

✦ place — Can the patient state his location correctly? For example, when looking around the room, can he conclude that he's in a health care facility? Or does he think he's at home?

ABNORMAL FINDINGS *A hospitalized patient disoriented to place most commonly confuses the health care facility's room with home or some other familiar surrounding; a nonhospitalized patient disoriented to place, such as a patient with Alzheimer's disease, may fail to recognize familiar home surroundings and may wander off in search of something familiar.*

Keep in mind that the patient oriented to place may not be able to name the health care facility, especially if he has been admitted through the emergency department. However, if a patient states the full name of the health care facility and later can't recall its name, he may be becoming disoriented to place.

Facts about orientation
(continued)

Abnormal findings: Orientation to person
✦ Inability of patient to remember his name
✦ Self-identity usually remains intact until late in decreasing LOC

Abnormal findings: Orientation to place
✦ A hospitalized patient may confuse health care facility with home
✦ A nonhospitalized patient (such as with Alzheimer's disease) may fail to recognize familiar home surroundings and wander

Facts about orientation
(continued)
Abnormal findings:
Orientation to time
✦ Disorientation to time may be first indicator of decreasing LOC

Facts about appearance
✦ Reveals patient's behavior, dress, and grooming
✦ Evaluates coloring, facial expressions, mobility, deformities, and nutritional state
✦ Detects impairments in gait, posture, and ability to rise

Abnormal findings
✦ Subtle changes in patient's behavior (new onset of chronic disease or more acute change, involving frontal lobe)
✦ Raccoon eyes (bleeding into periorbital tissue)
✦ Otorrhea (basilar skull fracture)

Facts about behavior
✦ Evaluates patient's thought content
✦ Indicates patient's ability to think abstractly and use judgment
✦ Reveals emotional status

Abnormal findings
✦ Disorderd thought patterns (delirium or psychosis); interpreting a common proverb literally (dementia)

Special points
✦ Non-English speaking patient may have difficulty interpreting a common proverb
✦ Ask a family member to explain a saying to the patient in his native language
✦ Symptoms of depression in elderly patients may be atypical (decreased function or increased agitation

✦ time—If oriented to time, most people can state the correct year, month and, usually, date. Most can also differentiate day from night if their environment provides enough information; for example, if the room has a window.

 ABNORMAL FINDINGS *Disorientation to time is one of the first indicators of decreasing LOC.*

Appearance
Also note how the patient behaves, dresses, and grooms himself. Does he look and act inappropriately? Is his personal hygiene poor? If so, discuss your findings with his family members to determine whether this is a change.

 ABNORMAL FINDINGS *Even subtle changes in a patient's behavior can signal a new onset of a chronic disease or a more acute change that involves the frontal lobe.*

Look at the patient's color, facial expressions, mobility, deformities, and nutritional state.

Observe the patient's gait, posture, and ability to rise from a chair. Does he need assistance to walk, rise from a chair, or get undressed? Can he hear and see you when you are talking? Does the patient have raccoon eyes?

 ABNORMAL FINDINGS *Raccoon eyes could indicate bleeding into the periorbital tissue.*

Does the patient have otorrhea (CSF leaking from the ears)?

 ABNORMAL FINDINGS *Otorrhea could indicate a basilar skull fracture. If the brain stem is lacerated or contused, immediate death can occur. Smaller leakages can resolve in 2 to 10 days.*

Behavior
Assess thought content by evaluating the clarity and cohesiveness of the patient's ideas. Is his conversation smooth, with logical transitions between ideas? Does he have hallucinations (sensory perceptions that lack appropriate stimuli) or delusions (beliefs not supported by reality)?

 ABNORMAL FINDINGS *Disordered thought patterns may indicate delirium or psychosis.*

Test the patient's ability to think abstractly by asking him to interpret a common proverb such as "A stitch in time saves nine."

 ABNORMAL FINDINGS *A patient with dementia may interpret a common proverb literally.*

 SPECIAL POINTS *If the patient's primary language isn't English, he'll probably have difficulty interpreting a common proverb. Engage the assistance of family members when English isn't the patient's primary language. Have them ask the patient to explain a saying in his native language.*

Test the patient's judgment by asking him how he would respond to a hypothetical situation. For example, what would he do if he were in a public building and the fire alarm sounded? Evaluate the appropriateness of his answer.

Throughout the interview, assess the patient's emotional status. Note his mood, his emotional stability or lability, and the appropriateness of his emotional responses. Also assess his mood by asking how he feels about himself and his future.

SPECIAL POINTS *Keep in mind that symptoms of depression in elderly patients may be atypical—for example, decreased function or increased agitation may occur rather than the usual sad effect.*

Communication

Assess the patient's ability to comprehend speech, writing, numbers, and gestures. Language skills include learning and recalling the parts of the language (such as words), organizing word relationships according to grammatical rules, and structuring message content logically. Speech involves neuromuscular actions of the mouth, tongue, and oropharynx.

Verbal responsiveness

During the interview and physical assessment, observe the patient when you ask a question. If you suspect a decreased LOC, call the patient's name or gently shake his shoulder to try to elicit a verbal response.

Note how much the patient says. Does he speak in complete sentences? In phrases? In single words? Does he communicate spontaneously? Or does he rarely speak?

Note the quality of the patient's speech. Is it unusually loud or soft? Does the patient articulate clearly, or are his words difficult to understand? What's the rate and rhythm of the patient's speech? What language does he speak? (If you can't speak this language, seek help from an interpreter or family member.)

Are the patient's verbal responses appropriate? Does he choose the correct words to express thoughts, or does he appear to have problems finding or articulating words? Does he use made-up words (neologisms)?

Can the patient understand and follow commands? When given a multistep command, does he forget what follows the first step?

If communication problems arise, is the patient aware of them? Does he appear frustrated or angry when communication fails, or does he continue to attempt to talk, unaware that you don't comprehend?

If you suspect a language difficulty, show the patient a common object, such as a cup or a book, and ask him to name it. Or, ask the patient to repeat a word that you say, such as dog or breakfast.

If the patient appears to have difficulty understanding spoken language, ask him to follow a simple instruction such as "Touch your nose." If the patient succeeds, then try a two-step command such as "Touch your right knee, then touch your nose."

Keep in mind that language performance tends to fluctuate with the time of day and changes in physical condition. A healthy individual may experience language difficulty when ill or fatigued.

 CLINICAL ALERT **Increasing language difficulties may indicate deteriorating neurologic status, warranting further evaluation and notification of the physician.**

ABNORMAL FINDINGS *Speech impairment or impaired language function can occur from:*
   ✦ dysphasia—impaired ability to use or understand language
✦ aphasia—inability to use or understand language, or both, that's caused by injury to the cerebral cortex. Several types of aphasia exist, including:

– expressive or Broca's aphasia — impaired fluency; difficulty finding words; impairment located in the frontal lobe, the anterior speech area
– receptive or Wernicke's aphasia — inability to understand written words or speech; use of made-up words; impairment located in the posterior speech cortex, which involves the temporal and parietal lobes
– global aphasia — lack of both expressive and receptive language; impairment of both speech areas.
◆ *facial muscle paralysis — difficulty in articulation and slurred speech*
◆ *dysarthria — impairment of neuromuscular speech*
◆ *dysphonia — impairment of voice.*

Formal language skills evaluation

The formal language skills evaluation identifies the extent and characteristics of the patient's language deficits. Usually performed by a speech pathologist, it may help pinpoint the site of a CNS lesion. For example, identifying expressive aphasia (the patient knows what he wants to say but can't speak the words) may help diagnose a frontal lobe lesion.

If you'll be evaluating the patient's language skills, include:

◆ spontaneous speech — After showing the patient a picture, ask him to describe what's going on.

◆ comprehension — Ask the patient a series of simple yes-or-no questions and evaluate his answers. Use questions with obvious answers. For example: "Does it snow in July?"

◆ naming — Show the patient various common objects, one at a time, and then ask him to name each one. Typical objects include a comb, ball, cup, and pencil.

◆ repetition — Ask him to repeat words or phrases such as "no ifs, ands, or buts."

◆ vocabulary — Have the patient explain the meaning of each of a series of words.

◆ reading — Ask him to read printed words on cards and perform the action described. For example: "Raise your hand."

◆ writing — Ask the patient to write something, perhaps a story describing a scene or a picture.

◆ copying figures — Show the patient several figures, one at a time, and then ask him to copy them. The figures usually become increasingly complex, starting with a circle, an X, and a square and proceeding to a triangle and a star.

Cognitive function

Assessing cognitive function involves testing the patient's memory, orientation, attention span, calculation ability, thought content, abstract thinking, judgment, insight, and emotional status.

To test your patient's orientation, memory, and attention span, use the mental status screening questions discussed previously.

Always consider the patient's environment and physical condition when assessing orientation. Also, when the person is intubated and unable to speak, ask questions that require only a nod, such as "Do you know you're in the hospital?" and "Are we in Pennsylvania?"

The patient with an intact short-term memory can generally repeat five to seven nonconsecutive numbers right away and again 10 minutes later. Remember that short-term memory is commonly affected first in patients with neurologic disease.

When testing attention span and calculation skills, keep in mind that lack of mathematical ability and anxiety can affect the patient's performance. If he has difficulty with numerical computation, ask him to spell the word "world" backward. While he's performing these functions, note his ability to pay attention.

Constructional ability

Constructional disorders affect the patient's ability to perform simple tasks and use various objects. Assess constructional ability by asking the patient to draw a clock or a square. Apraxia and agnosia are two types of constructional disorders.

 ABNORMAL FINDINGS *Commonly associated with parietal lobe dysfunction, apraxia is the inability to perform purposeful movements and make proper use of objects. It can appear in any of four types:*

✦ *ideomotor apraxia—loss of ability to understand the effect of motor activity; ability to perform simple activities but without awareness of performing them; inability to perform actions on command*
✦ *ideational apraxia—awareness of actions that need to be done but inability to perform them*
✦ *constructional apraxia—inability to copy a design such as the face of a clock*
✦ *dressing apraxia—inability to understand the meaning of various articles of clothing or the sequence of actions required to get dressed.*

The inability to identify common objects—called agnosia*—may indicate a lesion in the sensory cortex. Types include:*
✦ *visual—inability to identify common objects unless they're touched*
✦ *auditory—inability to identify common sounds*
✦ *body image—inability to identify body parts by sight or touch, inability to localize a stimulus, or denial of existence of half of the body.*

ASSESSING CRANIAL NERVE FUNCTION

There are 12 pairs of cranial nerves (CNs). These nerves transmit motor or sensory messages, or both, primarily between the brain and brain stem and the head and neck. Cranial nerve assessment provides valuable information about the condition of the CNS, particularly the brain stem.

Olfactory (CN I)

To assess the olfactory nerve, first check the patency of both nostrils, then instruct the patient to close his eyes. Occlude one nostril and hold a familiar, pungent-smelling substance—such as coffee, tobacco, soap, or peppermint—under his nose and ask its identity. Repeat this technique with the other nostril.

If the patient reports detecting the smell but can't name it, offer a choice such as "Do you smell lemon, coffee, or peppermint?"

The patient should be able to detect and identify the smell correctly. The location of the olfactory nerve makes it especially vulnerable to damage from facial fractures and head injuries.

 ABNORMAL FINDINGS *Damage to CN I may be due to disorders of the base of the frontal lobe, such as tumors or arteriosclerotic changes. The sense of smell remains intact as long as one of the two olfactory nerves exists; it's permanently lost (anosmia) if both nerves are affected. Anosmia can also result from nonneurologic causes, such as nasal congestion, sinus infection, smoking, and cocaine use, and impair the sense of taste. A complaint about food taste may signal CN I damage.*

Optic (CN II) and oculomotor (CN III)

To assess the optic nerve, check visual acuity, visual fields, and the retinal structures. To assess the oculomotor nerve, check pupil size, pupil shape, and pupillary response to light.

To test visual acuity quickly and informally, have the patient read a newspaper, starting with large headlines and moving to small print.

Visual field defects

Here are some examples of visual field defects. The black areas represent vision loss.

	LEFT	RIGHT
Blindness of right eye	○	●
Bitemporal hemianopsia, or loss of half the visual field	◑	◐
Left homonymous hemianopsia	◑	◑
Left homonymous hemianopsia, superior quadrant	◴	◴

Assessing CN II and CN III
(continued)

+ Use confrontation, when testing visual fields
+ Look for trends when assessing pupil size

Abnormal findings

+ Visual field defect may signal stroke, head injury, or brain tumor
+ Pupil size may be affected by increased ICP, hippus phenomenon, optic and oculomotor nerve damage, or anisocoria

Test visual fields with a technique called *confrontation*. To do this, stand 2′ (0.6 m) in front of the patient, and have him cover one eye. Then close one of your eyes and bring your moving fingers into the patient's visual field from the periphery. Ask him to tell you when he sees the object. Test each quadrant of the patient's visual field, and compare his results with your own. Chart defects you find. (See *Visual field defects.*)

 ABNORMAL FINDINGS *A visual field defect may signal stroke, head injury, or brain tumor. The area and extent of the loss depend on the location of the lesion.*

When assessing pupil size, look for trends. For example, watch for a gradual increase in the size of one pupil or the appearance of unequal pupils in a patient whose pupils were previously equal.

The pupils should be equal, round, and reactive to light.

 ABNORMAL FINDINGS *Pupil size can be affected by:*

+ *increased ICP—pressure on the oculomotor nerve causes a change in responsiveness or pupil size on the affected side that results in dilation of the pupil ipsilateral to the mass lesion; as the ICP rises, the other oculomotor nerve becomes affected, causing both pupils to become oval or react sluggishly to light shortly before dilating; but, without treatment, both pupils become fixed and dilated*
+ *the hippus phenomenon—brisk pupil constriction in response to light followed by a pulsating dilation and constriction (may be normal in some patients but may also reflect early oculomotor nerve compression)*
+ *optic and oculomotor nerve damage—pupillary response to light is affected, indicating neurologic demise*
+ *anisocoria (unequal pupils)—normal in about 20% of people; pupil size doesn't change with the amount of illumination. (See* Understanding pupillary changes.*)*

Understanding pupillary changes

Use this chart as a guide to pupillary changes.

PUPILLARY CHANGE	POSSIBLE CAUSES
Unilateral, dilated (4 mm), fixed, and nonreactive 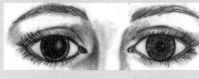	✦ Uncal herniation with oculomotor nerve damage ✦ Brain stem compression ✦ Increased intracranial pressure ✦ Tentorial herniation ✦ Head trauma with subdural or epidural hematoma ✦ May be normal in some people
Bilateral, dilated (4 mm), fixed, and nonreactive 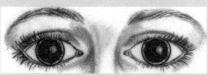	✦ Severe midbrain damage ✦ Cardiopulmonary arrest (hypoxia) ✦ Anticholinergic poisoning
Bilateral, midsize (2 mm), fixed, and nonreactive 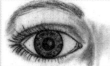	✦ Midbrain involvement caused by edema, hemorrhage, infarctions, lacerations, contusions
Bilateral, pinpoint (< 1 mm), and usually nonreactive 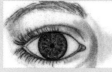	✦ Lesions of pons, usually after hemorrhage
Unilateral, small (1.5 mm), and nonreactive 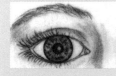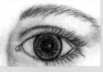	✦ Disruption of sympathetic nerve supply to the head caused by spinal cord lesion above the first thoracic vertebrae

SPECIAL POINTS *In a blind patient with a nonfunctional optic nerve, light stimulation will fail to produce either a direct or a consensual pupillary response. However, a legally blind patient may have some optic nerve function, which causes the blind eye to respond to direct light. In a patient who's totally blind in only one eye, the pupil of the eye with the intact optic nerve will react to direct light stimulation, whereas the blind eye, because it receives sensory messages from the functional optic nerve, will respond consensually.*

Assessing CN II and CN III
(continued)

Special points
✦ Blind patients — with a nonfunctional optic nerve, light stimulation fails to produce direct or consensual pupillary response
✦ Legally blind patient — has some optic nerve function
✦ Patient blind in one eye — with intact optic nerve, pupil reacts to direct light stimulation

Assessing CN III, CN IV, and CN VI

✦ Assess all three nerves simultaneously by evaluating extraocular eye movement
✦ Watch for nystagmus, disconjugate movement, and ophthalmoplegia; also note diplopia
✦ Eye movement should display smooth and coordinated function of all six directions of eye movement

Abnormal findings

✦ Ptosis
✦ Nystagmus

Assessing CN V

Sensory portion

✦ Involves patient's response to light and sharp touch of the right and left side of patient's forehead, cheek, and jaw
✦ Patient should feel light and sharp touch in all three areas

Motor portion

✦ Involves palpation of patient's clenched jaws, checking for symmetry; involves observation of patient opening and closing his mouth, checking for asymmetry
✦ Jaws should clench symmetrically and remained closed against resistance

Abnormal findings

✦ Loss of sensation in forehead, cheek, or jaw (peripheral nerve damage)
✦ Severe, piercing, or stabbing pain over one or more of facial dermatomes (trigeminal neuralgia)
✦ Impaired sensory and motor function (spinal cord lesion)
✦ Absent corneal reflex (peripheral nerve or brain stem damage)

Oculomotor (CN III), trochlear (CN IV), and abducens (CN VI)

To test the coordinated function of the oculomotor, trochlear, and abducens nerves, assess them simultaneously by evaluating the patient's extraocular eye movement.

Observe each eye for rapid oscillation (nystagmus), movement not in unison with that of the other eye (disconjugate movement), or inability to move in certain directions (ophthalmoplegia). Also, note complaints of double vision (diplopia).

The oculomotor nerve is also responsible for eyelid elevation and pupillary constriction.

 ABNORMAL FINDINGS *Drooping of the patient's eyelid, or ptosis, can result from a defect in the oculomotor nerve. To assess ptosis more accurately, have the patient sit upright.*

The patient's eyes should move smoothly and in a coordinated manner through all six directions of eye movement: left superior, left lateral, left inferior, right superior, right lateral, and right inferior.

 ABNORMAL FINDINGS *Nystagmus may indicate a disorder of the brain stem, the cerebellum, or the vestibular portion of CN VIII. It can also imply drug toxicity such as from the anticonvulsant phenytoin.*

Increased ICP can put pressure on CN IV, causing impaired extraocular eye movement inferiorly and medially, and CN VI, causing impaired extraocular eye movement laterally.

Trigeminal (CN V)

To assess the sensory portion of the trigeminal nerve, gently touch the right side and the left side of the patient's forehead with a cotton ball while his eyes are closed. Instruct him to state the moment the cotton touches the area. Compare his response on both sides. Repeat the technique on the right and left cheek and on the right and left jaw. Next, repeat the entire procedure using a sharp object. The cap of a disposable ballpoint pen can be used to test light touch (dull end) and sharp stimuli (sharp end). (If an abnormality appears, also test for temperature sensation by touching the patient's skin with test tubes filled with hot and cold water and asking the patient to differentiate between them.)

The patient should report feeling both light touch and sharp stimuli in all three areas (forehead, cheek, and jaw) on both sides of the face.

 ABNORMAL FINDINGS *Peripheral nerve damage can create a loss of sensation in any or all three regions supplied by the trigeminal nerve (forehead, cheek, jaw). Trigeminal neuralgia causes severe, piercing, or stabbing pain over one or more of the facial dermatomes. A lesion in the cervical spinal cord or brain stem can produce impaired sensory function in each of the three areas.*

To assess the motor portion of the trigeminal nerve, ask the patient to clench his jaws. Palpate the temporal and masseter muscles bilaterally, checking for symmetry. Try to open his clenched jaws. Next, watch the patient while he's opening and closing his mouth for asymmetry.

The jaws should clench symmetrically and remain closed against resistance.

 ABNORMAL FINDINGS *A lesion in the cervical spinal cord or brain stem can produce impaired motor function in regions supplied by the trigeminal nerve, weakening the patient's jaw muscles, causing the jaw to deviate toward the affected side when chewing, and allowing residual food to collect in the affected cheek.*

To assess the patient's corneal reflex, stroke a wisp of cotton lightly across a cornea. The lids of both eyes should close.

ABNORMAL FINDINGS *An absent corneal reflex may result from periph-eral nerve or brain stem damage. However, a diminished corneal reflex commonly occurs in patients who wear contact lenses.*

Facial (CN VII)

To test the motor portion of the facial nerve, ask the patient to wrinkle his forehead, raise and lower his eyebrows, smile to show teeth, and puff out his cheeks. Also, with the patient's eyes tightly closed, attempt to open the eyelids. With each of these movements, observe closely for symmetry.

Facial movements should be symmetrical.

 ABNORMAL FINDINGS *Unilateral facial weakness can reflect an upper motor neuron problem, such as a stroke or a tumor that has damaged neurons in the facial control area of the motor strip in the cerebral cortex. If the weakness originates in the cerebral cortex, the patient will retain the ability to wrinkle his forehead because the forehead receives motor messages from both hemispheres of the brain—which explains why when one side is damaged, such as in a stroke, the other side takes over.*

However, if CN VII is damaged, the weakness will extend to the forehead, and the eye on the affected side won't close.

To test the sensory portion of the facial nerve, which supplies taste sensation to the anterior two-thirds of the tongue, prepare four marked, closed containers: one containing salt; another sugar; a third, vinegar (or lemon); and a fourth, quinine (or bitters). Then, with the patient's eyes closed, place salt on the anterior two-thirds of his tongue using a cotton swab or dropper. Ask him to identify the taste as sweet, salty, sour, or bitter. Rinse his mouth with water. Repeat this procedure, alternating flavors and sides of the tongue, until all four flavors have been tested on both sides. Taste sensations to the posterior third of the tongue are supplied by the glossopharyngeal nerve (CN IX) and are usually tested at the same time.

The patient should have symmetrical taste sensations.

 ABNORMAL FINDINGS *An impaired sense of taste can signify damage to the patient's facial or glossopharyngeal nerve, or it may simply reflect a part of the normal aging process. Chemotherapy or head and neck radiation can also alter taste by damaging taste bud receptors.*

Acoustic (CN VIII)

To assess the acoustic portion of the acoustic nerve, test the patient's hearing acuity. To test hearing, ask the patient to cover one ear, and then stand on his opposite side and whisper a few words. See whether he can repeat what you said. Test the other ear the same way.

To assess the vestibular portion of this nerve, observe for nystagmus and disturbed balance and note reports of dizziness or the room spinning.

The patient should be able to hear a whispered voice, rubbing of fingers, or a watch ticking. He should have normal eye movement and balance and no dizziness or vertigo.

ABNORMAL FINDINGS *With sensorineural hearing loss, the patient may have trouble hearing high-pitched sounds, or he may have a total loss of hearing in the affected ear due to lesions of the cochlear branch of CN VIII. With nystagmus and vertigo, the patient may have a disturbance of the vestibular centers. If it's caused by a peripheral lesion, vertigo and nystagmus will occur 10 to 20 seconds after the patient changes position, and symptoms will gradually lessen with the repetition of the position change. If the vertigo is of central origin, there's no latent period, and the symptoms don't diminish with repetition.*

Assessing CN VII

Motor portion
+ Tests for symmetrical facial movements

Sensory portion
+ Tests for symmetrical taste sensation

Abnormal findings
+ Unilateral facial weakness (stroke)
+ Taste impairment (damage to facial or glossopharyngeal nerve)

Assessing CN VIII

+ Acoustic portion—test patient's hearing acuity
+ Vestibular portion—observe for nystagmus and disturbed balance and reports of dizziness or room spinning

Abnormal findings
+ With sensorineural hearing loss, the patient may have total hearing loss; with nystagmus and vertigo, he may have disturbance of the vestibular centers

Assessing CN IX and CN X

+ Involves assessing voice and gag reflex functions

Abnormal findings

+ Glossopharyngeal neuralgia or damage producing paroxysmal pain and impaired swallowing, or loss of gag reflex
+ Vagal damage affecting involuntary vital functions

Assessing CN XI

+ Tests patient's ability to overcome resistance applied to shoulders
+ Tests patient's ability to overcome resistance applied to his neck while his head is turned

Abnormal findings

+ Unilateral weakness, atrophy, or paralysis of the muscles (peripheral nerve lesion)

Assessing CN XII

+ Involves testing patient's tongue for movement, articulation, and response to pressure

Abnormal findings

+ Unilateral flaccid paralysis of tongue, atrophy of affected side, and deviation (peripheral nerve lesion)
+ Unilateral spastic paralysis produces dysarthria

Glossopharyngeal (CN IX) and vagus (CN X)

To assess the glossopharyngeal and vagus nerves, which have overlapping functions, first listen to the patient's voice for indications of a hoarse or nasal quality. Then watch his soft palate when he says "ah." Next, test the gag reflex after warning him. To evoke this reflex, touch the posterior wall of the pharynx with a cotton swab or tongue blade.

The patient's voice should sound strong and clear. The soft palate and the uvula should rise when he says "ah," and the uvula should remain midline. The palatine arches should remain symmetrical during movement and at rest. The gag reflex should be intact. If the gag reflex diminishes or the pharynx moves asymmetrically, evaluate each side of the posterior pharyngeal wall to confirm integrity of both cranial nerves.

 ABNORMAL FINDINGS Glossopharyngeal neuralgia produces paroxysmal pain, which radiates from the patient's throat to his ear. Damage to the CN IX or CN X impairs swallowing. Furthermore, during swallowing, the palate fails to rise and close off the nasal passageways, allowing nasal regurgitation of fluids.

A damaged CN X can also cause loss of the gag reflex and a hoarse or nasal-sounding voice. Finally, because the vagus nerve innervates most viscera through the parasympathetic nervous system, vagal damage can affect involuntary vital functions, producing tachycardia, other cardiac arrhythmias, and dyspnea.

Accessory (CN XI)

To assess the spinal accessory nerve, press down on the patient's shoulders while he attempts to shrug against this resistance. Note shoulder strength and symmetry while inspecting and palpating the trapezius muscle.

Then apply resistance to his turned head while he attempts to return to a midline position. Note neck strength while inspecting and palpating the sternocleidomastoid muscle. Repeat for the opposite side.

Both shoulders should be able to overcome the resistance equally well. The neck should overcome resistance in both directions.

ABNORMAL FINDINGS Unilateral weakness, atrophy, or paralysis of the muscles innervated by the spinal accessory nerve suggests a peripheral nerve lesion. Signs include a drooping shoulder or a scapula that appears displaced toward the affected side.

Hypoglossal (CN XII)

To assess the hypoglossal nerve, observe the patient's protruded tongue for any deviation from midline, atrophy, or fasciculations (very fine muscle flickering, which indicates lower motor neuron disease).

Next, instruct the patient to move his tongue rapidly from side to side with the mouth open, to curl his tongue up toward the nose, and to curl his tongue down toward the chin.

Then use a tongue blade or folded gauze pad to apply resistance to his protruded tongue and ask him to try to push the tongue blade to one side. Repeat this procedure on the other side and note the patient's tongue strength.

Listen to the patient's speech for the sounds d, n, and t, which require use of the tongue to articulate. If his general speech suggests a problem, have him repeat a phrase or a series of words that contain these sounds, such as "Round the rugged rock that ragged rascal ran."

The tongue should be midline, and the patient should be able to move it right and left equally. He also should be able to move the tongue up and down. Pressure exerted by the tongue on the tongue blade should be equal on either side. Speech should be clear.

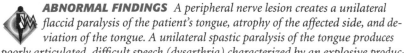 ***ABNORMAL FINDINGS*** *A peripheral nerve lesion creates a unilateral flaccid paralysis of the patient's tongue, atrophy of the affected side, and deviation of the tongue. A unilateral spastic paralysis of the tongue produces poorly articulated, difficult speech (dysarthria) characterized by an explosive production of words. The tongue deviates toward the affected side.*

ASSESSING SENSORY FUNCTION

Evaluation of the sensory system involves checking five areas of sensation: pain, light touch, vibration, position, and discrimination.

Pain

To test the patient for pain, have him close his eyes; then touch all the major dermatomes, first with the sharp end of a safety pin and then with the dull end. Proceed in this order: fingers, shoulders, toes, thighs, and trunk. Ask him to identify when he feels the sharp stimulus.

If the patient has major deficits, start in the area with the least sensation, and move toward the area with the most sensation. This helps you determine the level of deficit.

Light touch

To test for the sense of light touch, follow the same routine as above, but use a wisp of cotton. Lightly touch the patient's skin—don't swab or sweep the cotton, because you might miss an area of loss. A patient with a peripheral neuropathy might retain his sensation for light touch after he has lost pain sensation.

Vibration

To test vibratory sense, apply a tuning fork over certain bony prominences while the patient keeps his eyes closed. Start at the distal interphalangeal joint of the great toe, and move proximally. Test only until the patient feels the vibration, because everything above that level will be intact. (See *Evaluating vibration,* page 218.)

If vibratory sense is intact, you don't have to check position sense because the same pathway carries both.

Position

To assess position sense, have the patient close his eyes. Then grasp the sides of his big toe, move it up and down, and ask him what position it's in. To be tested for position sense, the patient needs intact vestibular and cerebellar function.

Perform the same test on the patient's upper extremities by grasping the sides of his index finger and moving it back and forth.

Discrimination

Discrimination testing assesses the ability of the cerebral cortex to interpret and integrate information. Stereognosis is the ability to discriminate the shape, size, weight, texture, and form of an object by touching and manipulating it. To test this, ask the patient to close his eyes and open his hand. Then place a common object, such as a key, in his hand, and ask him to identify it.

If he can't, test graphesthesia next. Have the patient keep his eyes closed and hold out his hand while you draw a large number on the palm. Ask him to identify the number. Both these tests assess the ability of the cortex to integrate sensory input.

To test point localization, have the patient close his eyes; then touch one of his limbs, and ask him where you touched him. Test two-point discrimination by

Assessing sensory function
- Evaluates the sensory system
- Checks five areas of sensation

Pain
- Test all major dermatomes with sharp and dull end of an object
- Start with area of least sensation and move toward area with most

Light touch
- Test with a wisp of cotton
- Start with area of least sensation and move toward area with most

Vibration
- Test with a tuning fork
- Start at distal interphalangeal joint of the great toe, move proximally

Position
- Grasp sides of patient's big toe, move it up and down, and ask him what position it's in
- Requires intact vestibular and cerebellar function

Discrimination
- Involves ability of cerebral cortex to interpret and integrate information
- Involves testing stereognosis, graphesthesia and point localization

Evaluating vibration

To evaluate the patient's vibratory sense, apply the base of a vibrating tuning fork to the interphalangeal joint of the great toe, as shown below.

Ask the patient what he feels. If he feels the sensation, he'll typically report a feeling of buzzing or vibration. If he doesn't feel the sensation at the toe, try the medial malleolus. Then continue moving proximally until he feels the sensation. Note where he feels it, and then repeat the process on the other leg.

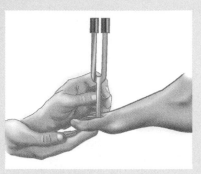

Discrimination (continued)

Abnormal findings: Sensory system

◆ Reduced sensory acuity
◆ Sensory deficit
◆ Tingling or dysesthesia
◆ Loss of sense of light touch, vibration, or position
◆ Impaired pain or temperature sensation
◆ Peripheral neuropathy
◆ Impaired discriminative sensation
◆ Impaired point localization

Assessing motor function

◆ Involves inspecting muscles and testing muscle tone and strength
◆ Tests cerebellar function for abnormal smooth-muscle movements

touching the patient simultaneously in two contralateral areas. He should be able to identify both touches.

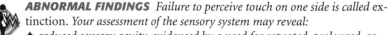

ABNORMAL FINDINGS *Failure to perceive touch on one side is called extinction. Your assessment of the sensory system may reveal:*
◆ reduced sensory acuity, evidenced by a need for repeated, prolonged, or excessive contact to evoke a response
◆ a sensory deficit, indicated by repeated failure to detect tactile stimuli in one body area or a difference in sensory acuity in the same extremity on opposite sides of the body
◆ damaged sensory nerve fibers, indicated by a complaint of tingling or dysesthesia in one area, even if the patient can correctly identify the tactile stimulus
◆ a disorder in the posterior tracts (dorsal columns) of the spinal cord or a peripheral nerve or root lesion, evidenced by a loss of the sense of light touch, vibration, and position
◆ a disorder in the spinothalamic tracts, indicated by impaired pain or temperature sensation
◆ developing peripheral neuropathy, commonly preceded by loss of the sense of vibration (a bilateral, symmetrical, distal sensory loss also suggests a peripheral neuropathy)
◆ a disorder in the dorsal columns or the sensory interpretive regions of the parietal lobe of the cerebral cortex, evidenced by an impaired ability to recognize the distance between two points (discriminative sensation)
◆ lesions of the sensory cortex, indicated by impaired point localization.

ASSESSING MOTOR FUNCTION

Assessing the patient's motor system includes inspecting the muscles and testing muscle tone and muscle strength. Cerebellar testing is also done because the cerebellum plays a role in abnormal smooth-muscle movements, such as tics, tremors, or fasciculation.

Muscle tone

Muscle tone represents muscular resistance to passive stretching. To test arm muscle tone, move the patient's shoulder through passive range-of-motion (ROM) exercises. You should feel a slight resistance. Then let the arm drop to the patient's side. It should fall easily.

To test leg muscle tone, guide the hip through passive ROM exercises; then let the leg fall to the bed. If it falls into an externally rotated position, this is an abnormal finding.

 ABNORMAL FINDINGS *Abnormal muscle movements include:*
◆ uncontrollable tics—sudden, uncontrolled movements of the face, shoulders, and extremities caused by abnormal neural stimuli; can be normal movements that appear repetitively and inappropriately, which include blinking, shoulder shrugging, and facial twitching
◆ involuntary tremors—repetitive, involuntary movements (like tics) usually seen in the fingers, wrist, eyelids, tongue, and legs that occur when the affected body part is at rest or with voluntary movement; for example, the patient with Parkinson's disease has a characteristic pill-rolling tremor, and the patient with cerebellar disease has an "intention tremor" when reaching for an object
◆ small muscle fasciculations—fine twitchings in small muscle groups; most commonly associated with lower motor neuron dysfunction.

Muscle strength

To perform a general examination of muscle strength, observe the patient's gait and motor activities.

ABNORMAL FINDINGS *During your assessment, you may identify gait abnormalities that may result from disorders of the cerebellum, posterior columns, corticospinal tract, basal ganglia, and lower motor neurons, including:*
◆ Hemiparetic gait—characteristics vary according to the amount of upper motor neuron damage. In severe cases, the patient walks with the affected upper extremity abducted and the elbow, wrist, and fingers flexed. The upper body is somewhat stooped, and he tilts slightly to the opposite side. As he walks, he extends his leg and inverts his foot at the ankle with the leg swinging in a circular motion.
◆ Ataxic gait—caused by cerebellar damage. The patient has a wide-based and reeling walk, commonly called drunken gait. If sensory loss occurs, the patient may not be able to feel where he's placing his foot so he partially flexes his hips and lifts up his legs and then slaps his feet down with each step.
◆ Steppage gait—associated with lower motor neuron disease and commonly accompanied by muscle weakness and atrophy. The patient purposely lifts up his legs and slaps them down on the floor.

To evaluate muscle strength, ask the patient to move major muscles and muscle groups against resistance. For instance, to test shoulder girdle strength, have him extend his arms with his palms up and maintain this position for 30 seconds.

If he can't maintain this position, test further by pushing down on his outstretched arms. If he does lift both arms equally, look for pronation of the hand and downward drift of the arm on the weaker side.

Cerebellum

Cerebellar testing looks at the patient's coordination and general balance. Can he sit and stand without support? If he can, observe him as he walks across the room, turns, and walks back. Note imbalances or abnormalities.

Assessing muscle tone
◆ Evaluates muscular resistance to passive stretching

Abnormal findings
◆ Uncontrollable tics, involuntary tremors, small muscle fasciculations

Assessing muscle strength
◆ Evaluates gait and motor activities
◆ Requires patient to move muscle groups against resistance

Abnormal findings
◆ Hemiparetic, ataxic, or steppage gait indicate disorders of the cerebellum, posterior columns, corticospinal tract, basal ganglia, and lower motor neurons

Assessing the cerebellum
◆ Testing evaluates patient's coordination and general balance
◆ Reveals patient's ability to walk heel to toe

Assessing the cerebellum
(continued)

Abnormal findings
+ Cerebellar dysfunction produces a wide-based, unsteady gait

Romberg's test
+ Used to assess balance
+ Result is positive if patient falls to one side while holding arms out on either side

Nose-to-finger test
+ Used to test for extremity coordination
+ Reveals accurate and smooth movements as patient touches his outstretched finger to his nose repeatedly

Other tests
+ Assesses patient for rapid alternating movements, which should be accurate and smooth

Assessing reflexes
+ Involves testing deep tendon and superficial reflexes
+ Observes for primitive reflexes

Assessing deep tendon reflexes
+ Tests reaction to sudden stimulus causing muscles to stretch
+ Compares reflexes on opposite body sides for symmetry of movement and muscle strength

 ABNORMAL FINDINGS *With cerebellar dysfunction, the patient will have a wide-based, unsteady gait. Deviation to one side may indicate a cerebellar lesion on that side.*

Ask the patient to walk heel to toe, and observe his balance. Then perform Romberg's test.

Romberg's test

Observe the patient's balance as he stands with his eyes open, feet together, and arms at his sides. Then ask him to close his eyes. Hold your arms out on either side of him to protect him if he sways. If he falls to one side, the result of Romberg's test is positive.

Nose-to-finger test

Test extremity coordination by asking the patient to touch his nose and then touch your outstretched finger as you move it. Have him do this faster and faster. His movements should be accurate and smooth.

Other tests

Other tests of cerebellar function assess rapid alternating movements. In these tests, the patient's movements should be accurate and smooth.

First, ask the patient to touch the thumb of his right hand to his right index finger and then to each of his remaining fingers. Observe the movements for accuracy and smoothness. Next, ask him to sit with his palms on his thighs. Tell him to turn his palms up and down, gradually increasing his speed.

Finally, have the patient lie in a supine position. Then stand at the foot of the table or bed and hold your palms near the soles of his feet. Ask him to alternately tap the sole of his right foot and the sole of his left foot against your palms. He should increase his speed as you observe his coordination.

ASSESSING REFLEXES

Evaluating the patient's reflexes involves testing deep tendon and superficial reflexes and observing for primitive reflexes.

Deep tendon reflexes

Deep tendon reflexes, also called *muscle-stretch reflexes,* occur when a sudden stimulus causes the muscle to stretch. Make sure the patient is relaxed and comfortable during assessment because tension or anxiety may diminish the reflex. Position the patient comfortably and encourage him to relax and become limp.

Ask the patient who seems to have depressed reflexes to perform these isometric muscle contractions:
+ To improve leg reflexes, have the patient clench his hands together and tense the arm muscles during the reflex assessment.
+ To improve arm reflexes, have him clench his teeth or squeeze one thigh with the hand not being evaluated.

These maneuvers force the patient to concentrate on something other than the reflexes being tested, which can help to eliminate unintentional inhibition of the reflexes. Hold the reflex hammer loosely, yet securely, between your thumb and fingers so that it can swing freely in a controlled direction. Place the patient's extremities in a neutral position, with the muscle you're testing in a slightly stretched position. Compare reflexes on opposite body sides for symmetry of movement and muscle strength. (See *Assessing deep tendon reflexes.*)

Grade deep tendon reflexes using the following scale:
+ *0*—absent impulses
+ *+1*—diminished impulses

Assessing deep tendon reflexes

During a neurologic examination, you'll assess the patient's deep tendon reflexes. Test the biceps, triceps, brachioradialis, patellar or quadriceps, and Achilles reflexes.

BICEPS REFLEX

Position the patient's arm so his elbow is flexed at a 45-degree angle and his arm is relaxed. Place your thumb or index finger over the biceps tendon and your remaining fingers loosely over the triceps muscle. Strike your finger with the pointed end of the reflex hammer, and watch and feel for the contraction of the biceps muscle and flexion of the forearm.

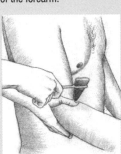

TRICEPS REFLEX

Have the patient adduct his arm and place his forearm across his chest. Strike the triceps tendon about 2″ (5 cm) above the olecranon process on the extensor surface of the upper arm. Watch for contraction of the triceps muscle and extension of the forearm.

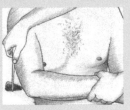

BRACHIORADIALIS REFLEX

Ask the patient to rest the ulnar surface of his hand on his abdomen or lap with the elbow partially flexed. Strike the radius, and watch for supination of the hand and flexion of the forearm at the elbow.

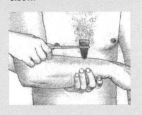

PATELLAR REFLEX

Have the patient sit with his legs dangling freely. If he can't sit up, flex his knee at a 45-degree angle, and place your nondominant hand behind it for support. Strike the patellar tendon just below the patella, and look for contraction of the quadriceps muscle in the thigh with extension of the leg.

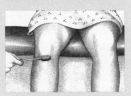

ACHILLES REFLEX

Have the patient flex his foot. Then support the plantar surface. Strike the Achilles tendon, and watch for plantar flexion of the foot at the ankle.

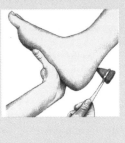

◆ *+2* — normal impulses
◆ *+3* — increased impulses, but may be normal
◆ *+4* — hyperactive impulses.

ABNORMAL FINDINGS *Deep tendon reflexes can display:*
◆ increased (hyperactive) reflexes — occur with upper motor neuron disorders, where damaged CNS neurons in the cerebral cortex or corticospinal tracts prevent the brain from inhibiting peripheral reflex activity thereby allowing a small stimulus to trigger reflexes, which then tend to overrespond. Examples of hyper-

active reflexes include spasticity associated with spinal cord injuries or other upper motor neuron disorders such as multiple sclerosis.

✦ *decreased (hypoactive or absent) reflexes — indicate a disorder of the lower motor neurons or the anterior horn of the spinal cord, where the peripheral nerve originates. Examples of lower motor neuron disorders characterized by hyporeflexia (or areflexia) include Guillain-Barré syndrome and amyotrophic lateral sclerosis.*

Remember that patients without a neurologic disorder may still display hypoactive reflexes but these reflexes should be symmetrical. For example, a compressed spinal nerve root, which can cause a herniated intervertebral disk at L3 or L4, may diminish the patient's reflex associated with that cord such as the knee jerk reflex.

Assessing superficial reflexes

✦ Involves stimulating skin or mucous membranes to test for responses

Superficial reflexes

Stimulating the skin or mucous membranes is a method of testing superficial reflexes. Because these are cutaneous reflexes, the more you try to elicit them in succession, the less of a response you'll get. So observe carefully the first time you stimulate.

Assessing Babinski's reflex

✦ Tests response of patient to stroking of sole from heel to great toe

Special points

✦ Can be elicited in normal infants until age 2; plantar flexion of the toes is seen in more than 90% of normal infants

Babinski's reflex

Using an applicator stick, tongue blade, or key, slowly stroke the lateral side of the patient's sole from the heel to the great toe. The normal response in an adult is plantar flexion of the toes.

Upward movement of the great toe and fanning of the little toes — called *Babinski's reflex* — is abnormal.

 SPECIAL POINTS *Babinski's reflex can be elicited in some normal infants — sometimes until age 2. However, plantar flexion of the toes is seen in more than 90% of normal infants.*

Assessing cremasteric reflex

✦ Tests male's reaction to stimulation of cremaster muscle of the inner thigh

Cremasteric reflex

The cremasteric reflex is tested in men by using an applicator stick to stimulate the inner thigh. Normal reaction is contraction of the cremaster muscle and elevation of the testicle on the side of the stimulus.

Assessing abdominal reflexes

✦ Tests response to brisk strokes of the abdomen above and below the umbilicus

Abdominal reflexes

Test the abdominal reflexes with the patient in the supine position with his arms at his sides and his knees slightly flexed. Briskly stroke both sides of the abdomen above and below the umbilicus, moving from the periphery toward the midline. Movement of the umbilicus toward the stimulus is normal.

Assessing primitive reflexes

✦ Reveals patient's grasp, snout, sucking, and glabella reflexes
✦ Grasping fingers between thumb and index finger may indicate cortical or premotor damage
✦ Pursing lips when lightly tapped indicates frontal lobe damage

Primitive reflexes

The primitive reflexes you'll check for are the grasp, snout, sucking, and glabella reflexes.

Assess the grasp reflex by applying gentle pressure to the patient's palm with your fingers. If the patient grasps your fingers between his thumb and index finger, suspect cortical or premotor cortex damage.

The snout reflex is assessed by lightly tapping on the patient's upper lip. If the patient's lip purses when lightly tapped, this is a positive snout reflex indicating frontal lobe damage.

Observe the patient while you're feeding him or if he has an oral airway or endotracheal tube in place. A sucking motion while the patient is being fed indicates cortical damage. This reflex is commonly seen in patients with advanced dementia.

The glabella response is elicited by repeatedly tapping the bridge of the patient's nose. If the patient responds with persistent blinking after being repeatedly tapped on the bridge of his nose, this indicates diffuse cortical dysfunction.

 SPECIAL POINTS *Primitive reflexes are abnormal in adults but normal in infants, whose central nervous systems are immature. As the patient's neurologic system matures these reflexes disappear.*

INTERPRETING YOUR FINDINGS

Your assessment will reveal a group of findings that may lead you to suspect a particular disorder. (See *The neurologic system: Interpreting your findings,* pages 224 and 225.)

NEUROLOGIC SYSTEM DISORDERS

STROKE

Commonly known as a *cerebrovascular accident* or *brain attack,* stroke is a sudden impairment of cerebral circulation in one or more of the blood vessels supplying the brain. It interrupts or diminishes oxygen supply, causing serious damage or necrosis in brain tissues. Physical findings depend on the artery affected and the portion of the brain it supplies, the severity of the damage, and the extent of collateral circulation that develops to help the brain compensate for a decreased blood supply.

MULTIPLE SCLEROSIS

Multiple sclerosis results from progressive demyelination of the white matter of the brain and spinal cord, leading to widespread neurologic dysfunction. The structures typically involved are the optic and oculomotor nerves and the spinal nerve tracts. This disorder doesn't affect the peripheral nervous system.

Signs and symptoms depend on the extent of myelin destruction, the site of the myelin destruction, the extent of remyelination, and the adequacy of subsequent restored synaptic transmission.

MYASTHENIA GRAVIS

Myasthenia gravis produces sporadic, progressive weakness and abnormal fatigue of voluntary skeletal muscles. These effects are exacerbated by exercise and repeated movement.

Signs and symptoms, which vary depending on the muscles involved and the severity of the disease, include extreme muscle weakness; fatigue; ptosis; diplopia; difficulty chewing and swallowing; sleepy, masklike expression; drooping jaw; bobbing head; and arm and hand muscle weakness.

PARKINSON'S DISEASE

Parkinson's disease is a slowly progressive movement disorder, characterized by muscle rigidity, loss of muscle movement (akinesia), and involuntary tremors. The disease isn't fatal, but death may result from aspiration pneumonia or some other

The neurologic system: Interpreting your findings

This chart shows some common groups of findings for signs and symptoms of the neurologic system, along with their probable causes.

SIGN OR SYMPTOM AND FINDINGS	PROBABLE CAUSE
Aphasia	
◆ Wernicke's, Broca's, or global aphasia ◆ Decreased level of consciousness (LOC) ◆ Right-sided hemiparesis ◆ Homonymous hemianopsia ◆ Paresthesia and loss of sensation	Stroke
◆ Any type of aphasia occurring suddenly, may be transient or permanent ◆ Blurred or double vision ◆ Headache ◆ Cerebrospinal otorrhea and rhinorrhea ◆ Disorientation ◆ Behavioral changes ◆ Signs of increased intracranial pressure	Head trauma
◆ Any type of aphasia occurring suddenly and resolving within 24 hours ◆ Transient hemiparesis ◆ Hemianopsia ◆ Paresthesia ◆ Dizziness and confusion	Transient ischemic attack
Decreased LOC	
◆ Slowly decreasing LOC, from lethargy to coma ◆ Apathy, behavior changes ◆ Memory loss ◆ Decreased attention span ◆ Morning headache ◆ Sensorimotor disturbances	Brain tumor
◆ Slowly decreasing LOC, from lethargy to possible coma ◆ Malaise ◆ Tachycardia ◆ Tachypnea ◆ Orthostatic hypotension ◆ Skin is hot, flushed, and diaphoretic	Heatstroke
◆ Lethargy progressing to coma ◆ Confusion, anxiety, and restlessness ◆ Hypotension ◆ Tachycardia ◆ Weak pulse with narrowing pulse pressure ◆ Dyspnea ◆ Oliguria ◆ Cool, clammy skin	Shock

The neurologic system: Interpreting your findings
(continued)

SIGN OR SYMPTOM AND FINDINGS	PROBABLE CAUSE
Headache	
✦ Excruciating headache ✦ Acute eye pain ✦ Blurred vision ✦ Halo vision ✦ Nausea and vomiting ✦ Moderately dilated, fixed pupil	Acute angle-closure glaucoma
✦ Slightly throbbing occipital headache on awakening that decreases in severity during the day ✦ Atrial gallop ✦ Restlessness ✦ Blurred vision ✦ Nausea and vomiting	Hypertension
✦ Severe generalized or frontal headache beginning suddenly ✦ Stabbing retro-orbital pain ✦ Weakness, diffuse myalgia ✦ Fever, chills ✦ Coughing ✦ Rhinorrhea	Influenza
Paralysis	
✦ Transient, unilateral, facial muscle paralysis, with sagging muscles and failure of eyelid closure ✦ Increased tearing ✦ Diminished or absent corneal reflex	Bell's palsy
✦ Transient paralysis that gradually becomes more persistent ✦ May include weak eye closure, ptosis, diplopia, lack of facial mobility, and dysphagia ✦ Neck muscle weakness ✦ Possible respiratory distress	Myasthenia gravis
✦ Permanent spastic paralysis below the level of back injury ✦ Absent reflexes may or may not return	Spinal cord injury

infections. Important signs of Parkinson's disease are muscle rigidity, akinesia, and a unilateral pill-rolling tremor.

AMYOTROPHIC LATERAL SCLEROSIS

Amyotrophic lateral sclerosis (ALS) causes progressive physical degeneration but leaves the patient's mental status intact, enabling him to perceive every change. The most common motor neuron disease of muscular atrophy, ALS results in degeneration of upper motor neurons in the medulla oblongata and lower motor neurons in the spinal cord.

Facts about ALS
✦ Causes progressive physical degeneration but leaves patient's mental status intact

SPECIAL POINTS *Onset of ALS usually occurs between ages 40 and 70. Most patients die within 3 to 10 years after onset, usually due to aspiration pneumonia or respiratory failure.*

Characteristic clinical features indicate a combination of upper and lower motor neuron involvement without sensory impairment. These features include atrophy and weakness, especially in the muscles of the forearms and the hands; impaired speech; difficulty chewing and swallowing; difficulty breathing; normal mental status; and possible choking and excessive drooling.

EPILEPSY

Patients affected with epilepsy are susceptible to recurrent seizures—paroxysmal events associated with abnormal electrical discharge of neurons in the brain. Seizures are among the most commonly observed neurologic dysfunctions in children and can occur with widely varying CNS conditions.

Accurate description of seizure activity is a vital part of assessment and can assist in correct classifications. Use these criteria to correctly identify seizure types:
+ *simple partial seizure*—patient will remain conscious but may experience unusual feelings or sensations
+ *complex partial seizure*—patient experiences a change in or loss of consciousness
+ *absence seizure*—the patient may appear to be staring into space, he may have jerking or twitching muscles
+ *tonic seizure*—causes stiffening of muscles of the body
+ *clonic seizure*—causes repeated jerking movements of muscles on both sides of the body
+ *myoclonic seizure*—causes jerks or twitches of the upper body, arms, or legs
+ *atonic seizure*—causes a loss of normal muscle tone; the patient will fall down or may nod his or her head involuntarily
+ *tonic-clonic seizure*—causes a mixture of symptoms, including stiffening of the body and repeated jerks of the extremities as well as loss of consciousness.

GUILLAIN-BARRÉ SYNDROME

An acute, rapidly progressive, and potentially fatal form of polyneuritis, Guillain-Barré syndrome causes segmental demyelination of the peripheral nerves. Signs of sensory and motor losses occur simultaneously.

Along with a history of febrile illness (usually a respiratory tract infection), look for paresthesia and muscle weakness. The major neurologic symptom, muscle weakness, usually appears in the legs first (ascending type), then extends to the arms and facial nerves in 24 to 72 hours. It sometimes develops in the arms first (descending type) or in the arms and legs simultaneously. In milder forms of this disease, muscle weakness may be absent.

Other possible features include facial diplegia (possibly with ophthalmoplegia [ocular paralysis]), dysphagia or dysarthria and, less commonly, weakness of the muscles supplied by the 11th cranial (spinal accessory) nerve. Hypotonia and areflexia may also be present.

MENINGITIS

In meningitis, the brain and the spinal meninges become inflamed as a result of bacterial or other type of infection. Such inflammation may involve all three meningeal membranes—the dura mater, arachnoid, and pia mater.

Diagnosing meningitis

A positive response, called *Brudzinski's* or *Kernig's sign,* to either of the tests described here, helps establish a diagnosis of meningitis.

BRUDZINSKI'S SIGN

Place the patient in a dorsal recumbent position, and then put your hands behind his neck and bend it forward. Pain and resistance may indicate neck injury or arthritis. However, if the patient also flexes his hips and knees, chances are that he has meningeal irritation and inflammation, a sign of meningitis.

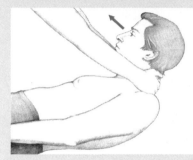

KERNIG'S SIGN

Place the patient in a supine position. Flex his leg at the hip and knee, and then straighten the knee. Pain or resistance suggests meningitis.

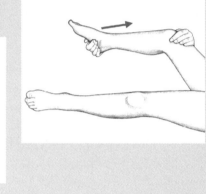

Findings may include fever, chills, malaise, headache, vomiting, nuchal rigidity, positive Brudzinski's and Kernig's signs, exaggerated and symmetrical deep tendon reflexes, and opisthotonos. (See *Diagnosing meningitis.*)

Other possible findings include sinus arrhythmias; irritability; photophobia, diplopia, and other vision problems; delirium, deep stupor, and coma; twitching; and seizures.

Facts about meningitis

+ Inflammation of brain and spinal meninges caused by bacterial or other type of infection
+ Findings including positive Brudzinski's and Kernig's signs

Musculoskeletal system

A LOOK AT THE MUSCULOSKELETAL SYSTEM

During a musculoskeletal assessment, you'll use sight, hearing, and touch to determine the health of the patient's muscles, bones, joints, tendons, and ligaments. These structures give the human body its shape and ability to move. Your sharp assessment skills will help uncover musculoskeletal abnormalities and evaluate the patient's ability to perform activities of daily living (ADLs).

The musculoskeletal system consists of muscles, tendons, ligaments, bones, cartilage, joints, and bursae. These structures work together to produce skeletal movement.

MUSCLES

The body contains three major muscle types: visceral (involuntary, smooth), skeletal (voluntary, striated), and cardiac. This chapter discusses only skeletal muscle, which is attached to bone.

Viewed through the microscope, skeletal muscle looks like long bands or strips (striations). Skeletal muscle is voluntary; its contraction can be controlled at will.

Muscle develops when existing muscle fibers hypertrophy. Exercise, nutrition, gender, and genetic constitution account for variations in muscle strength and size among individuals.

TENDONS

Tendons are bands of fibrous connective tissue that attach muscles to the periosteum (fibrous membrane covering the bone). They enable bones to move when skeletal muscles contract.

LIGAMENTS

Ligaments are dense, strong, flexible bands of fibrous connective tissue that tie bones to other bones. The ligaments of concern in a musculoskeletal system assessment connect the joint (articular) ends of bones, serving to limit or facilitate movement as well as provide stability.

BONES

Classified by shape and location, bones may be long (such as the humerus, radius, femur, and tibia), short (such as the carpals and tarsals), flat (such as the scapula, ribs, and skull), irregular (such as the vertebrae and mandible), or sesamoid (such as the patella). Bones of the axial skeleton (the head and trunk) include the facial and cranial bones, hyoid bone, vertebrae, ribs, and sternum; bones of the appendicular skeleton (the extremities) include the clavicle, scapula, humerus, radius, ulna, metacarpals, pelvic bone, femur, patella, fibula, tibia, and metatarsals. (See *The skeletal system*, pages 230 and 231.)

Bone function

Bones perform these anatomic (mechanical) and physiologic functions:
+ protect internal tissues and organs (for example, the 33 vertebrae surround and protect the spinal cord)
+ stabilize and support the body
+ provide a surface for muscle, ligament, and tendon attachment
+ move through "lever" action when contracted
+ produce red blood cells in the bone marrow (hematopoiesis)
+ store mineral salts (for example, about 99% of the body's calcium).

Bone formation

Cartilage composes the fetal skeleton at 3 months in utero. By about 6 months, the fetal cartilage has been transformed into bony skeleton. However, some bones harden (ossify) after birth, most notably the carpals and tarsals. The change results from endochondral ossification, a process by which bone-forming cells (osteoblasts) produce a collagenous material (osteoid) that ossifies.

Two types of osteocytes, osteoblasts and osteoclasts, are responsible for remodeling—the continuous process whereby bone is created and destroyed. Osteoblasts deposit new bone and osteoclasts increase long-bone diameter through reabsorption of previously deposited bone. These activities promote longitudinal bone growth, which continues until the epiphyseal growth plates, located at the bone ends, close in adolescence.

Researchers are currently studying the role of the endocrine system in bone formation. Estrogen secretion plays a significant role not only in calcium uptake and release but also in osteoblastic activity regulation. Researchers think that decreased estrogen levels lead to diminished osteoblastic activity.

SPECIAL POINTS   A patient's age, race, and gender affect bone mass, structural integrity (ability to withstand stress), and bone loss. For example, Blacks commonly have denser bones than Whites, and men commonly have denser bones than women. Bone density and structural integrity decrease after age 30 in women and age 45 in men. Thereafter, a relatively steady quantitative loss of bone matrix occurs.

CARTILAGE

Cartilage is a dense connective tissue that consists of fibers embedded in a strong, gel-like substance. It's avascular and lacks innervation.

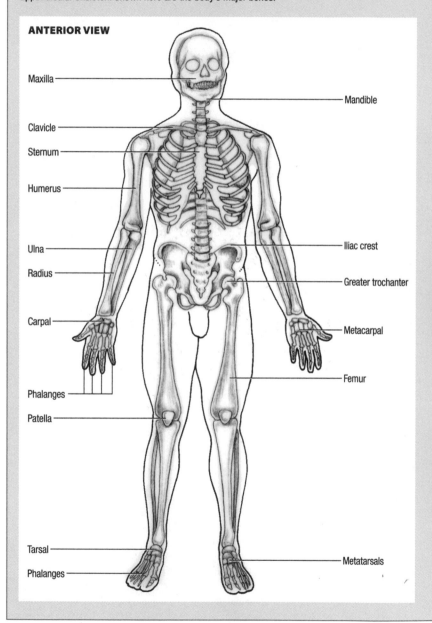

The skeletal system

Of the 206 bones in the human skeletal system, 80 form the axial skeleton and 126 form the appendicular skeleton. Shown here are the body's major bones.

ANTERIOR VIEW

- Maxilla
- Mandible
- Clavicle
- Sternum
- Humerus
- Ulna
- Radius
- Iliac crest
- Greater trochanter
- Carpal
- Metacarpal
- Phalanges
- Femur
- Patella
- Tarsal
- Phalanges
- Metatarsals

Facts about cartilage
(continued)

✦ Is fibrous, hyaline, or elastic
✦ Supports and shapes various structures
✦ Cushions and absorbs shock

Cartilage may be fibrous, hyaline, or elastic. Fibrous cartilage forms the symphysis pubis and the intervertebral disks. Hyaline cartilage covers the articular bone surfaces (where one or more bones meet at a joint); connects the ribs to the sternum; and appears in the trachea, bronchi, and nasal septum. Elastic cartilage is located in the auditory canal, external ear, and epiglottis.

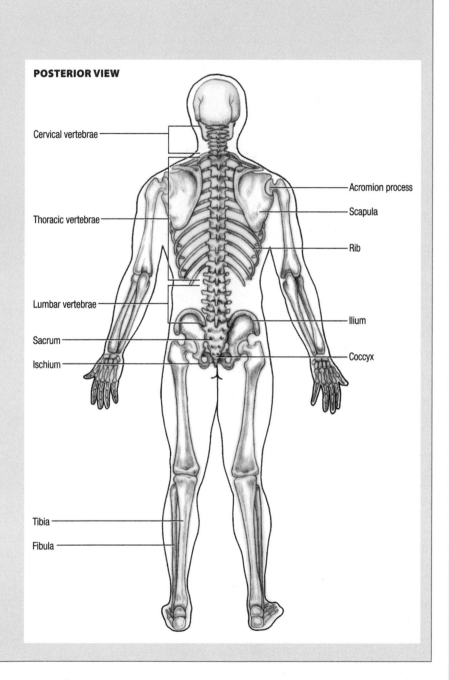

POSTERIOR VIEW

Cervical vertebrae

Thoracic vertebrae

Lumbar vertebrae

Sacrum

Ischium

Acromion process

Scapula

Rib

Ilium

Coccyx

Tibia

Fibula

Cartilage supports and shapes various structures, such as the auditory canal, and other structures such as the intervertebral disks. It also cushions and absorbs shock, preventing direct transmission to the bone.

Synovial joint
+ Cushions ends of bones
+ Synovial fluid lubricates joint, easing movement

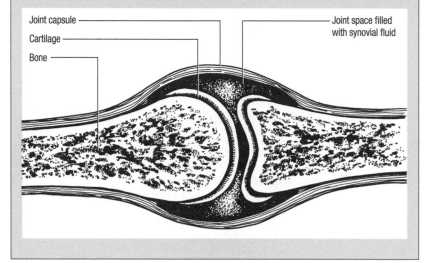

Synovial joint

In synovial joints, a layer of resilient cartilage covers the surface of opposing bones. This cartilage cushions the bones and allows full joint movement by making the surfaces of the bones smooth. The synovial joint cushions the end of each bone and the joint space is filled with synovial fluid, which lubricates the joint and eases movement.

Joint capsule

Cartilage

Bone

Joint space filled with synovial fluid

Facts about joints
+ Involve the junction of two or more bones
+ Stabilize bones and allow a specific type of movement
+ Include immovable nonsynovial joints, which connect bones by fibrous tissue or cartilage; and synovial joints, which move freely

JOINTS

The junction of two or more bones is called a *joint*. Joints stabilize the bones and allow a specific type of movement. The two types of joints are nonsynovial and synovial. In nonsynovial joints, the bones are connected by fibrous tissue or cartilage. The bones may be immovable, like the sutures in the skull, or slightly movable, like the vertebrae.

Synovial joints move freely; the bones are separate from each other and meet in a cavity filled with synovial fluid, a lubricant. (See *Synovial joint.*)

Synovial joints come in several types, including ball-and-socket joints and hinge joints.

+ Ball-and-socket joints — the shoulders and hips are the only examples — allow for flexion, extension, adduction, and abduction. These joints also rotate in their sockets and are assessed by their degree of internal and external rotation.

+ Hinge joints, such as the knee and elbow, normally move in flexion and extension only.

Synovial joints are surrounded by a fibrous capsule that stabilizes the joint structures. The capsule also surrounds the joint's ligaments — the tough, fibrous bands that join one bone to another.

BURSAE

Facts about bursae
+ Small synovial fluid sacs that act as cushions
+ Decrease stress to adjacent structures

Located at friction points around joints between tendons, ligaments, and bones, bursae are small synovial fluid sacs that act as cushions, thereby decreasing stress to adjacent structures. Examples of bursae include the subacromial bursa, located in the shoulder, and the prepatellar bursa, located in the knee.

SKELETAL MOVEMENT

Although skeletal movement results primarily from muscle contractions, other musculoskeletal structures also play a role. To contract, skeletal muscle, which is richly supplied with blood vessels and nerves, needs an impulse from the nervous system along with oxygen and nutrients from the circulatory system.

When a skeletal muscle contracts, force is applied to the tendon (the cordlike structure that connects the muscle to the bone). Then one bone is pulled toward, moved away from, or rotated around a second bone, depending on the type of muscle contracted. Usually, one bone moves less than the other. The muscle tendon attachment to the more stationary bone is called the *origin.* The muscle tendon attachment to the more movable bone is called the *insertion site.* The origin usually lies on the proximal end of the bone and the insertion site on the distal end.

In skeletal movement, the bones act as levers and the joints act as fulcrums, or fixed points. Each bone's function is partially determined by the location of the fulcrum, which establishes the relation between resistance (a force to be overcome) and effort (a force to be resisted). Most movement uses groups of muscles rather than one muscle. (See *Basics of body movement,* pages 234 and 235.)

OBTAINING A HEALTH HISTORY

Musculoskeletal assessment typically represents a small part of an overall physical assessment, especially when the patient's chief complaint involves a different body system. However, when the patient's health history or physical findings suggest musculoskeletal involvement, you'll need to perform a complete assessment of this system, beginning with a thorough history.

During your patient interview, use open-ended questions to assess broad areas quickly and identify specific problems that require further attention. Ask questions systematically to avoid missing important data. Keep in mind that you don't have to complete the entire history at once; as long as you obtain all the necessary information and incorporate it into your plan of care, you can break up the interview and complete it as time permits. Also take into account your patient's emotional and physical condition when conducting your interview.

During the interview, cover these main areas:
+ chief complaint
+ current health
+ past health
+ family history
+ psychosocial history.

CHIEF COMPLAINT

Ask your patient what made him seek medical care. Encourage him to describe his problem in detail. Patients with musculoskeletal problems commonly complain of joint pain and swelling, stiffness, deformity, immobility, muscle aches, and general systemic problems, such as fever and malaise.

Analyze the patient's chief complaint. Ask him to describe its onset, location, duration, timing, and quality. Also ask about exacerbating and alleviating factors and associated symptoms.

Onset

When did the symptom first occur? Did it begin suddenly or gradually? What circumstances surrounded its occurrence? For instance, did the patient hurt himself

---

Facts about skeletal movement
+ Results primarily from muscle contractions
+ Requires impulse from nervous system to contract
+ Bones act as levers and joints act as fulcrums, or fixed points

Obtaining a health history
+ Tracks relevant signs and symptoms over time
+ Includes chief complaint, current and past health, body system review, and family and psychosocial history

Exploring the chief complaint
+ Ask about onset, location, duration, timing, and quality; what exacerbates or alleviates it; and associated symptoms
+ Joint pain and swelling, stiffness, and deformity; immobility and muscle aches; and fever and malaise

Onset
+ Ask when symptoms first occurred
+ Find out if they began suddenly or gradually

Basics of body movement

- ✦ Diarthrodial joints allow 13 angular and circular movements
- ✦ Forms basis of musculoskeletal assessment

Basics of body movement

Diarthrodial joints allow 13 angular and circular movements that form the basis of musculoskeletal assessment. The jaw demonstrates retraction and protraction; the hip, external and internal rotation; the shoulder, abduction and adduction; the ankle, dorsiflexion and plantar flexion; the foot, eversion and inversion; the arm, circumduction; the hand, supination and pronation; and the wrist, extension and flexion.

RETRACTION AND PROTRACTION
Moving backward and forward

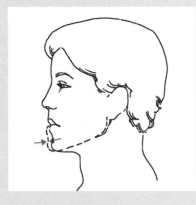

ABDUCTION AND ADDUCTION
Moving away from midline, and moving toward midline

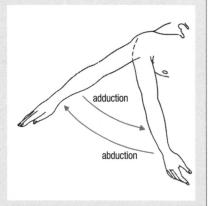

EXTERNAL ROTATION
Turning away from midline

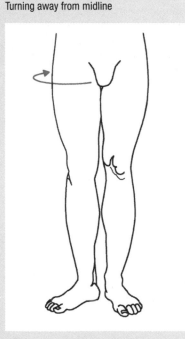

INTERNAL ROTATION
Turning toward midline

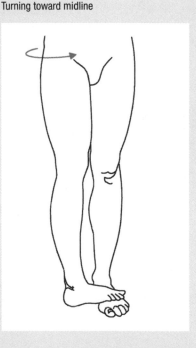

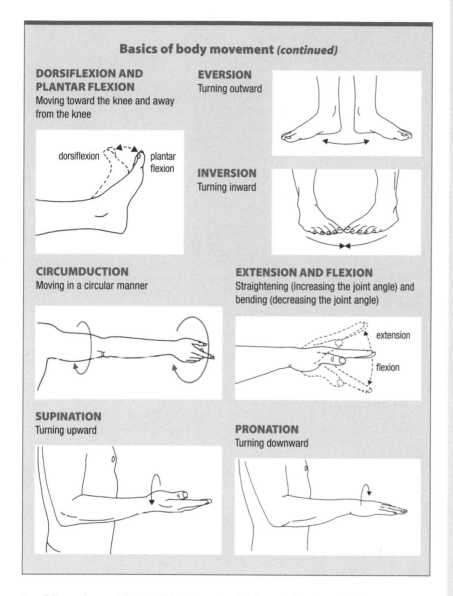

Basics of body movement *(continued)*

DORSIFLEXION AND PLANTAR FLEXION
Moving toward the knee and away from the knee

EVERSION
Turning outward

INVERSION
Turning inward

CIRCUMDUCTION
Moving in a circular manner

EXTENSION AND FLEXION
Straightening (increasing the joint angle) and bending (decreasing the joint angle)

SUPINATION
Turning upward

PRONATION
Turning downward

in a fall or other accident? With joint pain, did the pain begin suddenly or gradually?

Joint pain that begins suddenly may indicate gout, pseudogout, infection, or trauma. Whereas joint pain that begins gradually may indicate rheumatoid arthritis, rheumatic fever, or degenerative joint disease.

Location

Where does the patient experience the symptom? Can he point to the exact area? With joint pain, does the pain involve one joint or multiple joints? Try to determine whether joint involvement is symmetrical, asymmetrical, or migratory.

Pain that's located in one joint may indicate trauma, gout, pseudogout, or infectious arthritis. Pain that's located in multiple joints may indicate rheumatoid disease, juvenile-onset arthritis, or psoriatic arthritis. Symmetrical joint pain may indicate rheumatoid arthritis while asymmetrical joint pain may indicate psoriatic

Onset
(continued)

✦ Sudden — may indicate gout, pseudogout, infection, or trauma
✦ Gradual — may indicate rheumatoid arthritis, rheumatic fever, or degenerative joint disease

Location

✦ With joint pain, find out if it involves one or multiple joints
✦ Determine whether joint involvement is symmetrical, asymmetrical, or migratory
✦ Pain in one joint (trauma, gout, pseudogout, infectious arthritis)
✦ Pain in multiple joints (rheumatoid arthritis, juvenile-onset arthritis, psoriatic arthritis)

Location
(continued)

✦ Symmetrical joint pain (rheumatoid arthritis); asymmetrical, (psoriatic arthritis, spondyloarthropathies, polyarticular osteoarthritis); migratory (rheumatic fever, gonococcal arthritis, Reiter's syndrome)

Duration

✦ Joint pain for 1 to 2 days (gout, pseudogout, infection); joint pain for several weeks (rheumatoid arthritis, degenerative joint disease)

Timing

✦ Find out if pain occurs more in morning on arising (suggesting rheumatoid arthritis) or after activity (suggesting simple joint dysfunction)

Quality

✦ Deep, throbbing, or aching pain indicates bone or joint disease
✦ Sharp and intermittent pain indicates mild joint problem

Exacerbating and alleviating factors

✦ Ask what makes symptom worse and what relieves it
✦ Find out if medication, rest, and activity have an effect

Current health history

✦ ADLs affected
✦ Use of ice, heat, or other remedies for relief

Past health history

✦ Previous major illnesses, recurrent minor illnesses, accidents or injuries

arthritis, spondyloarthropathies, or polyarticular osteoarthritis. Pain that migrates through the joint may indicate rheumatic fever, gonococcal arthritis or, sometimes, Reiter's syndrome.

Duration

How long has the patient had this symptom? With joint pain, has the pain lasted for 1 to 2 days or for several weeks? Joint pain lasting 1 to 2 days may indicate gout, pseudogout, or infection. Joint pain that lasts for several weeks may indicate rheumatoid arthritis or degenerative joint disease.

Timing

When is the symptom worst? With joint pain or stiffness, does it hurt more in the morning on arising or after activity? Joint pain or stiffness that's worse in the morning suggests rheumatoid arthritis. Whereas, joint pain or stiffness that's worse after activity suggests simple joint dysfunction.

Quality

Does the patient have deep, throbbing, aching pain or is the pain sharp and intermittent? Deep, throbbing, aching pain suggests serious bone or joint disease; sharp and intermittent pain suggests a relatively mild joint problem.

Exacerbating and alleviating factors

What makes the symptom worse? What relieves it? With pain, do medication, rest, and activity have any effect?

Associated symptoms

Do other symptoms occur along with the primary symptom? Remember, associated symptoms may be wide ranging, depending on the primary disease involved.

During a general review of your patient's body systems, you may uncover such associated symptoms as dry eyes and mouth (Sjögren's syndrome), dysphagia (connective tissue disorders), colitis symptoms (enteropathic arthritis), dysuria and urinary frequency (gonococcal arthritis and Reiter's syndrome), cutaneous genital lesions (Reiter's syndrome and Behçet's syndrome), and generalized cutaneous lesions (psoriatic arthritis).

CURRENT HEALTH HISTORY

Are the patient's ADLs affected? Ask if he has noticed grating sounds when he moves certain parts of his body. Does he use ice, heat, or other remedies to treat the problem?

PAST HEALTH HISTORY

Inquire whether the patient has had gout, arthritis, tuberculosis, or cancer, which may have bony metastasis. Has the patient been diagnosed with osteoporosis? Ask if he has had a sexually transmitted infection. If yes, what kind and when?

Ask whether he has had a recent blunt or penetrating trauma. If so, how did it happen? For example, did he suffer knee and hip injuries after being hit by a car, or did he fall from a ladder and land on his coccyx? This information will help guide your assessment and predict hidden trauma.

Also ask the patient whether he uses an assistive device, such as a cane, walker, or brace. If he does, watch him use the device to assess how he moves.

Also note a history of allergies, hay fever, or asthma and ask about drug use (including prescription, illicit, herbal supplements, and over-the-counter drugs). Many drugs can affect the musculoskeletal system. Corticosteroids, for example, can cause muscle weakness, myopathy, osteoporosis, pathologic fractures, and avascular necrosis of the heads of the femur and humerus.

FAMILY HISTORY

Ask the patient if any family member suffers from joint disease. Disorders with a hereditary component include:
+ gout
+ osteoarthritis of the distal interphalangeal joints
+ spondyloarthropathies (such as ankylosing spondylitis, Reiter's syndrome, psoriatic arthritis, and enteropathic arthritis)
+ rheumatoid arthritis.

PSYCHOSOCIAL HISTORY

Determine factors in your patient's lifestyle that influence his musculoskeletal status. Start with a general review of your patient's background (including his age, gender, marital status, occupation, education, and ethnic background), and then focus on his specific problems.

Ask the patient about his job, hobbies, and personal habits. Knitting, playing football or tennis, working at a computer, or doing construction work can all cause repetitive stress injuries or injure the musculoskeletal system in other ways. Even carrying a heavy knapsack or purse can cause injury or increase muscle size.

ASSESSING THE MUSCULOSKELETAL SYSTEM

Because the central nervous system (CNS) and the musculoskeletal system are interrelated, you should assess them together.

To assess the musculoskeletal system, use the techniques of inspection and palpation to test all the major bones, joints, and muscles. Perform a complete examination if the patient has generalized symptoms such as aching in several joints. Perform an abbreviated examination if he has pain in only one body area such as his ankle.

Before starting your assessment, have the patient undress down to his underwear and put on a hospital gown. Explain each procedure as you perform it. The only special equipment you'll need is a tape measure.

Begin your examination with a general observation of the patient. Then systematically assess the whole body, working from head to toe and from proximal to distal structures. Because muscles and joints are interdependent, interpret these findings together. As you work your way down the body, follow these general rules:
+ Note the size and shape of joints, limbs, and body regions.
+ Inspect and palpate the skin and tissues around the joint, limbs, and body regions.
+ Have the patient perform active range-of-motion (ROM) exercises of a joint, if possible. If he can't, use passive ROM.

✦ During passive ROM exercises, support the joint firmly on either side, and move it gently to avoid causing pain or spasm.

ASSESSING POSTURE, GAIT, AND COORDINATION

Assessment begins the instant you see the patient. Good observation skills enable you to obtain a wealth of information, such as approximate muscle strength, facial muscle movement, body symmetry, and obvious physical or functional deformities or abnormalities. They also help you assess children who are unable or unwilling to follow directions.

Assess the patient's overall body symmetry as he assumes different postures and makes diverse movements. Note marked dissimilarities in side-to-side size, shape, and motion.

Posture

Evaluating posture—the attitude, or position, that body parts assume in relation to other body parts and to the external environment—includes inspecting spinal curvature and knee positioning.

Spinal curvature

To assess spinal curvature, instruct the patient to stand as straight as possible. Standing to the patient's side, back, and front, respectively, inspect the spine for alignment and the shoulders, iliac crests, and scapulae for symmetry of position and height. Then have the patient bend forward from the waist with arms relaxed and dangling. Standing behind him, inspect the straightness of the spine, noting flank and thorax position and symmetry. Normally, convex curvature characterizes the thoracic spine and concave curvature characterizes the lumbar spine in a standing patient.

Other normal findings include a midline spine without lateral curvatures; a concave lumbar curvature that changes to a convex curvature in the flexed position; and iliac crests, shoulders, and scapulae at the same horizontal level.

 SPECIAL POINTS *Be aware that race can lead to differences in spinal curvature; for example, some blacks have pronounced lumbar lordosis.*

Knee positioning

To assess knee positioning, have the patient stand with his feet together. Note the relation of one knee to the other. They should be bilaterally symmetrical and located at the same height in a forward-facing position. Normally, the knees are less than 1″ (2.5 cm) apart and the medial malleoli (ankle bones) are less than 1⅛″ (2.9 cm) apart.

Gait

Direct the patient to walk away, turn around, and walk back. Observe and evaluate his posture, movement (such as pace and length of stride), foot position, coordination, and balance. During the stance phase, the foot on the floor should flatten completely and be able to bear the weight of the body. As the patient pushes off, the toes should be flexed. In the swing phase, the foot in midswing should clear the floor and pass the opposite leg in its stance phase. When the swing phase ends, the patient should be able to control the swing as it stops, as the foot again contacts the floor.

Other normal findings include smooth, coordinated movements, the head leading the body when turning, and erect posture with approximately 2″ to 4″ (5 to

10 cm) of space between the feet. Be sure to remain close to an elderly or infirm patient, and be ready to help if he should stumble or start to fall.

 ABNORMAL FINDINGS *Abnormal gait results from joint stiffness and pain, muscle weakness, deformities, and orthopedic devices such as leg braces. Other abnormal gait findings you may also observe include an abnormally wide support base (which, in adults, may indicate CNS dysfunction), toeing in or out, arms held out to the side or in front, jerky or shuffling motions, and the ball of the foot, rather than the heel, striking the floor first.*

Coordination

Evaluate how well a patient's muscles produce movement. Coordination results from neuromuscular integrity; a lack of muscular or nervous system integrity, or both, impairs the ability to make voluntary and productive movements.

Assess gross motor skills by having the patient perform any body action involving the muscles and joints in natural directional movements, such as lifting the arm to the side and other ROM exercises. Assess fine motor coordination by asking the patient to pick up a small object from a desk or table.

 ABNORMAL FINDINGS *Examples of coordination problems associated with voluntary movement include ataxia (impaired movement coordination, which is characterized by unusual or erratic muscular activity), spasticity (awkward, jerky, and stiff movements), and tremors (muscular quivering).*

ASSESSING THE BONES AND JOINTS

Perform a head-to-toe evaluation of your patient's bones and joints using inspection and palpation. Then perform ROM exercises to help you determine whether the joints are healthy.

Head, jaw, and neck

First, inspect the patient's face for swelling, symmetry, and evidence of trauma. The mandible should be in the midline, not shifted to the right or left.

Next, evaluate ROM in the temporomandibular joint (TMJ). Place the tips of your first two or three fingers in front of the middle of the ear. Ask the patient to open and close his mouth. Then place your fingers into the depressed area over the joint, and note the motion of the mandible. The patient should be able to open and close his jaw and protract and retract his mandible easily, without pain or tenderness.

 ABNORMAL FINDINGS *If you hear or palpate a click as the patient's mouth opens, suspect an improperly aligned jaw. TMJ dysfunction may also lead to swelling of the area, crepitus, or pain.*

Inspect the front, back, and sides of the patient's neck, noting muscle asymmetry or masses. Palpate the spinous processes of the cervical vertebrae and supraclavicular fossae for tenderness, swelling, or nodules.

To palpate the neck area, stand facing the patient with your hands placed lightly on the sides of the neck. Ask him to turn his head from side to side, flex his neck forward, and then extend it backward. Feel for lumps or tender areas.

As the patient moves his neck, listen and palpate for crepitus. This is an abnormal grating sound, not the occasional "crack" we hear from our joints.

 ABNORMAL FINDINGS *Crepitus is a crunching or grating sound that you can hear and feel when a joint with roughened articular surfaces moves. It occurs in patients with rheumatoid arthritis or osteoarthritis or when broken pieces of bone rub together.*

Assessing gait
(continued)

Abnormal findings
- ✦ Abnormal gait results from joint stiffness and pain, muscle weakness, deformities, and leg braces
- ✦ Other findings include abnormally wide suport base, toeing in or out, arms held out to the side or in front, jerky or shuffling motions, and ball of foot rather than heel striking floor first

Assessing coordination
- ✦ Involves muscle movement
- ✦ Reveals gross motor skills and fine motor coordination

Abnormal findings
- ✦ Ataxia, spasticity, tremors

Assessing the bones and joints
- ✦ Involves patient performing ROM exercises to help determine whether joints are healthy

Assessing the head, jaw, and neck
- ✦ Reveals facial swelling, symmetry, and trauma
- ✦ Evaluates ROM in TMJ
- ✦ Detects tenderness, swelling, or nodules in cervical vertebrae and supraclavicular fossae

Abnormal findings
- ✦ A click (as mouth opens) may indicate an improperly aligned jaw
- ✦ Crepitus occurs with rheumatoid arthritis or osteoarthritis

Kyphosis and lordosis

These illustrations show the difference between kyphosis and lordosis.

KYPHOSIS
If the patient has a pronounced kyphosis, the thoracic curve is abnormally rounded, as shown.

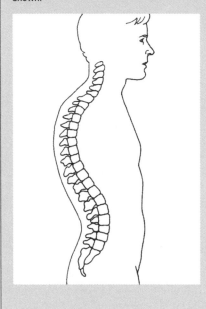

LORDOSIS
If the patient has a pronounced lordosis, the lumbar spine is abnormally concave, as shown. Lordosis (as well as a waddling gait) is normal in pregnant women and young children.

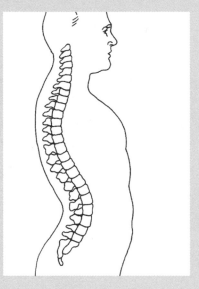

Now, check ROM in the neck. Ask the patient to try touching his right ear to his right shoulder and his left ear to his left shoulder. The usual ROM is 40 degrees on each side. Next, ask him to touch his chin to his chest and then to point his chin toward the ceiling. The neck should flex forward 45 degrees and extend backward 55 degrees.

To assess rotation, ask the patient to turn his head to each side without moving his trunk. His chin should be parallel to his shoulders. Finally, ask him to move his head in a circle — normal rotation is 70 degrees.

Spine

Ask the patient to remove his hospital gown so you can observe his spine. First check his spinal curvature as he stands in profile. In this position, the spine has a reverse S shape. (See *Kyphosis and lordosis*.)

Next, observe the spine posteriorly. It should be in midline position, without deviation to either side. Lateral deviation suggests scoliosis. You also may notice that one shoulder is lower than the other.

To assess for scoliosis, have the patient bend at the waist. This position makes deformities more apparent. Normally, the spine remains at midline. (See *Testing for scoliosis.*)

Next, assess the range of spinal movement. Ask the patient to straighten up, and use the measuring tape to measure the distance from the nape of his neck to his

Assessing the spine
+ Reveals spinal curvature as patient stands in profile and then posteriorly
+ Lateral deviation suggests scoliosis
+ Reveals range of spinal movement
+ Identifies tenderness, swelling, or spasm in spinal processes and areas lateral to spine

KNOW-HOW

Testing for scoliosis

When testing for scoliosis, have the patient remove the hospital gown and stand as straight as possible with her back to you. Look for:

✦ uneven shoulder height and shoulder blade prominence
✦ unequal distance between the arms and the body
✦ asymmetrical waistline
✦ uneven hip height
✦ sideways lean.

BENT OVER
Then have her bend forward, keeping her head down and palms together. Look for:

✦ asymmetrical thoracic spine or promi-nent rib cage (rib hump) on either side
✦ asymmetrical waistline.

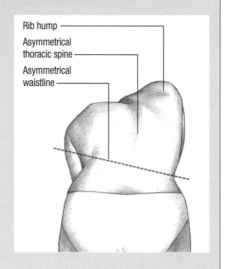

Rib hump

Asymmetrical thoracic spine

Asymmetrical waistline

---

waist. Then ask him to bend forward at the waist. Continue to hold the tape at his neck, letting it slip through your fingers slightly to accommodate the increased dis-tance as the spine flexes.

The length of the spine from neck to waist usually increases by at least 2″ (5 cm) when the patient bends forward. If it doesn't, the patient's mobility may be im-paired, and you'll need to assess him further.

Finally, palpate the spinal processes and the areas lateral to the spine. Have the patient bend at the waist and let his arms hang loosely at his sides. Palpate the spine with your fingertips. Then repeat the palpation using the side of your hand, lightly striking the areas lateral to the spine. Note tenderness, swelling, or spasm.

Shoulders and elbows

Start by observing the patient's shoulders, noting asymmetry, muscle atrophy, or deformity.

 ABNORMAL FINDINGS *Swelling or loss of the normal rounded shape could mean that one or more bones are dislocated or out of alignment.*

Remember, if the patient's chief complaint is shoulder pain, the problem may not have originated in the shoulder.

 CLINICAL ALERT Shoulder pain may be referred from other sources and may be due to a heart attack or ruptured ectopic pregnancy. Either of these situations requires emergency intervention.

Palpate the shoulders with the palmar surfaces of your fingers to locate bony landmarks; note crepitus or tenderness. Using your entire hand, palpate the shoul-der muscles for firmness and symmetry of size. Also palpate the elbow and the ulna for subcutaneous nodules that occur with rheumatoid arthritis. Palpate the acromion process and biceps tendon and assess for tenderness.

Assessing the shoulders and elbows

✦ Assesses symmetry, muscle tone, and alignment

Abnormal findings
✦ Dislocation
✦ Crepitus or tenderness
✦ Subcutaneous nodules

Alert!

✦ Shoulder pain may be due to a heart attack or ruptured ectopic pregnancy, each requiring emer-gency intervention

Assessing the shoulders and elbows
(continued)

+ Evaluates rotation, flexion and extension, abduction and adduction, and supination and pronation

Abnormal findings

+ Pain in the greater humeral tuberosity area (calcium deposits or trauma-related inflammation)
+ Pain upon palpation in the deltoid muscle or over the supraspinatus tendon insertion site (rotator cuff tear)

Assessing the wrists and hands

+ Reveals contour and symmetry
+ Detects nodules, redness, swelling, deformities, and webbing between fingers
+ Assesses ROM in wrists
+ Evaluates extension and flexion of metacarpophalangeal joints

Special points

+ To avoid causing pain, be gentle with elderly patients and those who have arthritis

Abnormal findings

+ Pain or numbness (carpal tunnel syndrome)

 ABNORMAL FINDINGS *If shoulder joint palpation produces pain in the greater humeral tuberosity area, calcium deposits or trauma-related inflammation may be the cause. If you have difficulty abducting the patient's arm and pain occurs in the deltoid muscle or over the supraspinatus tendon insertion site during palpation, this may indicate a rotator cuff tear.*

If the patient's shoulders don't appear dislocated, assess rotation. Start with the patient's arm straight at his side — the neutral position. Ask him to lift his arm straight up from his side to shoulder level and then to bend his elbow horizontally until his forearm is at a 90-degree angle to his upper arm. His arm should be parallel to the floor, and his fingers should be extended with palms down.

To assess external rotation, have him bring his forearm up until his fingers point toward the ceiling. To assess internal rotation, have him lower his forearm until his fingers point toward the floor. Normal ROM is 90 degrees in each direction.

To assess flexion and extension, start with the patient's arm in the neutral position (at his side). To assess flexion, ask him to move his arm anteriorly over his head, as if reaching for the sky. Full flexion is 180 degrees. To assess extension, have him move his arm from the neutral position posteriorly as far as possible. Normal extension ranges from 30 to 50 degrees.

To assess abduction, ask the patient to move his arm from the neutral position laterally as far as possible. Normal ROM is 180 degrees.

To assess adduction, have the patient move his arm from the neutral position across the front of his body as far as possible. Normal ROM is 50 degrees.

Next, assess the elbows for flexion and extension. Have the patient rest his arm at his side. Ask him to flex his elbow from this position and then extend it. Normal ROM is 90 degrees for both flexion and extension.

To assess supination and pronation of the elbow, have the patient place the side of his hand on a flat surface with the thumb on top. Ask him to rotate his palm down toward the table for pronation and upward for supination. The normal angle of elbow rotation is 90 degrees in each direction.

Wrists and hands

Inspect the wrists and hands for contour, and compare them for symmetry. Also check for nodules, redness, swelling, deformities, and webbing between fingers.

Use your thumb and index finger to palpate both wrists and each finger joint. Note tenderness, nodules, or bogginess.

 SPECIAL POINTS *To avoid causing pain, be especially gentle with elderly patients and those with arthritis.*

Assess ROM in the wrist. Ask the patient to rotate his wrist by moving his entire hand — first laterally, then medially — as if he's waxing a car. Normal ROM is 55 degrees laterally and 20 degrees medially.

Observe the wrist while the patient extends his fingers up toward the ceiling and down toward the floor, as if he's flapping his hand. He should be able to extend his wrist 70 degrees and flex it 90 degrees.

 ABNORMAL FINDINGS *If these movements cause pain or numbness, the patient may have carpal tunnel syndrome. (See* Testing for carpal tunnel syndrome.*)*

To assess extension and flexion of the metacarpophalangeal joints, ask the patient to keep his wrist still and move only his fingers — first up toward the ceiling, then down toward the floor. Normal extension is 30 degrees; normal flexion, 90 degrees.

Testing for carpal tunnel syndrome

To diagnose carpal tunnel syndrome, perform these two tests—Tinel's signs and Phalen's sign—as described here.

TINEL'S SIGN

Lightly percuss the transverse carpal ligament over the median nerve where the patient's palm and wrist meet. If this action produces discomfort, such as numbness and tingling shooting into the palm and finger, the patient has Tinel's sign, which suggests carpal tunnel syndrome.

PHALEN'S SIGN

If flexing the patient's wrist for about 30 seconds causes pain or numbness in his hand or fingers, he has Phalen's sign. The more severe the carpal tunnel syndrome, the more rapidly the symptoms develop.

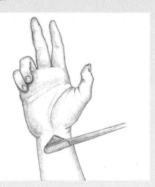

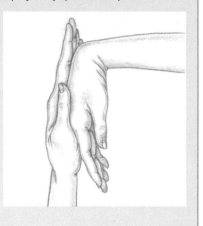

Next, ask the patient to touch his thumb to the little finger of the same hand. He should be able to fold or flex his thumb across the palm of his hand so that it touches or points toward the base of his little finger.

To assess flexion of all of the fingers, ask the patient to form a fist. Then have him spread his fingers apart to demonstrate abduction and draw them back together to demonstrate adduction.

If you suspect that one arm is longer than the other, take measurements. Put one end of the measuring tape at the acromial process of the shoulder and the other on the tip of the middle finger. Drape the tape over the outer elbow. The difference between the left and right extremities should be no more than ⅜" (1 cm).

Hips and knees

Inspect the hip area for contour and symmetry. Inspect the position of the knees, noting whether the patient is bowlegged, with knees that point out, or knock-kneed, with knees that turn in. Then watch the patient walk.

Palpate both knees. They should feel smooth, and the tissues should feel solid.

ABNORMAL FINDINGS *Swelling over the patella suggests prepatellar bursitis. (See* Assessing for bulge sign, *page 244.)*

Assess ROM in the hip. These exercises are usually done with the patient in the supine position.

Testing for carpal tunnel syndrome

✦ Tinel's sign—numbness and tingling shooting into the palm and finger occur upon percussing transverse carpal ligament
✦ Phalen's sign—pain or numbness in hand or fingers occur upon flexing wrist for about 30 seconds

Assessing the hips and knees

✦ Reveals hip contour and symmetry and knee position
✦ Assesses patient's walk
✦ Evaluates ROM in hip
✦ Knees should feel smooth and tissues solid; however, swelling over patella suggests prepatellar bursitis

Assessing for bulge sign

+ Indicates excess fluid in the joint
+ Upon palpation, reveals displacement of excess fluid
+ Reveals a fluid wave on the medial aspect with a lateral check

Assessing the hips and knees
(continued)

+ Assesses hip flexion and extension, abduction and adduction, and internal and external rotation
+ Evaluates ROM in knee

Abnormal findings

+ Arthritis of hip if restriction of internal rotation occurs
+ Degenerative disease of the knee signaled by pronounced crepitus
+ Sudden buckling indicates ligament injury of the knee

KNOW-HOW

Assessing for bulge sign

The bulge sign indicates excess fluid in the joint. To assess the patient for this sign, ask him to lie down so that you can palpate his knee. Then give the medial side of his knee two to four firm strokes, as shown, to displace excess fluid.

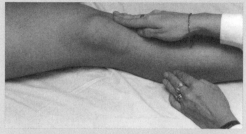

LATERAL CHECK
Next, tap the lateral aspect of the knee while checking for a fluid wave on the medial aspect, as shown.

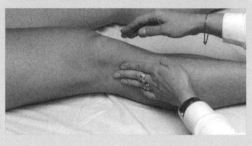

To assess hip flexion, have the patient bend each knee up to the chest and pull it firmly against the abdomen. You should have your hand under the patient's lumbar spine. Note when the back touches your hand. To assess hip extension, extend the thigh toward you in a posterior direction while the patient is lying face down.

To assess abduction, stabilize the pelvis by pressing down on the opposite anterior superior iliac spine with one hand. With the other hand, grasp the ankle and abduct the extended leg. To assess adduction, stabilize the pelvis and move the leg medially across the body while holding the ankle. Normal ROM is about 45 degrees for abduction and 30 degrees for adduction.

To assess internal and external rotation of the hip, flex the leg to 90 degrees at the hip and knee, stabilize the thigh with one hand, and swing the lower leg medially and laterally. Normal ROM for internal rotation is 40 degrees; for external rotation, 45 degrees.

 ABNORMAL FINDINGS *Restriction of internal rotation is a sensitive indicator of arthritis in the hip.*

Assess ROM in the knee. If the patient is standing, ask him to bend his knee as if trying to touch his heel to his buttocks. Normal ROM for flexion is 120 to 130 degrees. If the patient is lying down, have him draw his knee up to his chest. His calf should touch his thigh.

Knee extension returns the knee to a neutral position of 0 degrees; however, some knees may normally be hyperextended 15 degrees.

 ABNORMAL FINDINGS *If the patient can't extend his leg fully or if his knee "pops" audibly and painfully, consider the response abnormal. Other abnormalities included pronounced crepitus, which may signal a degenera-*

tive disease of the knee, and sudden buckling, which may indicate a ligament injury.

Ankles and feet

Inspect the ankles and feet for swelling, redness, nodules, and other deformities. Check the arch of the foot and look for toe deformities. Also note edema, calluses, bunions, corns, ingrown toenails, plantar warts, trophic ulcers, hair loss, or unusual pigmentation.

Use you fingertips to palpate the bony and muscular structures of the ankles and feet. Palpate each toe joint by compressing it with your thumb and fingers.

To examine the ankle, have the patient sit in a chair or on the side of a bed. To test plantar flexion, ask him to point his toes toward the floor. Test dorsiflexion by asking him to point his toes toward the ceiling. Normal ROM for plantar flexion is about 45 degrees; for dorsiflexion, 20 degrees.

Next, assess ROM in the ankle. Ask the patient to demonstrate inversion by turning his feet inward, and eversion by turning his feet outward. Normal ROM for inversion is 45 degrees; for eversion, 30 degrees.

To assess the metatarsophalangeal joints, ask the patient to flex his toes and then straighten them.

If you suspect that one leg is longer than the other, take measurements. Put one end of the tape at the medial malleolus at the ankle and the other end at the anterior iliac spine. Cross the tape over the medial side of the knee. A difference of more than ⅜″ (1 cm) in one leg is abnormal.

ASSESSING THE MUSCLES

Start by inspecting all major muscle groups for tone, strength, asymmetry, and other abnormalities. If a muscle appears atrophied or hypertrophied, measure it by wrapping a tape measure around the largest circumference of the muscle on each side of the body and comparing the two numbers.

 ABNORMAL FINDINGS *Abnormalities of muscle appearance include contracture and abnormal movements, such as spasms, tics, tremors, or fasciculation.*

Muscle tone describes muscular resistance to passive stretching. To test the patient's arm muscle tone, move his shoulder through passive ROM exercises. You should feel a slight resistance. Then let his arm drop. It should fall easily to his side.

Test leg muscle tone by putting the patient's hip through passive ROM exercises and then letting the leg fall to the examination table or bed. Like the arm, the leg should fall easily.

 ABNORMAL FINDINGS *Muscle rigidity indicates increased muscle tone, possibly caused by an upper motor neuron lesion such as from a stroke. Muscle flaccidity may result from a lower motor neuron lesion.*

Observe the patient's gait and movements to form an idea of his general muscle strength. To test specific muscle groups, ask him to move the muscles while you apply resistance; then compare the contralateral muscle groups. (See *Testing muscle strength*, page 246.)

Grade muscle strength on a scale of 0 to 5, with 0 representing no strength and 5 representing maximum strength. Document the results as a fraction, with the score as the numerator and maximum strength as the denominator. (See *Grading muscle strength*, page 247.)

Shoulder, arm, wrist, and hand strength

Test the strength of the patient's shoulder girdle by asking him to extend his arms with the palms up and hold this position for 30 seconds.

Assessing the ankles and feet

+ Reveals swelling, redness, and nodules
+ Checks arch of the foot and detects toe deformities
+ Notes edema, calluses, bunions, corns, ingrown toenails, plantar warts, trophic ulcers, hair loss, or unusual pigmentation
+ Evaluates bony and muscular structures of the ankles, feet, and toes
+ Assesses ROM in the ankle and metatarsophalangeal joints

Assessing the muscles

+ Inspects for tone, strength, and asymmetry
+ Tests arm muscle tone, moving patient's shoulder through passive ROM exercises
+ Tests leg muscle tone, putting patient's hip through passive ROM exercises
+ Evaluates gait and movements to assess general muscle strength

Abnormal findings

+ Spasms, tics, tremors, fasciculation, muscle rigidity and flaccidity

Techniques for testing muscle strength

- ◆ Biceps strength
- ◆ Triceps strength
- ◆ Ankle strength: plantar flexion
- ◆ Ankle strength: dorsiflexion

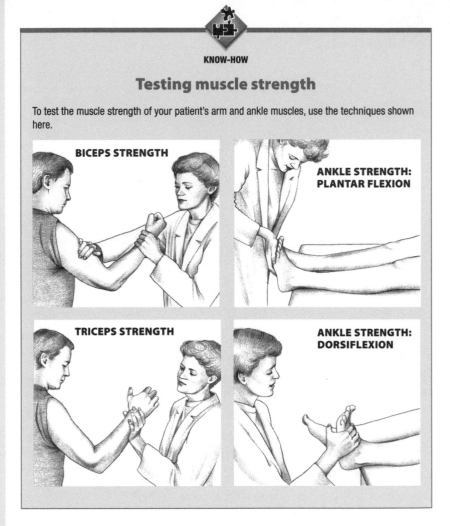

KNOW-HOW

Testing muscle strength

To test the muscle strength of your patient's arm and ankle muscles, use the techniques shown here.

BICEPS STRENGTH

ANKLE STRENGTH: PLANTAR FLEXION

TRICEPS STRENGTH

ANKLE STRENGTH: DORSIFLEXION

Assessing shoulder, arm, wrist, and hand strength

- ◆ Evaluates patient's shoulder girdle strength
- ◆ Tests his biceps and triceps strength
- ◆ Assesses strength of his flexed wrist, finger abduction, thumb opposition, and handgrip

Abnormal findings

- ◆ If patient can't lift both arms equally and keep palms up, or if one arm drifts down (shoulder girdle weakness on that side)

 ABNORMAL FINDINGS *If the patient can't lift both of his arms equally and keep his palms up, or if one arm drifts down, he probably has shoulder girdle weakness on that side.*

If he passes the first part of the test, gauge his strength by lacing your hands on his arms and applying downward pressure as he resists you.

Next, have the patient hold his arm in front of him with the elbow bent. To test biceps strength, pull down on the flexor surface of his forearm as he resists. To test triceps strength, have him try to straighten his arm as you push upward against the extensor surface of his forearm.

Assess the strength of the patient's flexed wrist by pushing against it. Test the strength of the extended wrist by pushing down on it. Test the strength of finger abduction, thumb opposition, and handgrip the same way. (See *Testing handgrip strength,* page 248.)

Leg strength

Ask the patient to lie in a supine position on the examination table or bed and lift both legs at the same time. Note whether he lifts both legs at the same time and to

Grading muscle strength

Grade muscle strength on a scale of 0 to 5, as follows:

◆ *5/5*—normal; patient moves joint through full range of motion (ROM) and against gravity with full resistance

◆ *4/5*—good; patient completes ROM against gravity with moderate resistance

◆ *3/5*—fair; patient completes ROM against gravity only

◆ *2/5*—poor; patient completes full ROM with gravity eliminated (passive motion)

◆ *1/5*—trace; patient's attempt at muscle contraction is palpable but without joint movement

◆ *0/5*—zero; no evidence of muscle contraction.

the same distance. To test quadriceps strength, have him lower his legs and raise them again while you press down on his anterior thighs.

Then ask the patient to flex his knees and put his feet flat on the bed. Assess lower-leg strength by pulling his lower leg forward as he resists and then by pushing it backward as he extends his knee.

Finally, assess ankle strength by having the patient push his foot down against your resistance and then pull his foot up as you try to hold it down.

INTERPRETING YOUR FINDINGS

Your assessment will reveal a group of findings that may lead you to suspect a particular disorder. (See *The musculoskeletal system: Interpreting your findings,* pages 249 and 250.)

MUSCULOSKELETAL SYSTEM DISORDERS

RHEUMATOID ARTHRITIS

Rheumatoid arthritis is a chronic, systemic, inflammatory disease that attacks peripheral joints and surrounding muscles, tendons, ligaments, and blood vessels. Spontaneous remissions and unpredictable exacerbations mark the course of rheumatoid arthritis. Potentially crippling, rheumatoid arthritis usually requires lifelong treatment and sometimes surgery.

In most patients, the disease follows an intermittent course and allows normal activity, although 10% suffer total disability from severe articular deformity and associated extra-articular symptoms, or both. Prognosis worsens with the development of nodules, vasculitis, and high titers of rheumatoid factor.

Initial symptoms may include fatigue, malaise, anorexia, persistent low-grade fever, weight loss, and lymphadenopathy. The patient may also experience vague articular symptoms.

Later, the patient may develop joint pain, tenderness, warmth, and swelling. Usually, joint symptoms occur bilaterally and symmetrically. Other symptoms may include morning stiffness; paresthesia in the hands and feet; and stiff, weak, or painful muscles. The patient may also develop rheumatoid nodules — subcuta-

Assessing leg strength

◆ Notes whether the patient can lift both legs at the same time and to the same distance

◆ Uses resistance techniques to test quadriceps strength, lower-leg strength, and ankle strength.

Musculoskeletal system disorders

Facts about rheumatoid arthritis

◆ Chronic, systemic, inflammatory disease attacking peripheral joints and surrounding muscles, tendons, ligaments, and blood vessels

◆ Includes initial symptoms of fatigue, malaise, anorexia, persistent low-grade fever, weight loss, and lymphadenopathy

Testing handgrip strength

When testing your patient's handgrip strength, face him and extend the first and second fingers of each hand. Then ask him to grasp your fingers and squeeze. Don't extend fingers with rings on them; a strong handgrip on those fingers can be painful.

neous, round or oval, nontender masses, usually on pressure areas such as the elbow. Advanced signs include joint deformities and diminished joint function.

OSTEOARTHRITIS

Osteoarthritis is the most common form of arthritis. This chronic condition causes deterioration of the joint cartilage and formation of reactive new bone at the margins and subchondral areas of the joints. Degeneration results from a breakdown of chondrocytes, most commonly in the hips and knees. Early symptoms usually begin in middle-age and may progress with age. A thorough physical examination confirms typical symptoms, and lack of systemic symptoms rules out an inflammatory joint disorder such as rheumatoid arthritis.

Disability depends on the site and severity of involvement and can range from minor limitation of the fingers to severe disability in people with hip or knee involvement. The rate of progression varies, and joints may remain stable for years in an early stage of deterioration.

The severity of the following signs and symptoms increases with poor posture, obesity, and occupational stress:
✦ joint pain (the most common symptom) that occurs particularly after exercise or weight bearing and is usually relieved by rest
✦ stiffness in the morning and after exercise that's usually relieved by rest
✦ achiness during changes in weather
✦ "grating" of the joint during motion
✦ limited movement.

In addition, irreversible changes in the distal joints (Heberden's nodes) and proximal joints (Bouchard's nodes) occur in osteoarthritis of the interphalangeal joints. Nodes may be painless at first but eventually become red, swollen, and tender, causing numbness and loss of dexterity. (See *Heberden's and Bouchard's nodes*, page 251.)

GOUT

With gout, urate deposits lead to painfully arthritic joints. It can strike any joint but favors those in the feet and legs.

 SPECIAL POINTS *Primary gout usually occurs in men age 30 and older and in postmenopausal women; secondary gout occurs in elderly patients.*

Gout follows an intermittent course and commonly leaves patients totally free from symptoms for years between attacks. Gout can lead to chronic disability or in-

Facts about osteoarthritis

✦ Disability depending on site and severity of involvement, ranging from minor limitation of the fingers to severe disability with hip or knee involvement
✦ Signs and symptoms (increase with poor posture, obesity, and occupation stress) include joint pain, stiffness, achiness, grating, and limited movement
✦ Rate of progression varies, with joints remaining stable for years in an early stage of deterioration
✦ Causes irreversible changes in the distal and proximal joints

Facts about gout

✦ Caused by urate deposits
✦ Leads to painfully arthritic joints

Special points
✦ Primary gout—occurring in men age 30 and older and postmenopausal women
✦ Secondary gout—occurring in elderly patients

The musculoskeletal system: Interpreting your findings

This chart shows some common groups of findings for signs and symptoms of the musculo-skeletal system, along with their probable causes.

SIGN OR SYMPTOM AND FINDINGS	PROBABLE CAUSE
Arm pain	
✦ Pain radiating through the arm ✦ Pain worsens with movement ✦ Crepitus, felt and heard ✦ Deformity (if bones are misaligned) ✦ Local ecchymosis and edema ✦ Impaired distal circulation ✦ Paresthesia	Fracture
✦ Left arm pain ✦ Deep and crushing chest pain ✦ Weakness ✦ Pallor ✦ Dyspnea ✦ Diaphoresis ✦ Apprehension	Myocardial infarction
✦ Severe arm pain with passive muscle stretching ✦ Impaired distal circulation ✦ Muscle weakness ✦ Decreased reflex response ✦ Paresthesia ✦ Edema ✦ Ominous signs: paralysis and absent pulse	Compartment syndrome
Leg pain	
✦ Severe, acute leg pain, particularly with movement ✦ Ecchymosis and edema ✦ Leg unable to bear weight ✦ Impaired neurovascular status distal to injury ✦ Deformity, crepitus, and muscle spasms	Fracture
✦ Shooting, aching, or tingling pain that radiates down the leg ✦ Pain exacerbated by activity and relieved by rest ✦ Limping ✦ Difficulty moving from a sitting to a standing position	Sciatica
✦ Discomfort ranging from calf tenderness to severe pain ✦ Edema and a feeling of heaviness in the affected leg ✦ Warmth ✦ Fever, chills, malaise, muscle cramps ✦ Positive Homans' sign	Thrombophlebitis

(continued)

The musculoskeletal system: Interpreting your findings *(continued)*

SIGN OR SYMPTOM AND FINDINGS	PROBABLE CAUSE
Muscle spasm	
✦ Spasms and intermittent claudication ✦ Loss of peripheral pulses ✦ Pallor or cyanosis ✦ Decreased sensation ✦ Hair loss ✦ Dry or scaling skin ✦ Edema ✦ Ulcerations	Arterial occlusive disease
✦ Localized spasms and pain ✦ Swelling ✦ Limited mobility ✦ Bony crepitation	Fracture
✦ Tetany (muscle cramps and twitching, carpopedal and facial muscle spasms, and seizures) ✦ Positive Chvostek's and Trousseau's signs ✦ Paresthesia of the lips, fingers, and toes ✦ Choreiform movements ✦ Hyperactive deep tendon reflexes ✦ Fatigue ✦ Palpitations ✦ Cardiac arrhythmias	Hypocalcemia
Muscle weakness	
✦ Unilateral or bilateral weakness of the arms, legs, face, or tongue ✦ Dysarthria ✦ Aphasia ✦ Paresthesia or sensory loss ✦ Vision disturbances ✦ Bowel and bladder dysfunction	Stroke
✦ Muscle weakness, disuse, and possible atrophy ✦ Altered level of consciousness ✦ Personality changes ✦ Severe low back pain, possibly radiating to buttocks, legs, and feet (usually unilateral) ✦ Diminished reflexes ✦ Sensory changes	Herniated disk
✦ Muscle weakness in one or more limbs which may lead to atrophy, spasticity, and contractures ✦ Diplopia, blurred vision, or vision loss ✦ Hyperactive deep tendon reflexes ✦ Paresthesia or sensory loss ✦ Incoordination ✦ Intention tremors	Multiple sclerosis

Heberden's and Bouchard's nodes

Heberden's and Bouchard's nodes are typically seen in patients with osteoarthritis.

HEBERDEN'S NODES
Heberden's nodes appear on the distal inter-phalangeal joints. Usually hard and painless, these bony and cartilaginous enlargements typically occur in middle-aged and elderly patients with osteoarthritis.

BOUCHARD'S NODES
Bouchard's nodes are similar but less common and appear on the proximal interpha-langeal joints.

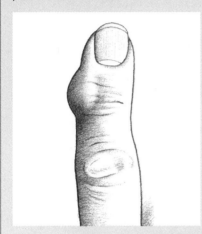

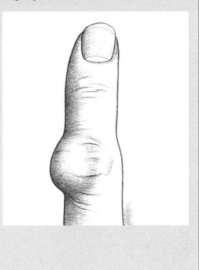

Heberden's and Bouchard's nodes

✦ Typically occurring in patients with osteoarthritis.
✦ Heberden's nodes appear on the distal interphalangeal joints and are usually hard and painless.
✦ Bouchard's nodes are similar but less common and appear on the proximal interphalangeal joints.

capacitation and, rarely, severe hypertension and progressive renal disease. Prognosis is good with treatment.

Gout develops in four stages: asymptomatic, acute, intercritical, and chronic.

In asymptomatic gout, serum urate levels rise but produce no symptoms. As the disease progresses, it may cause hypertension or nephrolithiasis, with severe back pain.

The first acute attack strikes suddenly and peaks quickly. Although it usually involves only one or a few joints, this initial attack is extremely painful. Affected joints appear hot, tender, inflamed, dusky red, or cyanotic. The metatarsopha-langeal joint of the great toe usually be comes inflamed first (podagra), then the instep, ankle, heel, knee, or wrist joints. Sometimes a low-grade fever is present. Mild acute attacks often subside quickly but tend to recur at irregular intervals. Severe attacks may persist for days or weeks. Intercritical periods are the symptom-free intervals between gout attacks. Most patients have a second attack within 6 months to 2 years; however, in some the second attack is delayed for 5 to 10 years. Delayed attacks are more common in those who are untreated and tend to be longer and more severe than initial attacks. Such attacks are also polyarticular, invariably affecting joints in the feet and legs, and are sometimes accompanied by fever. A migratory attack sequentially strikes various joints and the Achilles' tendon and is associated with either subdeltoid or olecranon bursitis.

Eventually, chronic polyarticular gout sets in. This final, unremitting stage of the disease (chronic or tophaceous gout) is marked by persistent painful polyarthritis, with large, subcutaneous tophi in cartilage, synovial membranes, tendons, and soft

Stages of gout

✦ Asymptomatic
✦ Acute
✦ Intercritical
✦ Chronic
✦ Pseudogout

tissue. Tophi form in the fingers, hands, knees, feet, ulnar sides of the forearms, helix of the ear, Achilles' tendons and, rarely, in internal organs, such as the kidneys and myocardium. The skin over the tophus may ulcerate and release a chalky, white exudate or pus. Chronic inflammation and tophaceous deposits precipitate secondary joint degeneration, with eventual erosions, deformity, and disability. Kidney involvement, with associated tubular damage, leads to chronic renal dysfunction. Hypertension and albuminuria occur in some patients and urolithiasis is common.

Pseudogout also causes abrupt joint pain and swelling but results from an accumulation of calcium pyrophosphate in periarticular joint structures.

TENDINITIS AND BURSITIS

Caused by stress on a tendon or joint, tendinitis is the inflammation of the tendons and muscle attachments to bone, especially in the hip, shoulder, Achilles' tendon, and elbow. Fluid may accumulate in the joint, causing swelling, limited movement, and pain.

Bursitis involves the bursae surrounding a joint and results from trauma or inflammatory joint disease. It causes pain and limited movement.

OSTEOPOROSIS

In osteoporosis, the rate of bone resorption accelerates while the rate of bone formation slows down, causing a loss of bone mass. Bones lose calcium and phosphate salts and become porous, brittle, and abnormally vulnerable to fracture. Osteoporosis may be primary or secondary to an underlying disease.

 SPECIAL POINTS *Primary osteoporosis most commonly develops in postmenopausal women. It's called* postmenopausal osteoporosis *if it occurs in women ages 50 to 75 and* senile osteoporosis *between ages 70 and 85.*

Risk factors include inadequate intake or absorption of calcium, estrogen deficiency, and sedentary lifestyle.

Osteoporosis primarily affects the weight-bearing vertebrae, ribs, femurs, and wrist bones. Vertebral and wrist fractures are common.

Although osteoporosis develops insidiously, discovery of the disease usually occurs suddenly. An elderly person typically becomes aware of the disorder when he bends to lift something, hears a snapping sound, then feels a sudden pain in the lower back. Any movement or jarring aggravates the backache. Other signs and symptoms include pain in the lower back that radiates around the trunk, deformity, kyphosis, loss of height, and a markedly aged appearance.

HERNIATED DISK

A herniated disk occurs when all or part of the nucleus pulposus (the soft, gelatinous, central portion of an intervertebral disk) forces through the weakened or torn outer ring (anulus fibrosus). The extruded disk may impinge on spinal nerve roots as they exit from the spinal canal or on the spinal cord itself, resulting in back pain and other signs of nerve root irritation. Most herniation occurs in the lumbar and lumbosacral regions.

The overriding symptom of lumbar herniated disk is severe lower back pain that radiates to the buttocks, legs, and feet (usually unilaterally) and intensifies with Valsalva's maneuver, coughing, sneezing, or bending.

The patient may also experience motor and sensory loss in the area innervated by the compressed spinal nerve root and, in later stages, weakness and atrophy of leg muscles.

ROTATOR CUFF INJURY

The rotator cuff—powerful muscles and tendons that surround the ball and socket of the shoulder—supports and stabilizes the shoulder joint and rotates the arm. An injury to the rotator cuff causes shoulder pain, weakness, spasm, and limited ROM. It also causes sudden dropping of the arm after the patient has abducted it. A rotator cuff injury may result from a fall on the shoulder or from activities like throwing and heavy lifting.

CARPAL TUNNEL SYNDROME

Carpal tunnel syndrome, the most common nerve entrapment syndrome, results from compression of the median nerve at the wrist, within the carpal tunnel (formed by the carpal bones and the transverse carpal ligament). The median nerve, along with blood vessels and flexor tendons, passes through this tunnel to the fingers and thumb. Compression neuropathy causes sensory and motor changes in the median distribution of the hand.

SPECIAL POINTS *Carpal tunnel syndrome usually occurs in women between ages 30 and 60 and poses a serious occupational health problem. Assembly-line workers, packers, and people who repeatedly use poorly designed tools are most likely to develop this disorder. Any strenuous use of the hands aggravates this condition.*

Signs and symptoms of carpal tunnel syndrome include weakness, pain, burning, numbness, or tingling in one or both hands. This paresthesia affects the thumb, forefinger, middle finger, and half of the fourth finger. Other indications include decreased sensation to light touch or pinpricks in the affected fingers; an inability to clench the hand into a fist; nail atrophy; dry, shiny skin; and pain, possibly spreading to the forearm and, in severe cases, as far as the shoulder.

Facts about rotator cuff injury

+ Causes shoulder pain, weakness, spasm, and limited ROM to muscles and tendons surrounding shoulder ball and socket
+ Sudden dropping of the arm after the patient has abducted it

Facts about carpal tunnel syndrome

+ Most common nerve entrapment syndrome
+ Results from compression of the median nerve at the wrist, within the carpal tunnel

Special points
+ Usually occurs in women between ages 30 and 60
+ Poses serious occupational health problem
+ Aggravated by strenuous use of hands

10

Breasts and axillae

A LOOK AT THE BREASTS AND AXILLAE

With breast cancer becoming increasingly prominent in the news, more women are aware of the disease's risk factors, treatments, and diagnostic measures. By staying informed and performing breast self-examinations regularly, women can take control of their health and seek medical care when they notice a change in their breasts.

No matter how informed a woman is, she can still feel anxious during breast examinations, even if she hasn't noticed a problem. That's because the social and psychological significance of the female breasts go far beyond their biological function. The breast is more than just a delicate structure; it's a delicate subject.

Keep this in mind during your assessment. It will help if you proceed carefully and professionally, helping your patient feel more at ease.

STRUCTURES OF THE BREAST

The breasts, also called *mammary glands* in women, lie on the anterior chest wall. (See *The female breast.*)

They're located vertically between the second or third and the sixth or seventh ribs over the pectoralis major muscle and the serratus anterior muscle, and horizontally between the sternal border and the midaxillary line.

Each breast has a centrally located nipple of pigmented erectile tissue ringed by an areola that's darker than the adjacent tissue. Sebaceous glands, also called *Montgomery's tubercles,* are scattered on the areola surface, along with hair follicles.

SPECIAL POINTS *The pigment of the nipple and areola vary among races, getting darker as skin tone darkens. Whites have light-colored nipples and areolae, usually pink or light beige. People with darker complexions, such as Blacks and Asians, have medium brown to almost black nipples and areolae.*

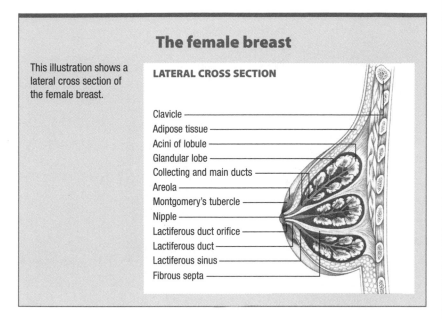

The female breast

This illustration shows a lateral cross section of the female breast.

LATERAL CROSS SECTION

Clavicle
Adipose tissue
Acini of lobule
Glandular lobe
Collecting and main ducts
Areola
Montgomery's tubercle
Nipple
Lactiferous duct orifice
Lactiferous duct
Lactiferous sinus
Fibrous septa

Support structures

Beneath the skin are glandular, fibrous, and fatty tissues that vary in proportion with age, weight, sex, and other factors such as pregnancy. A small triangle of tissue, called the *tail of Spence,* projects into the axilla. Attached to the chest-wall musculature are fibrous bands called *Cooper's ligaments* that support each breast.

Lobes and ducts

In women, each breast is surrounded by 12 to 25 glandular lobes containing alveoli that produce milk. The lactiferous ducts from each lobe transport milk to the nipple. In men, the breast has a nipple, an areola, and mostly flat tissue bordering the chest wall.

Lymph node chains

The breasts also hold several lymph node chains, each serving different areas. The pectoral lymph nodes drain lymph fluid from most of the breast and anterior chest. The brachial nodes drain most of the arm. The subscapular nodes drain the posterior chest wall and part of the arm. The midaxillary nodes, located near the ribs and the serratus anterior muscle high in the axilla, are the central draining nodes for the pectoral, brachial, and subscapular nodes.

In women, the internal mammary nodes drain the mammary lobes. The superficial lymphatic vessels drain the skin. In both men and women, the lymphatic system is the most common route of spread of cells that cause breast cancer. (See *Lymph node chains,* page 256.)

HOW THE BREASTS CHANGE WITH AGE

A woman's breasts make many transformations throughout the life cycle. Their appearance starts changing at puberty and continues changing during the reproductive years, pregnancy, and menopause. (See *Breast changes throughout life,* page 257.)

Support structures
+ Made up of glandular, fibrous, and fatty tissues
+ Include tail of Spence
+ Involve fibrous bands called *Cooper's ligaments*

Lobes and ducts
+ Each breast is surrounded by 12 to 25 glandular lobes containing alveoli
+ Lactiferous ducts from each lobe transport milk to the nipple

Lymph node chains
+ Pectoral nodes
+ Brachial nodes
+ Subscapular nodes
+ Midaxillary nodes
+ Mammary nodes
+ Superficial lymphatic vessels

Aging and breasts
+ Changes begin in puberty and continue through the reproductive years, pregnancy, and menopause

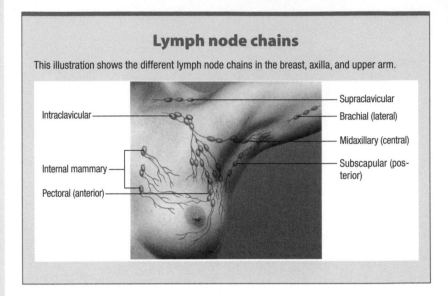

Lymph node chains

This illustration shows the different lymph node chains in the breast, axilla, and upper arm.

Intraclavicular

Internal mammary

Pectoral (anterior)

Supraclavicular

Brachial (lateral)

Midaxillary (central)

Subscapular (posterior)

Puberty

+ Breasts develop between ages 8 and 13; development before age 8 is abnormal

Reproductive years

+ During menstruation, full or tender due to hormonal fluctuations
+ During pregnancy, areola becomes deeply pigmented with increased diameter and nipple becomes darker and erect

After menopause

+ Glandular tissue atrophies, due to decreasing estrogen levels
+ Become flabbier, smaller; hang loosely
+ Nipple flattening; loss of some erectile quality

Obtaining a health history

+ Be sensitive to patient's concerns and feelings
+ Ask about current and past health and family and psychosocial history

Puberty

Breast development is an early sign of puberty in girls. It usually occurs between ages 8 and 13. Menarche, the start of the menstrual cycle, typically occurs about 2 years later. Development of breast tissue in girls younger than age 8 is abnormal, and the patient should be referred to a physician.

Breast development usually starts with the breast and nipple protruding as a single mound of flesh. The shape of the adult female breast is formed gradually. During puberty, breast development is commonly unilateral or asymmetrical.

Reproductive years

During the reproductive years, a woman's breasts may become full or tender in response to hormonal fluctuations during the menstrual cycle. During pregnancy, breast changes occur in response to hormones from the corpus luteum and the placenta.

The areola becomes deeply pigmented and increases in diameter. The nipple becomes darker, more prominent, and erect. The breasts enlarge due to the proliferation and hypertrophy of the alveolar cells and lactiferous ducts. As veins engorge, a venous pattern may become visible. Also, striae may appear as a result of stretching, and Montgomery's tubercles may become prominent.

After menopause

After menopause, estrogen levels decrease, causing glandular tissue to atrophy and be replaced with fatty deposits. The breasts become flabbier and smaller than they were before menopause. As the ligaments relax, the breasts hang loosely from the chest. The nipples flatten, losing some of their erectile quality. The ducts around the nipples may feel like firm strings.

OBTAINING A HEALTH HISTORY

During the interview, establish a rapport with the patient by explaining what you'll do. The quantity and quality of the information you gather depends on your relationship with the patient. Try to gain the patient's trust by being sensitive to con-

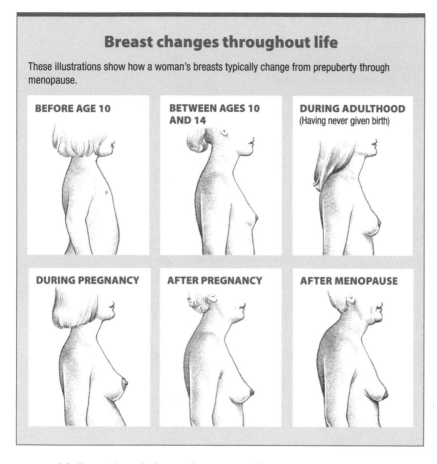

Breast changes throughout life

These illustrations show how a woman's breasts typically change from prepuberty through menopause.

BEFORE AGE 10

BETWEEN AGES 10 AND 14

DURING ADULTHOOD (Having never given birth)

DURING PREGNANCY

AFTER PREGNANCY

AFTER MENOPAUSE

ccrns and feelings. Also ask about other aspects of current and past health, and family and pscychosocial history.

CHIEF COMPLAINT

Common complaints about the breasts include breast pain, nipple discharge and rash, and lumps, masses, and other changes. Complaints such as these—whether they come from women or men—warrant further investigation.

To investigate these complaints, ask about onset, duration, and severity. For women, what day of the menstrual cycle do the signs or symptoms appear? What relieves or worsens them?

An unreliable indicator of cancer, breast pain (also known as mastalgia) commonly results from benign breast disease. It may occur during rest or movement and may be aggravated by manipulation or palpation. Breast tenderness refers to pain elicited by physical contact. If your patient has breast pain, it may be unilateral or bilateral; cyclic, intermittent, or constant; and dull or sharp.

Breast pain may result from surface cuts, furuncles, contusions, and similar lesions (superficial pain); nipple fissures and inflammation in the papillary ducts and areolae (severe, localized pain); stromal distention in the breast parenchyma (tenderness); a tumor that affects nerve endings (severe, constant pain); or inflammatory lesions that not only distend the stroma, but also irritate sensory nerve endings (severe, constant pain). The pain may also radiate to the back, the arms, and sometimes the neck.

Exploring the chief complaint

✦ Ask about onset, duration, and severity
✦ Breast pain, nipple discharge and rash, lumps, masses

Breast pain

✦ Also known as *mastalgia*
✦ May be unilateral or bilateral; cyclic, intermittent, or constant; and dull or sharp
✦ Unreliable indicator of cancer
✦ Commonly results from benign breast disease; may also occur before menstruation and during pregnancy

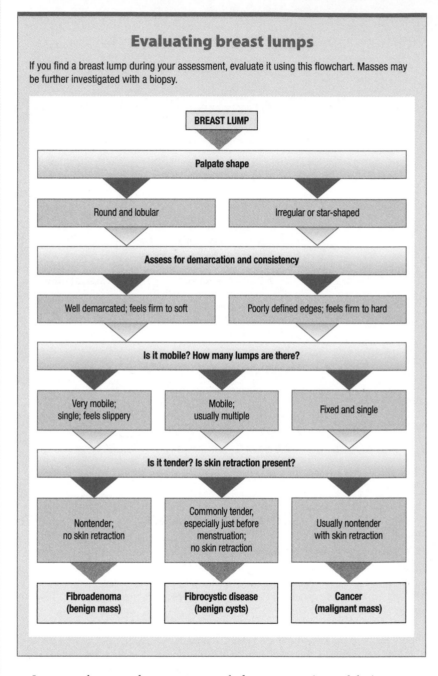

Evaluating breast lumps

If you find a breast lump during your assessment, evaluate it using this flowchart. Masses may be further investigated with a biopsy.

In women, breast tenderness may occur before menstruation and during pregnancy. Before menstruation, breast pain or tenderness stems from increased mammary blood flow due to hormonal changes. During pregnancy, breast tenderness and throbbing, tingling, or prickling sensations may occur, also from hormonal changes.

In men, breast pain may stem from gynecomastia (especially during puberty and senescence), reproductive tract anomalies, and organic disease of the liver or of the pituitary, adrenal cortex, and thyroid glands.

SPECIAL POINTS *In adolescent males, transient gynecomastia can cause breast pain during puberty.*

In postmenopausal women, breast pain secondary to benign breast disease is rare. Breast pain can also be caused by trauma from falls or physical abuse. Because of decreased pain perception and cognitive function, elderly patients may fail to report breast pain.

If your patient has a breast nodule, or lump, it may be found in any part of the breast, including in the axilla. Breast nodules are a commonly reported gynecologic sign that has two primary causes: benign breast disease and cancer. Benign breast disease, the leading cause of nodules, can stem from cyst formation in obstructed and dilated lactiferous ducts, hypertrophy or tumor formation in the ductal system, and inflammation or infection.

Although fewer than 20% of breast nodules are malignant, the signs of breast cancer aren't easily distinguished from those of benign breast disease. Breast cancer is a leading cause of death among women but can occur occasionally in men, with signs and symptoms mimicking those found in women. Thus, breast nodules in both sexes should always be evaluated.

A woman familiar with the feel of her breasts and who performs monthly breast self-examinations can detect a nodule that's 5 mm or less in size — considerably smaller than the 1-cm nodule that's readily detectable by an experienced examiner. However, a woman may fail to report a nodule for fear of breast cancer. (See *Evaluating breast lumps*.)

SPECIAL POINTS *In children and adolescent patients, most nodules reflect the normal response of breast tissue to hormonal fluctuations. For instance, the breasts of young teenage girls may normally contain cordlike nodules that become tender just before menstruation.*

In young boys — as well as women between ages 20 and 30 — a transient breast nodule may result from juvenile mastitis, which usually affects one breast. Signs of inflammation are present in a firm mass beneath the nipple.

In women age 70 and older, 75% of all breast lumps are malignant.

CURRENT HEALTH HISTORY

Because certain breast changes are a normal part of aging, ask the patient how old she is. If she has noticed breast changes, ask her to describe them in detail. When did the changes occur? Does she have breast pain, tenderness, discharge, or rash? Has she noticed changes or problems in her underarm area?

Ask the patient which medications she takes regularly — birth control pills with estrogen, for instance. Also, ask about other hormonal methods of birth control, such as contraceptive patches or vaginal rings. Ask about her diet, especially caffeine use. Hormonal contraceptives can cause breast swelling and tenderness, and ingestion of caffeine has been linked to fibrocystic disease of the breasts.

Ask the patient if she eats a high-fat diet, is under a lot of stress, and if she smokes or drinks alcohol. Discuss the possible link between those factors and breast cancer.

PAST HEALTH HISTORY

Ask the patient if she has ever had breast lumps, a breast biopsy, or breast surgery, including an enlargement or a reduction. If she has had breast cancer, fibroadenoma, or fibrocystic disease, ask for more information, such as when it occurred and any treatments she had.

Exploring the chief complaint
(continued)

Breast nodules
- Result from benign breast disease (leading cause of nodules) or cancer (fewer than 20% of nodules are malignant)

Special points: Breast pain
- In adolescent males, transient gynecomastia during puberty
- In postmenopausal women, secondary to benign breast disease

Special points: Breast nodules
- In children, normal due to hormonal fluctuations
- In young boys, transient breast nodule may occur due to juvenile mastitis
- In women over age 70, 75% of lumps are malignant

Current health history
- Reveals normal breast changes with aging
- Detects abnormal breast changes
- Tells about diet, caffeine use, stress level, smoking, and alcohol use

Past health history
- Previous breast lumps, biopsy, surgery, cancer; fibroadenoma, or fibrocystic disease

Scheduling breast examinations

The American Cancer Society and the American College of Radiology recommend the schedule shown here for regular breast examinations. Depending on their needs, some patients may follow a schedule that their physician has modified. Annual mammograms should be done earlier for women with family history, genetic predisposition, or a history of breast cancer.

AGE	BREAST SELF-EXAMINATION (OPTIONAL)	MAMMOGRAPHY	PHYSICAL EXAMINATION
20 to 39	Monthly, 7 to 10 days after menses begins	Not recommended	Every 3 years
40 and older	Monthly, 7 to 10 days after menses begins (Postmenopausal women should examine their breasts on the same date each month. Have them pick a date that's significant to them so they'll remember.)	Yearly	Yearly

Inquire about her menstrual cycle, and record the date of her last period. If the patient has been pregnant, ask about the number of pregnancies and live births that she has had. How old was she each time she became pregnant? Did she have complications? Did she breast-feed?

Family history
- Breast cancer
- Other types of cancer

Family history

Ask the patient if any family members have had breast disorders, especially breast cancer. Also, ask about the incidence of other types of cancer. Having a close relative with breast cancer greatly increases the patient's risk of having the disease. Teach the patient how to examine her breasts and about the importance of regular breast examinations and mammograms. (See *Scheduling breast examinations.*)

Psychosocial history
- Reveals smoking, alcohol and drug use habits
- Tells about support system

Psychosocial history

Ask the patient about psychosocial factors as well. Does she smoke? Does she drink alcohol or use drugs? What kind of support system does she have? Do family and friends live nearby? Does she have young children or older adults to care for? Determine any psychosocial concerns she has and address them as needed.

Assessing the breasts and axillae
- Reduce patient's level of anxiety by making her comfortable
- Explain what the examination involves

ASSESSING THE BREASTS AND AXILLAE

Having a breast examination can be stressful for a female patient. To reduce her anxiety, provide privacy, make her as comfortable as possible, and explain what the examination involves.

SPECIAL POINTS *Keep in mind that men also need breast examinations and that the incidence of breast cancer in males is rising. Men with breast disorders may feel uneasy or embarrassed about being examined because they see their condition as being unmanly. Remember that a man needs a gentle, professional manner as much as a woman does.*

Adolescent boys may have temporary stimulation of breast tissue due to the hormone estrogen, which is produced in males and females. Breast enlargement in boys usually stops when they begin producing adequate amounts of the male sex hormone testosterone.

Older men may have gynecomastia, or breast enlargement, due to age-related hormonal alterations or as an adverse effect of certain medications. It may also be caused by cirrhosis, leukemia, thyrotoxicosis, the administration of a hormone, or a hormonal imbalance. Be sure to examine a man's breasts thoroughly during a complete physical assessment. Don't overlook palpation of the nipple and areola in male patients; assess for the same changes you would in a female. Breast cancer in men usually occurs in the areolar area.

EXAMINING THE BREASTS

Before examining the breasts, make sure the room is well lit. Have the patient disrobe from the waist up and sit with her arms at her sides. Keep both breasts uncovered so you can observe them simultaneously to detect differences. Examine both breasts with your patient in supine, sitting, and forward-leaning positions.

Inspection

Observe the breast skin; it should be smooth, undimpled, and the same color as the rest of the skin. Check for edema, which can accompany lymphatic obstruction and may signal cancer. Note breast size and symmetry. Asymmetry may occur normally in some adult women, with the left breast usually larger than the right. Inspect the nipples, noting their size and shape. If a nipple is inverted (dimpled or creased), ask the patient when she first noticed the inversion.

 ABNORMAL FINDINGS *Prominent veins in the breast may indicate cancer in some patients but are normal in pregnant women due to engorgement. Acute mastitis, or breast inflammation, causes reddening of the skin and abrasions or cracking of the nipples. Fever and other signs of systemic infection may also occur. The condition is usually associated with lactation.*

Next, inspect the patient's breasts while she holds her arms over her head and then while she has her hands on her hips. Having the patient assume these positions will help you detect skin or nipple dimpling that might not have been obvious before. (*Note:* If the patient has large or pendulous breasts, have her stand with her hands on the back of a chair and lean forward. This position helps reveal subtle breast or nipple asymmetry.)

 ABNORMAL FINDINGS *Breast dimpling is the puckering or retraction of skin on the breast that results from abnormal attachment of the skin to underlying tissue. It suggests an inflammatory or malignant mass beneath the skin surface and usually represents a late sign of breast cancer; benign lesions usually don't produce this effect.*

Because breast dimpling occurs over a mass or induration, the patient usually discovers other signs before becoming aware of this one. However, a thorough breast examination may reveal dimpling and alert the nurse and physician to a possible problem.

Assessing the breasts and axillae
(continued)

Special points: Men and breast examinations
- Incidence of breast cancer in men rising
- Adolescent boys may have temporary stimulation of breast tissue due to estrogen
- Gynecomastia may occur in older men due to age-related hormonal alterations or certain medications

Examining the breasts
- Ensure that room is well-lit
- Have patient sit with arms at sides
- Observe breasts for differences
- Examine with patient in supine, sitting, and forward-leaning positions

Abnormal findings: Breast inspection
- Prominent veins
- Red skin with abrasions or cracking (acute mastitis)

Inspection
- Observe skin for smoothness and color
- Check for edema
- Observe size and symmetry
- Inspect nipples, noting size and shape
- Check for skin or nipple dimpling with patient in various positions

Abnormal findings: Breast dimpling
- Results from abnormal attachment of skin to underlying tissue
- Suggests an inflammatory or malignant mass beneath skin's surface

Dimpling and peau d'orange

These illustrations show two abnormalities in breast tissue: dimpling and peau d'orange.

DIMPLING
Dimpling usually suggests an inflammatory or malignant mass beneath the skin's surface. The illustration shows breast dimpling and nipple inversion caused by a malignant mass above the areola.

PEAU D'ORANGE
Peau d'orange is usually a late sign of breast cancer, but it can also occur with breast or axillary lymph node infection. The skin's orange-peel appearance comes from lymphatic edema around deepened hair follicles.

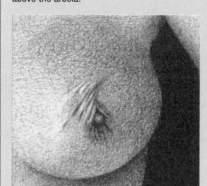
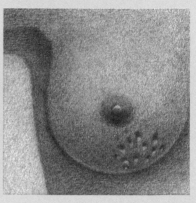

Inspection
(continued)

Special points: Breast dimpling
+ Extremely rare in children
+ In adolescents, may occur from fatty tissue necrosis
+ Usually affects women over age 40; may occasionally occur in men

Abnormal findings: Nipple retraction
+ Inward displacement of nipple
+ Indicates an inflammatory breast lesion or cancer
+ Results from scar tissue formation within a lesion or large mammary duct
+ Commonly confused with nipple inversion

Carefully inspect the dimpled area. Is it swollen or red? Do you see bruises or contusions? Ask the patient to tense her pectoral muscles by pressing her hips with both hands or by raising her hands over her head. Does puckering increase? Gently pull the skin upward toward the clavicle. Is dimpling exaggerated?

 SPECIAL POINTS Because breast cancer, the most likely cause of dimpling, is extremely rare in children, consider trauma a likely cause. As in adults, breast dimpling may occur in adolescents from fatty tissue necrosis caused by trauma.

Dimpling usually affects women older than age 40 but also occasionally occurs in men. (See Dimpling and peau d'orange.)

Observe the breast for nipple retraction. Do both nipples point in the same direction? Are the nipples flattened or inverted? Does the patient report nipple discharge? If so, ask her to describe the color and character of the discharge.

 ABNORMAL FINDINGS Nipple retraction, the inward displacement of the nipple below the level of surrounding breast tissue, may indicate an inflammatory breast lesion or cancer. It results from scar tissue formation within a lesion or large mammary duct. As the scar tissue shortens, it pulls adjacent tissue inward, causing nipple deviation, flattening, and finally, retraction.

Nipple retraction is commonly confused with nipple inversion, a common abnormality that's congenital in some patients and doesn't usually signal underlying disease. A retracted nipple appears flat and broad, whereas an inverted nipple can be pulled out from the sulcus where it hides.

SPECIAL POINTS Nipple retraction doesn't occur in prepubescent females.

KNOW-HOW

Palpating the breast

Use your three middle fingers to palpate the breast systematically. Rotating your fingers gently against the chest wall, move in concentric circles. Make sure you include the tail of Spence in your examination.

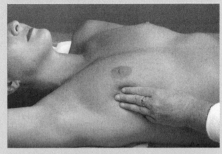

EXAMINING THE AREOLA AND NIPPLE

After palpating the breast, palpate the areola and nipple. Gently squeeze the nipple between your thumb and index finger to check for discharge.

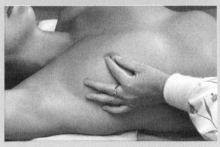

Palpation

Before palpating the breasts, ask the patient to lie in a supine position, and place a small pillow under her shoulder on the side you're examining. This causes the breast on that side to protrude.

Have the patient put her hand behind her head on the side you're examining. This spreads the breast more evenly across the chest and makes finding nodules easier. If her breasts are small, she can leave her arm at her side. (See *Palpating the breast.*)

To perform palpation, place your fingers flat on the breast and compress the tissues gently against the chest wall, palpating in concentric circles outward from the nipple. Palpate the entire breast, including the periphery, tail of Spence, and areola. For a patient with pendulous breasts, palpate down or across the breast with the patient sitting upright.

As you palpate, note the consistency of the breast tissue. Normal consistency varies widely, depending in part on the proportions of fat and glandular tissue. Check for nodules and unusual tenderness. Remember: Nodularity, fullness, and mild tenderness are premenstrual symptoms. Make sure you ask your patient where she is in her menstrual cycle.

Tenderness may also be related to cysts and cancer.

ABNORMAL FINDINGS *A lump or mass that feels different from the rest of the breast tissue may be a pathologic change and warrants further investigation by a physician. Hard, irregular, poorly circumscribed nodules that are fixed to the skin or underlying tissues, strongly suggest cancer. If you find what you think is an abnormality, check the other breast, too. Keep in mind that the inframam-*

Palpation

✦ Palpate with patient in supine position, with her hand behind her head on the side being examined
✦ Palpate entire breast, including periphery, tail of Spence, and areola
✦ Check for nodules and tenderness, noting that normal breast tissue consistency varies widely, depending on fat and glandular tissue
✦ Palpate nipple, noting elasticity; compress nipple and areola, checking for discharge

Abnormal findings

✦ Lump or mass; hard, irregular, poorly circumscribed nodules
✦ Inframammary ridge may be mistaken for a tumor

Palpation
(continued)

Documenting a mass
+ Shape and size in centimeters
+ Consistency and mobility
+ Degree of tenderness
+ Location

Abnormal findings
+ Well-defined, moveable lumps or cysts (fibrocystic disease)
+ Small, round, painless, well-defined, mobile lump that may be soft but is usually solid, firm, and rubbery (fibroadenoma)
+ Hard, immobile, irregular lump with nipple discharge and skin becoming edematous (malignant breast mass)

Abnormal findings: Breast discharge
+ Milky bilateral discharge in pregnancy (galactorrhea)
+ Nonmilky unilateral discharge (local breast disease)

Examining the axillae
+ Inspect for rashes, infections, or unusual pigmentation
+ Palpate high into the apex of the axilla and behind the pectoral muscles, pointing toward the midclavicle

Abnormal findings
+ Rash (sweat gland infection)
+ Deeply pigmented, velvety skin (internal malignancy)

---

mary ridge at the lower edge of the breast is normally firm and may be mistaken for a tumor.

Documenting a mass

If you palpate a mass, record the following characteristics:
+ size in centimeters
+ shape—round, discoid, regular, or irregular
+ consistency—soft, firm, or hard
+ mobility
+ degree of tenderness
+ location, using the quadrant or clock method. (See *Identifying locations of breast lesions.*)

 ABNORMAL FINDINGS *In a patient with fibrocystic breasts, you may palpate one or more well-defined, moveable lumps or cysts. Fibrocystic disease is a benign condition that results from excess fibrous tissue formation and hyperplasia of the linings of the mammary ducts.*

If the patient has fibroadenoma, which is also a benign condition, it produces a small, round, painless, well-defined, mobile lump that may be soft but is usually solid, firm, and rubbery.

In a patient with a malignant breast mass, it may occur in any part of the breast, though it's usually found in the upper outer quadrant as a hard, immobile, irregular lump. Nipple discharge may occur, and breast skin may become edematous with enlarged pores, discoloration, and an orange-peel appearance.

Finally, palpate the nipple, noting its elasticity. It should be rough, elastic, and round. The nipple also typically protrudes from the breast. Compress the nipple and areola to detect discharge. If discharge is present and the patient isn't pregnant or lactating, assess the color, consistency, and quantity of the discharge. If possible, obtain a cytologic smear.

To obtain a smear, put on gloves, place a glass slide over the nipple, and smear the discharge on the slide. Spray the slide with a fixative, label it with the patient's name and date, and send it to the laboratory, according to your facility's policy.

 ABNORMAL FINDINGS *If the patient has a milky bilateral discharge, called* galactorrhea, *this may reflect pregnancy or prolactin or other hormonal imbalance. A nonmilky unilateral discharge suggests local breast disease.*

EXAMINING THE AXILLAE

To examine the axillae, use the techniques of inspection and palpation. With the patient sitting or standing, inspect the skin of the axillae for rashes, infections, or unusual pigmentation.

 ABNORMAL FINDINGS *If the patient has a rash, this could suggest a sweat gland infection. Deeply pigmented skin that feels velvety could be associated with internal malignancy.*

Before palpating, ask the patient to relax her arm on the side you're examining. Support her elbow with one of your hands. Cup the fingers of your other hand, and reach high into the apex of the axilla. Place your fingers directly behind the pectoral muscles, pointing toward the midclavicle. (See *Palpating the axilla,* page 266.)

KNOW-HOW

Identifying locations of breast lesions

Mentally divide the breast into four quadrants and a fifth segment, the tail of Spence. Describe your findings according to the appropriate quadrant or segment. You can also think of the breast as a clock, with the nipple in the center. Then specify locations according to the time (2 o'clock, for example). Either way, specify the location of a lesion or other findings by the distance in centimeters from the nipple.

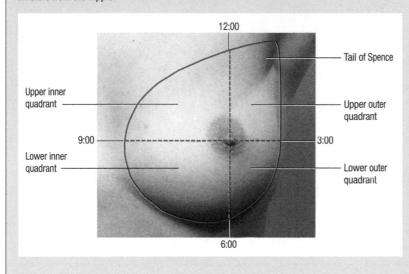

Identifying breast lesions

- ✦ Visualize four quadrants and the tail of Spence
- ✦ Specify locations according to time on a clock
- ✦ Record findings by distance in centimeters from nipple

Assessing the axillary nodes

First, try to palpate the central nodes by pressing your fingers downward and in toward the chest wall. You can usually palpate one or more of the nodes, which should be soft, small, and nontender. If you feel a hard, large, or tender lesion, try to palpate the other groups of lymph nodes for comparison.

To palpate the pectoral and anterior nodes, grasp the anterior axillary fold between your thumb and fingers and palpate inside the borders of the pectoral muscles. Palpate the lateral nodes by pressing your fingers along the upper inner arm. Try to compress these nodes against the humerus. To palpate the subscapular or posterior nodes, stand behind the patient and press your fingers to feel the inside of the muscle of the posterior axillary fold.

Assessing the neck nodes

If the axillary nodes appear abnormal, assess the nodes in the clavicular area. To do this, have the patient relax her neck muscles by flexing her head slightly forward. Stand in front of her and hook your fingers over the clavicle beside the sternocleidomastoid muscle. Rotate your fingers deeply into this area to feel the supraclavicular nodes.

Assessing the axillary nodes

- ✦ Palpate central, pectoral and anterior, lateral, and subscapular or posterior nodes

Assessing the neck nodes

- ✦ Assess for abnormal axillary nodes
- ✦ Palpate deeply into the sternocleidomastoid muscle to assess the supraclavicular nodes

Palpating the axilla

To palpate the axilla, have the patient sit or lie down. Wear gloves if an ulceration or discharge is present. Ask her to relax her arm, and support it with your nondominant hand.

Keeping the fingers of your dominant hand together, reach high into the apex of the axilla, as shown. Position your fingers so they're directly behind the pectoral muscles, pointing toward the midclavicle. Sweep your fingers downward against the ribs and serratus anterior muscle to palpate the midaxillary or central lymph nodes.

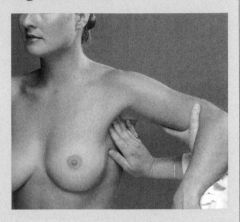

INTERPRETING YOUR FINDINGS

After you assess the patient, a group of findings may lead you to suspect a particular disorder. (See *The breasts and axillae: Interpreting your findings.*)

BREAST AND AXILLA DISORDERS

FIBROCYSTIC BREAST DISEASE

In a patient with fibrocystic breasts, you may palpate one or more well-defined, moveable lumps or cysts. Fibrocystic disease is a benign condition that results from excess fibrous tissue formation and hyperplasia of the linings of the mammary ducts.

Fibroadenoma, also a benign condition, produces a small, round, painless, well-defined, mobile lump that may be soft but is usually solid, firm, and rubbery.

BREAST CANCER

Breast cancer is the most common malignancy among females in the United States and ranks second only to lung cancer as the leading cause of cancer death in women ages 35 to 54. It also occurs in men, but rarely.

Although the cause of breast cancer is unknown, certain risk factors exist. Primary ones include gender (more than 90% of breast cancers occur in women), age (risk increases in patients over age 50), personal history of breast cancer (15% of women develop breast cancer in the opposite breast), and family history of breast cancer (women with a first-degree relative with breast cancer have a twofold to threefold increased risk). Genetically determined breast cancer accounts for less

Breast and axilla disorders

Facts about fibrocystic breast disease

+ Involves benign moveable lumps or cysts
+ Results from excess fibrous tissue formation and hyperplasia of linings of mammary ducts
+ Also results in fibroadenoma

Facts about breast cancer

+ Primary risk factors: gender, age, and personal and family history
+ Secondary risk factors: nulliparity or having first child after age 30; prolonged hormonal stimulation; exposure to excessive ionizing radiation; history of endometrial, ovarian, or colon cancer

The breasts and axillae: Interpreting your findings

This chart shows some common groups of findings for signs and symptoms of the breast and axillae, along with their probable causes.

SIGN OR SYMPTOM AND FINDINGS	PROBABLE CAUSE
Breast dimpling	
✦ Firm, irregular, nontender lump ✦ Nipple retraction, deviation, inversion, or flattening ✦ Enlarged axillary lymph nodes	Breast abscess
✦ History of trauma to fatty tissue of the breast (patient may not remember such trauma) ✦ Tenderness and erythema ✦ Bruising ✦ Hard, indurated, poorly delineated lump that's fibrotic and fixed to underlying tissue or overlying skin ✦ Signs of nipple retraction	Fat necrosis
✦ Heat ✦ Erythema ✦ Swelling ✦ Pain and tenderness ✦ Flulike signs and symptoms, such as fever, malaise, fatigue, and aching	Mastitis
Breast nodule	
✦ Single nodule that feels firm, elastic, and round or lobular, with well-defined margins ✦ Extremely mobile, "slippery" feel ✦ No pain or tenderness ✦ Size varies greatly from that of a pinhead to very large ✦ Grows rapidly ✦ Usually located around the nipple or on the lateral side of the upper outer quadrant	Fibroadenoma
✦ Hard, poorly delineated nodule ✦ Fixed to the skin or underlying tissue ✦ Breast dimpling ✦ Nipple deviation or retraction ✦ Usually located in the upper outer quadrant (almost one-half) ✦ Nontender ✦ Serous or bloody discharge ✦ Edema or peau d'orange of the skin overlying the mass ✦ Axillary lymphadenopathy	Breast cancer

(continued)

The breast and axillae:
Interpreting your findings *(continued)*

SIGN OR SYMPTOM AND FINDINGS	PROBABLE CAUSE
Breast nodule (continued)	
✦ Smooth, round, slightly elastic nodules ✦ Increase in size and tenderness just before menstruation ✦ Mobile ✦ Clear, watery (serous) discharge or sticky nipple ✦ Bloating ✦ Irritability ✦ Abdominal cramping	Fibrocystic breast disease
Breast pain	
✦ Tender, palpable abscesses on the periphery of the areola ✦ Fever ✦ Inflamed sebaceous Montgomery's glands	Areolar gland abscess
✦ Unilateral breast pain or tenderness ✦ Serous or bloody nipple discharge, usually only from one duct ✦ Small, soft, poorly delineated mass in the ducts beneath the areola	Intraductal papilloma
✦ Small, well-delineated nodule ✦ Localized erythema ✦ Induration	Infected sebaceous cyst
Nipple retraction	
✦ Poorly defined, rubbery nodule beneath the areola with a blue-green discoloration ✦ Areolar burning, itching, swelling, tenderness, and erythema ✦ Nipple pain with a thick, sticky, grayish, multiductal discharge	Mammary duct ectasia
✦ History of breast surgery that may have caused underlying scarring	Previous surgery

Facts about breast cancer
(continued)

✦ Signs and symptoms: painless lump or mass in the breast that feels hard and stony; changes in breast symmetry, size, skin, and nipples

than 5% of all cancers, but those who develop it seem to be younger and the cancer is more likely to be bilateral. The mutated BRCA-1 gene (on chromosome 17) is linked to an increased risk of breast and ovarian cancers; the BRCA-2 gene (on chromosome 13), an increased risk of breast cancer.

Secondary risk factors increase the risk of breast cancer in nulliparous women and women who had their first child after age 30. Prolonged hormonal stimulation is another risk factor—that is, menarche before age 12 and menopause after age 50. Other secondary risk factors include atypical hyperplasia on a previous breast biopsy, exposure to excessive ionizing radiation (Hodgkin's disease treatment), or a history of endometrial, ovarian, or colon cancer.

Women with a high-risk profile account for only one-third of breast cancer cases. Most women with breast cancer have no identifiable risk factors.

Signs and symptoms of breast cancer include a painless lump or mass in the breast—a hard, stony mass is usually malignant. (See *Breast tumor sites.*)

Breast tumor sites

This illustration shows the location and frequency of breast tumors.

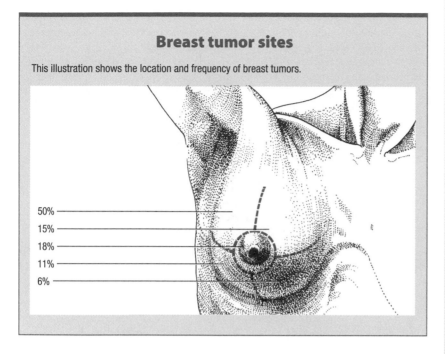

- 50%
- 15%
- 18%
- 11%
- 6%

Late signs and symptoms include changes in breast symmetry or size; changes in breast skin, such as thickening, dimpling, peau d'orange, edema, or ulceration; changes in nipples, such as itching, burning, erosion, or retraction; and changes in skin temperature (a warm, hot, or pink area).

Suspect cancer in a nonlactating woman past child-bearing age until proven otherwise. Investigate spontaneous discharge of any kind in a nonnursing, nonlactating woman. Metastatic disease may cause pain in the shoulders, hips, or pelvis; cough; anorexia; persistent dizziness; or enlarged axillary or supraclavicular lymph nodes.

MASTITIS AND BREAST ENGORGEMENT

Mastitis (parenchymatous inflammation of the mammary glands) occurs postpartum in about 1% of patients, mainly primiparas who are breast-feeding. It occurs occasionally in nonlactating females and rarely in males. All breast-feeding mothers develop some degree of engorgement (congestion), but it's especially likely to be severe in primiparas. Prognosis for both disorders is good.

Mastitis develops when a pathogen that typically originates in the nursing infant's nose or pharynx, invades breast tissue through a fissured or cracked nipple, and disrupts normal lactation. The most common pathogen of this type is *Staphylococcus aureus;* less commonly, it's *S. epidermidis* or beta-hemolytic Streptococcus. Rarely, mastitis may result from disseminated tuberculosis or the mumps virus. Predisposing factors include a fissure or abrasion on the nipple, blocked milk ducts, and an incomplete let-down reflex, usually from emotional trauma. Blocked milk ducts can result from a tight bra or prolonged intervals between breast-feedings.

Mastitis may develop anytime during lactation but usually begins 3 to 4 weeks postpartum, with fever (101° F [38.3° C] or higher in acute mastitis), malaise, and flulike symptoms. The breasts (or, occasionally, one breast) become tender, hard, swollen, and warm. Unless mastitis is treated adequately, it may progress to breast abscess.

Facts about mastitis and breast engorgement

Mastitis

- ✦ Also known as *parenchymatous inflammation of the mammary glands*
- ✦ Commonly occurs in breast-feeding patients; develops 3 to 4 weeks postpartum
- ✦ Results from nursing neonate transmitting a pathogen through a cracked nipple, which then invades tissue

Breast engorgement

- ✦ Usually starts 2 to 5 days postpartum; ranges from mild to severe pain
- ✦ May interfere with neonate's ability to feed
- ✦ Causes include venous and lymphatic stasis and alveolar milk accumulation

Breast engorgement generally starts with onset of lactation (days 2 to 5 postpartum). The breasts undergo changes similar to those in mastitis, and body temperature may be elevated. Engorgement may be mild and cause only slight discomfort, or severe and cause considerable pain. A severely engorged breast can interfere with the neonate's capacity to feed because of his inability to position his mouth properly on the swollen, rigid breast. Causes of breast engorgement include venous and lymphatic stasis and alveolar milk accumulation.

PAGET'S DISEASE

Paget's disease is a rare form of cancer of the mammary ducts. The cause of Paget's disease is unknown; however, it often results from malignant cells (from an underlying ductal carcinoma) invading the epidermis of the nipple, areola, and surrounding skin. Early signs include erythema and discharge from the nipple and areola. Nipple thickening, scaling, and erosion occur later. Another common sign of Paget's disease is a red, scaly, eczema-like rash over the affected nipple and areola.

SPECIAL POINTS *Clinical findings may appear to be similar to that of eczema, dermatitis, or psoriasis; therefore, this can lead to a delay in diagnosis.*

Paget's disease of the breast most commonly occurs in women ages 40 to 80; also occurs in men but is very rare.

Facts about Paget's disease

✦ Rare form of cancer of the mammary ducts
✦ Invades epidermis of the nipple, areola, and surrounding skin

Special points

✦ Diagnosis may be delayed due to similarities to eczema, dermatitis, and psoriasis
✦ Commonly occurs in women ages 40 to 80; rare in men

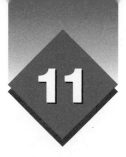

Female genitourinary system

A LOOK AT THE FEMALE GU SYSTEM

The female genitourinary (GU) system encompasses the urinary tract and the reproductive organs and structures. Disorders of this system can have wide-ranging effects on other body systems. For example, ovarian dysfunction can alter endocrine balance, and kidney dysfunction can affect the production of the hormone erythropoietin, which regulates the production of red blood cells (RBCs).

Assessing the female GU system can be a challenging task. Many patients with urinary disorders don't realize they're ill because they have only mild signs and symptoms; therefore, it's easy to overlook underlying problems.

More women seek health care for reproductive disorders than for anything else. Assessing those problems can be difficult because the reproductive system is complex and its functions have far-reaching psychosocial implications.

URINARY SYSTEM

The urinary system consists of the kidneys, ureters, bladder, and urethra. Working together, these structures remove wastes from the body, regulate acid-base balance by retaining or excreting hydrogen ions, and regulate fluid and electrolyte balance. (See *The urinary system,* page 272.)

Kidneys

The essential functions of the urinary system — such as forming urine and maintaining homeostasis — take place in the highly vascular kidneys. These bean-shaped organs are $4\frac{1}{2}''$ to $5''$ (11.5 to 12.5 cm) long and $2\frac{1}{2}''$ (6.5 cm) wide. Located retroperitoneally on either side of the lumbar vertebrae, the kidneys lie behind the abdominal organs and in front of the muscles attached to the vertebral column. The peritoneal fat layer protects them.

Crowded by the liver, the right kidney extends slightly lower than the left. Atop each kidney (suprarenal) lies an adrenal gland. At the hilus — an indentation in the kidney's medial aspect — the renal artery, renal vein, lymphatic vessels, and nerves

A look at the female GU system

+ Involves urinary tract and reproductive organs and structures
+ Disorders can cause wide-ranging effects on other body systems
+ Can produce mild symptoms; underlying problems are commonly overlooked

Urinary system

+ Consists of kidneys, ureters, bladder, and urethra
+ Removes wastes from the body
+ Regulates acid-base and fluid and electrolyte balance

Kidneys

+ Form urine and maintain homeostasis
+ Contain outer renal cortex with central renal medulla, internal calyces, and renal pelvis
+ Nephron serves as the kidney's functional unit

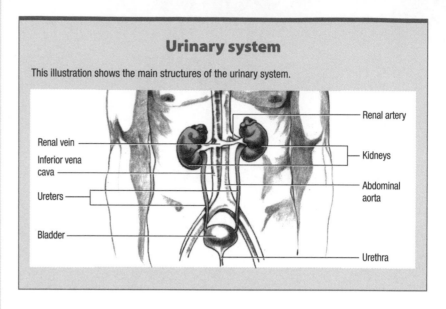

Urinary system

This illustration shows the main structures of the urinary system.

enter the kidney. The renal pelvis, a funnel-shaped ureter extension, also enters here.

A cross section of the kidney reveals the outer renal cortex, central renal medulla, internal calyces, and renal pelvis. At the microscopic level, the nephron serves as the kidney's functional unit.

Ureters

The ureters act as ducts to allow urine to pass from the kidneys to the bladder. They measure about 10″ to 12″ (25.5 to 30.5 cm) in adults and have a diameter varying from 2 to 8 mm, with the narrowest portion being at the ureteropelvic junction. The left kidney is higher than the right one, so the left ureter typically is slightly longer than the right one. Originating in the ureteropelvic junction of the kidneys, the ureters travel obliquely to the bladder, channeling urine via peristaltic waves that occur one to five times per minute.

Bladder

The bladder is a hollow, spherical, muscular organ in the pelvis that serves to store urine. It lies anterior and inferior to the pelvic cavity and posterior to the symphysis pubis. Bladder capacity ranges from 500 to 600 ml in a normal adult. If the amount of stored urine exceeds bladder capacity, the bladder distends above the symphysis pubis.

 SPECIAL POINTS *Children and elderly patients have bladders with a lower capacity.*

The base of the bladder contains three openings that form a triangular area called the *trigone*. Two ureteral orifices act as the posterior boundary of the trigone; one urethral orifice forms its anterior boundary.

Urination results from involuntary (reflex) and voluntary (learned or intentional) processes. When urine distends the bladder, the involuntary process begins:
✦ Parasympathetic nervous system fibers transmit impulses that make the bladder contract and the internal sphincter (located at the internal urethral orifice) relax.
✦ Then the cerebrum stimulates voluntary relaxation and contraction of the external sphincter (located about ½″ [1.5 cm] beyond the internal sphincter).

Ureters
✦ Ducts allowing urine to pass from kidneys to bladder
✦ Travel to the bladder, channeling urine by peristaltic waves, occurring 1 to 5 times per minute

Bladder
✦ Hollow, spherical, muscular organ, which stores urine
✦ Urination results from involuntary and voluntary processes
✦ Distends when stored urine exceeds bladder capacity
✦ Base contains three openings, forming a triangular area called the *trigone*

Special points
✦ Children and elderly patients have bladders with a lower capacity

Urethra

The urethra is a small duct that channels urine outside the body from the bladder. It has an exterior opening known as the *urinary (urethral) meatus.* In the female, the urethra ranges from 1″ to 2″ (2.5 to 5 cm) long, with the urethral meatus located anterior to the vaginal opening.

Urine formation

Three processes—glomerular filtration, tubular reabsorption, and tubular secretion—take place in the nephrons, ultimately leading to urine formation.

The kidneys can vary the amount of substances reabsorbed and secreted in the nephrons, changing the composition of excreted urine. Normal urine constituents include sodium, chloride, potassium, calcium, magnesium, sulfates, phosphates, bicarbonates, uric acid, ammonium ions, creatinine, and urobilinogen. A few leukocytes and RBCs may make their way into the urine as it passes from the kidneys to the ureteral orifice. Urine may also contain drugs if the patient is receiving drugs that undergo urinary excretion.

Varying with fluid intake and climate, total daily urine output averages 720 to 2,400 ml. For example, after a patient drinks a large volume of fluid, urine output increases as the body rapidly excretes excess water. If a patient restricts water intake or has an excessive intake of such solutes as sodium, urine output declines as the body retains water to restore normal fluid concentration.

Hormones

Hormones help regulate tubular reabsorption and secretion. For example, antidiuretic hormone (ADH) acts in the distal tubule and collecting ducts to increase water reabsorption and urine concentration. ADH deficiency decreases water reabsorption, causing dilute urine. Aldosterone affects tubular reabsorption by regulating sodium retention and helping to control potassium secretion by tubular epithelial cells.

By secreting the enzyme renin, the kidneys play a crucial role in blood pressure and fluid volume regulation. The distal tubules of the kidneys regulate potassium excretion. Responding to an elevated serum potassium level, the adrenal cortex increases aldosterone secretion. Through a poorly understood mechanism, aldosterone also affects the potassium-secreting capacity of distal tubular cells.

Other hormonal functions of the kidneys include secretion of the hormone erythropoietin and regulation of calcium and phosphorus balance. In response to low arterial oxygen tension, the kidneys produce erythropoietin, which travels to the bone marrow, then stimulates RBC production. To help regulate calcium and phosphorus balance, the kidneys filter and reabsorb about half of unbound serum calcium and activate vitamin D, a compound that promotes intestinal calcium absorption and regulates phosphate excretion.

REPRODUCTIVE SYSTEM

The female reproductive system consists of external and internal genitalia.

External genitalia

The external genitalia, collectively called the *vulva,* consist of the mons pubis, labia majora, labia minora, clitoris, vaginal introitus, urethral orifice, and Skene's and Bartholin's glands. (See *External genitalia,* page 274.)

Urethra

+ Small duct that channels urine outside the body from bladder
+ Includes an exterior opening called *urethral meatus*

Urine formation

+ Involves glomerular filtration, tubular reabsorption, and tubular secretion
+ Normal urine includes sodium, chloride, potassium, calcium, magnesium, sulfates, phosphates, bicarbonates, uric acid, ammonium ions, creatinine, and urobilinogen
+ Output declines as body retains water

Hormones

+ Regulate tubular reabsorption and secretion and blood pressure and fluid volume
+ Involve ADH, which increases water reabsorption and urine concentration
+ Include secretion of erythropoietin and regulation of calcium and phosphorus balance

External genitalia

+ Vulva, collective name for the external genitalia
+ Includes mons pubis, labia majora, labia minora, clitoris, vaginal introitus, urethral orifice, and Skene's and Bartholin's glands

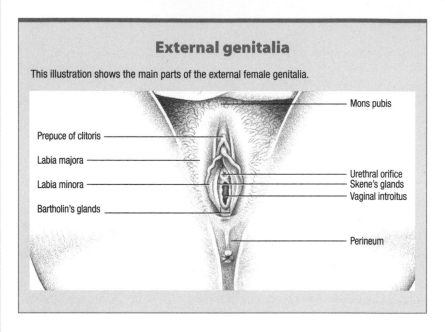

External genitalia

This illustration shows the main parts of the external female genitalia.

- Mons pubis
- Prepuce of clitoris
- Labia majora
- Labia minora
- Bartholin's glands
- Urethral orifice
- Skene's glands
- Vaginal introitus
- Perineum

Mons pubis
+ Mound of adipose tissue
+ Overlies the symphysis pubis and is covered with pubic hair in the adult

Labia majora
+ Outer vulval lips
+ Two rounded folds of adipose tissue
+ Covered with hair

Labia minora
+ Inner vulval lips
+ Joins the anterolateral and medial parts forming the prepuce

Clitoris, vestibule, and urethral opening
+ Clitoris contains erectile tissue located beneath mons pubis
+ Vestibule contains the urethral and vaginal openings
+ Urethral opening located below the clitoris

Vaginal opening and perineum
+ Introitus is posterior to urethral orifice
+ Perineum is bordered by anus and top of labial fold

Mons pubis

The mons pubis is a mound of adipose tissue overlying the symphysis pubis and is covered with pubic hair in the adult. Pubic hair typically appears at age 10½. It may become sparse after menopause due to hormonal changes.

 SPECIAL POINTS *Native Americans and Asians usually have less pubic hair than people of other races.*

Labia majora

The outer vulval lips, or labia majora, are two rounded folds of adipose tissue that extend from the mons pubis to the perineum. The labia majora are covered with hair.

Labia minora

The inner vulval lips are called the *labia minora.* The anterolateral and medial parts join to form the prepuce or hood, the folds of skin that cap the clitoris. The posterior union of the labia minora is called the *fourchette* or *frenulum.*

Clitoris, vestibule, and urethral opening

The clitoris is the small, protuberant organ located just beneath the arch of the mons pubis. The clitoris contains erectile tissue, venous cavernous spaces, and specialized sensory corpuscles that are stimulated during coitus. The clitoris lies between the labia minora at the top of the vestibule, which contains the urethral and vaginal openings. The urethral opening is a slit below the clitoris.

Vaginal opening and perineum

The vaginal opening, or *introitus,* is posterior to the urethral orifice. This opening is a thin vertical slit in women with intact hymens and a large opening with irregular edges in women whose hymens have been perforated. The hymen is a thin membranous fold that may cover the vaginal orifice or may be absent. The perineum is the area bordered anteriorly by the top of the labial fold and posteriorly by the anus.

Skene's and Bartholin's glands

Two types of glands have ducts that open into the vulva. Skene's glands are tiny structures just below the urethra, each containing 6 to 31 ducts. Bartholin's glands are found posterior to the vaginal opening. Neither of these glands can be seen, but they can be palpated if enlarged.

Skene's and Bartholin's glands produce fluids important for the reproductive process. They can become infected, usually with organisms known to cause sexually transmitted diseases (STDs).

Internal genitalia

The internal genitalia include the vagina, uterus, ovaries, and fallopian tubes. (See *Internal genitalia,* page 276.)

Vagina

The vagina, a highly elastic muscular tube, is located between the urethra and the rectum. Between 2½″ and 2¾″ (6.5 to 7 cm) long anteriorly and 3½″ (9 cm) long posteriorly, the vagina lies at a 45-degree angle to the long axis of the body. It's a pink, hollow, collapsed tube that extends up and back from the vulva to the uterus. The vagina is the route of passage for childbirth and menstruation.

Uterus

The uterus, a small, firm, pear-shaped, muscular organ, rests between the bladder and the rectum and usually lies at almost a 90-degree angle to the vagina. However, the position of the uterus in the pelvic cavity may vary, depending on bladder fullness. The uterus may also tip in different directions.

The mucous membrane lining the uterus is called the *endometrium;* the muscular layer, the myometrium. In pregnancy, the elastic, upper uterine portion (the fundus) accommodates most of the growing fetus until term. The uterine neck (isthmus) joins the fundus to the cervix, the uterine part extending into the vagina. The fundus and the isthmus make up the corpus, the main uterine body. The cervix contains mucus-secreting glands that help in reproduction and protect the uterus from pathogens. The function of the uterus is to nurture and then expel the fetus.

Ovaries

A pair of oval organs about 1¼″ (3 cm) long, the ovaries are usually found near the lateral pelvic wall at the height of the anterosuperior iliac spine. They produce ova and release the hormones estrogen and progesterone. The ovaries become fully developed after puberty and shrink after menopause.

Fallopian tubes

Two fallopian tubes attach to the uterus at the upper angles of the fundus. Usually nonpalpable, these 2¾″ to 5½″ (7- to 14-cm) long, narrow tubes of muscle fibers have fingerlike projections, called *fimbriae,* on the free ends that partially surround the ovaries, which help guide the ova to the uterus after expulsion from the ovaries. Fertilization of the ovum usually occurs in the outer third of the fallopian tube.

SPECIAL POINTS *During a woman's lifetime, the size of the uterine corpus and cervix changes, as does the percentage of space these parts occupy. For example, in a premenarchal female, the uterine corpus may occupy one-third of the uterus, and the cervix may occupy two-thirds; in an adult multiparous female, the distribution may be reversed.*

Skene's and Bartholin's glands

+ Contain ducts that open into the vulva
+ Skene's glands are tiny structures located just below urethra
+ Bartholin's glands lie posterior to the vaginal opening
+ Both produce fluids for reproductive process

Internal genitalia

+ Includes vagina, uterus, ovaries, and fallopian tubes

Vagina

+ Located between the urethra and rectum
+ Serves as passage for childbirth and menstruation

Uterus

+ Nurtures and expels fetus
+ Involves the endometrium and myometrium
+ Contains the cervix

Ovaries

+ Produce ova and release estrogen and progesterone
+ Develop fully after puberty and shrink after menopause

Fallopian tubes

+ Guide the ova to uterus after expulsion from ovaries
+ Serves as fertilization ground where the ovum rests

Special points

+ Over a woman's lifetime, the size of the uterine corpus and cervix changes

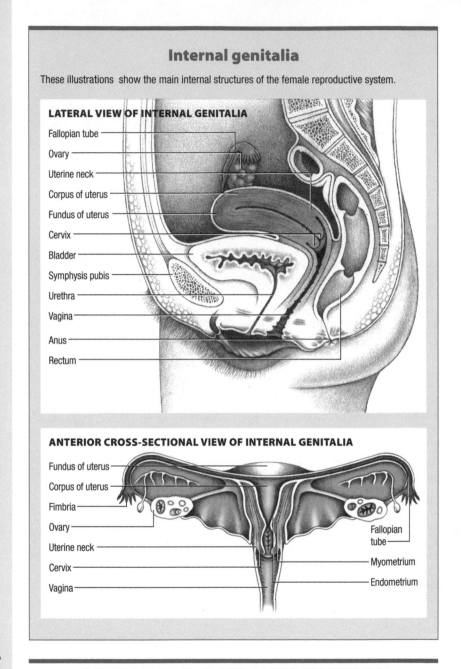

Internal genitalia

These illustrations show the main internal structures of the female reproductive system.

LATERAL VIEW OF INTERNAL GENITALIA

- Fallopian tube
- Ovary
- Uterine neck
- Corpus of uterus
- Fundus of uterus
- Cervix
- Bladder
- Symphysis pubis
- Urethra
- Vagina
- Anus
- Rectum

ANTERIOR CROSS-SECTIONAL VIEW OF INTERNAL GENITALIA

- Fundus of uterus
- Corpus of uterus
- Fimbria
- Ovary
- Uterine neck
- Cervix
- Vagina
- Fallopian tube
- Myometrium
- Endometrium

Obtaining a health history

- ✦ Tracks relevant signs and symptoms over time
- ✦ Includes chief complaint, current and past health, body system review, and family and psychosocial history

OBTAINING A HEALTH HISTORY

Because the urinary and reproductive systems are located so close together in women, you and your patient may have trouble differentiating signs and symptoms. Even if the patient's complaint seems minor, investigate it. Ask about its onset, duration, and severity, and about measures taken to treat it. The information you gain will help you formulate a more appropriate plan of care.

ASKING ABOUT THE URINARY SYSTEM

The most common complaints of the urinary system include output changes, such as polyuria, oliguria, and anuria; voiding pattern changes, such as hesitancy, frequency, urgency, nocturia, and incontinence; urine color changes; and pain.

Chief complaint

Ask the patient a general question such as, "What made you seek medical help?" If she mentions several complaints, ask which bothers her most. Document her responses in her own words.

As you gather information, remain objective. Don't let the patient's opinions about her condition distract you from a thorough investigation. For example, a patient with a history of abdominal aneurysm who's experiencing flank pain may assume that the aneurysm is to blame. Further investigation, however, could reveal renal calculi. You can usually detect renal dysfunction by assessing other related body symptoms.

Current health history

Find out how the patient's symptoms developed and progressed. Ask how long she has had the problem, how it affects her daily routine, when and how it began, and how often it occurs. Also ask about related signs and symptoms, such as nausea and vomiting. If she has had pain, ask about its location, radiation, intensity, and duration. Does anything precipitate, exacerbate, or relieve it? Which, if any, self-help remedies and over-the-counter (OTC) medications has she used?

Ask the patient if she has a history of diabetes or hypertension. Patients with diabetes have an increased risk of UTIs. Hypertension can contribute to renal failure and nephropathy. Ask the patient if she has noticed a change in the color or odor of her urine. Does she have problems with incontinence or frequency? Does she have allergies? Allergic reactions can cause tubular damage. A severe anaphylactic reaction can cause temporary renal failure and permanent tubular necrosis.

Past health history

Past illnesses and preexisting conditions can affect a patient's urinary tract health. For example, has the patient ever had a urinary tract infection (UTI), kidney trauma, or kidney stones? Kidney stones or trauma can alter the structure and function of the kidneys and bladder. Does she have difficulty controlling urine or does she notice that she leaks urine when she sneezes, laughs, coughs, or bears down?

For clues to the patient's present condition, explore past medical problems, including those she experienced as a child. If she has ever had a serious condition, such as kidney disease or a tumor, find out what treatment she received and its outcome. Ask similar questions about traumatic injuries, surgery, and other condition that required hospitalization.

Next, obtain an immunization and allergy history, including a history of medication reactions. Also, inquire about current medications (prescription and OTC), alcohol use, smoking habits, and illicit drug use.

Make a list of all medications and herbal preparations the patient takes. Some drugs can affect the appearance of urine; nephrotoxic drugs can alter urinary function.

Family history

For clues to risk factors, ask the patient if any blood relatives have ever been treated for renal or cardiovascular disorders, diabetes, cancer, or any other chronic illness.

Asking about the urinary system

+ Output changes
+ Voiding pattern changes
+ Urine color changes
+ Pain

Exploring the chief complaint

+ Record patient's responses
+ Don't let patient's opinions distract you
+ Assess other related body systems

Current health history

+ Reveals symptom onset, location, duration, timing, quality, and exacerbating or alleviating factors
+ Diabetes increases risk of UTI; hypertension contributes to renal failure and nephropathy

Past health history

+ Past UTIs, kidney trauma, kidney stones, loss of urine control, and urine leakage
+ Childhood medical problems and traumatic injuries
+ Immunization, allergy, medication, and surgical history
+ Alcohol and drug use and smoking habits

Family history

+ Renal or cardiovascular disorders, diabetes, cancer, or chronic illnesses

Psychosocial history

+ Reveals marital status, living conditions, and employment
+ Detects self-image and patient's fears and concerns

Sexual history

+ Identifies knowledge deficits and expectations
+ May suggest a need for psychological or sexual therapy
+ Guides treatment decisions

Key signs and symptoms

+ Polyuria, oliguria, anuria, hematuria, dysuria, and nocturia
+ Edema
+ Urine urgency and frequency
+ Pain
+ Pruritus
+ Fever and chills

Psychosocial history

Investigate psychosocial factors that may affect the way the patient deals with her condition. Marital problems, poor living conditions, job insecurity, and other such stresses can strongly affect how she feels.

Also, find out how the patient views herself. A disfiguring genital lesion or an STD can alter self-image. Try to determine what concerns she has about her condition. For example, does she fear that the disease or therapy will affect her sex life? If she can express her fears and concerns, you can develop appropriate nursing interventions more easily.

Sexual history

A complete sexual history helps you identify your patient's knowledge deficits and expectations. This information may suggest a need for psychological or sexual therapy. It can also guide treatment decisions. For example, pain or discomfort associated with intercourse or diminished sexual desire may reflect disease progression or depression.

Key signs and symptoms

Explore the patient's key signs and symptoms of her urinary system complaints.

 ABNORMAL FINDINGS Be alert for these abnormal signs and symptoms:
+ *polyuria — (urine volume exceeding 2,000 ml/24 hours), which may develop after heavy fluid intake, diuretic therapy, or removal of a urologic obstruction (postobstruction diuresis); underlying conditions that cause polyuria include diabetes mellitus and diabetes insipidus.*
+ *oliguria — (urine volume below 400 ml /24 hours), which can signal renal failure.*
+ *anuria — (no urine output), which can be fatal.*
+ *edema — when associated with fluid retention and electrolyte imbalance, it may indicate a renal dysfunction such as nephritis; however, a nonrenal condition such as heart failure could also be responsible.*
+ *hematuria — an important finding, it can indicate urologic disorders, allergic reactions, toxicity, and other problems. Ask about this sign and accompanying signs or symptoms, such as gross, painless hematuria, which may indicate genitourinary carcinoma; and early-stream hematuria (occurring at the start of urination), which may suggest a urethral lesion; late-stream hematuria (occurring at the end of urination), which may indicate a lesion at the bladder's base.*
+ *urine urgency — this sudden urge to urinate may indicate cystitis, neurogenic bladder, or bladder instability from early obstructive disease.*
+ *urine frequency — when documenting urinary patterns, remember to distinguish between frequency (frequent urination) and polyuria (excessive urination). Frequency can occur throughout the day or only at night. When frequency occurs both day and night, possible causes include infection, calculi, pregnancy, bladder hypertrophy, urethral stricture, and bladder cancer.*
+ *nocturia — urinary frequency at night; can be experienced in patients undergoing diuretic therapy. It's also common among elderly patients who accumulate fluid in their legs during the day. At night, when they lie down, the bloodstream returns much of this fluid to the kidneys, increasing urine production.*
+ *pain — it can be difficult to distinguish urinary pain from that of other disorders, such as appendicitis and biliary disease, so in order to accurately assess the patient's pain, first ask her to point to the painful area. Determine the character of the pain — for example, if it's sharp or dull. Also, determine if it's constant or intermittent and if it radiates. Different types of pain may include:*
–bladder pain, which typically occurs just above the pubic bone, whereas pain from

renal disease typically occurs in the lumbus under the costovertebral margin, lateral to the spine, or anteriorly near the tip of the ninth rib.
–dull ache in kidney area or colicky pain, which periodically radiates to the genital area or leg on the affected side that may indicate renal calculus.
–ureteral pain, which usually occurs between the costal margin and the pubic bone.
–continuous, nonradiating pain, which may indicate inflammation or a tumor.
–shifting pain, which may indicate appendicitis; whereas renal, bladder, and ureteral pain remain fixed.
–colicky pain, which may be caused by peristaltic waves moving from the kidney to a ureteral obstruction.
✦ *dysuria — pain associated with urination, which can originate in the perineum, bladder, or urethra and can occur before, during, or after urination with pyuria and urinary — may also suggest a lower UTI or obstruction.*
✦ *pruritus — itching, which may occur in chronic renal failure. Although the cause remains a mystery, researchers speculate that calcium deposition in the skin is the reason for the itching; it may disappear with dialysis.*
✦ *fever and chills — are caused by urologic infections, particularly pyelonephritis. (Patients with simple cystitis are an exception.)*

 CLINICAL ALERT Urine retention is a urologic emergency, which can result from obstruction, urethral stricture, extraurinary mass, neurogenic disease, drug effect, or pain; in some patients, psychological factors play a part. If left untreated, it can lead to kidney damage and failure as fluid backs up and creates pressure inside the kidneys. Because retained urine provides an ideal medium for bacterial growth, pyelonephritis or sepsis may develop. To identify urine retention early, monitor fluid intake and output, assess for bladder distention, and stay alert for complaints of bladder fullness.

ASKING ABOUT THE REPRODUCTIVE SYSTEM

Conduct your questioning in a comfortable environment that protects the patient's privacy. Avoid rushing her so you don't overlook important details. Use terms that the patient understands and explain technical terms.

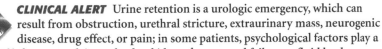 **SPECIAL POINTS** *Remember that in some cultures, discussing female physiologic functions or problems is taboo.*

Ideally, the patient should be allowed to remain seated and dressed until the physical assessment. Always ask health history questions before the patient is in the lithotomy position. In many busy medical practices or health clinics, the patient is asked to undress, get on the examination table, and wait for the physician to come in and begin the examination and interview. Some women find this demeaning as well as stressful.

Although you'll focus your questions on the reproductive system, maintain a holistic approach by inquiring about other physical and psychological concerns. Keep in mind that reproductive system problems may affect other aspects of the patient's life, including self-image and overall wellness.

Chief complaint
The most common reproductive system complaints are pain, vaginal discharge, abnormal uterine bleeding, pruritus, and infertility. To obtain the most complete data about those problems, focus on the patient's current complaints, and then explore her reproductive, psychosocial, and family history. Ask her to describe symptoms in her own words, encouraging her to speak freely. Use open-ended questions.

Types of urinary system pain
✦ Bladder pain
✦ Kidney pain (dull or colicky)
✦ Ureteral pain
✦ Continuous, nonradiating pain
✦ Shifting or fixed pain
✦ Colicky pain

Alert!
✦ Urine retention can result from obstruction, urethral stricture, extraurinary mass, neurogenic disease, drug effect, or pain
✦ Pyelonephritis or sepsis may develop due to retained urine

Asking about the reproductive system
✦ Provide a private, comfortable environment
✦ Explain technical terms to the patient
✦ Reproductive system problems may affect patient's life, self-image, and overall wellness

Special points
✦ Note that discussing female physiologic functions is taboo in some cultures

Chief complaint
✦ Pain
✦ Vaginal discharge
✦ Abnormal uterine bleeding
✦ Pruritus
✦ Infertility

Many patients feel uncomfortable answering questions about their sexual health or reproductive system. Start with the less personal questions and establish a rapport.

Menstrual and contraceptive history

Menstrual and contraceptive history

These questions can be used to assess the patient's menstrual and contraceptive history:

◆ Age the patient began menstruating

◆ First day of last menses, duration, and comparison of most recent with past ones

◆ Sexual practices and contraceptive use

◆ History of medication use, alcohol consumption, and smoking

◆ How old were you when you began menstruating? In girls, menses generally starts by age 14. If it hasn't, and if no secondary sex characteristics have developed, the patient should be evaluated by a physician.

◆ When was the first day of your last menses?

◆ Was that period normal compared with your previous periods?

◆ When was the first day of your previous menses?

◆ How often do your periods occur? The normal cycle for menstruation is one menses every 21 to 38 days.

◆ How long do your periods usually last? The normal duration is 2 to 8 days.

◆ How would you describe your menstrual flow? How many pads or tampons do you use on each day of your period?

◆ Do you experience pain during menstruation?

Abnormal findings: Dysmenorrhea

◆ Sharp, intermittent, or dull, aching pain

◆ Mild to severe cramping in pelvis or lower abdomen

◆ Radiating to the thighs and lower sacrum

 ABNORMAL FINDINGS *Affecting over 50% of menstruating women, dysmenorrhea (painful menstruation) is the leading cause of lost time from school and work among women of childbearing age. It can involve sharp, intermittent pain or dull, aching pain. Dysmenorrhea is usually characterized by mild to severe cramping or colicky pain in the pelvis or lower abdomen that may radiate to the thighs and lower sacrum. This pain may precede menses by several days or accompany it and gradually subsides as bleeding tapers off.*

Special points: Dysmenorrhea

◆ Rare during first year of menses

◆ Occurs more in adolescent girls than older women

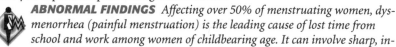 **SPECIAL POINTS** *Dysmenorrhea is rare during the first year of menses, before the cycle becomes ovulatory. However, in general, more adolescent girls experience dysmenorrhea than older women.*

◆ Are your sexual practices bisexual, homosexual, or heterosexual?

◆ Do you use a hormonal contraceptive? If so, what do you use? How long have you used it?

◆ If you don't use a hormonal contraceptive, what method of contraception do you use? How long have you used it? If it's a device, is it in good condition?

◆ What medications (including prescribed and OTC drugs and alternative medications) do you take? At what dosage and for what reason? Have you ever taken illicit drugs?

Abnormal findings: Drug effects

◆ Amenorrhea (androgens, antihypertensives, antipsychotics, cytotoxics, estrogens, progestins, and steroids)

◆ Libido changes (antidepressants, antihypertensives, beta-adrenergic blockers, and estrogens)

◆ Vaginal candidiasis (estrogens)

◆ Infertility (cytotoxics)

 ABNORMAL FINDINGS *Many drugs affect the female reproductive system. For example, androgens, antihypertensives, antipsychotics, cytotoxics, estrogens, progestins, and steroids can cause amenorrhea. Antidepressants and thyroid hormones can cause other menstrual irregularities. Antidepressants, antihypertensives, beta-adrenergic blockers, and estrogens can cause changes in libido. Estrogens can cause vaginal candidiasis and some cytotoxics can cause infertility.*

◆ How much alcohol do you drink? How long have you been drinking?

◆ Do you smoke? If so, how much do you smoke? How long have you smoked? Have you tried a smoking-cessation program?

◆ Do you have signs or symptoms of infection, such as discharge, itching, painful intercourse, sores or lesions, fever, chills, or swelling of the vagina or vulva?

◆ Do you ever bleed between periods? If so, how much and for how long? Spotting between periods, or metrorrhagia, may be normal in patients using low-dose hormonal contraceptives or progesterone; otherwise, spotting may indicate infection or cancer.

✦ Do you ever have vaginal bleeding after intercourse?

✦ Have you had uncomfortable signs and symptoms before or during your periods?

✦ How often do you visit the gynecologist?

Reproductive history

To collect data about the patient's reproductive history, ask these questions:

✦ Has anyone ever told you that something is wrong with your uterus or other female organs? Have you ever had a positive Papanicolaou (Pap) test? When was your last Pap test?

✦ Have you ever had an STD or other genital or reproductive system infection?

✦ Have you had surgery for a reproductive system problem?

✦ Have you ever been pregnant? If so, how many times, and how many times did you give birth? Did you have a vaginal delivery or cesarean birth?

✦ Have you ever had problems conceiving or been treated for infertility?

✦ Have you ever had an abortion or miscarriage?

Family history

Because some reproductive problems tend to be familial, ask about family reproductive history. Ask the patient if she or anyone in her family ever had reproductive problems, hypertension, diabetes mellitus (including gestational diabetes mellitus), obesity, heart disease, or gynecologic surgery. Next ask her if she's having any problems that she believes are related to her reproductive system or any other problems not yet covered during the interview. Finally, answer any questions she may have about her reproductive organs or sexual activity.

Psychosocial history

Ask the patient if she's sexually active. If so, ask her when she had intercourse last and if she's sexually active with more than one partner. Finally, ask if her sexual partner has signs or symptoms of infection, such as genital sores, warts, or penile discharge.

Menopausal history

To find out more about the menopausal signs and symptoms your patient is experiencing, ask her these questions: Does she have any abnormal vaginal discharge? Does she have external lesions or itching? Does she experience pain with intercourse? Does she douche, and if so, how often? When was her last Pap test and what was the result?

Ask for the date of her last menses. Ask if she's having hot flashes, mood swings, or flushing. Ask about vaginal dryness, itching, use of hormone replacement therapy or herbal or soy products to control symptoms. Also, ask her about bleeding, pelvic muscle weakening, and uterine prolapse.

ASSESSING THE FEMALE GU SYSTEM

To perform a physical assessment of the female GU system, you'll use the techniques of inspection, auscultation, percussion, and palpation to evaluate the urinary and reproductive systems. We'll look at the urinary system first.

EXAMINING THE URINARY SYSTEM

Begin the physical examination by documenting baseline vital signs and weighing the patient. Comparing subsequent weight measurements to this baseline may reveal a developing problem, such as dehydration or fluid retention. The urinary

---

Reproductive history

✦ Past uterine problems
✦ Date and results of last Pap test
✦ STD or infection
✦ Past surgeries or reproductive problems
✦ Pregnancies
✦ Infertility, abortion, and miscarriages

Family history

✦ Hypertension
✦ Diabetes mellitus or gestational diabetes mellitus
✦ Obesity
✦ Heart disease
✦ Gynecologic surgery

Psychosocial history

✦ Sexual activity and partners
✦ Last date of intercourse
✦ Infection, genital sores, warts, or penile discharge of partner

Menopausal history

✦ Discharge, lesions or itching, bleeding, or pain
✦ Date and result of last Pap test
✦ Date of last menses
✦ Hot flashes, mood swings, flushing, or vaginal dryness

Assessing the female GU system

✦ Inspection
✦ Auscultation
✦ Percussion
✦ Palpation

Examining the urinary system

✦ Document baseline vital signs and weight

Examining the urinary system
(continued)

+ Obtain a urine sample and assess it for color, odor, and clarity

Abnormal findings

+ Poor concentration, memory loss, or disorientation (kidney dysfunction)
+ Lethargy, confusion, disorientation, stupor, seizures, and coma (progressive, chronic kidney failure)

Inspection

+ Includes inspection of the abdomen and urethral meatus

Abdomen

+ May reveal gross enlargements or fullness
+ Should be smooth, flat or concave, and symmetrical
+ Skin should be free from scars, lesions, bruises, and discolorations

Abnormal findings: Abdomen

+ Extremely prominent veins (renal dysfunction)
+ Distention, skin tightness and glistening, and striae (fluid retention)

Urethral meatus

+ Assess last and explain beforehand how you'll assess this area
+ During assessment, wear gloves

Abnormal findings: Urethral meatus

+ Inflammation and discharge (urethral infection; ulceration [STD])

Auscultation

+ Includes auscultation of the renal arteries

Abnormal findings

+ In a patient with hypertension, systolic bruits suggests renal artery stenosis

---

system affects many body functions, so a thorough assessment includes examination of multiple, related body systems using inspection, auscultation, percussion, and palpation techniques.

Observing the patient's behavior can give you clues about her mental status. Does she have trouble concentrating, have memory loss, or seem disoriented? Ask the patient to urinate into a specimen cup. Assess the sample for color, odor, and clarity. Then have the patient undress, providing her with a gown and drapes, and proceed with a systematic physical examination.

 ABNORMAL FINDINGS *If the patient has kidney dysfunction she may experience poor concentration, memory loss, or disorientation. If she has progressive, chronic kidney failure her signs and symptoms may include lethargy, confusion, disorientation, stupor, seizures, and coma.*

Inspection

Urinary system inspection includes examination of the abdomen and urethral meatus.

Abdomen

Help the patient assume a supine position with her arms relaxed at her sides. Make sure she's comfortable and draped appropriately. Expose the patient's abdomen from the xiphoid process to the symphysis pubis and inspect the abdomen for gross enlargements or fullness by comparing the left and right sides, noting asymmetrical areas. In a normal adult, the abdomen is smooth, flat or concave, and symmetrical. Abdominal skin should be free from scars, lesions, bruises, and discolorations.

 ABNORMAL FINDINGS *If your patient has extremely prominent veins, other vascular signs associated with renal dysfunction, such as hypertension or renal artery bruits, may occur. Distention, skin tightness and glistening, and striae (streaks or linear scars caused by rapidly developing skin tension) may signal fluid retention. If you suspect ascites, which may suggest nephrotic syndrome, perform the fluid wave test.*

Urethral meatus

Help the patient feel more at ease during your inspection by examining the urethral meatus last and by explaining beforehand how you'll assess this area. Be sure to wash your hands and put on gloves (first, asking the patient if she has a latex allergy). Urethral meatus inspection may reveal several abnormalities.

 ABNORMAL FINDINGS *If your patient displays inflammation and discharge during inspection of the urethral meatus, these signs may signal urethral infection. Ulceration usually indicates a sexually transmitted disease.*

Auscultation

Auscultate the renal arteries in the left and right upper abdominal quadrants by pressing the stethoscope bell lightly against the abdomen and instructing the patient to exhale deeply. Begin auscultating at the midline and work to the left. Then return to the midline and work to the right.

 ABNORMAL FINDINGS *If your patient displays systolic bruits (whooshing sounds) or other unusual sounds during auscultation, these signs may alert you to potentially significant abnormalities. For example, in a patient with hypertension, the presence of systolic bruits suggests renal artery stenosis.*

Percussion

Kidney percussion checks for costovertebral angle tenderness that occurs with inflammation. To percuss over the kidneys, have the patient sit up. Place the ball of

KNOW-HOW

Palpating the kidneys

To palpate the kidneys, first have the patient lie in a supine position. To palpate the right kidney, stand on her right side. Place your left hand under her back and your right hand on her abdomen.

Instruct her to inhale deeply, so her kidney moves downward. As she inhales, press up with your left hand and down with your right, as shown.

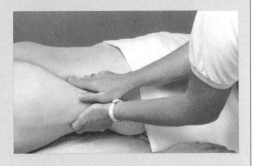

your nondominant hand on her back at the costovertebral angle of the 12th rib. Strike the ball of that hand with the ulnar surface of your other hand. Use just enough force to cause a painless but perceptible thud.

To percuss the bladder, first ask the patient to empty it. Then have her lie in the supine position. Start at the symphysis pubis and percuss upward toward the bladder and over it. You should hear tympany.

 ABNORMAL FINDINGS *If your patient experiences tenderness and pain during kidney percussion, these signs may suggest glomerulonephritis or glomerulonephrosis. A dull sound heard on bladder percussion in a patient who has just urinated may indicate urine retention, reflecting bladder dysfunction or infection.*

Palpation

Because the kidneys lie behind other organs and are protected by muscle, they normally aren't palpable unless they're enlarged. However, in very thin patients, you may be able to feel the lower end of the right kidney as a smooth round mass that drops on inspiration. (See *Palpating the kidneys.*)

 SPECIAL POINTS *In elderly patients, you may be able to palpate both kidneys because of decreased muscle tone and elasticity. If the kidneys feel enlarged, the patient may have hydronephrosis, cysts, or tumors.*

You won't be able to palpate the bladder unless it's distended. With the patient in a supine position, use the fingers of one hand to palpate the lower abdomen in a light dipping motion. A distended bladder will feel firm and relatively smooth.

 SPECIAL POINTS *In pregnant patients (12 weeks' gestation or more), you might actually be feeling the fundus of the uterus, palpable just above the symphysis pubis.*

 ABNORMAL FINDINGS *If your patient has a lump, mass, or tenderness during kidney palpation, these findings may indicate a tumor or cyst. A soft kidney may reflect chronic renal disease; a tender kidney, acute infection. Unequal kidney size may reflect hydronephrosis, a cyst, a tumor, or another disorder. Bilateral enlargement suggests polycystic kidney disease.*

If your patient has a lump or mass during bladder palpation, these findings may signal a tumor or cyst, or tenderness, which may stem from infection.

Percussion
+ Includes kidney percussion for costovertebral angle tenderness, occurring with inflammation and bladder percussion

Abnormal findings
+ Kidney percussion — tenderness and pain (glomerulonephritis or glomerulonephrosis)
+ Bladder percussion — dull sounds heard in the bladder in a patient who has just urinated (bladder dysfunction or infection)

Palpation
+ Kidneys aren't palpable unless enlarged
+ Bladder isn't palpable unless distended, in which case it will feel firm and smooth

Abnormal findings
+ Kidney palpation — lump, mass, or tenderness (tumor or cyst); soft kidney (chronic renal disease); tender kidney (acute infection) unequal size (hydronephrosis); bilateral enlargement (polycystic kidney disease)
+ Bladder palpation — lump or mass (tumor or cyst)

Examining the reproductive system

- ✦ Gather all necessary supplies
- ✦ Ensure that the room is comfortable
- ✦ Explain the procedure and what to expect
- ✦ Provide supportive assurances
- ✦ Ask patient to empty her bladder before beginning

Examination positions

- ✦ Lithotomy — normal positioning
- ✦ Sims' (left lateral) — if patient can't assume lithotomy position because of age, arthritis, or back pain

Privacy

- ✦ Ensure that the patient has privacy
- ✦ Provide adequate draping to give her a sense of security

EXAMINING THE REPRODUCTIVE SYSTEM

Before beginning the assessment, gather the necessary equipment and supplies. This includes gloves, several different sizes and types of specula, a lubricant, a spatula, swabs, an endocervical brush, glass slides and cover slips, a cytologic fixative, culture bottles or plates, a sponge, forceps, a mirror, and a light source.

The room should be comfortable, and no one other than the examiner, assistants, and the patient should be there.

Keep in mind that many women become anxious when undergoing a gynecologic assessment. Some feel uncomfortable or embarrassed exposing their genitalia. Others are afraid from their lack of knowledge about the examination, past painful examinations, or accounts of painful experiences.

It's almost impossible to accurately assess a very tense patient. Merely telling her to relax is ineffective. To help her calm down, ask if this is her first gynecologic assessment. If it is, explain the procedure so that she knows what to expect. If it isn't, ask her about previous assessment experiences, which may help her express her feelings. Consider using pictures and the equipment to explain the examination procedure, even if the patient has had previous gynecologic assessments. Provide supportive assurances. Stand next to the examination table, talk to her during the assessment, explain what's occurring and what will occur next, and avoid using such words as hurt and pain.

Ask the patient to empty her bladder before the examination begins.

The patient must assume the lithotomy position for the assessment. Her heels should be secure in the stirrups and her knees comfortably placed in the knee supports if they're used. Adjust the foot or knee supports so that the legs are equally and comfortably separated and symmetrically balanced.

The patient's buttocks must extend about 2½″ (6.5 cm) over the end of the table. Because this position is precarious, give the patient help, direction, and ample time to get ready. The hips and knees will be flexed and the thighs abducted. The patient should place her feet (or knees) in the stirrups and inch down to the proper position. A pillow placed beneath her head may help her to relax the abdominal muscles. Her arms should be at her side or over her chest; this also reduces abdominal muscle tension. The examiner will sit on a movable swivel stool an arm's length away from and between the patient's abducted legs. In this way, equipment can be reached and the genitalia seen and palpated easily.

If the patient can't assume the lithotomy position because of age, arthritis, back pain, or other reasons, place her in Sims' (left lateral) position instead. To assume this position, the patient should lie on her left side almost prone, with her buttocks close to the edge of the table, her left leg straight, and her right leg slightly bent in front of her left leg.

Privacy and adequate draping give the patient a sense of security. Positioning the drape low on the patient's abdomen allows her to see the examiner and exchange visual cues. If the patient prefers no draping, respect her choice. Raising the head of the examination table helps maintain eye contact and doesn't hinder the examination.

To help the patient relax, describe what she'll feel. For example, she'll feel her inner thigh being touched, then her labia, then a finger slightly in the vaginal opening pressing on the muscle (the bulbocavernous muscle) in the lower vaginal wall. Explain that it's normal to tighten this muscle when tense, and show the patient how to relax by inhaling slowly and deeply through the nose, exhaling through the mouth, and concentrating on breathing regularly to relax the muscle. If the patient begins to tense up and hold her breath, remind her to breathe and relax. A ceiling poster or mobile in the examination room may help distract her.

Assure the patient that the assessment takes little time and that she'll be told what to expect before each new step. Also, keep in mind that gentle words and actions soothe; jerky movements alarm. Idle conversation may also make the patient more tense.

If the patient is extremely nervous, more than one appointment may be needed to complete the assessment. The examiner will decide, based on the urgency of the patient's chief complaint and based on the patient's anxiety, whether to perform the assessment over two or three visits. A nervous patient can be coached during a difficult assessment, but a tranquilizer or even a general anesthetic may be necessary. The latter is especially true with young children or women who have been sexually abused.

If the examiner is male, a female assistant should be present during the examination for the patient's emotional comfort and the examiner's legal protection.

Inspecting the external genitalia

Sometimes only the patient's external genitalia need to be inspected to determine the origin of sores or itching. Wash your hands and put on gloves (first, ask the patient if she has a latex allergy), then follow these steps.

Place the patient in a supine position with the pubic area uncovered, and begin the assessment by determining sexual maturity. Inspect pubic hair for amount and pattern. It's usually thick and appears on the mons pubis as well as the inner aspects of the upper thighs.

 SPECIAL POINTS *Pubic hair changes in density, color, and texture throughout a woman's life. Before adolescence, the pubic area is covered only with body hair. In adolescence, this hair grows thicker, darker, coarser, and curlier. In full maturity, it spreads over the symphysis pubis and inner thighs. In later years, the hair grows thin, gray, and brittle.*

Using a gloved index finger and thumb, gently spread the labia majora and look for the labia minora. The labia should be pink and moist with no lesions. Normal cervical discharge varies in color and consistency It's clear and stretchy before ovulation, white and opaque after ovulation, and usually odorless and nonirritating to the mucosa. No other discharge should be present.

Examine the vestibule, especially the area around the Bartholin's and Skene's glands. Check for swelling, redness, lesions, discharge, and unusual odor. If you detect any of these conditions, notify the physician and obtain a specimen for culture. Finally, inspect the vaginal opening, noting whether the hymen is intact or perforated.

 ABNORMAL FINDINGS *If your patient displays a male pubic hair distribution pattern, note the clitoral size as well as any other masculinization signs such as a deepened voice. You may need to refer this patient to an endocrinologist.*

You may find other abnormalities including:
♦ *varicosities (distended superficial vessels on the labia), which can indicate increased pressure in the pelvic region, as seen in pregnant patients and in those with uterine tumors.*
♦ *lesions, such as ulcerations or wartlike growths, which can indicate human papillomavirus (HPV).*
♦ *edema of the mons pubis, labia majora, labia minora, urethral orifice, vaginal introitus, or the surrounding skin.*
♦ *organisms, such as Candida, a yeastlike infection that may cause an inflamed vulva with a cheeselike discharge;* Chlamydia trachomatis, *which may cause a heavy gray-white discharge;* Haemophilus *or* Trichomonas, *which may cause a frothy, malodorous, green or gray watery discharge;* Neisseria gonorrhoeae, *which may*

Inspecting the external genitalia

♦ Place patient in supine position
♦ Inspect pubic area for amount and pattern of hair
♦ Gently spread the labia majora and inspect labia minora (pink and moist with no lesions or discharge)
♦ Examine vestibule and area around Bartholin's and Skene's glands
♦ Check for swelling, redness, lesions, discharge, and unusual odor
♦ Inspect the vaginal opening

Special points: Pubic hair
♦ Adolescence — grows thicker, darker, coarser, curlier
♦ Full maturity — spreads over symphysis pubis and inner thighs
♦ Later years — grows thin, gray, and brittle

Abnormal findings: External genitalia
♦ Masculinization signs
♦ Varicosities
♦ Lesions
♦ Edema
♦ Organisms

Speculum types

Specula come in various shapes and sizes. A Graves' speculum is usually used; however, if the patient has an intact hymen, has never given birth through the vaginal canal, or has a contracted introitus from menopause, use a Pederson speculum. These illustrations show the parts of a typical speculum and three types of specula available.

PARTS OF A SPECULUM

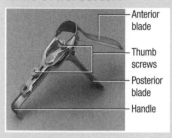

- Anterior blade
- Thumb screws
- Posterior blade
- Handle

TYPES OF SPECULA

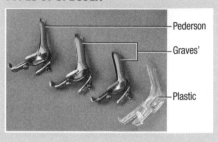

- Pederson
- Graves'
- Plastic

cause a purulent, green-yellow urethral or vaginal discharge; and Pediculus pubis (lice) or nits (minute white louse eggs attached to pubic hairs), which may be present without symptoms, or with symptoms of another infection.

Specimens of all discharges should be cultured or examined microscopically in the laboratory.

Palpating the external genitalia

Spread the labia with one hand and palpate with the other. The labia should feel soft. Note swelling, hardness, or tenderness. If you detect a mass or lesion, palpate it to determine its size, shape, and consistency.

If you find swelling or tenderness, see if you can palpate Bartholin's glands, which normally aren't palpable. To do this, insert your finger carefully into the patient's posterior introitus, and place your thumb along the lateral edge of the swollen or tender labium. Gently squeeze the labium.

 ABNORMAL FINDINGS *Swollen or tender Bartholin's glands, could indicate infection. Make sure to culture any glandular discharge.*

If the urethra is inflamed, milk it and the area of Skene's glands. First, moisten your gloved index finger with water. Then separate the labia with your other hand, and insert your index finger about 1¼″ (3 cm) into the anterior vagina. With the pad of your finger, gently press and pull outward. Continue palpating down to the introitus. This procedure shouldn't cause the patient discomfort. Culture the discharge.

Inspecting the internal genitalia

Nurses don't routinely inspect internal genitalia unless they're in advanced practice. However, you may be asked to assist with this examination. To start, select an appropriate speculum for your patient. (See *Speculum types.*)

Hold the speculum under warm, running water to lubricate and warm the blades. Don't use lubricants; many of them are bacteriostatic and can alter Pap test results.

Sit or stand at the foot of the examination table. Tell the patient she'll feel internal pressure and possibly some slight, transient discomfort as you insert and open the speculum.

Palpating the external genitalia
- ✦ Detects swelling, hardness, or tenderness
- ✦ May reveal a mass or lesion
- ✦ May reveal inflamed urethra

Abnormal findings
- ✦ Swollen or tender Bartholin's glands (infection)

Inspecting the internal genitalia
- ✦ Performed by physician or advanced practice nurse; however, nurses can assist
- ✦ Involves use of a speculum
- ✦ Allows observation of color, texture, and integrity of the vaginal lining

Inserting a speculum

Proper positioning and insertion of the speculum are important for the comfort of the patient and for proper visualization of the internal structures. These illustrations show the proper angle and hand position for insertion.

INITIAL INSERTION
Place the index and middle fingers of your nondominant hand about 1″ (2.5 cm) into the vagina and spread the fingers to exert pressure on the posterior vagina. Hold the speculum in your dominant hand, and insert the blades between your fingers as shown.

DEEPER INSERTION
Ask the patient to bear down to open the introitus and relax the perineal muscles. Point the speculum slightly downward, and insert the blades until the base of the speculum touches your fingers, inside the vagina.

ROTATE AND OPEN
Rotate the speculum in the same plane as the vagina, and withdraw your fingers. Open the blades as far as possible and lock them. You should now be able to view the cervix clearly.

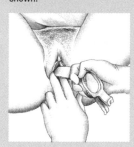
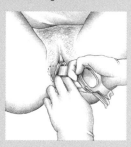
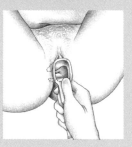

Using your dominant hand, hold the speculum by the base with the blades anchored between your index and middle fingers. This keeps the blades from accidentally opening during insertion. Encourage the patient to take slow, deep breaths during insertion to relax her abdominal muscles. (See *Inserting a speculum.*) Insert your fingers first and allow the pelvic floor muscles to relax, then insert the speculum. Ease insertion by asking the patient to bear down.

Using the thumb of the hand holding the speculum, press the lower lever to open the blades. Lock them in the open position by tightening the thumb screw above the lever.

Examine the cervix for color, position, size, shape, mucosal integrity, and discharge. It should be smooth and round. The central cervical opening, or cervical os, is circular in a woman who hasn't given birth vaginally and a horizontal slit in a woman who has. Expect to see a clear, watery cervical discharge during ovulation and a slightly bloody discharge just before menstruation. (See *The normal os,* page 289.)

ABNORMAL FINDINGS *During pregnancy the cervix is enlarged. A cyanotic cervix can indicate pelvic congestion from a tumor or pregnancy. Infection may give the cervix a bright red or spotted red appearance (erythema). A cervix projecting low into the vagina or visible at the introitus can indicate uterine prolapse (displacement of the uterus from its normal position) caused by weak pelvic muscles or ligaments. A less severe prolapse may occur when the patient bears down;*

Inserting a speculum
+ Begin with initial insertion
+ Continue with deeper insertion
+ Rotate and open for a clear view of the cervix

Inspecting the internal genitalia
(continued)

Abnormal findings: Cervix
+ Cyanotic cervix (pelvic congestion from tumor or pregnancy)
+ Bright red or spotted red appearance (infection)
+ Visible at introitus (uterine prolapse caused by weak pelvic muscles or ligaments)

Inspecting the internal genitalia
(continued)

Abnormal findings: Cervical inspection
+ Laterally place cervix (uterine tumor or adhesion to peritoneum)
+ Cervical cancer
+ Trichomoniasis
+ *Chlamydia trachomatis*
+ Ulcerations, masses, nodules, or surface irregularities
+ Cervical ectropion
+ Polyps
+ Purulent or malodorous discharge
+ Nabothian cysts

Abnormal findings: Vaginal lining
+ Painless, eroding lesion with raised, indurated border (syphilitic chancre, in early stages)
+ Painless warts beginning as shiny red or pink swellings that develop into a cauliflower appearance (genital warts)
+ Multiple, shallow vesicles, lesions, or crusts (genital herpes)

Special points: Vaginal mucosa
+ In postmenopausal patients, appears pale with rugae loss due to estrogen deficiency

---

if urine leakage occurs, this indicates stress incontinence. A laterally placed cervix can indicate a uterine tumor or uterine adhesion to the peritoneum.

Other abnormal cervical findings may include:

+ *cervical cancer, which, if visible, appears as hard, granular, friable lesions usually beginning near the os and growing outward irregularly.*
+ *trichomoniasis, which may cause an abundant malodorous discharge that's either yellow or green and frothy or watery, as well as redness, or red papules on the cervix and vaginal walls, commonly known as a "strawberry" cervix.*
+ Chlamydia trachomatis, *a common but in many cases subtle STD that causes a mucopurulent cervical discharge and cystitis. (It's important to note that three out of four women have no symptoms. Gonorrhea is commonly asymptomatic, but it may cause a purulent green-yellow discharge and cystitis. It's now recommended to screen all sexually active women regardless of symptoms.)*
+ *ulcerations, masses, nodules, or surface irregularities, which should be considered malignant until proven otherwise, and assessed carefully. Ulcerations may indicate trauma or infection. Herpes simplex virus, type 1 or 2, causes ulcerative lesions, whereas trichomonal infection usually produces strawberry spots (punctate hemorrhages).*
+ *endocervical lining that's turned outward on the cervical surface, which gives the area around the external os a velvety red appearance, is known as a* cervical ectropion *or eversion. This tissue is friable (bleeds easily) when the Pap test specimen is obtained. Because an early carcinoma may resemble an ectropion, evaluation is indicated.*
+ *polyps, which may be visible when they protrude from the external os, arise from the endometrium or the endocervical tissue and may bleed easily when the Pap test specimen is obtained. Areas where the mucosa has eroded bleed easily when touched. Bleeding from the os may also occur with menses or may signal another problem.*
+ *purulent or malodorous discharge, which indicates an infection, requires a culture or cytologic evaluation.*
+ *small, smooth, round, raised yellow cysts (nabothian cysts), which appear with or after chronic cervicitis or with cervical gland duct obstructions, are harmless but may signal an underlying problem.*

Obtain a specimen for a Pap test and perform any other tests at this time, including cultures for sexually transmitted infections. Finally, unlock and close the blades and withdraw the speculum.

As you slowly remove the speculum, observe the color, texture, and integrity of the vaginal lining.

 ABNORMAL FINDINGS *You may find abnormalities including:*
+ *syphilitic chancre (in the early stages), which causes a painless, eroding lesion with a raised, indurated border; lesions usually appear inside the vagina, but may also appear on the external genitalia*
+ *genital warts, which are caused by HPV, are painless warts on the vulva, vagina, and cervix; they begin as tiny red or pink swellings that grow and develop stemlike structures and can multiply, producing a cauliflower appearance*
+ *genital herpes, which produces multiple, shallow vesicles, lesions, or crusts inside the vagina, on the external genitalia, on the buttocks, and sometimes on the thighs.*

SPECIAL POINTS *In a postmenopausal patient, the vaginal mucosa may be pale with rugae loss due to estrogen deficiency.*

A thin, white, odorless discharge on the vaginal walls is normal.

ABNORMAL FINDINGS *In a patient with abnormal vaginal discharge you may find:*
+ *vaginitis, which usually results from an overgrowth of infectious organ-*

The normal os

These illustrations show the difference between the os of a woman who has never given birth vaginally (nulliparous) and the os of a woman who has (parous).

NULLIPAROUS

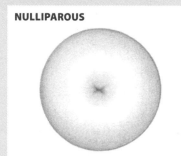

PAROUS

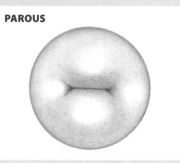

isms and causes redness, itching, dyspareunia (painful intercourse), dysuria, and a malodorous discharge
✦ *bacterial vaginosis, which causes a fishy odor and a thin, grayish white discharge*
✦ *Candida albicans, which causes pruritus and a thick, white, curdlike discharge that appears in patches on the cervix and vaginal walls and has a yeastlike odor.*

Palpating the internal genitalia

To palpate the internal genitalia, lubricate the index and middle fingers of your gloved dominant hand. Stand at the foot of the examination table and position the hand for insertion into the vagina by extending your thumb, index, and middle fingers and curling your ring and little finger toward your palm.

Use the thumb and index finger of your other hand to spread the labia majora. Insert your two lubricated fingers into the vagina, exerting pressure posteriorly to avoid irritating the anterior wall and urethra.

When your fingers are fully inserted, note tenderness or nodularity in the vaginal wall. Ask the patient to bear down so you can assess the support of the vaginal outlet.

 ABNORMAL FINDINGS *Bulging of the patient's vaginal wall may indicate a cystocele or a rectocele.*

To palpate the cervix, sweep your fingers from side to side across the cervix and around the os. The cervix should be smooth and firm and protrude ¼″ to 1¼″ (1 to 3 cm) into the vagina.

 ABNORMAL FINDINGS *If you palpate nodules or irregularities, the patient may have cysts, tumors, or other lesions.*

Next, place your fingers into the recessed area around the cervix. The cervix should move in all directions.

 ABNORMAL FINDINGS *If the patient reports pain during this part of the examination, she may have inflammation of the uterus or adnexa (ovaries, fallopian tubes, and ligaments of the uterus). A patient with pelvic inflammatory disease (PID) may experience severe pain when you manipulate her cervix.*

Inspecting the internal genitalia
(continued)

Abnormal findings: Vaginal discharge
✦ Redness, itching, dyspareunia, dysuria, and malodorous discharge (vaginitis)
✦ Fishy odor and thin, grayish white discharge (bacterial vaginosis)
✦ Thick, white, curdlike discharge (*Candida albicans*)

Palpating the internal genitalia
✦ Assesses the support of the vaginal wall
✦ Allows for evaluation of the cervix by sweeping fingers across os
✦ Normal cervix feels smooth and firm and protrudes into the vagina

Abnormal findings
✦ Bulging vaginal wall (cystocele or rectocele)
✦ Nodules or irregularities (cysts, tumors, or lesions)
✦ Pain during examination (inflammation of uterus or adnexa)

Bimanual examination
✦ Allows for palpation of the uterus and ovaries
✦ Performed by physicians or advanced practice nurses
✦ Palpation occurs inside and outside of the body, simultaneously

Rectovaginal palpation
✦ Assesses posterior part of uterus pelvic cavity
✦ Assesses rectal muscle and sphincter tone
✦ Assesses the posterior edge of the cervix and lower posterior wall of the uterus

Bimanual examination

A bimanual examination allows you to palpate the uterus and ovaries. Usually, only a physician or a nurse in advanced practice performs bimanual palpation. (See *Performing a bimanual examination.*)

 ABNORMAL FINDINGS *With hyperplasia and increasing blood supply, the pregnant patient's uterus softens and normally feels somewhat tender; however, when a tumor is suspected, the uterus may feel hard, especially if cancerous. Excessive tenderness usually indicates disease, particularly infection.*

A palpable ovary in a postmenopausal woman or prepubescent girl is abnormal. Any abnormal ovarian enlargement in a patient of any age calls for medical evaluation. Although common and usually benign in young fertile women, ovarian cysts should also be evaluated.

Rectovaginal palpation

Rectovaginal palpation, the last step in a genital assessment, examines the posterior part of the uterus and the pelvic cavity. Warn the patient that this procedure may be uncomfortable.

Put on a new pair of gloves and apply water-soluble lubricant to the index and middle fingers of your gloved dominant hand. Instruct the patient to bear down with her vaginal and rectal muscles; then insert your index finger a short way into her vagina and your middle finger into her rectum.

Use your middle finger to assess rectal muscle and sphincter tone. Insert your finger deeper into the rectum, and palpate the rectal wall with your middle finger. Sweep the rectum with your fingers, assessing for masses or nodules.

Palpate the posterior wall of the uterus through the anterior wall of the rectum, evaluating the uterus for size, shape, tenderness, and masses. The rectovaginal septum, the wall between the rectum and the vagina, should feel smooth and springy.

Place your nondominant hand on the patient's abdomen at the symphysis pubis. With your index finger in the vagina, palpate deeply to feel the posterior edge of the cervix and the lower posterior wall of the uterus.

When you're finished, discard the gloves and wash your hands. Help the patient to a sitting position, and provide privacy for dressing and personal hygiene.

INTERPRETING YOUR FINDINGS

After you assess the patient, a group of findings may lead you to suspect a particular disorder. (See *The female GU system: Interpreting your findings,* pages 292 and 293.)

Female GU system disorders

Facts about cervical cancer
✦ Preinvasive cancer ranging from minimal cervical dysplasia to carcinoma in situ
✦ Curable with early detection and treatment

FEMALE GU SYSTEM DISORDERS

CERVICAL CANCER

The third most common cancer of the female reproductive system after uterine and ovarian cancer, cervical cancer is classified as either preinvasive or invasive.

Preinvasive cancer ranges from minimal cervical dysplasia, in which the lower third of the epithelium contains abnormal cells, to carcinoma in situ, in which the full thickness of epithelium is involved. Preinvasive cancer is curable 75% to 90% of the time with early detection and proper treatment. If untreated (and depending on the form in which it appears), it may progress to an invasive cancer. In invasive

(Text continues on page 294.)

KNOW-HOW

Performing a bimanual examination

During a bimanual examination, you palpate the uterus and ovaries from the inside and the outside simultaneously. These illustrations show how to perform such an examination.

PROPER POSITION

After putting on gloves, place the index and third finger of your dominant hand in the patient's vagina and move them up to the cervix. Place the fingers of your other hand on the patient's abdomen between the umbilicus and the symphysis pubis, as shown.

Elevate the cervix and uterus by pressing upward with the two fingers inside the vagina. At the same time, press down and in with the hand on the abdomen. Try to grasp the uterus between your hands.

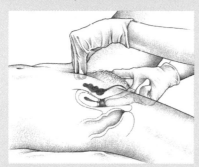

NOTE THE POSITION

Now move your fingers into the posterior fornix, pressing upward and forward to bring the anterior uterine wall up to your nondominant hand. Use your dominant hand to palpate the lower portion of the uterine wall. Note the position of the uterus.

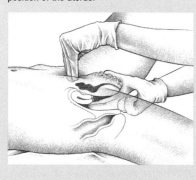

PALPATE THE WALLS

Slide your fingers farther into the anterior section of the fornix, the space between the uterus and cervix. You should feel part of the posterior uterine wall with this hand. You should feel part of the anterior uterine wall with the fingertips of your nondominant hand. Note the size, shape, surface characteristics, consistency, and mobility of the uterus as well as tenderness.

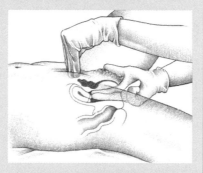

PALPATE THE OVARIES

After palpating the anterior and posterior walls of the uterus, move your nondominant hand toward the right lower quadrant of the abdomen. Slip the fingers of your dominant hand into the right fornix and palpate the right ovary. Then palpate the left ovary. Note the size, shape, and contour of each ovary. They should be unpalpable in postmenopausal women. Remove your hand from the patient's abdomen and your fingers from her vagina, and discard your gloves.

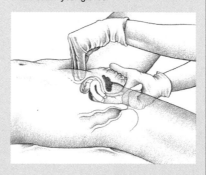

Performing a bimanual examination

✦ Ensure proper positioning of your hands
✦ Note the position of the uterus
✦ Palpate the cervix and uterine wall
✦ Palpate the ovaries

The female GU system: Interpreting your findings

This chart shows common groups of findings for the signs and symptoms of the female genitourinary (GU) system, along with their probable causes.

SIGN OR SYMPTOM AND FINDINGS	PROBABLE CAUSE
Dysmenorrhea	
✦ Steady, aching pain that begins before menses and peaks at the height of menstrual flow; may occur between menstrual periods ✦ Pain may radiate to the perineum or rectum ✦ Premenstrual spotting ✦ Dyspareunia ✦ Infertility ✦ Nausea and vomiting ✦ Tender, fixed adnexal mass palpable on bimanual examination	✦ Endometriosis
✦ Severe abdominal pain ✦ Fever ✦ Malaise ✦ Foul-smelling, purulent vaginal discharge ✦ Menorrhagia ✦ Cervical motion tenderness and bilateral adnexal tenderness on pelvic examination	✦ Pelvic inflammatory disease
✦ Cramping pain that begins with menstrual flow and diminishes with decreasing flow ✦ Abdominal bloating ✦ Breast tenderness ✦ Depression ✦ Irritability ✦ Headache ✦ Diarrhea	✦ Premenstrual syndrome
Dysuria	
✦ Urinary frequency ✦ Nocturia ✦ Straining to void ✦ Hematuria ✦ Perineal or lower-back pain ✦ Fatigue ✦ Low-grade fever	✦ Cystitis
✦ Dysuria throughout voiding ✦ Bladder distention ✦ Diminished urinary stream ✦ Urinary frequency and urgency ✦ Sensation of bloating or fullness in the lower abdomen or groin	✦ Urinary system obstruction

The female GU system:
Interpreting your findings *(continued)*

SIGN OR SYMPTOM AND FINDINGS	PROBABLE CAUSE

Dysuria (continued)

✦ Urinary urgency ✦ Hematuria ✦ Cloudy urine ✦ Bladder spasms ✦ Feeling of warmth or burning during urination	✦ Urinary tract infection

Urinary incontinence

✦ Urge or overflow incontinence ✦ Hematuria ✦ Dysuria ✦ Nocturia ✦ Urinary frequency ✦ Suprapubic pain from bladder spasms ✦ Palpable mass on bimanual examination	✦ Bladder cancer
✦ Overflow incontinence ✦ Painless bladder distention ✦ Episodic diarrhea or constipation ✦ Orthostatic hypotension ✦ Syncope ✦ Dysphagia	✦ Diabetic neuropathy
✦ Urinary urgency and frequency ✦ Vision problems ✦ Sensory impairment ✦ Constipation ✦ Muscle weakness ✦ Emotional lability	✦ Multiple sclerosis

Vaginal discharge

✦ Profuse, white, curdlike discharge with a yeasty, sweet odor ✦ Exudate may be lightly attached to the labia and vaginal walls ✦ Vulvar redness and edema ✦ Intense labial itching and burning ✦ External dysuria	✦ Candidiasis
✦ Yellow, mucopurulent, odorless, or acrid discharge ✦ Dysuria ✦ Dyspareunia ✦ Vaginal bleeding after douching or coitus	✦ Chlamydia infection
✦ Yellow or green, foul-smelling discharge that can be expressed from the Bartholin's or Skene's ducts ✦ Dysuria ✦ Urinary frequency and incontinence ✦ Vaginal redness and swelling	✦ Gonorrhea

cancer, cancer cells penetrate the basement membrane and may spread directly to adjacent pelvic structures or spread to distant sites via the lymph system.

 SPECIAL POINTS *Invasive cervical cancer usually occurs in women between ages 30 and 50 and rarely in those under age 20.*

The cause of cervical cancer is unknown. Risk factors include presence of selected viruses (HPV and herpes), initiation of sexual intercourse during teenage years, multiple sexual partners, and cigarette smoking.

For early detection, the American Cancer Society and the American College of Obstetricians and Gynecologists recommend that a woman should have her first Pap test by age 21 or within 3 years of her first sexual intercourse, whichever is first. Annual Pap tests should be performed until age 30; if at that point, a woman has had three consecutive normal Pap tests, the frequency may be decreased to every 2 to 3 years.

Preinvasive cervical cancer is asymptomatic. Abnormal vaginal bleeding, persistent vaginal discharge, and postcoital pain and bleeding may signal early invasive disease. Advanced disease may cause pelvic pain, vaginal leakage of urine and feces from a fistula, anorexia, weight loss, and fatigue.

FIBROIDS

Also known as *myomas, fibromyomas,* and *uterine leiomyomas,* fibroids are the most common benign tumors in women. They usually occur in the uterine corpus, although they may appear on the cervix or on the round or broad ligament.

 SPECIAL POINTS *Fibroids are usually multiple and occur in about 20% of all women over age 35; they affect Blacks three times more commonly than Whites. They become malignant (leiomyosarcoma) in only 0.1% of patients.*

The cause of fibroids is unknown, but excessive levels of estrogen and human growth hormone (hGH) probably influence tumor formation by stimulating susceptible fibromuscular elements. Large doses of estrogen and the later stages of pregnancy increase tumor size and hGH levels. Conversely, fibroids usually shrink or disappear after menopause, when estrogen production decreases.

Signs and symptoms include submucosal hypermenorrhea and possibly other forms of abnormal endometrial bleeding, dysmenorrhea, and pain.

If the tumor is large, the patient may develop a feeling of heaviness in the abdomen, pain, intestinal obstruction, constipation, urinary frequency or urgency, and irregular uterine enlargement.

OVARIAN CANCER

Primary ovarian cancer ranks as the fourth most common cause of cancer deaths among women in the United States, after cancer of the breast, the colon, and the lung. In women who have been treated for breast cancer, metastatic ovarian cancer is more common than cancer at any other site. Incidence is higher in women between ages 40 and 65 who have a family history of breast, colon, and ovarian cancers, and in nulliparous women and women with a history of early menarche and late menopause. The disease may occur anytime, including during childhood or pregnancy.

The three main types of ovarian cancer are primary epithelial tumors (90% of all ovarian cancers), germ cell tumors, and sex cord (stromal) tumors. Ovarian tumors spread rapidly intraperitoneally by local extension or surface seeding and, occasionally, through the lymphatic system and the bloodstream. Generally, the tumor spreads extraperitoneally through the diaphragm into the chest cavity, which may cause pleural effusions. Other metastasis is rare. Diagnosis of ovarian cancer requires clinical evaluation, complete patient history, surgical exploration, and histologic studies.

Prognosis varies with the histologic type and staging of the disease but is generally poor because ovarian tumors tend to progress rapidly. About 25% of women with ovarian cancer survive for 5 years, but prognosis may be improving because of recent advances in chemotherapy. The cause of ovarian cancer is unknown.

Women with localized disease have symptoms similar to and as frequently as women with advanced disease. Only 10% of the patients are without symptoms. The most common ones are abdominal pain and swelling, intestinal symptoms, and vaginal bleeding. Almost all of these signs and symptoms are nonspecific. Therefore, all providers should consider the possibility of ovarian neoplasm when these signs and symptoms persist. Other signs and symptoms include urinary frequency, constipation, pelvic discomfort, distention, and weight loss.

In some types of tumors, signs and symptoms include feminizing effects (such as bleeding between periods in premenopausal women) and virilizing effects — and, in advanced ovarian cancer, ascites, postmenopausal bleeding (rarely), pain, and symptoms related to metastatic sites (most commonly pleural effusion).

OVARIAN CYSTS

Ovarian cysts are nonneoplastic sacs that contain fluid or semisolid material. Although they're usually small and produce no symptoms, ovarian cysts should be thoroughly investigated as possible sites of malignant change. Common types include follicular cysts, which are usually very small, semitransparent, and fluid-filled; and lutein cysts, including corpus luteum cysts, which are functional, nonneoplastic enlargements of the ovaries; and theca-lutein cysts, which are commonly bilateral and filled with clear, straw-colored fluid. Polycystic (or sclerocystic) ovary disease is part of the Stein-Leventhal syndrome.

Ovarian cysts can develop any time between puberty and menopause, including during pregnancy. Corpus luteum cysts occur infrequently, usually during early pregnancy. The prognosis for nonneoplastic ovarian cysts is excellent.

Follicular cysts arise from follicles that overdistend instead of going through the atretic stage of the menstrual cycle. Corpus luteum cysts are caused by excessive accumulation of blood during the hemorrhagic phase of the menstrual cycle. Theca-lutein cysts are commonly associated with hydatidiform mole, choriocarcinoma, or hormone therapy (with hCG or clomiphene citrate). Polycystic ovary disease results from endocrine abnormalities.

Small cysts usually produce no symptoms, unless torsion or rupture causes signs of an acute abdomen. General signs and symptoms include mild pelvic discomfort, lower back pain, dyspareunia, abnormal uterine bleeding (secondary to a disturbed ovulatory pattern), and acute abdominal pain similar to that of appendicitis (in ovarian cysts with torsion).

With corpus luteum cysts appearing early in pregnancy, the patient may develop unilateral pelvic discomfort and (with rupture) massive intraperitoneal hemorrhage.

With polycystic ovary disease, the patient may develop amenorrhea, oligomenorrhea, or infertility secondary to the disorder as well as bilaterally enlarged ovaries.

PYELONEPHRITIS

One of the most common renal diseases, acute pyelonephritis is a sudden bacterial inflammation. It primarily affects the interstitial area and the renal pelvis and, less

Facts about pyelonephritis

+ Sudden bacterial inflammation affecting renal pelvis and renal tubules
+ With treatment and follow-up care, prognosis is good
+ Results from ascending infection and infecting organisms
+ Risk factors include catheterization, cystoscopy, or urologic surgery

commonly, the renal tubules. With treatment and continued follow-up care, the prognosis is good. Extensive permanent damage is rare.

Pyelonephritis most commonly results from an ascending infection, less commonly from hematogenous or lymphatic spread. The most common infecting organism is *Escherichia coli*. Others are *Proteus, Pseudomonas, Staphylococcus aureus,* and *Streptococcus faecalis* (enterococcus). Risk factors can include diagnostic and therapeutic use of instruments, as in catheterization, cystoscopy, or urologic surgery. Inability to empty the bladder (for example, in patients with neurogenic bladder), urine stasis, and urinary obstruction from tumors or strictures can also lead to pyelonephritis.

Other risk factors include sexual activity in women, use of diaphragms and condoms with spermicidal gel, pregnancy (about 5% of pregnant women develop asymptomatic bacteriuria; if untreated, about 40% develop pyelonephritis), diabetes (glycosuria may support bacterial growth in the urine), and other renal diseases.

Signs and symptoms of pyelonephritis include urinary urgency and frequency, burning during urination, dysuria, nocturia, hematuria, possibly cloudy urine with an ammonia or fishy odor, temperature of 102° F (38.9° C) or higher, shaking chills, flank pain, anorexia, and general fatigue.

Facts about urinary incontinence

+ Uncontrollable passage of urine
+ Results from either bladder abnormality or neurologic disorder
+ May be transient or permanent
+ Can be classified as stress, overflow, urge, or total

URINARY INCONTINENCE

Incontinence, the uncontrollable passage of urine, results from either a bladder abnormality or a neurologic disorder. A common urologic sign, incontinence may be transient or permanent and may involve large volumes of urine or scant dribbling.

Urinary incontinence can be classified as stress, overflow, urge, or total incontinence. Stress incontinence refers to intermittent leakage resulting from a sudden physical strain, such as a cough, sneeze, or quick movement. Overflow incontinence is a dribble resulting from urine retention, which fills the bladder and prevents it from contracting with sufficient force to expel a urinary stream. Urge incontinence refers to the inability to suppress a sudden urge to urinate. Total incontinence is continuous leakage resulting from the bladder's inability to retain urine.

Assessment findings may include inflammation or anatomic defect of the urethral meatus. Leakage may be observed while asking the patient to bear down. Bladder distention signals urine retention.

Facts about uterine cancer

+ Most common gynecologic cancer
+ Early signs include uterine enlargement and bleeding

Special points
+ Affects postmenopausal women between ages 50 and 60; uncommon in women between ages 30 and 40

UTERINE CANCER

Also known as *cancer of the endometrium,* uterine cancer is the most common gynecologic cancer.

 SPECIAL POINTS *Usually, uterine cancer affects postmenopausal women between ages 50 and 60. It's uncommon in those between ages 30 and 40, and it's extremely rare in those under age 30.*

Most premenopausal women who develop uterine cancer have a history of anovular menstrual cycles or other hormonal imbalance.

Uterine cancer is usually caused by adenocarcinoma. Other causes include adenoacanthoma, endometrial stromal sarcoma, lymphosarcoma, mixed mesodermal tumors (including carcinosarcoma), and leiomyosarcoma.

Risk factors include obesity, hypertension, nulliparity, history of exogenous estrogen therapy, and hormonal imbalance.

Early signs include uterine enlargement and unusual premenopausal or postmenopausal bleeding (discharge may be watery and blood-streaked at first, but gradually becomes more bloody). Late signs and symptoms include pain and weight loss (cancer is well advanced when these appear).

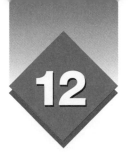

12

Male genitourinary system

A LOOK AT THE MALE GU SYSTEM

Disorders of the male urinary tract or reproductive system can have far-reaching consequences and influence other body systems. There exists a great potential to challenge a man's quality of life, self-esteem, and sense of well-being.

Despite these potential compromises and general changes in social behavior, men remain reluctant to discuss their GU system problems with nurses or other health care professionals. You must gain insight into the cultural background of your patient and conduct yourself in a professional manner at all times. Providing a setting where patient and nurse are comfortable in the examination will allow openness in the evaluation of the patient's needs.

To thoroughly and accurately assess your patient's GU system, you'll need to review the organs and structure of the urinary and reproductive systems and how they work.

URINARY SYSTEM

The urinary system helps maintain homeostasis by regulating fluid and electrolyte balance. It consists of the kidneys, ureters, bladder, and urethra. The essential functions of the system, such as forming urine and maintaining homeostasis, occur in the highly vascular kidneys. This process involves filtration, reabsorption, and secretion.

Although the male and female urinary systems function in the same way, a man's urethra is 6″ (15.2 cm) longer than a woman's. That's because it must pass through the erectile tissue of the penis. In the male, the urethra is about 8″ (20 cm) long, with the urethral meatus located at the end of the glans penis.

REPRODUCTIVE SYSTEM

In men, the urethra is also part of the reproductive system, carrying semen as well as urine. Contraction of the muscle fibers that surround the urethra inhibits the

Male reproductive system

This illustration shows the important structures of the male reproductive system.

- Seminal vesicle
- Common ejaculation duct
- Prostate gland
- Bladder
- Symphysis pubis
- Vas deferens
- Urethra
- Corpus cavernosum
- Penis
- Glans penis
- Corona
- Prepuce
- Urethral meatus
- Scrotum
- Testicle
- Epididymis

Reproductive system
(continued)

✦ Includes penis, scrotum, testicles, epididymis, vas deferens, seminal vesicles, and prostate gland

Penis

✦ Consists of shaft, glans, urethral meatus, corona, and prepuce
✦ Shaft contains three columns of vascular erectile tissue
✦ Glans located at end of penis where urethral meatus is located
✦ During sexual activity, sperm and semen are ejaculated

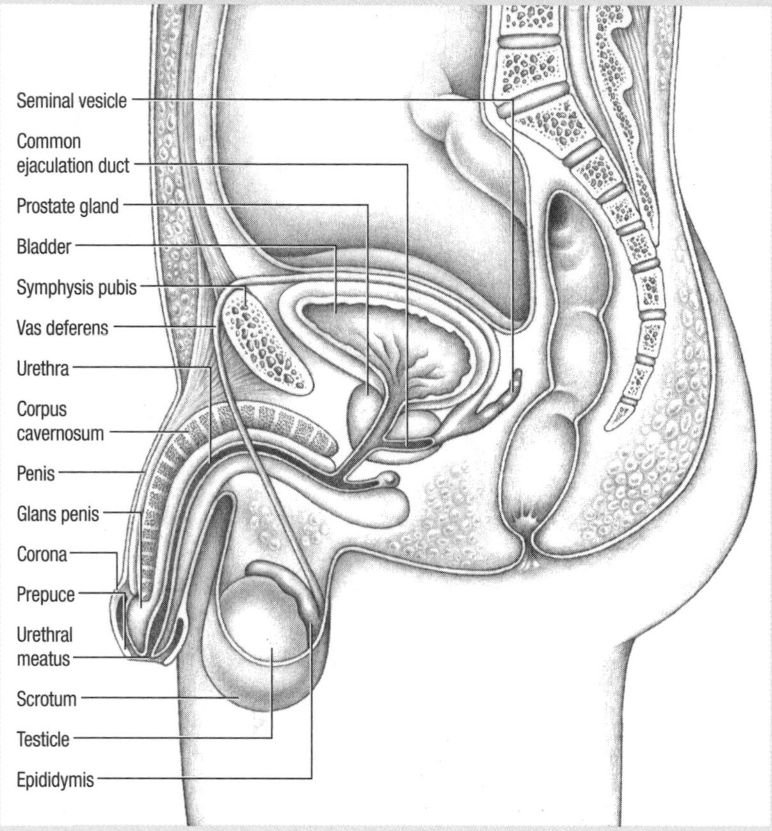

retrograde flow of semen into the bladder during ejaculation. The male reproductive system also includes the penis, scrotum, testicles, epididymis, vas deferens, seminal vesicles, and prostate gland. (See *Male reproductive system.*)

Penis

The penis consists of the shaft, glans, urethral meatus, corona, and prepuce. The skin of the penis is hairless and usually darker than the skin on other parts of the body.

The shaft contains three columns of vascular erectile tissue. The glans is located at the end of the penis. The urethral meatus, a slitlike opening, is located ventrally at the tip of the glans. The corona is formed by the junction of the glans and the shaft. The prepuce, the loose skin covering the glans, is commonly removed shortly after birth in a surgical procedure called *circumcision.*

When the penile tissues are engorged with blood, the erect penis can discharge sperm. During sexual activity, sperm and semen are forcefully ejaculated from the urethral meatus.

Scrotum

The scrotum is located at the base of the penis. It's a loose, wrinkled, deeply pigmented pouch that consists of a muscle layer covered by skin. Each of its two compartments contains a testicle, epididymis, and portions of the spermatic cord. The left side of the scrotum is usually lower than the right because the left spermatic cord is longer.

Testicles

The testicles are oval, rubbery structures suspended vertically and slightly forward in the scrotum. They produce testosterone and sperm.

Testosterone stimulates the changes that occur during puberty, which starts between ages 9½ and 13½. The testicles enlarge, pubic hair grows, and penis size increases. Secondary sex characteristics appear, such as facial and body hair, muscle development, and voice changes.

 SPECIAL POINTS *In boys, the first sign of pubescent changes is the enlargement of the testicles, along with pubic hair and increased size of the penis. These stages of development are documented in Tanner's sexuality ratings.*

Epididymis

The epididymis is a reservoir for maturing sperm. It curves over the posterolateral surface of each testicle, creating a visible bulge on the surface. In a small number of men, the epididymis is located anteriorly.

Vas deferens

The vas deferens—a storage site and the pathway for sperm—begins at the lower end of the epididymis, climbs the spermatic cord, travels through the inguinal canal, and ends in the abdominal cavity where it rests on the fundus of the bladder.

Seminal vesicles

A pair of saclike glands, the seminal vesicles are found on the lower posterior surface of the bladder in front of the rectum. Secretions from the seminal vesicles help form seminal fluid.

Prostate gland

A walnut-shaped gland about 2½″ (6.5 cm) long, the prostate surrounds the urethra like a doughnut, just below the bladder. It produces a thin, milky, alkaline fluid that mixes with seminal fluid during ejaculation. During sexual activity, prostatic fluid adds volume to the semen and enhances sperm motility and possibly fertility by neutralizing the acidity of the urethra and of the woman's vagina.

Urinary problems may develop from cancerous growths or from a condition known as benign prostatic hyperplasia (BPH).

Inguinal structures

The spermatic cord travels from the testis through the inguinal canal, exits the scrotum through the external inguinal ring and enters the abdominal cavity through the internal inguinal ring. The external inguinal ring is located just above and lateral to the pubic tubercle; the internal ring, about ½″ (1 cm) above the midpoint of the inguinal ligament, between the pubic tubercle of the symphysis pubis and the anterior superior iliac spine. Between the two rings lies the inguinal canal. Lymph nodes from the penis, scrotal surface, and anus drain into the inguinal lymph nodes. Lymph nodes from the testes drain into the lateral aortic and preaortic lymph nodes in the abdomen.

Scrotum

✦ Two compartments, each containing a testicle, epididymis, and portions of spermatic cord

Testicles

✦ Produce testosterone and sperm
✦ Testosterone stimulates changes during puberty
✦ Enlarged testicles, along with pubic hair and increased penis size occur in puberty

Epididymis

✦ Serves as a reservoir for maturing sperm
✦ Creates visible bulge on the surface of each testicle

Vas deferens

✦ Serves as a storage site and pathway for sperm
✦ Ends in the abdominal cavity; rests on bladder

Seminal vesicles

✦ Help to form seminal fluid

Prostate gland

✦ Produces thin, milky, alkaline fluid; mixes with seminal fluid
✦ During sexual activity, prostatic fluid adds volume to semen, enhancing sperm motility
✦ Urinary problems may develop from growths or BPH

Inguinal structures

✦ Spermatic cord travels from testis through inguinal canal, exits the scrotum through the external inguinal ring
✦ Enters the abdominal cavity through the internal inguinal ring

Obtaining a health history

+ Common urinary complaints include pain during urination and changes in urine output, voiding pattern, and urine color
+ Common reproductive complaints include penile discharge, impotence, infertility, and scrotal masses or pain

Exploring the chief complaint

+ Record patient's responses
+ Ask specific questions about current and past health

Current health history

+ Identifies changes in color of skin of penis or scrotum
+ Reveals ability to retract and replace the foreskin, if uncircumcised

Abnormal findings

+ Phimosis (inability to retract the foreskin); paraphimosis (inability to replace it); impairs local circulation and leads to edema, even gangrene
+ Sores, lumps, or ulcers (STD)
+ Discharge or bleeding from the urethra, or a swollen scrotum (inguinal hernia, hematocele, epididymitis, testicular tumor)

OBTAINING A HEALTH HISTORY

Common complaints about the urinary system include pain during urination and changes in urine output, voiding pattern, and urine color. The most common complaints about the reproductive system are penile discharge, impotence, infertility, and scrotal or inguinal masses, pain, and tenderness.

Men can be sensitive when questioned about sexual performance; they tend to equate sexual and reproductive functioning with manhood and may view sexual problems as signs of diminished masculinity.

 SPECIAL POINTS *Older men may view declining sexual ability as a sign of lost youth and declining health.*

A patient with sexual dysfunction may feel uncomfortable discussing it. Assure him that his replies to your questions will be kept strictly confidential. To put him at ease, begin the interview with general questions about his health as it relates to the male reproductive system. Reserve questions about sexual function until the end of the health history.

Remember that the patient has his own view of sexuality and reproduction, largely influenced by his cultural and religious background. Take these views into account and remain nonjudgmental and supportive.

During the assessment, use terminology that the patient can understand. Medical terminology may be confusing, especially to a younger patient. On the other hand, using too much slang may render the interview process too informal to be effective. (See *Putting your patient at ease.*)

CHIEF COMPLAINT

Ask the patient about his chief complaint. Document his answer using his own words. If he can't identify a single reason, ask more specific questions about his current and past health status.

CURRENT HEALTH HISTORY

Ask the patient these questions:
+ Have you noticed changes in the color of the skin on your penis or scrotum?
+ If you're uncircumcised, can you retract and replace the foreskin easily?

 ABNORMAL FINDINGS *An inability to retract the prepuce (foreskin) is called* phimosis; *an inability to replace it is called* paraphimosis. *Untreated, these conditions can impair local circulation and lead to edema and even gangrene.*

+ Have you noticed sores, lumps, or ulcers on your penis?

 ABNORMAL FINDINGS *Sores, lumps, or ulcers on a patient's penis can signal a sexually transmitted disease (STD).*

+ Have you noticed discharge or bleeding from the opening where urine comes out?
+ Have you noticed swelling in your scrotum?

 ABNORMAL FINDINGS *Discharge or bleeding from the urethra, or a swollen scrotum, can indicate an inguinal hernia, a hematocele, epididymitis, or a testicular tumor.*

+ Are you experiencing pain in the penis, testes, or scrotal sac? If so, where? How long have you been experiencing this pain? Is the pain constant or intermittent and

KNOW-HOW

Putting your patient at ease

Here are some tips for helping your patient feel more comfortable during the health history:

✦ Make sure that the room is private and that there are no interruptions.

✦ Phrase your questions in a clear and tactful manner.

✦ Tell the patient that his answers are and will remain confidential.

✦ Begin with less sensitive questions about his urinary function, and lead up to more sensitive areas such as sexual function.

✦ Don't rush or omit important facts because the patient seems embarrassed.

✦ Be sensitive to the patient's responses during the interview. Decreases in sexual prowess as a sign of declining health may interfere with the interview.

✦ When asking questions, keep in mind that many male patients view sexual problems as a sign of diminished masculinity. Phrase your questions carefully and offer reassurance as needed.

✦ Consider the patient's educational and cultural background. If he uses slang or euphemisms to talk about his sexual organs or sexual function, make sure you're both talking about the same subject.

how long does it last? Does the pain radiate? If so, to where? What measures aggravate or relieve the pain? When does it occur?

✦ Have you felt a lump, painful sore, or tenderness in the groin?

✦ Do you get up during the night to urinate?

 ABNORMAL FINDINGS *Excessive urination at night, or nocturia, is a common sign of renal or lower urinary tract disorders. It may also result from BPH, when significant urethral obstruction develops, or from prostate cancer.*

✦ Do you have urinary frequency, hesitancy, or dribbling; or pain in the area between your rectum and penis, hips, or lower back?

 ABNORMAL FINDINGS *Urinary frequency and urgency are classic symptoms of a urinary tract infection (UTI). Urinary frequency also occurs with BPH, urethral stricture, and a prostate tumor, which can put pressure on the bladder.*

Urinary hesitancy is most common in older patients who have an enlarged prostate gland, which can partially obstruct the urethra.

Urinary incontinence may be caused by BPH, prostate infection, and prostate cancer.

✦ Do you have blood in your urine?

 ABNORMAL FINDINGS *A patient with hematuria may have brown or bright red urine. Bleeding at the end of urination signals a disorder of the bladder neck, urethra, or prostate gland.*

✦ What does your urine look like?

 ABNORMAL FINDINGS *If the patient has noticed changes in the color of his urine, use this list to help interpret the changes:*

✦ *pale and diluted — diabetes insipidus, diuretic therapy, excessive fluid intake*

✦ *dark yellow or amber and concentrated — acute febrile disease, inadequate fluid intake, severe diarrhea or vomiting*

Current health history
(continued)

Abnormal findings: Urine color

+ Blue-green (methylene blue ingestion)
+ Green-brown (bile duct obstruction)
+ Dark brown or black (acute glomerulonephritis, intake of chlorpromazine)
+ Orange-red or orange-brown (obstructive jaundice, urobilinuria, or intake of rifampin or phenazopyridine)
+ Red or red-brown (hemorrhage, porphyria, intake of phenazopyridine)

Abnormal findings: Priapism

+ Erection unrelated to sexual activity (infections, lesions, drug use, CNS injury, acute leukemia, sickle cell anemia)

Abnormal findings: Sexual activity and drugs

+ Impotence (anticonvulsants, antidepressants, antihypertensives, beta-adrenergic blockers, antipsychotics)
+ Changes in libido (antidepressants, antihypertensives, benzodiazepines, adrenergic steroids)
+ Ejaculatory failure (antidepressants, beta-adrenergic blockers)
+ Priapism (antidepressants, antihypertensives, antipsychotics)

Past health history

+ Past illnesses, reproductive system problems or dysfunctions in other body systems
+ Surgery or traumatic injury of GU tract
+ Exposure to STDs
+ Diabetes mellitus, cardiovascular disease, neurologic disease, cancer of GU tract

+ blue-green — methylene blue ingestion
+ green-brown — bile duct obstruction
+ dark brown or black — acute glomerulonephritis, intake of such drugs as chlorpromazine
+ orange-red or orange-brown — obstructive jaundice, urobilinuria, or intake of such drugs as rifampin or phenazopyridine
+ red or red-brown — hemorrhage, porphyria, intake of such drugs as phenazopyridine.

+ Do you have difficulty achieving and maintaining an erection during sexual activity? If so, do you have erections at other times such as on awakening?
+ Do you have difficulty with ejaculation?
+ Do you ever experience pain from erection or ejaculation?

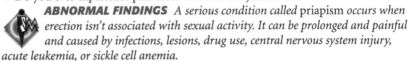 **ABNORMAL FINDINGS** *A serious condition called* priapism *occurs when erection isn't associated with sexual activity. It can be prolonged and painful and caused by infections, lesions, drug use, central nervous system injury, acute leukemia, or sickle cell anemia.*

+ What medications (including prescribed and over-the-counter drugs and alternative medications) do you take? At what dosage and for what reason? Have you ever taken illicit drugs?

ABNORMAL FINDINGS *Many drugs affect the male reproductive system. For example, anticonvulsants, antidepressants, antihypertensives, beta-adrenergic blockers, antipsychotics, anticholinergics, and androgenic steroids can cause impotence. Antidepressants, antihypertensives, antipsychotics, beta-adrenergic blockers, benzodiazepines, and androgenic steroids can cause changes in libido. Antidepressants and beta-adrenergic blockers can cause ejaculatory failure. Antidepressants, antihypertensives, and antipsychotics can cause priapism.*

PAST HEALTH HISTORY

Information about the patient's past illnesses is important; past reproductive system problems or dysfunctions in other body systems may affect present reproductive function. Important questions include:

+ Have you fathered any children? If so, how many and what are their ages? Have you had a problem with infertility? Is it a current concern? Have you been diagnosed with a low sperm count? If so, hot baths, frequent bicycle riding, and tight underwear or athletic supporters can elevate scrotal temperature and temporarily decrease sperm count.
+ Have you had surgery on the GU tract? If so, where, when, and why? Did you experience any postoperative complications?
+ Have you experienced trauma to the GU tract? If so, what happened, when did it occur, and what — if any — symptoms developed as a result?
+ Have you experienced blood in the urine, difficulty urinating, an excessive urge to urinate, dribbling, or difficulty maintaining the urine stream?
+ Have you been diagnosed as having an STD or other infection in the GU tract? If so, what was the specific problem? How long did it last? What treatment was provided? Did any associated complications develop? Have you been tested for human immunodeficiency virus (HIV), the virus that causes acquired immunodeficiency syndrome (AIDS)?
+ Have you had diabetes mellitus, cardiovascular disease, neurologic disease, or cancer of the GU tract?
+ Do you have a history of undescended testes or an endocrine disorder? Have you had mumps? If so, did the disease affect your testes?

KNOW-HOW

Teaching about testicular self-examination

To help your patient detect testicular abnormalities early, urge him to examine his testicles once each month. Explain that eventually he'll be able to recognize anything abnormal. Tell him that testicular cancer, the most common cancer in men ages 20 to 35, can be treated successfully when it's detected early.

CHECKING APPEARANCE

Instruct the patient to precede the examination with a warm shower. Cold hands or cold air will cause the scrotum to retract (cremasteric reflex) making an effective examination difficult. Tell him to stand in front of a mirror and lift his penis, checking his scrotum for changes in shape or size and for red, distended veins. Inform him that the scrotum's left side naturally hangs slightly lower than the right.

PALPATING FOR LUMPS AND MASSES

Tell the patient to palpate each testicle with both hands. Cup the index and middle fingers under the testicle and place the thumbs on top. Roll the testicle gently between the thumbs and fingers. One testicle may be larger than the other. Tell him that this is normal, but to be concerned about lumps or areas of pain. The testicles should move freely and feel rubbery. The epididymis is a soft, tubelike structure that should be palpable at the back of the testicle. There should be no lumps or tenderness. If a firm, painless lump or an enlarged testicle is noted, have him notify his physician Immediately. Explain that as he ages, there may be a decrease in penile size, and a more pendulous scrotal sac with less rugae.

✦ Do you examine your testes periodically? Have you been taught the proper procedure?

Provide information for testicular self-examination at this time with follow-up demonstration during physical examination if conducted. (See *Teaching about testicular self-examination.*)

FAMILY HISTORY

Questions about family health history can provide clues to disorders with known familial tendencies. Ask the patient if anyone in his family has had infertility problems or a hernia. Also ask him if anyone in his family has ever had cancer of the reproductive tract.

PSYCHOSOCIAL HISTORY

Obtain information about the patient's lifestyle and relationships with others. Ask these questions:
✦ If you're sexually active, do you have more than one partner? How many partners have you had during the last month?

Multiple partners can lead to increased incidence of STDs, hepatitis, and AIDS.

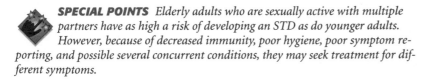

SPECIAL POINTS *Elderly adults who are sexually active with multiple partners have as high a risk of developing an STD as do younger adults. However, because of decreased immunity, poor hygiene, poor symptom reporting, and possible several concurrent conditions, they may seek treatment for different symptoms.*

Teaching about testicular self-examination

✦ Urge patients to examine their testicles monthly
✦ Instruct patient to check scrotum for appearance
✦ Tell patient to palpate each testicle with both hands
✦ If he notes a firm, painless lump or an enlarged testicle, advise him to notify his physician

Family history

✦ Infertility
✦ Hernia
✦ Cancer of the reproductive tract

Psychosocial history

✦ Reveals information about patient's lifestyle and relationships with others
Special points
✦ Elderly adults having multiple partners risk developing STDs

✦ Are your sexual practices homosexual, bisexual, or heterosexual?

✦ Do you take precautions to prevent contracting an STD or AIDS? If so, what do you do?

✦ What's your job?

✦ Are you now or have you ever been exposed to radiation or toxic chemicals?

✦ Do you engage in sports or other activities that require heavy lifting or straining? If so, do you wear protective or supportive devices, such as a jock strap, protective cup, or truss?

✦ Would you describe yourself as being under a lot of stress?

✦ What's your self-image? Do you consider yourself attractive to others?

✦ What's your cultural and religious background? Do any cultural or religious factors affect your beliefs or practices regarding sexuality and reproduction?

✦ Do you have a supportive relationship with another person?

✦ If you're experiencing sexual difficulty, is it affecting your emotional and social relationships?

Assessing the male GU system

✦ Inspection
✦ Percussion
✦ Palpation
✦ Auscultation

Examining the urinary system

✦ Document baseline vital signs and weight
✦ Observe patient's behavior
✦ Obtain a urine specimen and assess it for color, odor, and clarity

Inspection

✦ Abdomen should be smooth, flat or concave, symmetrical, and free from lesions, bruises, and prominent veins

Abnormal findings

✦ Tight, glistening skin and striae (ascites)
✦ Edema, increased urine protein levels, and decreased serum albumin levels (nephrotic syndrome)

ASSESSING THE MALE GU SYSTEM

To perform a physical assessment of the male GU system, use the techniques of inspection, percussion, palpation, and auscultation. Assessment of the urinary system may be done now or as part of the GI assessment.

EXAMINING THE URINARY SYSTEM

In many ways, assessing the male urinary system is similar to assessing the female urinary system. Before examining specific structures, obtain a urine specimen, check the patient's blood pressure and weight, and observe the patient's skin.

 ABNORMAL FINDINGS *A patient with decreased renal function may be pale because of a low hemoglobin level or may even have uremic frost— snowlike crystals on the skin from metabolic wastes. Also, look for signs of fluid imbalance, such as dry mucous membranes, sunken eyeballs, edema, or ascites.*

Before performing an assessment, ask the patient to urinate. If a urinalysis has been ordered, obtain the specimen at this time. Then help him into the supine position with his arms at his sides. As you proceed, expose only the areas being examined.

Inspection

First, inspect the patient's abdomen. When he's supine, his abdomen should be smooth, flat or concave, and symmetrical. The skin should be free from lesions, bruises, discolorations, and prominent veins.

Watch for abdominal distention with tight, glistening skin and striae—silvery streaks caused by rapidly developing skin tension.

ABNORMAL FINDINGS *Abdominal distention with tight, glistening skin and striae, are signs of ascites, which may accompany nephrotic syndrome. This syndrome is characterized by edema, increased urine protein levels, and decreased serum albumin levels.*

Percussion and palpation

First, tell the patient what you're going to do; otherwise, he may be startled, and you could mistake his reaction for a feeling of acute tenderness. Next, percuss the kidneys to check for pain or tenderness and the bladder to elicit tympany or dullness.

KNOW-HOW

Performing fist percussion

To assess the kidneys by indirect fist percussion, ask the patient to sit up with his back to you. Tell the patient that he'll feel a "blow to the kidneys." Place one hand at the costovertebral angle and strike it with the ulnar surface of your other hand, as shown.

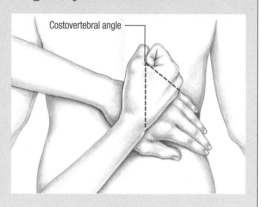

Costovertebral angle

 ABNORMAL FINDINGS *If a patient experiences pain or tenderness upon kidney percussion and palpation, this may suggest a kidney infection. (See* Performing fist percussion.*)*
Remember to percuss both sides of the body to assess both kidneys.

 ABNORMAL FINDINGS *If you hear a dull sound instead of the normal tympany, this may indicate urine retention in the bladder caused by bladder dysfunction or infection.*
You can also palpate the bladder to check for distention. Because the kidneys aren't usually palpable, detecting an enlarged kidney may prove to be important.

ABNORMAL FINDINGS *Kidney enlargement may accompany hydronephrosis, a cyst, or a tumor.*

Auscultation
Auscultate the renal arteries to rule out bruits, which signal renal artery stenosis. You can do this now or as part of an abdominal assessment.

EXAMINING THE REPRODUCTIVE SYSTEM
Before examining the reproductive system, or any part of the body, first wash your hands, put on examination gloves (first, asking the patient if he has a latex allergy), and make the patient as comfortable as possible. At this time make sure that the privacy curtain is drawn and the door is closed.

Inspection
Inspect the penis, scrotum, and testicles as well as the inguinal and femoral areas.

Penis
Start by examining the penis. Penis size depends on the patient's age and overall development.

Percussion and palpation
✦ Percuss kidneys for pain or tenderness; usually not palpable
✦ Percuss bladder to elicit tympany or dullness; palpate for distention

Abnormal findings
✦ Pain or tenderness (kidney infection)
✦ Dull sound (bladder dysfunction, infection)
✦ Kidney enlargement (hydronephrosis, cyst, tumor)

Auscultation
✦ Auscultate renal arteries to rule out bruits, which signal renal artery stenosis

Examining the reproductive system
✦ Wash your hands
✦ Ensure that patient is comfortable, and provide privacy

Inspection
✦ Penis, scrotum, testicles, and inguinal and femoral areas

Inspecting the penis
✦ Size depends on patient's age and overall development

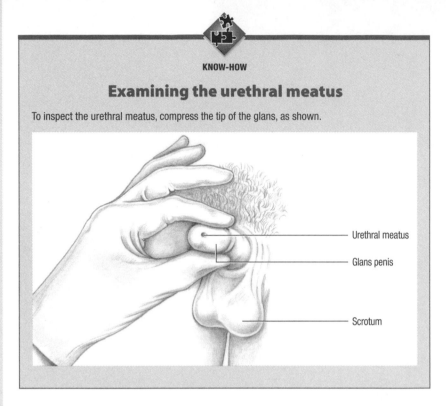

Examining the urethral meatus

To inspect the urethral meatus, compress the tip of the glans, as shown.

Urethral meatus

Glans penis

Scrotum

Inspecting the penis
(continued)

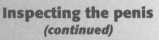

+ Check penile shaft and glans for lesions, nodules, inflammation, or swelling
+ Check glans for smegma

Special points: Penis
+ Skin should be slightly wrinkled
+ Pink to light brown in Whites
+ Light brown to dark brown in Blacks

Abnormal findings: Penis
+ Inflammation of the glans
+ Inflammation of the glans and prepuce
+ Lesions
+ Discharge

 SPECIAL POINTS *The penile skin should be slightly wrinkled and the color should be pink to light brown in Whites and light brown to dark brown in Blacks.*

Ask an uncircumcised patient to retract his prepuce, or foreskin, to expose the glans penis. Normally, he can do this easily to reveal a glans with no ulcers or lesions and then easily replace it over the glans after inspection.

Check the penile shaft and glans for lesions, nodules, inflammation, and swelling. Also check the glans for smegma, a cheesy secretion commonly found beneath the prepuce.

Then gently compress the tip of the glans to open the urethral meatus. It should be located in the center of the glans and be pink and smooth. Inspect it for swelling, discharge, lesions, inflammation and, especially, genital warts. If you note discharge, obtain a culture specimen. (See *Examining the urethral meatus.*)

ABNORMAL FINDINGS *Upon examining your patient, you may find these abnormalities:*
+ *inflammation of the glans* (balanitis); *inflammation of the glans and prepuce* (balanoposthitis).
+ *penile lesions—lesions on the penis can vary in appearance. A hard, nontender nodule, especially in the glans or inner lip of the prepuce, may indicate penile cancer.* (See Male genital lesions.)
+ *penile discharge—a profuse, yellow discharge from the penis suggests gonococcal urethritis. Other symptoms include urinary frequency, burning, and urgency. Without treatment, the prostate gland, epididymis, and periurethral glands will become inflamed. A copious, watery, purulent urethral discharge may indicate chlamydial infection; a bloody discharge may indicate infection or cancer in the urinary or reproductive tract.*

Male genital lesions

Several types of lesions may affect the male genitalia. Some of the more common lesions are described here.

PENILE CANCER

Penile cancer causes a painless, ulcerative lesion on the glans or foreskin, possibly accompanied by discharge. It's generally associated with genital herpes viral infections. The cancer presents as a local mass or bleeding ulcer and metastasizes early.

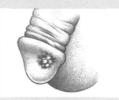

GENITAL HERPES

Genital herpes causes a painful, reddened group of small vesicles or blisters on the foreskin, shaft, or glans. Lesions eventually disappear but tend to recur. The vesicles are associated with itching or pain. Because the virus can remain latent in the nervous tissues, stress may activate their recurrence.

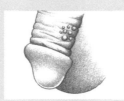

GENITAL WARTS

Genital warts present as small, soft, moist, pink or red swollen papillary growths that may be painless and appear as cauliflower-like groups. They are caused by the human papillomavirus and are sexually transmitted. Atypical warts may possibly be related to carcinoma.

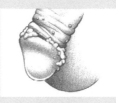

SYPHILIS

Syphilis causes a hard, round papule—usually on the glans penis. When palpated, this syphilitic chancre may feel like a button. Eventually, the papule erodes into an ulcer. You may also note swollen lymph nodes in the inguinal area. Syphilis occurs in three stages: the primary stage produces a bloodless ulcer known as a *chancre,* which contains spirochetes. This lesion spontaneously heals in 10 to 40 days and may not be of concern to the patient; the secondary and tertiary stages involve other body systems and become more debilitating with the disease's progress.

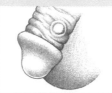

Male genital lesions
✦ Penile cancer — painless, ulcerative lesion
✦ Genital herpes — painful, reddened group of small vesicles or blisters
✦ Genital warts — small, soft, moist, pink or red swollen papillary growths
✦ Syphilis — hard, round papule

✦ *paraphimosis—the prepuce is so tight that, when retracted, it gets caught behind the glans and can't be replaced. Edema can result. Instruct uncircumcised men to retract the prepuce each time they clean the glans, and then to replace it afterward. Frequent retraction and cleaning of the prepuce prevents excessive tightness, which in turn prevents the prepuce from closing off the urinary meatus and constricting the glans. Causes of paraphimosis include rigorous cleaning, masturbation, sexual intercourse, catheter insertion, or cystoscopy.*

✦ *displacement of the urethral meatus—when the urethral meatus is located on the underside of the penis, the condition is called* hypospadias. *When the urethral meatus is located on the top of the penis, it's called* epispadias. *Both conditions are congenital.*

Inspecting the penis
(continued)

Abnormal findings
✦ Paraphimosis
✦ Displacement of the urethral meatus

Inspecting the scrotum and testicles

✦ Inspect for amount, distribution, color, and texture of pubic hair
✦ Assess general size and appearance, check for swelling, nodules, redness, ulceration, distended veins, pitting edema, lesions, and parasites

Abnormal findings

✦ Lesions, ulcers, induration, or reddened areas (inflammation)
✦ Lack of pubic hair (vascular or hormonal problem)
✦ In boys younger than age 2, enlarged scrotum (scrotal extension of an inguinal hernia or a hydrocele)

Inspecting the inguinal and femoral areas

✦ Check for obvious bulges
✦ Inspect for increased intra-abdominal pressure

Abnormal findings

✦ Enlarged lymph nodes (infection)

Palpation

✦ Penis, testicles, epididymis, spermatic cords, inguinal and femoral areas, and prostate gland

Palpating the penis

✦ Note swelling, nodules, or indurations

Palpating the testicles

✦ Assess size, shape, and response to pressure
✦ If you note hard, irregular areas, transilluminate and compare findings

Scrotum and testicles

To inspect the scrotum, first evaluate the amount, distribution, color, and texture of pubic hair. Hair should cover the symphysis pubis and scrotum.

 ABNORMAL FINDINGS *The absence of pubic hair or presence of bald spots is abnormal. So are lesions, ulcers, induration, or reddened areas, which may indicate infection or inflammation. Lack of pubic hair may indicate a vascular or hormonal problem.*

Have the patient hold his penis away from his scrotum so you can observe the scrotum's general size and appearance. The skin here is darker than on the rest of the body. Spread the surface of the scrotum, and examine the skin for swelling, nodules, redness, ulceration, and distended veins.

Sebaceous cysts — firm, white to yellow, nontender cutaneous lesions — are a normal finding. Also check for pitting edema, a sign of cardiovascular disease. Spread the pubic hair and check the skin for lesions and parasites.

 SPECIAL POINTS *Before palpating a boy's scrotum for a testicular examination, explain what you'll be doing and why. Make sure he's comfortably warm and as relaxed as possible. Cold and anxiety may cause his testicles to retract so that you can't palpate them. Having a parent in the room may offer him support.*

 ABNORMAL FINDINGS *If you see an enlarged scrotum in a boy younger than age 2, suspect a scrotal extension of an inguinal hernia, a hydrocele, or both. Hydroceles, commonly associated with inguinal hernias, are common in children of this age-group. To differentiate between the two, remember that hydroceles transilluminate and aren't tender or reducible.*

An adolescent boy who's obese may appear to have an abnormally small penis. You may have to retract the fat over the symphysis pubis to properly assess penis size. Have the child hold up any excessive adipose tissue, or have him lay down on the examination table.

Inguinal and femoral areas

Have the patient stand. Check the inguinal area for obvious bulges — a sign of hernias. Then ask the patient to bear down as you inspect again. This maneuver increases intra-abdominal pressure, which pushes any herniation downward and makes it more easily visible. Also, check for enlarged lymph nodes.

 ABNORMAL FINDINGS *Enlarged lymph nodes in a patient could be a sign of infection.*

Palpation

Palpate the penis, testicles, epididymis, spermatic cords, inguinal and femoral areas, and prostate gland.

Penis

Use your thumb and forefinger to palpate the entire penile shaft. It should be somewhat firm, and the skin should be smooth and movable. Note swelling, nodules, or indurations.

Testicles

Gently palpate both testicles between your thumb and first two fingers. Assess their size, shape, and response to pressure. A normal response is a deep visceral pain. The testicles should be equal in size, move freely in the scrotal sac, and feel firm, smooth, and rubbery.

If you note hard, irregular areas or lumps, transilluminate them by darkening the room and pressing the head of a flashlight against the scrotum, behind the lump. The testicle and any lumps, masses, warts, or blood-filled areas will appear as opaque shadows.

Transilluminate the other testicle to compare your findings. This is also a good time to reinforce the methods and importance of doing a monthly testicular self-examination.

 ABNORMAL FINDINGS *Scrotal swelling occurs when a condition affecting the testicles, epididymis, or scrotal skin produces edema or a mass; the penis may not be involved. Scrotal swelling can affect males at any age. It can be unilateral or bilateral and painful or painless and can result from inguinal hernia, hydrocele, or trauma to the scrotum.*

 CLINICAL ALERT The sudden onset of painful scrotal swelling suggests torsion of a testicle or testicular appendages, especially in a prepubescent male. This emergency requires immediate surgery to untwist and stabilize the spermatic cord or to remove the appendage.

 SPECIAL POINTS *In children up to age 1, a hernia or hydrocele of the spermatic cord may stem from abnormal fetal development. In infants, scrotal swelling may stem from ammonia-related dermatitis, if diapers aren't changed often enough.*

Other disorders that can produce scrotal swelling in children include epididymitis (rare in those younger than age 10), orchitis from contact sports, and mumps, which usually occurs after puberty.

 ABNORMAL FINDINGS *A painless scrotal nodule that can't be transilluminated may be a testicular tumor. This disorder is most common in men ages 20 to 35. The tumor can grow, enlarging the testicle.*

In a patient with an enlarged scrotum, this may be a sign of hydrocele, or a collection of fluid in the testicle. Hydrocele is associated with conditions that cause poor fluid reabsorption, such as cirrhosis, heart failure, and testicular tumor. A hydrocele can be transilluminated.

The absence of a testis may result from temporary migration. The cremaster muscle surrounding the testes contracts in response to such stimuli as cold air, cold water, or touching the inner thigh. This contraction raises the contents of the scrotum toward the inguinal canal. When the muscle relaxes, the scrotal contents resume their normal position. This temporary migration is normal and may occur at any time during the assessment.

Epididymis
Next, palpate the epididymis, which is usually located in the posterolateral area of the testicle. It should be smooth, discrete, nontender, and free from swelling and induration.

Spermatic cords
Palpate both spermatic cords, which are located above each testicle. Palpate from the base of the epididymis to the inguinal canal. The vas deferens is a smooth, movable cord inside the spermatic cord. If you feel swelling, irregularity, or nodules, transilluminate the problem area as described earlier. If serous fluid is present, you won't see this glow.

 ABNORMAL FINDINGS *Palpation of multiple tortuous veins in the spermatic cord area, usually on the left, suggests a varicocele.*

Inguinal area
To assess the patient for a direct inguinal hernia, place two fingers over each external inguinal ring and ask the patient to bear down.

Palpating the testicles
(continued)

Abnormal findings
+ Scrotal swelling (inguinal hernia, hydrocele, trauma)
+ Painless scrotal nodules that can't be transilluminated (tumor)

Special points
+ In children up to age 1, abnormal fetal development may cause hernia or hydrocele of the spermatic cord
+ In infants, ammonia-related dermatitis may cause scrotal swelling
+ Epididymitis, orchitis, mumps produce scrotal swelling

Alert!
+ Sudden onset of painful scrotal swelling suggests torsion of testicle or testicular appendages
+ Immediate surgery to stabilize the spermatic cord or remove the appendage is required

Palpating the epididymis
+ Should be smooth, discrete, nontender, and free from swelling and induration

Palpating the spermatic cords
+ Palpate from the base of the epididymis to the inguinal cord for swelling, irregularity, or nodules

Abnormal findings
+ Multiple tortuous veins on left side (varicocele)

Palpating the inguinal area
+ Palpate for a direct inguinal hernia

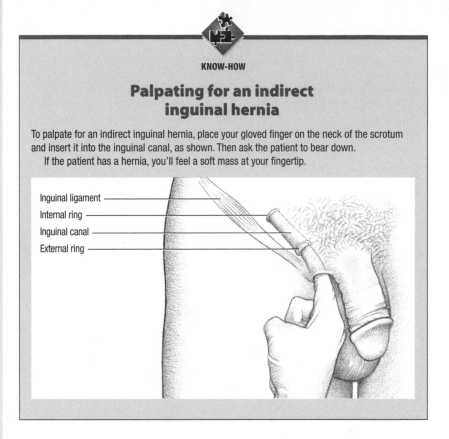

Palpating for an indirect inguinal hernia

To palpate for an indirect inguinal hernia, place your gloved finger on the neck of the scrotum and insert it into the inguinal canal, as shown. Then ask the patient to bear down. If the patient has a hernia, you'll feel a soft mass at your fingertip.

Inguinal ligament

Internal ring

Inguinal canal

External ring

Palpating the inguinal area
(continued)

Abnormal findings

+ Hernia presence indicated by a bulge; feels like a mass of tissue and withdraws when it meets the finger
+ Direct inguinal hernia emerges from behind the external inguinal ring and protrudes through it
+ Indirect inguinal hernia most common and occurs in men of all ages

Palpating the femoral area

+ Estimate femoral canal's location to help detect a femoral hernia, which feels like a soft tumor below the inguinal ligament

 ABNORMAL FINDINGS *If the patient has a hernia, you'll feel a bulge. It also feels like a mass of tissue that withdraws when it meets the finger.*

To assess the patient for an indirect inguinal hernia, examine him while he's standing and then while he's in a supine position with his knee flexed on the side you're examining. (See *Palpating for an indirect inguinal hernia.*)

Place your index finger on the neck of the scrotum and gently push upward into the inguinal canal. The inguinal ring should feel like a triangular, opening. You may be able to place your finger into the canal. If you can insert your finger, do so as far as possible and then ask the patient to bear down or cough.

 ABNORMAL FINDINGS *A direct inguinal hernia emerges from behind the external inguinal ring and protrudes through it. This type of hernia seldom descends into the scrotum and usually affects men older than age 40.*

An indirect inguinal hernia is the most common type of hernia, and it occurs in men of all ages. It can be palpated in the internal inguinal canal with its tip in or beyond the canal, or the hernia may descend into the scrotum.

Femoral area

Although you can't palpate the femoral canal, you can estimate its location to help detect a femoral hernia. Place your right index finger on the right femoral artery with your finger pointing toward the patient's head. Keep your other fingers close together. Your middle finger will rest on the femoral vein; your ring finger, on the femoral canal. Note tenderness or masses. Use your left hand to check the patient's left side.

Recognizing common skin disorders

On this page and the pages that follow, you'll find photos of common skin disorders along with brief descriptions of each. Use the photos to guide your assessment of abnormal skin findings.

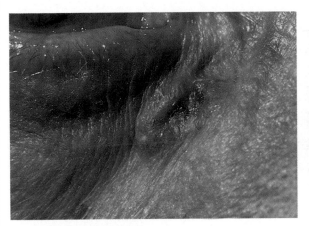

BASAL CELL CARCINOMA

The most common type of skin cancer, basal cell carcinoma results from sun exposure. It usually appears as a small waxy-looking nodule that ulcerates and forms a central depression. Basal cell carcinoma typically starts as a skin-colored papule (may be deeply pigmented) with a translucent top and overlying telangiectases. It rarely metastasizes and commonly appears on the head and neck.

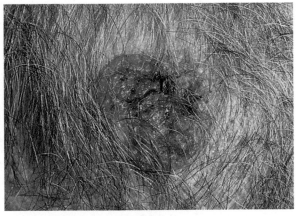

SQUAMOUS CELL CARCINOMA

Squamous cell carcinoma results from sun exposure and can metastasize. It appears as a raised border with a central ulcer and may be rough, thickened, or scaly. It most commonly appears on the face and neck as an erythematous scaly patch with sharp edges.

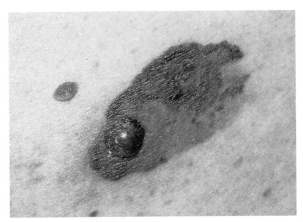

MALIGNANT MELANOMA

Malignant melanoma can occur anywhere on the body and can arise from a preexisting mole. Its border, color, and surface are usually irregular. The lesion is usually black or purple (although some may be pink, red, or whitish-blue) and may be accompanied by scaling, flaking, or oozing. Melanoma spreads through the lymphatic and vascular systems and can metastasize to the regional lymph nodes liver, lungs, and central nervous system.

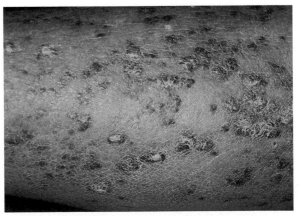

KAPOSI'S SARCOMA

Kaposi's sarcoma commonly appears first on the lower legs; however, the lesions may develop anywhere. Initially, you'll note multiple brown or bluish-red nodules of varying shapes and sizes. These nodules develop into larger plaques that may open and drain or cause edema of the legs.

(continued)

Recognizing common skin disorders *(continued)*

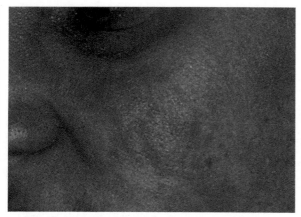

LUPUS ERYTHEMATOSUS (DISCOID OR SYSTEMIC)
The typical sign of lupus erythematosus, a butterfly-shaped rash, appears as a red, scaly, sharply demarcated rash over the cheeks and nose. The rash may extend to other areas of the face or to other exposed areas, such as the ears and neck.

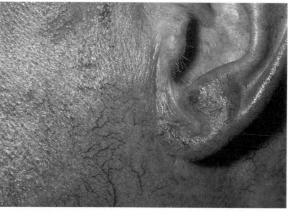

TELANGIECTASIA
Formed by dilation of small blood vessels, telangiectasia blanches when pressure is applied. This type of lesion may be a normal finding in an elderly person or may be associated with cirrhosis or lupus erythematosus.

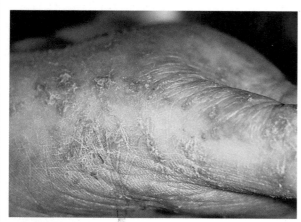

SCABIES
Mites, which can be picked up from an infested person, burrow under the skin and cause scabies lesions. The lesions appear in a straight or zigzagging line about 1 cm long with a black dot at the end. Commonly seen between the fingers, at the bend of the elbow and knee, and around the groin or perineal area, scabies lesions itch and may cause a rash.

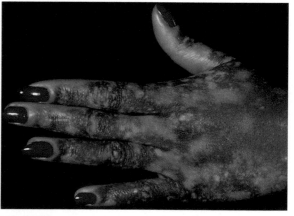

VITILIGO
Vitiligo is a slowly progressive disease of hypopigmentation that causes irregular areas of pigmented skin around milk-colored patches. These areas commonly appear on the face, hands, and feet.

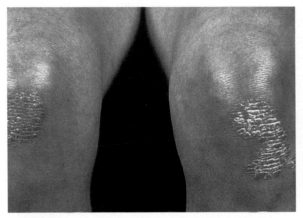

PSORIASIS

Psoriasis is a chronic disease of marked epidermal thickening and plaques that are symmetrical and that generally appear as red bases topped with silvery scales. The lesions, which may connect with one another, occur most commonly on the scalp, elbows, and knees.

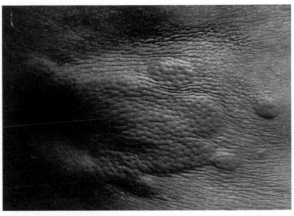

URTICARIA (HIVES)

Occurring as an allergic reaction, urticaria appears suddenly as pink, edematous papules or wheals (round elevations of the skin) that cause intense itching. The lesions may become large and contain vesicles.

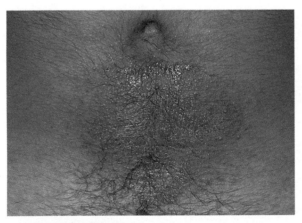

CONTACT DERMATITIS

Contact dermatitis is an inflammatory disorder that results from contact with an irritant. Primary lesions, including vesicles, large oozing bullae, and red macules that appear at localized areas of redness, may itch and burn.

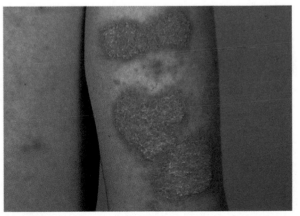

ECZEMA

Eczema may be acute or chronic and may be accompanied by severe itching. It appears as reddened papules, vesicles, or pustular lesions and typically affects the antecubital and popliteal areas. Blisters, oozing, and crusting may occur. Thickening, excoriation, and extreme dryness of the skin can also occur.

(continued)

Recognizing common skin disorders *(continued)*

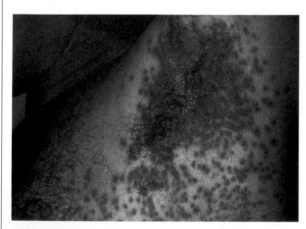

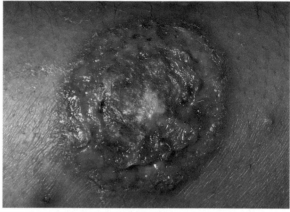

HERPES ZOSTER

Herpes zoster appears as a group of vesicles or crusted lesions along a nerve root. The vesicles are usually unilateral and typically appear on the face, hands, and neck. These lesions cause pain but not itching or rash.

TINEA CORPORIS (RINGWORM)

Tinea corporis are round, red, scaly lesions that are accompanied by intense itching. These lesions have slightly raised, red borders consisting of tiny vesicles. Individual rings may connect to form patches with scalloped edges. They usually appear on exposed areas of the body.

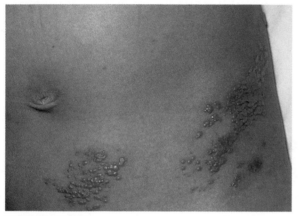

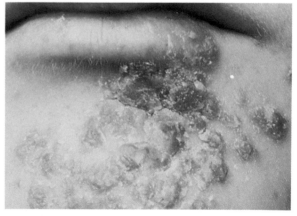

CANDIDIASIS

Candidiasis is a fungal infection that produces erythema and a scaly, papular rash. Because the fungus thrives in moist environments, it usually occurs under the breasts and in the axillae.

IMPETIGO

Impetigo is a rash that usually appears on the face. It's caused by a bacterial infection. When ruptured, fragile vesicles in the rash ooze a honey-colored fluid and crusts may form.

Middle ear conditions

OTITIS MEDIA

Otitis media is an inflammation of the middle ear. It can be caused by bacteria, viruses, allergies, or malfunctions of the eustachian tubes.

Inflammation may be accompanied by an accumulation of fluid in the middle ear that may restrict the movement of the eardrum and may result in hearing loss. Pain may occur if there's pressure from the fluid against the eardrum.

CLASSIFICATION AND COMMON COMPLICATIONS OF OTITIS MEDIA

The illustrations below show three of the classifications along with common complications of otitis media.

NORMAL RIGHT EARDRUM

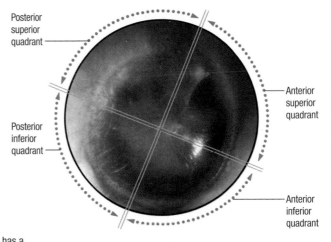

Posterior superior quadrant

Posterior inferior quadrant

Anterior superior quadrant

Anterior inferior quadrant

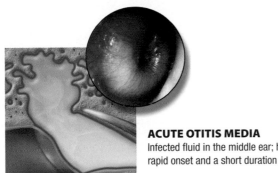

ACUTE OTITIS MEDIA

Infected fluid in the middle ear; has a rapid onset and a short duration

OTITIS MEDIA WITH EFFUSION

Fluid in the middle ear that may be acute, subacute, or chronic; produces relatively few symptoms

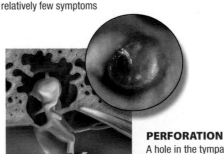

PERFORATION

A hole in the tympanic membrane caused by chronic negative middle ear pressure, inflammation, or trauma

Disorders of the eye

NORMAL OPTIC DISC

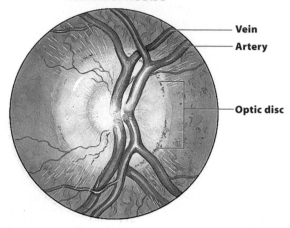

Vein

Artery

Optic disc

GLAUCOMA

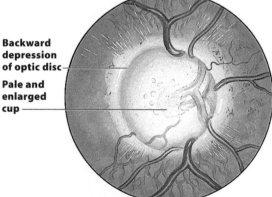

Backward depression of optic disc

Pale and enlarged cup

MALIGNANT MELANOMA

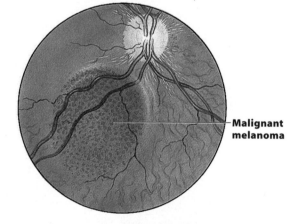

Malignant melanoma

DIABETIC RETINOPATHY

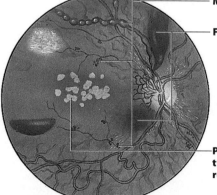

Microaneurysms

Flame-shaped hemorrhages

Puntate exudates typical of diabetic retinopathy

MACULAR DEGENERATION

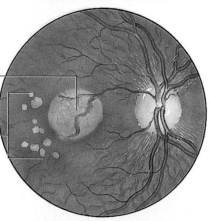

Macula

Altered pigmentation associated with macular degeneration of aging

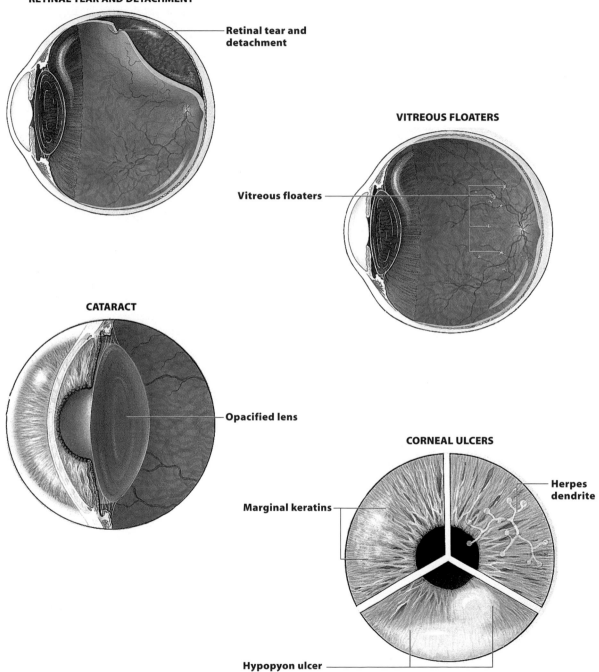

RETINAL TEAR AND DETACHMENT

Retinal tear and detachment

VITREOUS FLOATERS

Vitreous floaters

CATARACT

Opacified lens

CORNEAL ULCERS

Herpes dendrite

Marginal keratins

Hypopyon ulcer

The common cold

The common cold, an upper respiratory tract infection, is a contagious inflammation of the mucous membranes of the head and the throat. *Acute rhinitis* is one of the first discomforts of the common cold. It's characterized by swelling and increased discharge from the mucous membranes lining the nose.

PARANASAL SINUSES

Within the bones surrounding the nose are many air-filled sacs called *sinuses*. The mucous membranes lining these sinuses are continuous with the nasal lining, and infections may easily spread through the openings in the nose. If bacteria invade the sinuses, *sinusitis*—a painful infection with an associated gray, yellow, or green nasal discharge—results.

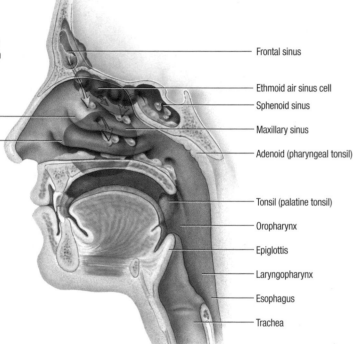

- Frontal sinus
- Ethmoid air sinus cell
- Sphenoid sinus
- Maxillary sinus
- Adenoid (pharyngeal tonsil)
- Tonsil (palatine tonsil)
- Oropharynx
- Epiglottis
- Laryngopharynx
- Esophagus
- Trachea

Middle turbinate

Inferior turbinate

THE THROAT AND TONSILS

Airborne particles, viruses, and bacteria that aren't trapped in the nose or in the mouth may land on the pharynx. As shown in the illustration at right, a circle of lymphatic tissue surrounds the pharynx and serves as a first line of defense. Inflammation affecting the throat and tonsils causes swelling, redness, and pain with swallowing and is commonly called a *sore throat*. Bacteria (most frequently *Streptococcus*) may cause a more severe infection called *strep throat*. An infection of the palatine tonsils is called *tonsillitis* and their enlargement may cause discomfort.

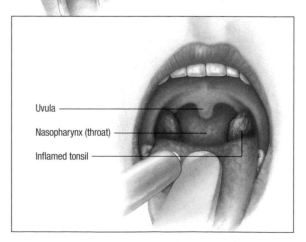

- Uvula
- Nasopharynx (throat)
- Inflamed tonsil

KNOW-HOW

Palpating the prostate gland

To palpate the prostate gland, insert your gloved, lubricated index finger into the rectum. Then palpate the prostate on the anterior rectal wall, just past the anorectal ring, as shown.

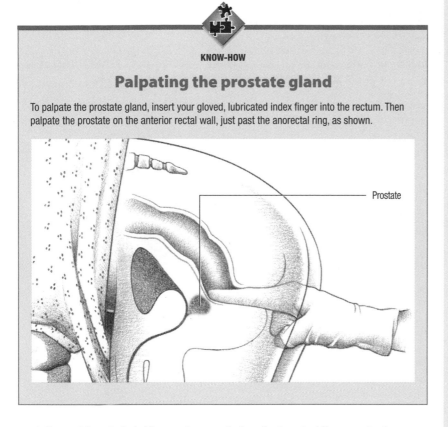

Prostate

A femoral hernia feels like a soft tumor below the inguinal ligament in the femoral area. It may be difficult to distinguish from a lymph node and is uncommon in men.

Prostate gland

Tell the patient that he'll feel some pressure or urgency during this examination. Have him stand and lean over the examination table. If he can't do this, have him lie on his left side, with his right knee and hip flexed or with both knees drawn toward his chest. Inspect the skin of the perineal, anal, and posterior scrotal areas. It should be smooth and unbroken, with no protruding masses.

Tell the patient that you are going to place your finger in his rectum. Have him relax as much as possible. If he maintains anal sphincter tension, have him bear down as if having a bowel movement and gently insert your finger into his rectum. With your finger, rotate and palpate the entire muscular ring. The canal should be smooth. There should be no pain, only mild discomfort with this examination. The prostate gland is on the anterior wall just past the anorectal ring. The gland should feel smooth, rubbery, and about the size of a walnut. A test for occult blood would be appropriate at this time. (See *Palpating the prostate gland*.)

ABNORMAL FINDINGS *If the patient's prostate gland protrudes into the rectal lumen, it's probably enlarged. The enlargement is classified from grades 1 (protruding less than ⅜" [1 cm] into the rectal lumen) to 4 (protruding more than 1¼" [3 cm] into the rectal lumen). Also note tenderness or nodules.*

Palpating the prostate gland
- ✦ Inspect the skin of the perineal, anal, and posterior scrotal areas
- ✦ Place your finger in the patient's rectum, asking him to bear down
- ✦ Palpate the prostate gland

Abnormal findings
- ✦ Prostate protruding into the rectal lumen (enlarged)
- ✦ Smooth, firm, symmetrical enlargement (BPH, nocturia, urinary hesitancy and frequency, and recurring UTIs)

A smooth, firm, symmetrical enlargement of the prostate gland indicates BPH, which typically starts after age 50. This finding may be associated with nocturia, urinary hesitancy and frequency, and recurring UTIs.

INTERPRETING YOUR FINDINGS

After you assess the patient, a group of findings may lead you to suspect a particular disorder. (See *The male GU system: Interpreting your findings.*)

MALE GU SYSTEM DISORDERS

BENIGN PROSTATIC HYPERPLASIA

In BPH, also known as *benign prostatic hypertrophy*, the prostate gland enlarges enough to compress the urethra and cause overt urinary obstruction. Depending on the size of the enlarged prostate, the age and health of the patient, and the extent of the obstruction, BPH is treated symptomatically or surgically.

The presenting signs and symptoms of BPH include:
+ reduced urinary stream caliber and force
+ urinary hesitancy
+ feeling of incomplete voiding, interrupted stream.
  As obstruction increases, findings may include:
+ frequent urination with nocturia
+ sense of urgency
+ retention, dribbling, and incontinence
+ possible hematuria.

EPIDIDYMITIS

Infection of the epididymis, the cordlike excretory duct of the testis, is one of the most common infections of the male reproductive tract. Usually, the causative organisms spread from an established UTI or prostatitis and reach the epididymis through the lumen of the vas deferens. Rarely, epididymitis is secondary to a distant infection, such as pharyngitis or tuberculosis that spreads through the lymphatic system or, less commonly, the bloodstream. It usually affects adults and is rare before puberty. Epididymitis may spread to the testis itself.

Epididymitis usually results from pyogenic organisms, such as *Staphylococci, Escherichia coli, Chlamydia trachomatis,* and S*treptococci.* Other causes include gonorrhea, trauma (which may reactivate a dormant infection or initiate a new one), prostatectomy, and chemical irritation resulting from extravasation of urine through the vas deferens.

Key signs and symptoms include unilateral pain, extreme tenderness, and swelling in the groin and scrotum. Other clinical effects include high fever, malaise, and a characteristic waddle (an attempt to protect the groin and scrotum when walking).

IMPOTENCE

Impotence, also known as *erectile dysfunction,* prevents a man from attaining or maintaining penile erection sufficient to complete intercourse. Primary impotence implies that the patient has never achieved a sufficient erection; secondary impotence, which is more common and less serious, implies that, despite the patient's

Male GU system disorders

Facts about BPH
+ Prostate gland enlarges enough to compress urethra, causing urinary obstruction
+ Treated symptomatically or surgically
+ Reduced urinary stream caliber and force, urinary hesitancy, and feeling of incomplete voiding

Facts about epididymitis
+ Infection of cordlike excretory duct of testis
+ Results from *Staphylococci, Escherichia coli, Chlamydia trachomatis,* and *Streptococci*
+ Unilateral pain, extreme tenderness, and swelling in groin and scrotum

Facts about impotence
+ Inability to attain or maintain penile erection

The male GU system: Interpreting your findings

This chart shows common groups of findings for the signs and symptoms of the male genitourinary (GU) system, along with their probable causes.

SIGN OR SYMPTOM AND FINDINGS	PROBABLE CAUSE
Male genital lesions	
✦ Fluid-filled vesicles on the glans penis, foreskin, or penile shaft ✦ Painful ulcers ✦ Tender inguinal lymph nodes ✦ Fever ✦ Malaise ✦ Dysuria	✦ Genital herpes
✦ Painless warts (tiny pink swellings that grow and become pedunculated) near the urethral meatus ✦ Lesions spread to the perineum and the perianal area ✦ Cauliflower appearance of multiple swellings	✦ Genital warts
✦ Sharply defined, slightly raised, scaling patches on the inner thigh or groin (bilaterally), or on the scrotum or penis ✦ Severe pruritus	✦ Tinea cruris (jock itch)
Scrotal swelling	
✦ Swollen scrotum that's soft or unusually firm ✦ Bowel sounds may be auscultated in the scrotum	✦ Hernia
✦ Gradual scrotal swelling ✦ Scrotum may be soft and cystic or firm and tense ✦ Painless ✦ Round, nontender scrotal mass on palpation ✦ Glowing when transilluminated	✦ Hydrocele
✦ Scrotal swelling with sudden and severe pain ✦ Unilateral elevation of the affected testicle ✦ Nausea and vomiting	✦ Testicular torsion
Urethral discharge	
✦ Purulent or milky urethral discharge ✦ Sudden fever and chills ✦ Lower back pain ✦ Myalgia ✦ Perineal fullness ✦ Arthralgia ✦ Urinary frequency and urgency ✦ Cloudy urine ✦ Dysuria ✦ Tense, boggy, very tender, and warm prostate palpated on digital rectal examination	✦ Prostatitis

(continued)

The male GU system: Interpreting your findings (continued)

SIGN OR SYMPTOM AND FINDINGS	PROBABLE CAUSE
Urethral discharge (continued)	
✦ Opaque, gray, yellowish, or blood-tinged discharge that's painless ✦ Dysuria ✦ Eventual anuria	✦ Urethral neoplasm
✦ Scant or profuse urethral discharge that's either thin and clear, mucoid, or thick and purulent ✦ Urinary hesitancy, frequency, and urgency ✦ Dysuria ✦ Itching and burning around the meatus	✦ Urethritis
Urinary hesitancy	
✦ Reduced caliber and force of urinary stream ✦ Perineal pain ✦ A feeling of incomplete voiding ✦ Inability to stop the urine stream ✦ Urinary frequency ✦ Urinary incontinence ✦ Bladder distention	✦ Benign prostatic hyperplasia
✦ Urinary frequency and dribbling ✦ Nocturia ✦ Dysuria ✦ Bladder distention ✦ Perineal pain ✦ Constipation ✦ Hard, nodular prostate palpated on digital rectal examination	✦ Prostate cancer
✦ Dysuria ✦ Urinary frequency and urgency ✦ Hematuria ✦ Cloudy urine ✦ Bladder spasms ✦ Costovertebral angle tenderness ✦ Suprapubic, lower back, pelvic, or flank pain ✦ Urethral discharge	✦ Urinary tract infection

Facts about impotence
(continued)

Special points
✦ Affects men of all age-groups but more common in older men

present inability to maintain a penile erection for intercourse, he has done so in the past.

Transient periods of impotence aren't considered dysfunctional and probably occur in 50% of adult males. The prognosis depends on the severity and duration of impotence and on the underlying cause.

 SPECIAL POINTS *Erectile dysfunction affects men of all age-groups but is more common in older men.*

Psychogenic factors cause 50% to 60% of erectile dysfunction; organic factors underlie the rest. In some patients, psychogenic and organic factors coexist, hampering isolation of the primary cause.

Psychogenic causes may be intrapersonal, reflecting personal sexual anxieties, or interpersonal, reflecting a disturbed sexual relationship. Intrapersonal factors usually involve guilt, fear, depression, or feelings of inadequacy resulting from previous traumatic sexual experience, rejection by parents or peers, exaggerated religious orthodoxy, abnormal mother-son intimacy, or homosexual experiences. Interpersonal factors may stem from differences in sexual preferences between partners, lack of communication, insufficient knowledge of sexual function, or nonsexual personal conflicts. Situational impotence, a temporary condition, may develop in response to stress.

Organic causes may include chronic disorders, such as cardiopulmonary disease, diabetes, multiple sclerosis, or renal failure; spinal cord trauma; complications of surgery; drug- or alcohol-induced dysfunction; and, rarely, genital anomalies or defects of the central nervous system.

Secondary erectile dysfunction is classified as:
+ partial — the patient can't achieve a full erection
+ intermittent — the patient is sometimes potent with the same partner
+ selective — the patient is potent only with certain partners.

Some patients lose erectile function suddenly; others lose it gradually. If the cause isn't organic, erection may still be achieved through masturbation.

Patients with psychogenic impotence may appear anxious, with sweating and palpitations, or they may become totally disinterested in sexual activity. Patients with psychogenic or drug-induced impotence may suffer extreme depression, which may cause the impotence or result from it.

PROSTATE CANCER

SPECIAL POINTS *Prostate cancer is the most common cancer in men over age 50 and is the second leading cause of cancer death among males. Incidence is highest among Blacks and men with blood type A and is lowest in Asians. However, its occurrence is unaffected by socioeconomic status or fertility. To detect this cancer early, all males over age 40 should undergo a digital rectal examination and annual serum prostate-specific antigen (PSA) determination as part of their annual physical examination.*

Signs and symptoms of prostate cancer appear only in the advanced stages of the disease. They include difficult urination, dribbling, urine retention, unexplained cystitis, and hematuria (rare). A hard nodule may appear on rectal examination. This may be felt before other signs and symptoms develop.

PROSTATITIS

An inflammation of the prostate gland, prostatitis may be acute or chronic. Acute prostatitis most commonly results from gram-negative bacteria and is easy to recognize and treat. However, chronic prostatitis, the most common cause of recurrent UTI in men, isn't easily recognizable. As many as 35% of men over age 50 have chronic prostatitis.

Prostatitis results primarily from infection by *Escherichia coli*. It also results from infection by *Klebsiella, Enterobacter, Proteus, Pseudomonas, Streptococcus,* or *Staphylococcus.*

Signs and symptoms of acute prostatitis include sudden fever, chills, lower back pain, myalgia, perineal fullness, arthralgia, urgency, possibly dysuria, nocturia, some degree of urinary obstruction, and cloudy urine. Rectal palpation of the prostate reveals tenderness, induration, swelling, firmness, and warmth.

Chronic prostatitis may be asymptomatic, or it may involve less severe forms of the symptoms that characterize acute prostatitis. These include painful ejaculation, hemospermia, persistent urethral discharge, and sexual dysfunction.

TESTICULAR CANCER

 SPECIAL POINTS *Testicular cancer is the leading cause of death from solid tumors in men between ages 15 and 34. With testicular tumors that occur in children (which are rare), 50% are detectable before age 5. Nearly all testicular tumors arise in the gonadal cells.*

Prognosis varies with the cancer cell type and staging. When treated with surgery and radiation — provided the cancer hasn't metastasized beyond regional lymph nodes — 100% of patients with seminomas and 90% of those with non-seminomas survive beyond 5 years. Prognosis is poor if the cancer has advanced beyond regional lymph nodes at diagnosis.

Whites and men with a history of cryptorchidism (even after surgical correction) are at increased risk for testicular cancer, but its cause is unknown.

Signs and symptoms of testicular cancer include a firm, painless, smooth testicular mass; testicular heaviness; and gynecomastia and nipple tenderness. In later stages, ureteral obstruction, abdominal mass, cough, hemoptysis, shortness of breath, weight loss, fatigue, pallor, and lethargy, with lymph node involvement and distant metastases, are possible.

TESTICULAR TORSION

Testicular torsion is the abnormal twisting of the spermatic cord that results from rotation of a testis or the mesorchium (a fold in the area between the testis and epididymis), which causes strangulation and, if untreated, eventual infarction of the involved testis. This condition is almost always unilateral. The prognosis is good with early detection and prompt treatment.

 SPECIAL POINTS *Most common between ages 12 and 18, testicular torsion may occur at any age.*

Normally, the tunica vaginalis envelops the testis and attaches to the epididymis and spermatic cord. With intravaginal torsion (the most common type of testicular torsion in adolescents), testicular twisting may result from an abnormality of the tunica, in which the testis is abnormally positioned, or from a narrowing of the mesentery support. With extravaginal torsion (most common in neonates), loose attachment of the tunica vaginalis to the scrotal lining causes spermatic cord rotation above the testis. A sudden forceful contraction of the cremaster muscle may precipitate this condition.

Torsion produces excruciating pain in the affected testis or iliac fossa.

Facts about testicular cancer

+ Prognosis varies with cancer cell type and staging
+ Treatment includes surgery and radiation
+ Firm, painless, smooth testicular mass; testicular heaviness; gynecomastia and nipple discharge

Special points

+ In men ages 15 to 34, leading cause of death from solid tumors
+ In children, 50% of tumors detectable before age 5

Facts about testicular torsion

+ Abnormal twisting of the spermatic cord that results from rotation of a testis or the mesorchium
+ Prognosis good with early detection and prompt treatment

Special points

+ Most commonly occurs between ages 12 and 18, but may occur at any age

Integumentary system

A LOOK AT SKIN, HAIR, AND NAILS

The skin covers the body's internal structures and protects them from the external world. Along with hair and nails, the skin provides a window for viewing changes taking place inside the body. As a nurse, you observe a patient's skin, hair, and nails regularly, so it's likely that you would be the first to detect abnormalities. Your sharp assessment skills will help supply a reliable picture of the patient's overall health.

To perform an accurate physical assessment, you'll need to understand the anatomy and physiology of the skin, hair, and nails.

SKIN

Also called the *integumentary system*, the skin is the body's largest organ and can be divided into several layers.

Layers of the skin

The skin consists of two distinct layers: the epidermis and the dermis. Subcutaneous tissue lies beneath these layers.

Epidermis

The epidermis — the outer layer which is thin and avascular — consists of squamous epithelial tissue. The two major layers of the epidermis are the stratum corneum — the most superficial layer — and the deeper basal cell layer, or stratum germinativum. (See *Structure of the skin*, page 318.)

Stratum corneum

After mitosis occurs in the germinal layer, epithelial cells undergo a series of changes as they migrate to the outermost part of the epidermis called the *stratum corneum*, which is made up of tightly arranged layers of cellular membranes and keratin.

A look at skin, hair, and nails

+ The skin covers the body's internal structures and protects them from the external world
+ Helps detect abnormalities and changes in overall health

Layers of the skin

+ Epidermis and dermis
+ Subcutaneous tissue lies beneath

Epidermis

+ Outer layer, which is thin and avascular
+ Consists of squamous epithelial tissue

Stratum corneum

+ Made up of tightly arranged layers of cellular membranes and keratin
+ Superficial layer of epidermis

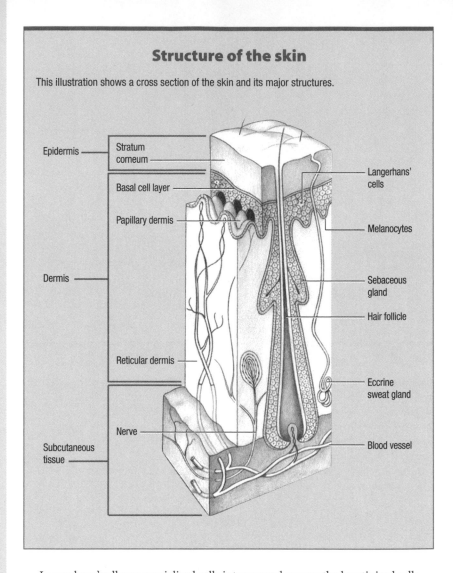

Structure of the skin

This illustration shows a cross section of the skin and its major structures.

Epidermis

Stratum corneum

Basal cell layer

Papillary dermis

Dermis

Reticular dermis

Nerve

Subcutaneous tissue

Langerhans' cells

Melanocytes

Sebaceous gland

Hair follicle

Eccrine sweat gland

Blood vessel

Langerhans' cells are specialized cells interspersed among the keratinized cells below the stratum corneum. Langerhans' cells have an immunologic function and assist in the initial processing of antigens that enter the epidermis. Epidermal cells are usually shed from the surface as epidermal dust. Differentiation of cells from the basal layer to the stratum corneum takes up to 28 days.

Basal layer

The basal layer produces new cells to replace the superficial keratinized cells that are continuously shed or worn away.

The basal layer also contains specialized cells known as *melanocytes*, which produce the brown pigment melanin and disperse it to the surrounding epithelial cells. Melanin primarily serves to filter ultraviolet radiation (light). Exposure to ultraviolet light can stimulate melanin production. Hormones, the environment, and heredity influence melanocyte production. Because melanocyte production is greater in some people than others, skin color varies considerably.

Basal layer

✦ Produces new cells interspersed below the stratum corneum
✦ Differentiation of cells occurs here and moves to stratum corneum in up to 28 days
✦ Contains melanocytes, which produce melanin to filter ultraviolet radiation

Dermis

Also called the *corium,* the dermis is an elastic system that contains and supports blood vessels, lymphatic vessels, nerves, and epidermal appendages such as the hair, nails, and glands — eccrine and apocrine. The dermis itself is made up of two layers: the superficial papillary dermis and the reticular dermis.

The papillary dermis is studded with fingerlike projections (papillae) that nourish the epidermal cells. The epidermis lies over these papillae and bulges downward to fill the spaces. A collagenous membrane known as the *basement membrane* lies between the epidermis and dermis, holding them together.

The reticular dermis covers a layer of subcutaneous tissue (adipose layer), a specialized layer primarily made up of fat cells. It insulates the body to conserve heat, acts as a mechanical shock absorber, and provides energy.

Extracellular material called *matrix* makes up most of the dermis; matrix contains connective tissue fibers called collagen, elastin, and reticular fibers. *Collagen,* a protein, gives strength to the dermis; *elastin* makes the skin pliable; and *reticular fibers* bind the collagen and elastin fibers together.

The matrix and connective tissue fibers are produced by spindle-shaped connective tissue cells (dermal fibroblasts), which become part of the matrix as it forms. Fibers are loosely arranged in the papillary dermis, but more tightly packed in the deeper reticular dermis.

Epidermal appendages

The sebaceous, eccrine, and apocrine glands are all epidermal appendages.

Sebaceous glands

Sebaceous glands occur on all parts of the skin except for the palms and soles. The glands are most prominent on the scalp, face, upper torso, and anogenital region. Sebum, a lipid substance, is produced within the lobule and secreted into the hair follicle via the sebaceous duct; it then exits through the hair follicle opening to reach the skin surface. Sebum may help waterproof the hair and skin and promote the absorption of fat-soluble substances into the dermis. It may also be involved in the production of vitamin D and have some antibacterial function.

Eccrine glands

Eccrine glands are widely distributed, coiled glands that produce an odorless, watery fluid with a sodium concentration equal to that of plasma. A duct from the secretory coils passes through the dermis and epidermis and opens onto the skin surface. Eccrine glands in the palms and soles secrete fluid primarily in response to emotional stress, such as that from taking a test. The remaining 3 million eccrine glands respond primarily to thermal stress, effectively regulating temperature.

Apocrine glands

Located primarily in the axillary and anogenital areas, apocrine glands have a coiled secretory portion that lies deeper in the dermis than the eccrine glands. A duct connects the apocrine glands to the upper portion of the hair follicle. Apocrine glands, which begin to function at puberty, have no known biological function. Bacterial decomposition of the fluid produced by these glands causes body odor.

 SPECIAL POINTS *As people age, all skin functions decline and normal skin changes occur as a result. Because of that decline, elderly patients are more prone to skin disease, infection, problems in wound healing, and tissue atrophy. (See* Skin and the aging process, *page 320.)*

Dermis

+ Also called the *corium*
+ Contains and supports blood vessels, lymphatic vessels, nerves, and epidermal appendages
+ Includes superficial papillary dermis and reticular dermis
+ Consists of matrix (extracellular material) made of collagen, elastin, and reticular fibers

Epidermal appendages

+ Include sebaceous, eccrine, and apocrine glands

Sebaceous glands

+ Occur in all parts of the skin, except for palms and soles
+ Produces sebum

Eccrine glands

+ Widely distributed, coiled glands produce an odorless, watery fluid
+ Secrete fluid in palms and soles from emotional stress

Apocrine glands

+ Coiled secretory portion lies deep in dermis
+ Duct connects glands to hair follicles
+ Bacterial decomposition of gland fluid produces body odor

Special points

+ Functions decline and change with age; elderly patients more prone to skin disease, infections, problems in wound healing, and tissue atrophy

Skin and the aging process

This table lists skin changes that normally occur with aging.

SKIN CHANGE	FINDINGS
Pigmentation	✦ Pale skin color
Thickness	✦ Wrinkling, especially on the face, arms, and legs ✦ Parchmentlike appearance, especially over bony prominences and on the dorsal surfaces of the hands, feet, arms, and legs
Moisture	✦ Dry, flaky, and rough
Turgor	✦ "Tented" position when squeezed, especially if the patient is dehydrated
Texture	✦ Numerous creases and lines

Skin functions

✦ Performs protection, sensory perception, temperature and blood pressure regulation, vitamin synthesis, and excretion

Protection

✦ Epidermis protects against trauma, noxious chemicals, and invasion of microorganisms

Sensory perception

✦ Nerve fibers carry impulses to the CNS and transmit sensations including temperature, touch, pressure, pain, and itching

Temperature and blood pressure regulation

✦ Nerves, blood vessels, and eccrine glands help thermoregulation
✦ Blood vessels constrict when body temperature falls
✦ Small arteries dilate when body temperature rises
✦ Dermal blood vessels regulate systemic blood pressure by vasoconstriction

Skin functions

The skin performs many functions, including protection, sensory perception, temperature and blood pressure regulation, vitamin synthesis, and excretion.

Protection

The epidermis protects against trauma, noxious chemicals, and invasion by microorganisms. Langerhans' cells enhance the immune response by helping lymphocytes process antigens entering the epidermis. Melanocytes protect the skin by producing melanin to help filter ultraviolet light (irradiation). The intact skin also protects the body by limiting excretion of water and electrolytes.

Sensory perception

Sensory nerve fibers carry impulses to the central nervous system, and autonomic nerve fibers carry impulses to smooth muscles in the walls of the dermal blood vessels, to the muscles around the hair roots, and to the sweat glands. Sensory nerve fibers originate in dorsal nerve roots and supply specific areas of the skin known as *dermatomes*. Through these fibers, the skin can transmit various sensations, including temperature, touch, pressure, pain, and itching.

Temperature and blood pressure regulation

Abundant nerves, blood vessels, and eccrine glands within the dermis help with thermoregulation. When the skin is exposed to cold or when internal body temperature falls, the blood vessels constrict in response to stimuli from the autonomic nervous system. This decreases blood flow through the skin and conserves body heat. When the skin is too hot or internal body temperature rises, the small arteries in the dermis dilate. Increased blood flow through these vessels reduces body heat. If this doesn't adequately lower temperature, the eccrine glands act to increase sweat production; subsequent evaporation cools the skin.

Dermal blood vessels also help with the regulation of systemic blood pressure by vasoconstriction.

Hair structure

The illustration below shows a hair shaft and its associated glands.

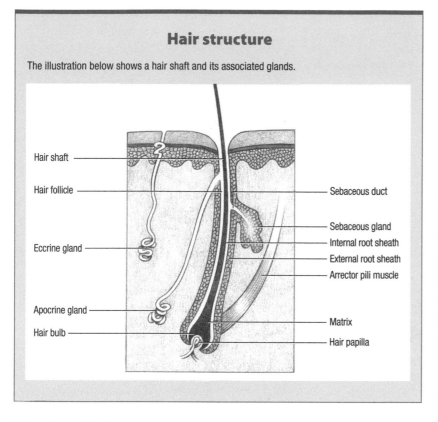

Hair shaft
Hair follicle
Eccrine gland
Apocrine gland
Hair bulb

Sebaceous duct
Sebaceous gland
Internal root sheath
External root sheath
Arrector pili muscle
Matrix
Hair papilla

Vitamin synthesis

The skin synthesizes vitamin D or cholecalciferol, when stimulated by ultraviolet light.

Excretion

The skin is also an excretory organ: The sweat glands excrete sweat, which contains water, electrolytes, urea, and lactic acid. The skin maintains body surface integrity by migration and shedding. It can repair surface wounds by intensifying normal cell replacement mechanisms. However, regeneration won't occur if the dermal layer is destroyed. The sebaceous glands produce sebum—a mixture of keratin, fat, and cellulose debris. Combined with sweat, sebum forms a moist, oily, acidic film that's mildly antibacterial and antifungal and that protects the skin surface.

HAIR

Hair consists of long, slender shafts made up of keratin. Each hair shaft has an expanded lower end (bulb or root) indented on its undersurface. Each hair lies within an epithelial-lined sheath called a *hair follicle* and receives nourishment from the papilla—a cluster of connective tissue and blood vessels at the base of the follicle. A bundle of smooth-muscle fibers (arrector pili) extends through the dermis to attach to the base of the hair follicle. Contraction of these muscles during emotional stress or exposure to cold causes hair to stand on end. Hair follicles also have a rich blood and nerve supply. The hair bulb contains melanocytes, which determine hair color. (See *Hair structure*.)

Vitamin synthesis

✦ When stimulated by ultraviolet light, skin synthesizes vitamin D or cholecalciferol

Excretion

✦ Sweat glands excrete sweat containing water, electrolytes, urea, and lactic acid
✦ Skin maintains body surface integrity by migration and shedding
✦ Sebaceous glands produce sebum, which forms moist, oily, acidic film to protect skin when mixed with sweat

Hair

✦ Long, slender shafts made up of keratin
✦ Follicle provides rich blood and nerve supply
✦ Hair bulb contains melanocytes, determining hair color

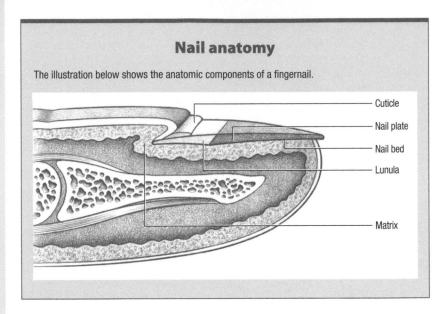

Nail anatomy

The illustration below shows the anatomic components of a fingernail.

- Cuticle
- Nail plate
- Nail bed
- Lunula
- Matrix

Hair
(continued)

Special points
- ✦ In neonates, lanugo covers skin
- ✦ As a person ages, melanocyte function declines, producing light or gray hair
- ✦ Aging resulting in balding

Nails

- ✦ Form when epidermal cells are converted into hard plates of keratin
- ✦ Comprise nail root, nail plate, nail bed, lunula, nail folds, and cuticle
- ✦ Nail matrix is site of nail growth

Special points
- ✦ Aging process produces brittle, splitting, and thin nails, which lose luster and become yellowed

Obtaining a health history

- ✦ Includes chief complaint; medical, family, psychological history; and patterns of daily living

SPECIAL POINTS *In neonates, the skin is covered with lanugo (fine, soft and lightly pigmented fetal hair) and the hair on the scalp may be lost several weeks after birth, especially at the temple and occiput, but it slowly grows back. As the person ages, melanocyte function declines, producing light or gray hair, and the hair follicle itself becomes drier as sebaceous gland function decreases. Hair growth also declines, decreasing the amount of body hair. In addition, balding, genetically determined in younger people, occurs as a normal result of aging.*

NAILS

Nails are formed when the epidermal cells are converted into hard plates of keratin. The nails consist of a nail root (or nail matrix), nail plate, nail bed, lunula, nail folds, and cuticle. (See *Nail anatomy*.)

The nail plate is the visible, hardened layer attached to and covering the fingertip. The plate is clear with fine longitudinal ridges. The pink color results from blood vessels underlying vascular epithelial cells.

The nail matrix is the site of nail growth and is protected by the cuticle. At the end of the matrix is the white, crescent-shaped area, the lunula, that extends beyond the cuticle.

SPECIAL POINTS *The aging process slows down nail growth, resulting in brittle and thin nails. Longitudinal ridges in the nail plate become much more pronounced, making the nails prone to splitting. In addition, they lose their luster and become yellowed.*

OBTAINING A HEALTH HISTORY

When assessing a problem related to skin, hair, or nails, you'll need to thoroughly explore the patient's chief complaint, medical history, family history, psychological history, and patterns of daily living. Keep in mind that skin, hair, and nail abnormalities commonly result from a medical problem unrelated to the patient's chief complaint, so the patient may overlook or minimize them.

Asking about the skin

Most complaints about the skin involve problems with itching, rashes, lesions, pigmentation abnormalities, or changes in existing lesions.

Typical questions to ask about changes in a patient's skin include:
+ How and when did the skin changes occur?
+ Are the changes in the form of a skin rash or lesion?
+ When did you first notice the change and when did it spread?
+ Is the change confined to one area or has the condition spread?
+ Is there bleeding or drainage from the area?
+ Does the area itch?

ABNORMAL FINDINGS *If the patient reports pruritus — an unpleasant itching sensation that usually provokes scratching to gain relief — have him describe its onset, frequency, and intensity. Pruritus affects the skin, certain mucous membranes, and the eyes. Most severe at night, it may be exacerbated by increased skin temperature, poor skin turgor, local vasodilation, dermatoses, and stress. If the patient experiences pruritus at night, ask him whether it prevents him from falling asleep or awakens him. (Generally, pruritus related to dermatoses prevents — but doesn't disturb — sleep.)*

Ask if the itching is localized or generalized. When is it most severe? How long does it last? Is there a relationship to such activities as physical exertion, bathing, makeup application, or use of perfume?

Ask the patient how he cleans his skin. In particular, does he bathe excessively, use harsh soaps or hot water, and have contact with allergens? Does he have occupational exposure to known skin irritants, such as glass fiber insulation or chemicals? Ask about the patient's general health and the medications he takes; new medications are suspect. Has he recently traveled abroad? Does he have pets? Does anyone else in the house report itching? Ask about contact with skin irritants, previous skin disorders, and related symptoms. Then obtain a complete medication history.

SPECIAL POINTS *In primigravidas late in the third trimester, physiologic pruritus, such as pruritic urticarial papules and plaques of pregnancy, may occur.*

Many adult disorders also cause pruritus in children, but they may affect different parts of the body. For instance, scabies may affect the head in infants, but not in adults. Pityriasis rosea may affect the face, hands, and feet of adolescents.

Some childhood diseases, such as measles and chickenpox, can cause pruritus. Hepatic diseases can also produce pruritus in children as bile salts accumulate on the skin.

+ How much time do you spend in the sun, and how do you protect your skin from ultraviolet rays?
+ Do you have allergies?

ABNORMAL FINDINGS *If the patient reports urticaria — a vascular skin reaction also known as hives — he'll have an eruption of transient pruritic wheals (smooth, slightly elevated patches with well-defined erythematous margins and pale centers) that are produced by the local release of histamine or other vasoactive substances as part of a hypersensitivity reaction.*

If the patient isn't in distress, obtain a complete history. Ask him:
+ Does the urticaria follow a seasonal pattern?
+ Do certain foods or drugs seem to aggravate it?
+ Is there any relationship to physical exertion?
+ Is he routinely exposed to chemicals on the job or at home?

Also obtain a detailed medication history, including use of prescription and over-the-counter drugs, and note any history of chronic or parasitic infections, skin disease, or GI disorders.

Asking about the skin
+ Complaints involve problems with itching, rashes, lesions, pigmentation abnormalities, or changes in existing lesions

Abnormal findings
+ Pruritus, an unpleasant itching sensation, provokes scratching to gain relief
+ Urticaria (hives) causes an eruption of transient pruritic wheals due to a hypersensitivity reaction

Special points
+ In primigravidas late in third trimester, physiologic pruritus occurs as urticarial papules and plaques

Asking about the skin
(continued)

Special points

✦ In pediatric patients, urticaria includes acute papular urticaria occurring after an insect bite; urticaria pigmentosa, which is rare; and hereditary angioedema, which may be causative

Asking about the hair

✦ Common concerns are hair loss or hirsutism
✦ Ask patient about onset, location, duration, aggravating factors, and past illnesses

Abnormal findings

✦ Alopecia usually affects the scalp; classified as diffuse or patchy, and scarring or nonscarring

Special points

✦ In children, common causes of alopecia include chemotherapy or radiation therapy, seborrheic dermatitis, alopecia mucinosa, tinea capitis, and hypopituitarism

SPECIAL POINTS *In pediatric patients, forms of urticaria include acute papular urticaria, which usually occurs after an insect bite, and urticaria pigmentosa, which is rare. Hereditary angioedema may be causative.*

✦ Do you have a family history of skin cancer or other significant diseases?
✦ Do you have a fever or joint pain, or have you lost weight?
✦ Have you recently been bitten by an insect?
✦ Do you take any medications? If yes, which ones?
✦ What changes in your skin have you observed in the past few years?

ASKING ABOUT THE HAIR

The most common concerns about hair refer to either to hair loss or to an increased growth and distribution of body hair, called *hirsutism*. Psychological factors — such as skin infections, ovarian or adrenal tumors, increased stress, or systemic diseases, such as hypothyroidism or malignancies — can cause either of these hair disorders.

To identify the cause of your patient's hair problem, ask:

✦ When did you first notice the loss (or gain) of hair? Was it sudden or gradual?
✦ Did the change occur in just a few spots or all over your body?
✦ What was happening in your life when the problem started?
✦ Are you taking any medications?
✦ Are you experiencing itching, pain, discharge, fever, or weight loss?
✦ What serious illnesses, if any, have you had?

ABNORMAL FINDINGS *If the patient reports alopecia, it usually affects the scalp and develops gradually. It can be classified as diffuse or patchy, and scarring or nonscarring. Scarring alopecia, or permanent hair loss, results from hair follicle destruction, which smooths the skin surface, erasing follicular openings. Nonscarring alopecia, or temporary hair loss, results from hair follicle damage that spares follicular openings, allowing future hair growth.*

If the patient isn't receiving chemotherapeutic drugs or radiation therapy, begin by asking when he first noticed the hair loss or thinning. Does it affect the scalp alone or occur elsewhere on the body? Is it accompanied by itching or rashes? Then carefully explore other signs and symptoms to help distinguish between normal and pathologic hair loss. Ask about recent weight change, anorexia, nausea, vomiting, and altered bowel habits. Also ask about urine changes, such as hematuria or oliguria. Has the patient been especially tired or irritable? Does he have a cough or difficulty breathing? Ask about joint pain or stiffness and about heat or cold intolerance. Inquire about exposure to insecticides.

If the patient is female, find out if she has had menstrual irregularities, and note her pregnancy history. If the patient is male, ask about sexual dysfunction, such as decreased libido or impotence.

Next, ask about hair care. Does the patient frequently use a hot blow dryer or electric curlers? Does he periodically dye, bleach, or perm his hair? Ask the black patient if he uses a hot comb to straighten his hair or a long-toothed comb to achieve an "Afro". Does he ever braid the hair in cornrows?

Check for a family history of alopecia, and ask what age relatives were when they started experiencing hair loss. Also ask about nervous habits, such as pulling the hair or twirling it.

SPECIAL POINTS *In children, common causes of alopecia include use of chemotherapy or radiation therapy, seborrheic dermatitis (known as* cradle cap *in infancy), alopecia mucinosa, tinea capitis, and hypopituitarism. Tinea capitis may produce a kerion lesion — a boggy, raised, tender, and hairless lesion. Trichotillomania, a psychological disorder more common in children than*

adults, may produce patchy baldness with stubby hair growth due to habitual hair pulling. Other causes include progeria and congenital hair shaft defects such as trichorrhexis nodosa.

ASKING ABOUT THE NAILS

The most common complaints about the nails concern changes in growth or color. Either of these problems can be caused by infection, nutritional deficiencies, systemic illnesses, or stress.

Typical questions to ask about changes in a patient's nails include:
+ When did you first notice the changes in your nails?
+ What types of changes have you noticed (for example, in nail shape, color, or brittleness)?
+ Were the changes sudden or gradual?
+ Do you have other signs or symptoms, such as bleeding, pain, itching, or discharge?
+ What's the normal condition of your nails?
+ Do you have a history of serious illness?
+ Do you have a history of nail problems?
+ Do you bite your nails?
+ Have you had nail tips attached?

ASSESSING SKIN, HAIR, AND NAILS

To assess skin, hair, and nails, you'll use the techniques of inspection and palpation. Before beginning the examination, make sure the room is well lit and comfortably warm. Wear gloves during your examination.

Systematically assess all of the skin, hair, nails, and mucous membranes, even if the patient reports only a local lesion. The patient may not recognize subtle skin changes or skin disturbances that don't produce symptoms, such as an early melanoma located on the back. Also, the patient may feel too embarrassed to mention a lesion in the genital area. Failure to assess the entire skin surface can lead to incorrect diagnosis and care planning.

During the assessment, look for variations in lesion color, vascular supply, and pattern compared with other lesions. Also, check for lesion distribution over the whole body.

ASSESSING THE SKIN

Before you begin your skin assessment, gather the following equipment: clear millimeter/centimeter ruler, tongue blade, penlight or flashlight, Wood's lamp, and magnifying glass. This equipment will enable you to measure and closely inspect skin lesions and other abnormalities.

Inspect and palpate the skin area by area, focusing on color, texture, turgor, moisture, and temperature.

Skin color

Look for localized areas of bruising, cyanosis, pallor, or erythema. Check for uniformity of color and hypopigmented or hyperpigmented areas. Places exposed to the sun may show a darker pigmentation than other areas. Color changes may vary depending on skin pigmentation. (See *Detecting color variations in dark-skinned patients,* page 326, and *Evaluating skin color variations,* page 327.)

Asking about the nails
+ Common complaints concern changes in growth or color
+ Causes include infection, nutritional deficiencies, systemic illness, or stress

Assessing skin, hair, and nails
+ Includes inspection and palpation
+ Includes assessment of mucous membranes
+ Look for variations in skin lesion color, vascular supply, pattern, and distribution

Assessing the skin
+ Gather equipment
+ Inspect and palpate skin area by area
+ Focus on color, texture, turgor, moisture, and temperature

Skin color
+ Look for bruising, cyanosis, pallor, or erythema
+ Check for uniformity of color and hypopigmented or hyperpigmented areas

Skin texture and turgor
✦ Inspect and palpate for thickness and mobility
✦ Normally smooth and intact

Abnormal findings
✦ Rough, dry skin (hypothyroidism, psoriasis, or excessive keratinization)
✦ Poor skin turgor (dehydration and edema)

Special points
✦ In elderly patients, poor skin turgor occurs due to aging

Skin moisture
✦ Skin normally feels relatively dry, with minimal perspiration
✦ Skin-fold areas normally fairly dry

Abnormal findings
✦ Overly moist skin (anxiety, obesity, or too warm environment)
✦ Heavy sweating (fever, strenuous activity, cardiac and pulmonary diseases, or activity that elevates metabolic rate)

Skin temperature
✦ Palpation reveals cool to warm skin
✦ Warm skin suggests normal circulation
✦ Cool skin signals possible underlying disorder

> ### Detecting color variations in dark-skinned patients
>
> **CYANOSIS**
> Examine the conjunctiva, palms, soles, buccal mucosa, and tongue. Look for dull, dark color.
>
> **EDEMA**
> Examine the area for decreased color, and palpate for tightness.
>
> **ERYTHEMA**
> Palpate the area for warmth.
>
> **JAUNDICE**
> Examine the sclerae and hard palate. Look for a yellow color. If possible, perform this assessment in natural light, not fluorescent.
>
> **PALLOR**
> Examine the sclerae, conjunctiva, buccal mucosa, tongue, lips, nail beds, palms, and soles. Look for an ashen color.
>
> **PETECHIAE**
> Examine areas of lighter pigmentation, such as the abdomen. Look for tiny, purplish red dots.
>
> **RASHES**
> Palpate the area for skin texture changes.

Skin texture and turgor

Inspect and palpate the skin's texture, noting its thickness and mobility. It should look smooth and be intact.

 ABNORMAL FINDINGS *Rough, dry skin is a common sign that may indicate hypothyroidism, psoriasis, or excessive keratinization. Skin that isn't intact may indicate local irritation or trauma.*

Palpation will also help you evaluate the patient's hydration status. (See *Evaluating skin turgor,* page 328.)

 ABNORMAL FINDINGS *In patients who are dehydrated and have edema, poor skin turgor occurs. In patients who are overhydrated, the skin appears edematous and spongy. Localized edema can also result from trauma or systemic disease.*

 SPECIAL POINTS *In elderly patients, poor skin turgor occurs due to aging, so it may not be a reliable indicator of hydration status.*

Skin moisture

Observe the moisture content of the patient's skin. It should be relatively dry, with a minimal amount of perspiration. Skin-fold areas should also be fairly dry.

 ABNORMAL FINDINGS *Overly dry skin appears red and flaky. Overly moist skin can be caused by anxiety, obesity, or an environment that's too warm. Heavy sweating, or diaphoresis, usually accompanies fever, strenuous activity, cardiac and pulmonary diseases, and any activity or illness that elevates the metabolic rate.*

Skin temperature

Palpate the skin for temperature, which can range from cool to warm. Warm skin suggests normal circulation; cool skin, a possible underlying disorder. Make sure to distinguish between generalized and localized coolness and warmth. Make sure to check skin temperature bilaterally. When you're trying to compare subtle temperature differences in one area of the body with another, use the dorsal surface of your hands and fingers. They're the most sensitive to changes in temperature.

Evaluating skin color variations

To interpret your findings faster, refer to this chart.

COLOR	DISTRIBUTION	POSSIBLE CAUSE
Absent	✦ Small circumscribed areas ✦ Generalized	✦ Vitiligo ✦ Albinism
Blue	✦ Around lips or generalized	✦ Cyanosis (Note: In blacks, blue gingivae are normal.)
Deep red	✦ Generalized	✦ Polycythemia vera (increased red blood cell count)
Pink	✦ Local or generalized	✦ Erythema (superficial capillary dilation and congestion)
Tan to brown	✦ Facial patches	✦ Chloasma of pregnancy; butterfly rash of lupus erythematosus
Tan to brown-bronze	✦ Generalized (not related to sun exposure)	✦ Addison's disease
Yellow to yellowish brown	✦ Sclera or generalized	✦ Jaundice from liver dysfunction. (Note: In blacks, yellowish brown pigmentation of sclera is normal.)
Yellow-orange	✦ Palms, soles, and face; not sclera	✦ Carotenemia (carotene in the blood)

 ABNORMAL FINDINGS *In patients with areas of localized skin coolness, suspect vasoconstriction associated with cold environments or impaired arterial circulation to a limb. General coolness can result from such conditions as shock or hypothyroidism.*

In patients with areas of localized warmth, suspect infection, inflammation, or a burn. Generalized warmth occurs with fever or systemic diseases such as hyperthyroidism.

Skin lesions

During your inspection, you may see normal variations in the patient's skin texture and pigmentation.

 ABNORMAL FINDINGS *Red, pigmented lesions can be caused by vascular changes including hemangiomas, telangiectases, petechiae, purpura, and ecchymoses, and may indicate disease.*

Other normal variations include birthmarks, freckles, and nevi or moles. Birthmarks are generally flat and range from tan to red or brown. They can be found on all areas of the body. Freckles are small, flat macules located primarily on the face, arms, and back and are usually red-brown to brown. Nevi are either flat or raised and may be pink, tan, or dark brown. Like birthmarks, they can be found on all areas of the body.

Skin temperature
(continued)

Abnormal findings
✦ Vasoconstriction can cause localized skin coolness
✦ Shock or hypothyroidism result in general coolness
✦ Infection, inflammation, or burn can cause areas of warmth

Skin lesions
✦ Inspect for normal variations in skin texture and pigmentation
Abnormal findings
✦ Hemangiomas, telangiectases, petechiae, purpura, and ecchymoses signaled by red, pigmented lesions indicate possible disease

Evaluating skin turgor

+ Gently squeeze patient's skin on forearm, then release it
+ Normal turgor — skin returns to original shape
+ Poor turgor — skin maintains a tented position

Skin lesions
(continued)

Abnormal findings

+ Solid (macules, papules, nodules, wheals, and hives)
+ Fluid-filled (vesicles, bullae, pustules, and cysts)
+ Bluish green (fungal infection)
+ Asymmetrical lesion with an irregular border (malignancy)

KNOW-HOW

Evaluating skin turgor

To assess skin turgor in an adult, gently squeeze the skin on the forearm or sternoclavicular junction between your thumb and forefinger as shown. In an infant, roll a fold of loosely-adherent abdominal skin between your thumb and forefinger. Then release the skin.

If the skin quickly returns to its original shape, the patient has normal turgor. If it returns to its original shape slowly over 30 seconds, or maintains a tented position as shown, the skin has poor turgor.

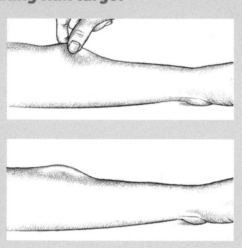

Whenever you see a lesion, evaluate it to determine its origin. Start by classifying it as primary or secondary. A primary lesion is the initial lesion that develops. Changes in a primary lesion then constitute a secondary lesion. Examples of secondary lesions include fissures, scales, crusts, scars, and excoriations. (See *Recognizing skin lesions*.)

Determine if the lesion is solid or fluid-filled by using a flashlight or penlight. (See *Illuminating lesions*, page 331.)

 ABNORMAL FINDINGS *Macules, papules, nodules, wheals, and hives are solid lesions. Vesicles, bullae, pustules, and cysts are fluid-filled lesions.*

To identify lesions that fluoresce, use a Wood's lamp, which gives out specially filtered ultraviolet light. Darken the room and shine the light on the lesion.

 ABNORMAL FINDINGS *If the patient's lesion looks bluish green, he has a fungal infection.*

After you've identified the type of lesion, you'll need to describe its characteristics, pattern, location, and distribution. A detailed description will help you determine whether the lesion is a normal or pathologic skin change.

Examine the lesion to see if it looks the same on both sides. Also, check the borders to see if they're regular or irregular.

 ABNORMAL FINDINGS *An asymmetrical lesion that has an irregular border may indicate malignancy.*

Lesions occur in various colors and can change color over time. Therefore, watch for such changes in your patient.

KNOW-HOW

Recognizing skin lesions

The illustrations below depict the most common primary and secondary lesions.

PRIMARY LESIONS

Bulla — Fluid-filled lesion that's more than ¾″ (2 cm) in diameter (also called a blister) — for example, severe poison oak or ivy dermatitis, bullous pemphigoid, second-degree burn

Comedo — Plugged pilosebaceous duct, exfoliative, formed from sebum and keratin — for example, blackhead (open comedo), whitehead (closed comedo)

Cyst — Semisolid or fluid-filled encapsulated mass extending deep into dermis (sebaceous cyst, cystic acne)

Macule — Flat, pigmented, circumscribed area that's less than ⅜″ (1 cm) in diameter — for example, freckle, rubella

Nodule — Firm, raised lesion that's deeper than a papule, that extends into the dermal layer, and that's ¼″ to ¾″ (0.5 to 2 cm) in diameter — for example, intradermal nevus

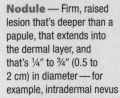

Papule — Firm, inflammatory, raised lesion that's up to ¼″ in diameter and may be the same color as skin or pigmented — for example, acne papule, lichen planus

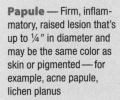

Patch — Flat, pigmented, circumscribed area that's more than ¾″ in diameter — for example, herald patch (pityriasis rosea)

Plaque — Circumscribed, solid, elevated lesion that's more than ⅜″ in diameter — for example, psoriasis (Elevation above skin surface occupies larger surface area in comparison with height.)

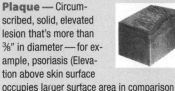

Pustule — Raised, circumscribed lesion that's usually less than ⅜″ in diameter and contains purulent material, making it a yellow-white color — for example, acne pustule, impetigo, furuncle

Tumor — Elevated solid lesion more than 2 cm in diameter, extending into dermal and subcutaneous layers (dermatofibroma)

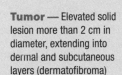

Vesicle — Raised, circumscribed, fluid-filled lesion that's less than ¼″ in diameter; for example, chickenpox, herpes simplex

Wheal — Raised, firm lesion (with intense localized skin edema) that varies in size, shape, and color (from pale pink to red) and disappears within hours — for example, hive (urticaria), insect bite

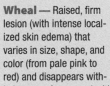

(continued)

Recognizing primary skin lesions

- ✦ Bulla — fluid-filled; also called a *blister*
- ✦ Patch — flat, pigmented, circumscribed
- ✦ Comedo — plugged pilosebaceous duct
- ✦ Plaque — circumscribed, solid, elevated
- ✦ Cyst — semisolid or fluid-filled
- ✦ Pustule — raised, circumscribed
- ✦ Macule — flat, pigmented, circumscribed
- ✦ Tumor — elevated, solid; extends into dermal and subcutaneous layer
- ✦ Nodule — firm, raised; deeper than papule into dermal layer
- ✦ Vesicle — raised, circumscribed, fluid-filled
- ✦ Papule — firm, inflammatory, raised; same color as skin or pigmented
- ✦ Wheal — raised, firm

Recognizing secondary skin lesions

+ Atrophy — thinning of skin surface
+ Lichenification — thickened, prominent markings
+ Crust — dried sebum, serous, sanguineous, or purulent exudate
+ Scale — thin, dry flakes; shedding
+ Erosion — circumscribed; loss of skin
+ Scar — red, raised, and fibrous tissue
+ Excoriation — linear scratched or abraded area
+ Ulcer — epidermal and dermal destruction
+ Fissure — linear cracking

Skin lesions
(continued)

Abnormal findings: Moles
+ Changing from tan or brown to multiple shades of tan, dark brown, black, or a mixture of red, white, and blue (malignancy)
+ Foul odor (superimposed infection)

Recognizing skin lesions *(continued)*

SECONDARY LESIONS

Atrophy — Thinning of skin surface at the site of the disorder — for example, striae, aging skin

Crust — Dried sebum, serous, sanguineous, or purulent exudate, overlying an erosion or weeping vesicle, bulla, or pustule — for example, impetigo

Erosion — Circumscribed lesion involving loss of superficial epidermis — for example, rug burn, abrasion

Excoriation — Linear scratched or abraded areas, commonly self-induced — for example, abraded acne lesions, eczema

Fissure — Linear cracking of the skin extending into the dermal layer — for example, hand dermatitis (chapped skin)

Lichenification — Thickened, prominent skin markings caused by constant rubbing — for example, chronic atopic dermatitis

Scale — Thin, dry flakes of shedding skin — for example, psoriasis, dry skin, neonate desquamation

Scar — Fibrous tissue (caused by trauma, deep inflammation, or surgical incision) that's red and raised when it's new, pink and flat for up to 6 weeks, and pale and depressed when it's old — for example, a healed surgical incision

Ulcer — Epidermal and dermal destruction that may extend into subcutaneous tissue and that usually heals with scarring — for example, pressure ulcer or stasis ulcer

---

ABNORMAL FINDINGS *If the patient has a lesion, such as a mole, that has changed from tan or brown to multiple shades of tan, dark brown, black, or a mixture of red, white, and blue, the lesion might be malignant.*

Pay close attention as well to the configuration and distribution of the lesion. Many skin diseases often have typical configuration patterns. Identifying those patterns will help you determine the cause of the problem. (See *Recognizing common lesion configurations,* page 332.)

Measure the exact diameter of the lesion using a centimeter/millimeter ruler. If you estimate the diameter, you may not be able to determine subtle changes in size. An increase in the size or elevation of a mole over a period of many years is common and probably normal. Still, be sure to note moles that change size rapidly.

If you note drainage, document the type, color, and amount.

KNOW-HOW

Illuminating lesions

Illuminating a lesion will enable you to assess it more clearly and learn more about its characteristics. Use these techniques when illuminating lesions.

MACULE OR PAPULE?
To determine whether a lesion is a macule or a papule, use this technique: Reduce direct light and shine a penlight or flashlight at a right angle to the lesion. If the light casts a shadow, the lesion is a papule. Macules are flat and don't produce a shadow.

SOLID OR FLUID-FILLED?
To determine whether a lesion is solid or fluid-filled, use this technique: Place the tip of a flashlight or penlight against the side of the lesion. Solid lesions don't transmit light. Fluid-filled lesions will transilluminate with a red glow.

 ABNORMAL FINDINGS *Note if the patient's lesion has a foul odor, which can indicate a superimposed infection.*

ASSESSING THE HAIR

Start by inspecting and palpating the hair over the patient's entire body, not just on his head. To palpate the patient's hair, rub a few strands between your index finger and thumb. Note the distribution, quantity, texture, and color. The quantity and distribution of head and body hair varies among patients. However, hair should be evenly distributed over the entire body.

 ABNORMAL FINDINGS *Sparse hair may indicate hypothyroidism; fine silky hair is seen in patients with hyperthyroidism.*

Check for patterns of hair loss and growth. If you notice patchy hair loss, look for regrowth. Also, examine the scalp for erythema, scaling, and encrustation. The only way to detect scalp-crusting is by using a Wood's lamp.

 ABNORMAL FINDINGS *Excessive hair loss with scalp-crusting may indicate ringworm infestation.*

Also, note areas of excessive hair growth.

 ABNORMAL FINDINGS *Excessive hair growth may indicate a hormone imbalance or be a systemic disorder such as Cushing's syndrome.*

The texture of scalp hair also varies among patients. As a rule, hair should be shiny and smooth, not dry or brittle. Differences in grooming and hairstyling may affect the texture and quality of the hair. Dryness or brittleness can result from the use of harsh hair treatments or hair care products, or it might be due to a systemic illness.

 ABNORMAL FINDINGS *Extremely oily hair is usually related to an excessive production of sebum or poor grooming habits.*

Illuminating lesions
+ Macule — doesn't cast a shadow
+ Papule — casts a shadow
+ Solid — doesn't transmit light
+ Fluid-filled — transilluminates with red glow

Assessing the hair
+ Inspect and palpate patient's hair (by rubbing a few strands between index finger and thumb) over his entire body
+ Note distribution, quality, texture, distribution, and color

Abnormal findings
+ Sparse hair (hypothyroidism)
+ Fine, silky hair (hyperthyroidism)
+ Excessive hair loss with scalp crusting (ringworm infestation)
+ Excessive hair growth (systemic disorder or Cushing's syndrome)
+ Extremely oily hair (excessive sebum production or poor grooming habits)

Recognizing common lesion configurations

- ✦ Discrete — separate and distinct
- ✦ Annular — single ring or circle
- ✦ Grouped — clusters
- ✦ Polycyclic — multiple circles
- ✦ Confluent — merging
- ✦ Arciform — arcs or curves
- ✦ Linear — line
- ✦ Reticular — meshlike network

KNOW-HOW

Recognizing common lesion configurations

Identify the configuration of your patient's skin lesion by matching it to one of these diagrams.

DISCRETE
Individual lesions are separate and distinct.

ANNULAR
Lesions are arranged in a single ring or circle.

GROUPED
Lesions are clustered together.

POLYCYCLIC
Lesions are arranged in multiple circles.

CONFLUENT
Lesions merge so that individual lesions aren't visible or palpable.

ARCIFORM
Lesions form arcs or curves.

LINEAR
Lesions form a line.

RETICULAR
Lesions form a meshlike network.

Assessing the nails

- ✦ Indicate systemic illness
- ✦ Reveal patient's grooming habits and self-care ability
- ✦ Detects color, shape, thickness, consistency, and contour

Special points
- ✦ Light-skinned patients generally have pinkish nails
- ✦ Dark-skinned patients generally have brown nails

ASSESSING THE NAILS

Assessing the nails is vital for two reasons: The appearance of nails can be a critical indicator of systemic illness, and their overall condition tells you a lot about the patient's grooming habits and self-care ability. Examine the nails for color, shape, thickness, consistency, and contour.

First, look at the color of the nails.

 SPECIAL POINTS *Light-skinned patients generally have pinkish nails. Dark-skinned patients generally have brown nails. Brown-pigmented bands in the nail beds are normal in dark-skinned people and abnormal in light-skinned people.*

KNOW-HOW

Evaluating clubbed fingers

In a patient whose fingers are clubbed, suspect hypoxia. When examining a patient's fingers for early clubbing, gently palpate the bases of the nails. Normally, they'll feel firm, but in early clubbing, they'll feel springy.

To evaluate clubbing, have the patient place the first phalanges of the forefingers together. Normal nail bases are concave and create a small, diamond-shaped space when the first phalanges are opposed, as shown.

LATE CLUBBING

In late clubbing, however, the now convex nail bases can touch without leaving a space, as shown. This condition is associated with pulmonary or cardiovascular disease. When you spot clubbed fingers, think about the possible causes, such as emphysema, chronic bronchitis, lung cancer, or congestive heart failure.

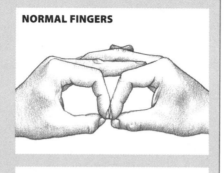

NORMAL FINGERS

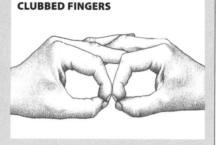

CLUBBED FINGERS

ABNORMAL FINDINGS *In patients who smoke cigarettes, yellow nails may occur as a result of nicotine stains.*

Nail beds can be used to assess a patient's peripheral circulation (capillary refill). Press on the nail bed and then release, noting how long the color takes to return. It should return immediately, or at most within 3 seconds.

Next inspect the shape and contour of the nails. The surface of the nail bed should be either slightly curved or flat. The edges of the nail should be smooth, rounded, and clean.

The normal angle of the nail base is 160 degrees.

ABNORMAL FINDINGS *An increase in the nail angle may suggest clubbing. With clubbed fingers, the proximal edge of the nail elevates so the angle is greater than 180 degrees. The nail is also thickened and curved at the end, and the distal phalanx looks rounder and wider than normal. To check for clubbing, view the index finger in profile and note the angle of the nail base. (See Evaluating clubbed fingers.)*

Clubbing is typically a sign of pulmonary or cardiovascular disease, such as emphysema, chronic bronchitis, lung cancer, or heart failure. Although it may also result from such hepatic and GI disorders as cirrhosis, Crohn's disease, and ulcerative colitis, it occurs only rarely in these disorders. So, first check the patient for more common signs and symptoms.

SPECIAL POINTS *In children, clubbing is most common in those with cyanotic congenital heart disease and cystic fibrosis. Surgical correction of heart defects may reverse clubbing.*

Evaluating clubbed fingers

- ✦ Palpate base of nails; springy nails signal clubbing
- ✦ Evaluate by having patient place the first phalanges of the forefingers together
- ✦ Late clubbing reveals increase in nail angle

Assessing the nails
(continued)

Abnormal findings
- ✦ Increased nail angle suggests clubbing
- ✦ Thickened and curved nail; distal phalanx looks round and wide
- ✦ Results from pulmonary or cardiovascular disease; less commonly from hepatic and GI disorders

Special points
- ✦ In children, clubbing most commonly occurs with cyanotic congenital heart disease and cystic fibrosis
- ✦ In elderly patients, arthritic deformities may disguise clubbing

In elderly patients, arthritic deformities of the fingers or toes may disguise the presence of clubbing.

Curved nails are a normal variation. They may appear to be clubbed until you determine that the nail angle is still 160 degrees or less.

Finally, palpate the nail bed to check the thickness of the nail and the strength of its attachment to the bed.

INTERPRETING YOUR FINDINGS

After you assess the patient, a group of findings may lead you to suspect a particular disorder. (See *The skin, hair, and nails: Interpreting your findings.*)

SKIN, HAIR, AND NAIL DISORDERS

Skin, hair, and nail disorders are classified according to cause, location, or type of lesion. Sometimes, two patients with the same diagnosis will have very different signs and symptoms, and two patients with the same signs and symptoms will have different diagnoses. Carefully document all signs and symptoms, pertinent health history, and as much information as possible from the physical examination.

SKIN DISORDERS

The signs and symptoms you detect during your assessment may be caused by a wide variety of skin disorders. This section describes the most common dermatoses, infestations, pigmentation disorders, skin lesions, and viral, bacterial, and fungal infections.

Allergic disorders

These disorders result from allergic reactions and include atopic eczema, contact dermatitis, and urticaria.

Atopic eczema

Also known as *atopic dermatitis*, atopic eczema occurs in infants and adults. Generally, the patient has a family history of allergies and may have a single episode or chronic occurrences. Lesions usually appear on the scalp, forehead, cheeks, backs of the knees, and the arms, especially on the antecubital flexure.

Primary lesions include erythematous papules and vesicles that weep and ooze. Crusting may also occur. In chronic occurrences, a thickening, or lichenification, may occur in the antecubital fossa and the popliteal fossae. Primary signs and symptoms include itching and extreme irritability.

Contact dermatitis

Contact dermatitis is an inflammation of the skin resulting from contact with certain irritants or allergenic substances. It can develop on any area of the body as a result of contact with soaps, deodorants, creams, shampoos, clothing, jewelry, or plants.

Primary lesions include red macules that appear as localized areas of redness, vesicles, and large, oozing bullae. Secondary lesions, such as crusting and excoriations, can result from bacterial infections. Primary symptoms include itching and burning.

Skin, hair, and nail disorders

Skin disorders

+ Most common include dermatoses, infestations, pigmentation disorders, skin lesions, and viral, bacterial, and fungal infections

Facts about allergic disorders

+ Atopic eczema, contact dermatitis, urticaria

Atopic eczema

+ Occurs in infants and adults
+ Family history of allergies, single episodes, or chronic occurrences
+ Itching and extreme irritability

Contact dermatitis

+ Inflammation of skin resulting from contact with irritants or allergenic substances
+ Develops on any area of the body
+ Causes primary and secondary lesions

The skin, hair, and nails:
Interpreting your findings

The chart below shows common groups of findings for the signs and symptoms of disorders of the hair, skin, and nails, along with their probable causes.

SIGN OR SYMPTOM AND FINDINGS	PROBABLE CAUSE
Alopecia	
✦ Patchy alopecia, typically on the lower extremities ✦ Thin, shiny, atrophic skin ✦ Thickened nails ✦ Weak or absent peripheral pulses ✦ Cool extremities ✦ Paresthesia	✦ Arterial insufficiency
✦ Translucent, charred, or ulcerated skin ✦ Pain	✦ Burns
✦ Loss of the outer one-third of the eyebrows ✦ Thin, dull, coarse, brittle hair on the face, scalp, and genitals ✦ Fatigue ✦ Constipation ✦ Cold intolerance ✦ Weight gain ✦ Puffy face, hands, and feet	✦ Hypothyroidism
Clubbing	
✦ Anorexia ✦ Malaise ✦ Dyspnea ✦ Tachypnea ✦ Diminished breath sounds ✦ Pursed-lip breathing ✦ Barrel chest ✦ Peripheral cyanosis	✦ Emphysema
✦ Wheezing ✦ Dyspnea ✦ Fatigue ✦ Neck vein distention ✦ Palpitations ✦ Unexplained weight gain ✦ Dependent edema ✦ Crackles on auscultation	✦ Heart failure
✦ Hemoptysis ✦ Dyspnea ✦ Wheezing ✦ Chest pain ✦ Fatigue ✦ Weight loss ✦ Fever	✦ Lung and pleural cancer

(continued)

The skin, hair, and nails: Interpreting your findings *(continued)*

SIGN OR SYMPTOM AND FINDINGS	PROBABLE CAUSE
Pruritus	
✦ Intense, severe pruritus ✦ Erythematous rash on dry skin at flexion points ✦ Possible edema, scaling, and pustules	✦ Atopic dermatitis
✦ Scalp excoriation from scratching ✦ Matted, foul-smelling, lusterless hair ✦ Occipital and cervical lymphadenopathy ✦ Oval, gray-white nits on hair shafts	✦ Pediculosis capitis (head lice)
✦ Gradual or sudden pruritus ✦ Ammonia breath odor ✦ Oliguria or anuria ✦ Fatigue ✦ Irritability ✦ Muscle cramps	✦ Chronic renal failure
Urticaria	
✦ Rapid eruption of diffuse urticaria and angioedema, with wheals ranging from pinpoint to palm-size or larger ✦ Pruritic, stinging lesions ✦ Profound anxiety ✦ Weakness ✦ Shortness of breath ✦ Nasal congestion ✦ Dysphagia ✦ Warm, moist skin	✦ Anaphylaxis
✦ Nonpitting, nonpruritic edema of an extremity or the face ✦ Possibly acute laryngeal edema	✦ Hereditary angioedema
✦ Erythema chronicum migrans that results in urticaria ✦ Constant malaise and fatigue ✦ Fever ✦ Chills ✦ Lymphadenopathy ✦ Neurologic and cardiac abnormalities ✦ Arthritis	✦ Lyme disease

Facts about allergic disorders *(continued)*

Urticaria
✦ Commonly known as *hives*
✦ Caused by allergies, cancer, hyperthyroidism, and juvenile rheumatoid arthritis

Urticaria

Commonly known as *hives*, urticaria is typically acute, though you may also see the chronic form in patients. Commonly caused by allergies, chronic and acute urticaria can also result from cancer, hyperthyroidism, and juvenile rheumatoid arthritis.

Primary lesions range from small, red papules to larger circular patterns with red borders. In severe cases, you may see vesicles and bullae. The lesions usually subside on their own, though treatment may be necessary.

Vascular disorders

Vascular disorders can occur in many forms, each of which produces some type of lesion. The most common vascular disorders are cherry angioma, port-wine hemangioma, purpuric lesions, and telangiectases.

Cherry angioma

Cherry angiomas are tiny, bright red, round papules that may become brown with time. Cherry angiomas commonly occur on the trunk, but may also appear on the extremities.

 SPECIAL POINTS *Cherry angiomas are clinically insignificant lesions that occur in virtually everyone older than age 30 and increase in number with age.*

Port-wine hemangioma

Port-wine hemangioma, commonly called *port-wine stains,* are usually present at birth and commonly appear on the face and upper body as flat purple marks.

Purpuric lesions

Purpuric lesions are caused by red blood cells and blood pigments in the skin, so they don't blanch under pressure. The three types of purpuric lesions are:
+ petechiae — red or brown pinpoint lesions generally caused by capillary fragility
+ ecchymoses — bluish discolorations resulting from blood accumulation in the skin after injury to the vessel walls
+ hematoma — masses of blood that accumulate in a tissue, organ, or body space after a break in a blood vessel.

Purpuric lesions also produce deep red or reddish purple bruising that may be caused by bleeding disorders such as disseminated intravascular coagulation.

Telangiectases

Permanently dilated, small blood vessels, telangiectases typically form a weblike pattern. For example, spider hemangiomas, a type of telangiectasis, are small, red lesions arranged in a weblike configuration. They usually appear on the face, neck, and chest and may be normal or associated with pregnancy or cirrhosis.

Bacterial infections

Two bacterial infections associated with the skin are impetigo and cellulitis.

Impetigo

The bacterial infection you'll observe most often is impetigo. It's a superficial infection caused by bacteria from group A beta-hemolytic streptococci or *Staphylococcus.* Primary lesions range from small vesicles to large bullae that, when ruptured, ooze a honey-colored serous fluid that can become purulent.

Crusts typically form as secondary lesions. These lesions usually occur on the face, especially near the nose and mouth, though they may also occur in the creases of the hands and elsewhere.

Impetigo is contagious and may spread to other parts of the patient's body or to other family members through primary or secondary contact.

SPECIAL POINTS *Impetigo usually affects children.*

Facts about vascular disorders

+ Cherry angioma, port-wine hemangioma, purpuric lesions, and telangiectases

Cherry angioma
+ Tiny, bright red, round papules
+ May become brown with time
+ Occur on the trunk and extremities
+ Occurring in virtually everyone over age 30; numbers increase with age

Port-wine hemangioma
+ Present at birth
+ Appear on the face and upper body as flat, purple marks

Purpuric lesions
+ Caused by red blood cells and blood pigments
+ Three types — petechiae, ecchymoses, and hematoma

Telangiectases
+ Permanently dilated, small blood vessels
+ Form a weblike pattern
+ Appear on face, neck, and chest

Facts about bacterial infections

+ Include impetigo and cellulitis

Impetigo
+ Superficial infection caused by bacteria from group A beta-hemolytic streptococci or *Staphylococcus*
+ Primary lesions range from small vesicles to large bullae
+ Contagious, spread through primary or secondary contact
+ Usually affects children

Facts about bacterial infections
(continued)

Cellulitis
- ✦ Diffuse inflammation of subcutaneous tissue
- ✦ Appears around a break in the skin
- ✦ Tender, warm, erythematous, swollen area

Facts about fungal infections
- ✦ Most commonly include candidiasis and tinea infection

Candidiasis
- ✦ Occur in the mouth as thrush and on skin, resulting in scalding, red, moist patches
- ✦ Occur in the vagina, causing milklike discharge

Tinea infections
- ✦ Include tinea corporis, cruris, capitis, pedis, and unguium
- ✦ Appear as papular, pustular, vesicular, erythematous, or scaling lesions

Facts about viral infections
- ✦ Herpes simplex, herpes zoster, and warts

Herpes simplex
- ✦ Recurrent virus with eruption of vesicles or fever blister
- ✦ Two strains including Type 1 (mouth) and Type 2 (genital)

Herpes zoster
- ✦ Also known as *shingles*
- ✦ Severe deep pain, pruritus, and paresthesia or hyperesthesia develop
- ✦ Caused by same virus as chickenpox

Cellulitis

A diffuse inflammation of the subcutaneous tissue, cellulitis commonly appears around a break in the skin—usually around fresh wounds or small puncture sites. Infection spreads rapidly through the lymphatic system and destroys the skin.

This disorder usually results from infection by group A beta-hemolytic streptococci. It may also result from infection by other streptococci, *S. aureus,* or *Haemophilus influenzae.*

Signs and symptoms include a tender, warm, erythematous, swollen area, which is usually well-demarcated. A warm, red, tender streak that follows the course of a lymph vessel may appear. The patient may experience fever, chills, headache, and malaise.

Fungal infections

Candidiasis and tinea infections are the most common fungal infections.

Candidiasis

Candidiasis causes lesions in the mouth, vagina, and the diaper area in infants. Candidiasis of the mouth, or thrush, appears as whitish flakes on reddened mucous membranes. You may also note fissures in the corners of the patient's mouth.

Candidiasis of the skin, or diaper rash, occurs as scalding, red, moist patches with sharply demarcated borders and loose scales in the genital area. Candidiasis of the vagina, or vulvovaginitis, causes the same signs and symptoms plus a milklike discharge.

Tinea infections

Tinea infections are noncandidal fungal infections that involve the stratum corneum, nails, and hair. The lesions are usually classified according to anatomic location and can occur on:
- ✦ nonhairy parts of the body (tinea corporis)
- ✦ the groin and inner thigh (tinea cruris)
- ✦ the scalp (tinea capitis)
- ✦ the feet (tinea pedis)
- ✦ the nails (tinea unguium).

The lesions vary in appearance and may be papular, pustular, vesicular, erythematous, or scaling. They usually develop into circular or oval lesions with scaling borders.

Viral infections

The viral infections you're mostly likely to see include herpes simplex, herpes zoster, and warts.

Herpes simplex

Herpes simplex is a recurrent virus characterized by an acute, moderately painful eruption of a single group of vesicles or a fever blister. The vesicles progress to pustules and then crust. The patient may experience tingling and sensitivity around the mouth before the vesicles erupt or blister.

Herpes simplex occurs in two strains: Type 1 and Type 2. If the patient has a fever blister near his mouth, he has Type 1; if the lesion appears in the genital area, he has Type 2, a sexually transmitted infection.

Herpes zoster

Herpes zoster, or *shingles,* is probably caused by the same virus that causes chickenpox, the varicella virus. Onset of herpes zoster is characterized by fever and malaise. Within 2 to 4 days, severe deep pain, pruritus, and paresthesia or hyperesthesia develop, usually on the trunk and occasionally on the arms and legs. Pain may be continuous or intermittent. Small, red, nodular skin lesions then usually erupt on the painful areas and commonly spread unilaterally around the thorax or vertically over the arms and legs. They quickly become vesicles filled with clear fluid or pus. About 10 days after they appear, the vesicles dry and form scabs.

Warts

The growths known as *warts,* or *verrucae,* are caused by papillomavirus. The clinical diagnosis of warts varies, depending on their appearance and location.
+ Common wart — Also called a *verruca vulgaris,* this rough, elevated wart appears most commonly on the extremities, particularly the hands and fingers.
+ Condyloma acuminatum — Also called *genital warts,* this sexually transmitted infection appears on the penis, scrotum, vulva, and anus.
+ Filiform wart — This stalklike, horny projection commonly occurs around the face and neck.
+ Flat wart — these warts are common on the face, neck, chest, knees, dorsa of hands, wrists, and flexor surfaces of the forearms.
+ Periungual wart — This rough wart occurs around the edges of fingernails and toenails.
+ Plantar wart — This wart appears on the foot, and can be slightly elevated or flat.

Skin tumors

Common skin tumors include basal cell carcinoma, squamous cell carcinoma, malignant melanomas, and Kaposi's sarcoma.

Basal cell carcinoma

Basal cell carcinoma, which is the most common skin cancer, grows slowly and doesn't metastasize. It's caused by sun exposure and usually occurs on the head and neck. The most common type of basal cell carcinoma, nodulo-ulcerative, produces a small, waxy-looking nodule that ulcerates, forming a central depression. Histologic studies should be done whenever basal cell carcinoma is suspected.

Squamous cell carcinoma

Squamous cell carcinoma, a malignant skin cancer, is usually caused by direct exposure to the sun. Characterized by a raised border and a central ulcer, squamous cell carcinomas vary from fast-growing lesions to slowly developing raised growths. The degree of metastasis and malignancy also varies. This cancer can develop on any area, but it's especially common on the face and neck.

Malignant melanoma

Malignant melanomas usually appear as black or purple nodules, though some are pink or red. They may have irregular or notched borders and a scaling, flaking, or oozing texture. They can develop anywhere on the body.

Some melanomas result from repeated sun exposure, but they're more common in patients who have had a single, severe, blistering sunburn as children. Because most melanomas develop from preexisting nevi, always document changes in the size, symmetry, border, and color of nevi as well as associated erythema.

It's important to remember the "ABCDEs" for melanoma:
+ A for asymmetry
+ B for irregular borders
+ C for color variation or change
+ D for diameter larger than 6 mm
+ E for elevation.

**Facts about
skin tumors**
(continued)

Kaposi's sarcoma
✦ Multiple hemorrhagic sarcoma
✦ Appears as multiple bluish red or brown nodules and plaques
✦ Patients infected with HIV have significantly different pattern

**Facts about other
skin disorders**
✦ Most common include acne, psoriasis, scabies, seborrheic keratoses, and vitiligo

Acne
✦ Most common skin problem of adolescence
✦ Results from oversecretion of sebaceous glands
✦ Appears on face, chest, back, and shoulders
✦ Cystic acne produces scars

Psoriasis
✦ Papulosquamous disorder
✦ Chronic, recurrent disease of keratin synthesis
✦ Appears on elbows, knees, and scalp

Scabies
✦ Caused by mite burrowing under skin
✦ Results in extreme itching interfering with sleep
✦ Common in school-age children

Seborrheic keratoses
✦ Pigmented, raised, wartlike lesions
✦ Can become malignant
✦ Common in elderly people; caused by skin changes due to aging

Vitiligo
✦ Complete absence of melanin pigment

Kaposi's sarcoma

This multiple hemorrhagic sarcoma usually begins on the feet and ankles. Initially, you'll notice multiple bluish red or brown nodules and plaques. Visceral lesions may develop later.

Patients infected with human immunodeficiency virus have a significantly different pattern of Kaposi's sarcoma. In these patients, the lesions are small, pink papules that usually occur on the temple or beard area, but can occur anywhere. Lesions develop into raised papules or thickened, oval plaques that vary from red to brown. In advanced stages, violet-colored tumors cover the nose and face.

Other skin disorders

Other common skin disorders you might encounter include acne, psoriasis, scabies, seborrheic keratoses, and vitiligo.

Acne

Acne, which results from oversecretion of the sebaceous glands, is the most common skin problem in adolescents. It usually appears on the face, chest, back, and shoulders. The appearance of acne varies. If the acne plug doesn't protrude from the follicle and is covered by the epidermis, it may appear as a closed comedo, or whitehead. If the acne plug protrudes and isn't covered by the epidermis, it may appear as an open comedo, or blackhead. The patient may develop characteristic acne pustules, papules, or in severe forms, acne cysts or abscesses. Cystic acne produces scars. (See *Understanding acne.*)

Psoriasis

The most common papulosquamous disorder you're likely to detect during your assessment is psoriasis. A chronic, recurrent disease of keratin synthesis, psoriasis commonly appears on the patient's elbows, knees, and scalp. Primary lesions consist of well-circumscribed, dry, silvery, scaling papules and plaques. About one-half of all patients with psoriasis also have pitting or thickening of the skin on the elbows and knees. The tendency to develop psoriasis is genetically determined.

Scabies

Scabies is caused by a mite that burrows under the skin.

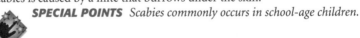 **SPECIAL POINTS** *Scabies commonly occurs in school-age children.*

It causes extreme itching that intensifies at night and is characterized by vesicles and excoriation over the burrow sites. The most common areas for infestation are the finger webs, flexor surface of the wrists, and antecubital fossae.

Seborrheic keratoses

Seborrheic keratoses are pigmented, raised, wartlike lesions that appear primarily on the face and trunk. They must be distinguished from actinic keratoses, which are faint red and scaly. Seborrheic keratoses, which gradually enlarge and occur mainly on sun-exposed areas, can become malignant.

 SPECIAL POINTS *Seborrheic keratoses are common in elderly people and are caused by changes in the skin due to aging.*

Vitiligo

Vitiligo is the complete absence of melanin pigment and leads to patchy areas of white or light skin. It most commonly appears on the face, neck, hands, feet, body folds, and around orifices. It can occur in any patient but is usually seen in dark-skinned people.

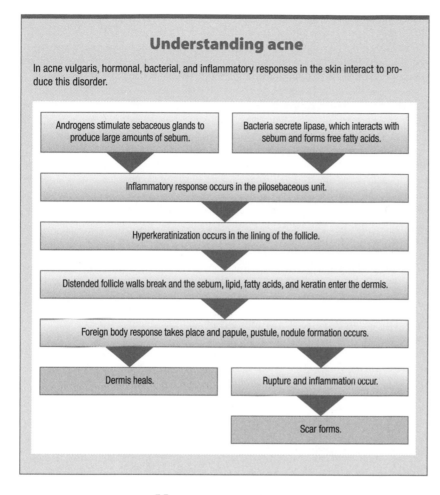

Understanding acne

In acne vulgaris, hormonal, bacterial, and inflammatory responses in the skin interact to produce this disorder.

Androgens stimulate sebaceous glands to produce large amounts of sebum.

Bacteria secrete lipase, which interacts with sebum and forms free fatty acids.

Inflammatory response occurs in the pilosebaceous unit.

Hyperkeratinization occurs in the lining of the follicle.

Distended follicle walls break and the sebum, lipid, fatty acids, and keratin enter the dermis.

Foreign body response takes place and papule, pustule, nodule formation occurs.

Dermis heals.

Rupture and inflammation occur.

Scar forms.

Understanding acne
+ Occurs from hormonal, bacterial, and inflammatory responses
+ Distended follicle walls break with sebum entering dermis
+ Androgens stimulate sebaceous glands
+ Nodules form
+ Dermis heals or ruptures
+ Scar forms

Hair disorders
+ Stem from other problems, causing emotional distress
+ Include alopecia, folliculitis, hirsutism, pediculosis, and tinea capitis

Facts about alopecia
+ Known as *hair loss,* usually affects the scalp
+ In nonscarring form, hair follicle generally regrows
+ Scarring form destroys hair follicle (irreversible)

HAIR DISORDERS

Commonly stemming from other problems, hair disorders can cause patients emotional distress. Among the most common hair abnormalities are alopecia, folliculitis, hirsutism, pediculosis, and tinea capitis.

Alopecia

Also known as *hair loss,* alopecia usually affects the scalp. It's rarer and less conspicuous elsewhere on the body. In the nonscarring form of this disorder (noncicatricial alopecia), the hair follicle can generally regrow hair. However, scarring alopecia usually destroys the hair follicle, making hair loss irreversible.

The most common form of nonscarring alopecia, male pattern alopecia, appears to be related to androgen levels, aging, and genetic predisposition.

Other forms of nonscarring alopecia include alopecia areata, physiologic alopecia, and trichotillomania.

+ Alopecia areata — an idiopathic form of alopecia that's usually reversible and self-limiting. It occurs most commonly in young and middle-aged adults of both sexes.
+ Physiologic alopecia — usually temporary, occurring as sudden hair loss in infants, loss of straight hairline in adolescents, and diffuse hair loss after childbirth.

✦ Trichotillomania—compulsive pulling out of one's own hair, most common in children.

Scarring alopecia may result from physical or chemical trauma or chronic tension on a hair shaft, such as braiding or rolling the hair. Diseases that produce scarring alopecia include destructive skin tumors, granulomas, lupus erythematosus, scleroderma, follicular lichen planus, and severe bacterial or viral infections, such as folliculitis or herpes simplex.

In male pattern alopecia, hair loss is gradual and usually affects the thinner, shorter, and less pigmented hairs of the scalp's frontal and parietal portions. In women, hair loss is generally more diffuse; completely bald areas are uncommon but may occur.

Alopecia areata affects small patches of the scalp but may also occur as alopecia totalis, which involves the entire scalp, or as alopecia universalis, which involves the entire body. Although mild erythema may occur initially, affected areas of scalp or skin appear normal. "Exclamation point" hairs occur at the periphery of new patches. Regrowth initially appears as fine, white, downy hair, which is replaced by normal hair.

In trichotillomania, patchy, incomplete areas of hair loss with many broken hairs appear on the scalp but may occur on other areas, such as the eyebrows.

Folliculitis

Facts about folliculitis

✦ Superficial infection of the hair follicle caused by staphylococci
✦ Infects hair bulb; characterized by multiple pustules

A superficial infection of the hair follicle, folliculitis is usually caused by staphylococci. This infection can extend to the hair bulb and is characterized by multiple pustules with hair visible at the center and an erythematous base. It usually occurs on the arms, legs, face, and buttocks.

Hirsutism

Facts about hirsutism

✦ Excessive hairiness in women
✦ Develops on body and face

Excessive hairiness in women, or hirsutism, can develop on the body and face, affecting the patient's self-image. Localized hirsutism may occur on pigmented nevi. Generalized hirsutism can result from drug therapy or from endocrine problems, such as Cushing's syndrome and acromegaly.

Pediculosis

Facts about pediculosis

✦ Lice infestation usually occurring on the scalp
✦ Causes itching and scratching
✦ Common in children; spreads easily in school and day-care centers

Pediculosis, or lice infestation, usually occurs on the scalp but can occur anywhere that the patient has hair. Although you may not see the mites themselves, you'll most likely see their eggs (nits) in the patient's hair. This disorder causes itching and scratching and affects people of all ages. It usually results from crowded living conditions or lack of cleanliness.

 SPECIAL POINTS *In children, head lice is particularly common and spreads easily in schools and day-care centers.*

Tinea capitis

Facts about tinea capitis

✦ Fungal infection involving hair
✦ Causes rounded, patchy hair loss on scalp

Tinea capitis, a fungal infection that involves the hair, causes rounded, patchy hair loss on the scalp and leaves broken hairs, pustules, and scales on the skin.

NAIL DISORDERS

Nail disorders

✦ Point to serious underlying problems

Although many nail abnormalities are harmless, some point to serious underlying problems. Common nail problems include Beau's lines, koilonychia, onycholysis, paronychia, and Terry's nails.

Beau's lines

Beau's lines are transverse depressions in the nail that extend to the nail bed. They occur with acute illness, malnutrition, anemia, and trauma that temporarily impairs nail function. A dent appears first at the cuticle and then moves forward as the nail grows.

Koilonychia

Koilonychia refers to thin, spoon-shaped nails with lateral edges that tilt upward, forming a concave profile. The nails are white and opaque. This condition is associated with hypochromic anemia, chronic infections, Raynaud's disease, and malnutrition.

Onycholysis

Onycholysis is the loosening of the nail plate with separation from the nail bed, which begins at the distal groove. It's associated with minor trauma to long fingernails and disease processes, such as psoriasis, contact dermatitis, hyperthyroidism, and *Pseudomonas* or fungal infections.

Paronychia

Causing red, swollen, tender inflammation of the nail folds, acute paronychia is usually caused by a bacterial infection. Chronic paronychia is usually caused by a fungal infection that results from a break in the cuticle; it's an occupational hazard of people whose jobs involve frequently submerging their hands in water.

Terry's nails

Terry's nails are characterized by transverse bands of white that cover the nail, except for a narrow zone at the distal end. Terry's nails are associated with hypoalbuminemia.

Facts about Beau's lines
- Transverse depressions in nail
- Occurs with acute illness, malnutrition, anemia, and trauma

Facts about koilonychia
- Thin, spoon-shaped nails with lateral edges that tilt upward
- Associated with hypochromic anemia, chronic infections, Raynaud's disease, and malnutrition

Facts about onycholysis
- Loosening of nail plate with separation from nail bed
- Associated with minor trauma to long fingernails and disease processes or fungal infections

Facts about paronychia
- Causes red, swollen, tender inflammation of nail folds
- Usually caused by bacterial infection

Facts about Terry's nails
- Transverse bands of white covering the nail
- Associated with hypoalbuminemia

Eyes

A LOOK AT THE EYES

About 70% of all sensory information reaches the brain through the eyes. Disorders in vision can interfere with a patient's ability to function independently, perceive the world, and enjoy beauty.

A thorough assessment of your patient's eyes and vision can help you identify vision problems that can affect the patient's health and quality of life. In many cases, early detection can lead to successful, sight-saving treatment.

Fewer people lose their sight from infections or injuries today than in the past. Still, the overall incidence of blindness is rising as the population ages. Primary causes of vision loss include diabetic retinopathy, glaucoma, cataracts, and macular degeneration—conditions more common in elderly patients than younger ones.

Younger people can lose their sight due to opportunistic infections associated with human immunodeficiency virus and acquired immunodeficiency syndrome. The opportunistic infections toxoplasmosis and cytomegalovirus retinitis commonly cause blindness. Other vision disorders that may limit a person's ability to function include strabismus, amblyopia, and refractory errors.

EYE STRUCTURES

The sensory organ of sight, the eye transmits visual images to the brain for interpretation. The eyeball is about 1″ (2.5 cm) in diameter and occupies the bony orbit, a skull cavity formed anteriorly by the frontal, maxillary, zygomatic, acromial, sphenoid, ethmoid, and palatine bones. Nerves, adipose tissue, and blood vessels cushion and nourish the eye posteriorly.

Extraocular (external) and intraocular (internal) structures form the eye, and extraocular muscles and nerves control it.

Extraocular nerves, muscles, and structures

Six cranial nerves—the optic (II), oculomotor (III), trochlear (IV), trigeminal (V), abducens (VI), and facial (VII)—innervate the eye, ocular muscles, and lacrimal apparatus.

Reviewing extraocular muscles and structures

The extraocular muscles and structures work together to support and protect the eyes.

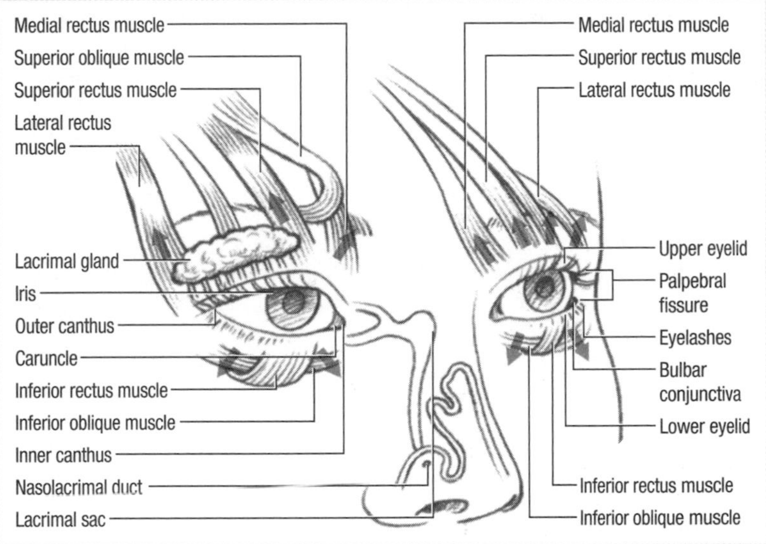

Medial rectus muscle
Superior oblique muscle
Superior rectus muscle
Lateral rectus muscle
Lacrimal gland
Iris
Outer canthus
Caruncle
Inferior rectus muscle
Inferior oblique muscle
Inner canthus
Nasolacrimal duct
Lacrimal sac

Medial rectus muscle
Superior rectus muscle
Lateral rectus muscle
Upper eyelid
Palpebral fissure
Eyelashes
Bulbar conjunctiva
Lower eyelid
Inferior rectus muscle
Inferior oblique muscle

The coordinated action of six eye muscles—the superior, inferior, medial, and lateral rectus muscles, and the superior and inferior oblique muscles—controls eye movement. Extraocular structures—the eyelids, conjunctivae, and lacrimal apparatus—protect and lubricate the eye. (See *Reviewing extraocular muscles and structures.*)

Extraocular muscles

By functioning together, the extraocular muscles hold both eyes parallel and create binocular vision. The superior and inferior rectus muscles move the eye up and down on a transverse axis; the medial and lateral rectus muscles move the eye toward the nose and toward the temple on an anteroposterior axis; and the superior and inferior oblique muscles move the eye to the right and left on a vertical axis.

Extraocular structures

The eyelids, conjunctivae, and lacrimal apparatus form the eye's extraocular structures.

Eyelids

Also called *palpebrae*, the eyelids are loose folds of skin covering the anterior eye. The eyelids protect the eye from foreign bodies, regulate the entrance of light, and distribute tears over the eye by blinking. The lid margins contain hair follicles, which in turn contain eyelashes and sebaceous glands. When closed, the upper and lower eyelids cover the eye completely. When open, the upper eyelid extends beyond the limbus (the junction of the cornea and the sclera) and covers a small portion of the iris. The lower lid margin lies even with, or just below, the limbus. The

Extraocular nerves, muscles, and structures
(continued)

✦ Action of six eye muscles controls movement
✦ Extraocular structures protect and lubricate eye

Extraocular muscles
✦ Hold eyes parallel, creating binocular vision
✦ Move eye up and down; toward nose and temple; and right to left

Extraocular structures
✦ Include eyelids, conjunctivae, and lacrimal apparatus

Eyelids
✦ Loose folds of skin covering the anterior eye
✦ Protect eye from foreign bodies
✦ Regulate light
✦ Distribute tears

Conjunctivae
◆ Transparent mucous membranes protect eye
◆ Glands secrete sebum, retain tears, and keep eye lubricated

Lacrimal apparatus
◆ Lubricates and protects the cornea and conjunctivae
◆ Tears drain through the punctum, then into the nose

Intraocular structures
◆ Easily visible structures include the sclera, cornea, anterior chamber, iris, and pupil
◆ Ophthalmoscope reveals aqueous humor, lens, ciliary body, vitreous humor, retina, and choroid

Sclera, choroid, and vitreous humor
◆ Sclera — white coating maintains eye size and shape
◆ Choroid — arteries and veins maintains blood supply
◆ Vitreous humor — gelatinous material maintains retina's placement and eyeball's shape

Bulbar conjunctiva and cornea
◆ Bulbar conjunctiva — transparent membrane protects anterior portion of the white sclera
◆ Cornea — avascular, transparent tissue refracts light rays

palpebral fissure, which is the distance between the lid margins, should be equal in both eyes.

Conjunctivae

Serving to protect the eye from foreign bodies, the conjunctivae are transparent mucous membranes extending from the lid margins. The palpebral conjunctiva lines the highly vascular eyelids and, therefore, appears shiny pink or red. The bulbar conjunctiva, which contains many small, normally visible blood vessels, joins the palpebral portion and covers the sclera up to the limbus.

A small, fleshy elevation called the *caruncle* sits at the nasal aspect of the conjunctivae. The tarsal plates are lined posteriorly by conjunctivae and contain meibomian glands in vertical columns, which create the appearance of light yellow streaks. These glands secrete sebum (made up of keratin, fat, and cellular debris) onto the posterior lid margins to retain tears and keep the eye lubricated.

Lacrimal apparatus

The lacrimal apparatus (which consists of the lacrimal glands, the punctum, the lacrimal sac, and the nasolacrimal duct) lubricates and protects the cornea and the conjunctivae by producing and absorbing tears.

After washing across the eyeball, the tears drain through the punctum. The punctum, which is the only visible portion of the lacrimal apparatus, is a tiny opening at the medial junction of the upper and lower eyelids. From there, the tears flow through the lacrimal canals into the lacrimal sac. They then drain through the nasolacrimal duct and into the nose.

Intraocular structures

Easily visible anterior intraocular structures include the sclera, cornea, anterior chamber, iris, and pupil. Other intraocular structures are visible only with the use of an ophthalmoscope or other instrument. These include the aqueous humor, lens, ciliary body, vitreous humor, retina, and choroid. The eye must be surgically rotated in order to see the posterior sclera. (See *Anatomic structures of the eye.*)

With ophthalmoscopic (funduscopic) examination of the posterior portion of the eye (the fundus), you can view the retinal blood vessels, the optic disk, the physiologic cup of the optic disk, the macula, and the fovea centralis.

Sclera, choroid, and vitreous humor

The white coating on the outside of the eyeball, the sclera, maintains the eye's size and shape. The choroid, which lines the recessed portion of the eyeball beneath the sclera, contains a network of arteries and veins that maintain blood supply to the eye. The vitreous humor is a thick, gelatinous material that fills the space directly behind the lens and maintains the retina's placement and the eyeball's spherical shape.

Bulbar conjunctiva and cornea

A thin, transparent membrane, the bulbar conjunctiva lines the eyelids and covers and protects the anterior portion of the white sclera. The cornea is a smooth, avascular, transparent tissue that merges with the sclera at the limbus. It refracts, or bends, light rays entering the eye.

The cornea, which is located in front of the pupil and iris, is fed by the ophthalmic branch of cranial nerve V (the trigeminal nerve). Stimulation of this nerve initiates a protective blink, the corneal reflex.

Iris

The iris is a circular, contractile diaphragm that contains smooth and radial muscles and is perforated in the center by the pupil. Varying amounts of pigment gran-

Anatomic structures of the eye

This cross section details important anatomic structures of the eye.

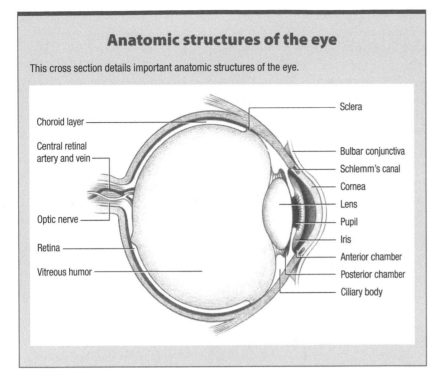

ules within the smooth muscle fibers give it color. Its posterior portion contains involuntary muscles that control pupil size and regulate the amount of light entering the eye.

Pupil
The iris's central opening, the pupil is normally round and equal in size to the opposite pupil. The pupil permits light to enter the eyes. Depending on the patient's age, pupil diameter can range from 0.3 to 0.5 cm.

 SPECIAL POINTS *At birth, the pupil is small and unresponsive to light. It enlarges during childhood, and then progressively decreases in size throughout adulthood.*

Anterior and posterior chambers
The posterior chamber, located directly behind the lens, is filled with a watery fluid called *aqueous humor.* This fluid bathes the lens capsule as it flows through the pupil into the anterior chamber.

The anterior chamber is filled with the clear, aqueous humor. The amount of fluid in the chamber varies in an effort to maintain pressure in the eye. Fluid drains from the anterior chamber through collecting channels into Schlemm's canal.

Ciliary body and choroid
The iris, ciliary body, and choroid make up the eyeball's middle layer. Suspensory ligaments attached to the ciliary body control the lens's shape, for close and distant vision. The pigmented, vascular choroid supplies the outer retina's blood supply, and then drains blood through its remaining vasculature.

Iris
◆ Circular, contractile diaphragm gives eye color
◆ Involuntary muscles control pupil size and regulate amount of light entering the eye

Pupil
◆ Central opening of the iris

Anterior and posterior chambers
◆ Anterior — filled with clear, aqueous humor maintaining pressure
◆ Posterior — filled with aqueous humor that bathes the lens as it flows through the pupil in the anterior chamber

Ciliary body and choroid
◆ Make up eyeball's middle layer, with iris
◆ Ciliary body controls lens shape, for close and distant vision
◆ Choroid supplies the outer retina's blood supply

Lens

+ Consists of avascular transparent fibrils in lens capsule
+ Refracts and focuses light onto the retina

Vitreous chamber

+ Filled with vitreous humor, which maintains shape of eyeball

Retina

+ Receives visual stimuli and transmits images to brain for processing

Optic disc and physiologic cup

+ Optic disc — well-defined, round or oval area within retina; called the *blind spot*
+ Physiologic cup — light-colored depression where blood vessels enter the retina

Photoreceptor neurons

+ Make up retina's visual receptors
+ Shaped like rods and cones
+ Responsible for vision

Macula and fovea centralis

+ Macula — contains no visible retinal vessels
+ Fovea centralis — acts as eye's clearest vision and color receptor

Physiology of vision

+ To perceive an object clearly, eye must intercept reflected light
+ Image then passes through cornea, anterior chamber, pupil, lens, and vitreous humor
+ Lens focuses light as image on retina, sending nerve impulses to optic nerve and occipital lobe, finally interpreting image

Lens

Located directly behind the iris at the pupillary opening, the lens consists of avascular transparent fibrils in an elastic membrane called the *lens capsule*. The lens refracts and focuses light onto the retina.

Vitreous chamber

The vitreous chamber, located behind the lens, occupies four-fifths of the eyeball. This chamber is filled with vitreous humor, an avascular gelatinous substance that maintains the shape of the eyeball.

Retina

The innermost region of eyeball, the retina receives visual stimuli and transmits images to the brain for processing. Four sets of retinal blood vessels — the superonasal, inferonasal, superotemporal, and inferotemporal — are visible through an ophthalmoscope.

Each set of vessels contains a transparent arteriole and vein. As these vessels leave the optic disc, they become progressively thinner, intertwining as they extend to the periphery of the retina.

Optic disc and physiologic cup

A well-defined, round or oval area measuring less than ⅛" (0.2 cm) within the retina's nasal portion, the optic disc is the opening through which the ganglion nerve axons (fibers) exit the retina to form the optic nerve. This area is called the *blind spot* because no light-sensitive cells (photoreceptors) are located there.

The physiologic cup is a light-colored depression within the temporal side of the optic disc where blood vessels enter the retina. It covers one-fourth to one-third of the disc but doesn't extend completely to the margin.

Photoreceptor neurons

Photoreceptor neurons make up the retina's visual receptors. Not visible through the ophthalmoscope, these receptors — some shaped like rods and some like cones — are responsible for vision. Rods respond to low-intensity light, but they don't provide sharp images or color vision. Cones respond to bright light and provide high-acuity color vision.

Macula and fovea centralis

Located laterally from the optic disc, the macula is slightly darker than the rest of the retina and contains no visible retinal vessels. Because its borders are poorly defined, the macula is difficult to see on an ophthalmologic examination. It's best identified by having the patient look straight at the ophthalmoscope's light.

The fovea centralis, a slight depression in the macula, appears as a bright reflection when examined with an ophthalmoscope. Because the fovea contains the heaviest concentration of cones, it acts as the eye's clearest vision and color receptor.

PHYSIOLOGY OF VISION

Every object reflects light. For an individual to perceive an object clearly, this reflected light must be intercepted by the eye and pass through numerous intraocular structures, including the cornea, anterior chamber, pupil, lens, and vitreous humor. The lens focuses the light into an upside-down and reversed image on the retina. Reacting to the light, specialized photoreceptor cells (rods and cones) in the retina send nerve impulses via the optic nerve and optic tract to the visual cortex of the occipital lobe, which then interprets the image.

OBTAINING A HEALTH HISTORY

Now that you're familiar with the normal anatomy and physiology of the eyes, you're ready to obtain a health history of them. The most common eye-related complaints are double vision (diplopia), visual floaters, photophobia (light sensitivity), vision loss, and eye pain.

Other complaints include decreased visual acuity or clarity, defects in color vision, and difficulty seeing at night. Even if a patient's chief complaint or previous diagnosis isn't eye-related, you'll need to question him about his eyes and vision. Keep in mind that poor vision can affect the patient's ability to comply with treatment. (See *Common eye complaints,* page 350.)

To obtain an accurate and complete patient history, adjust questions to the patient's specific complaint and compare the answers with the results of the physical assessment.

SPECIAL POINTS *Further modify questions according to the patient's age, for example, by asking a child if the writing on the school chalkboard is readable or by asking an elderly patient about peripheral vision, visual acuity, glaucoma testing, problems with glare, and abnormal tearing. (See* Examining the eyes of children and elderly patients, *page 351.)*

CURRENT HEALTH HISTORY

Begin by asking about the patient's current eye health status. Carefully document the patient's chief complaint (using the patient's own words.) Ask for a complete description of this problem and any others. During the interview, observe the patient's eye movements and focusing ability for clues to visual acuity and eye muscle coordination. To investigate further, ask the following questions about eye function:

✦ Do you have any problems with your eyes? Besides indicating visual disturbances, problems with the eyes can result from other conditions, such as diabetes, hypertension, or neurologic disorders.

✦ Do you wear or have you ever worn corrective lenses? If so, for how long? This establishes how long the patient has had a vision disorder and informs the nurse of the patient's need to wear corrective lenses during the visual acuity check.

✦ If you wear corrective lenses, are they glasses or hard or soft contact lenses? Improperly fitted contact lenses or prolonged wear can cause eye inflammation and corneal abrasions. Those who wear of soft lenses are especially vulnerable to conjunctival inflammation and infection because the lenses, worn for long periods, can irritate the eye.

✦ For what eye condition do you wear corrective lenses? Besides providing information about any existing eye condition, the answer allows adjustment of the diopters for ophthalmoscopic examination of nearsightedness or farsightedness.

✦ If you wear corrective lenses, do you wear them all the time or just for certain activities, such as reading or driving? The answer provides information about the severity and type of visual disturbance.

✦ If you once wore corrective lenses and have stopped wearing them, why and when did you stop? Eyestrain or excessive tearing may occur if the patient isn't wearing necessary lenses.

PAST HEALTH HISTORY

During the next part of the health history, ask the following questions to gather additional information about the patient's eyes:

Obtaining a health history
◆ Common eye complaints include diplopia, visual floaters, photophobia, vision loss, and eye pain
◆ Adjust questions to patient's specific complaint, comparing answers with those of physical assessment

Special points
◆ In children, modify questions; for example, to situations in school
◆ In elderly patients, ask about peripheral vision, visual acuity, glaucoma testing, problems with glare, and abnormal tearing

Current health history
◆ Uncovers chief complaint
◆ Allows for observation of patient's eyes during interview
◆ Detects eye problems resulting from other conditions, such as diabetes, hypertension, or neurologic disorders
◆ Reveals information about eye function, including wearing corrective or contact lenses

Past health history
◆ Corrective lenses; blurred vision; spots, floater, or halos; eye infections or inflammation; eye surgery or injury; sties; high blood pressure; diabetes; and prescription eye medication or other medications

Common eye complaints

- ✦ Decreased visual acuity
- ✦ Diplopia
- ✦ Eye pain
- ✦ Visual halos or bright light rings
- ✦ Night blindness
- ✦ Vision loss
- ✦ Visual floaters

Common eye complaints

If your patient is seeking medical attention for a vision problem, his chief complaint will probably be one of the following disorders.

DECREASED VISUAL ACUITY

Lack of visual acuity—the ability to see clearly—is commonly associated with refractive errors. In nearsightedness, or myopia, the eye focuses the visual image in front of the retina, causing objects in close view to be seen clearly and those at a distance to be blurry. In farsightedness, or hyperopia, the eye focuses the visual image behind the retina, causing objects in close view to be blurry and those at a distance to be clear. Both of these problems are caused by an abnormally shaped eyeball.

DIPLOPIA

Also called double vision, diplopia is caused by extraocular muscle misalignment. It occurs when the visual axes aren't directed at the object of sight at the same time.

EYE PAIN

A complaint of eye pain needs immediate attention because it may signal an emergency. Ask the patient what the quality, duration, frequency, and onset of the pain is; what causes it (for example, bright light); whether headaches accompany it; and what he does to relieve it.

Diseases that can cause eye pain include coma, acute angle-closure glaucoma, corneal damage (foreign body, abrasions), trauma to eye, and conjunctivitis.

VISUAL HALOS OR BRIGHT LIGHT RINGS

Increased intraocular pressure, (IOP) as occurs in glaucoma, causes the patient to see halos and rainbows around bright lights. It can be caused by corneal edema, as a result of prolonged contact lens wear, or fluctuation in blood glucose levels in undiagnosed diabetic patients.

NIGHT BLINDNESS

The patient may complain of poor vision when darkness descends. Night blindness, or the inability to adapt to dim light or darkness, is caused by retinal degeneration, such as retinitis pigmentosa, optic nerve disease, glaucoma, or vitamin A deficiency related to malnutrition or chronic alcoholism.

VISION LOSS

Your patient may complain of central or peripheral vision loss, or he may report a scotoma—a blind spot in the visual field that's surrounded by an area of normal vision. Disease in any structure of the eye can result in vision loss. The degree and location of blindness depends on the disease causing the problem and the lesion's location. The major causes of blindness in the United States are glaucoma, untreated cataracts, retinal disease, and macular degeneration.

VISUAL FLOATERS

Visual floaters are specks of varying shape and size that float through the visual field and disappear when the patient tries to look at them. They're caused by small cells floating in the vitreous humor. Visual floaters require further investigation because they may indicate vitreous hemorrhage and retinal separation. A large, black floater that appears suddenly may indicate vitreous detachment.

Past health history
(continued)

Abnormal findings
- ✦ Blurred vision (need for corrective lenses or suggesting a neurologic or endocrine disorder)

✦ When did you last have your corrective lenses changed? A recent lens change with continued visual disturbances could indicate an underlying health problem, such as a brain tumor.

✦ Have you ever had blurred vision?

 ABNORMAL FINDINGS Blurred vision can indicate a need for corrective lenses or suggest a neurologic disorder, such as a brain tumor, or an endocrine disorder, such as diabetic retinopathy.

If the patient isn't in distress, ask him how long he has had the visual blurring. Does it occur only at certain times? Ask about associated symptoms, such as pain or

Examining the eyes of children and elderly patients

If your patient is a child, ask a parent or guardian these additional questions:

✦ Was the child delivered vaginally or by cesarean delivery? If he was delivered vaginally, did his mother have a vaginal infection at the time? (Inform the parents that infections — such as chlamydia, gonorrhea, genital herpes, or candidiasis — can cause eye problems in infants.)

✦ Did he have erythromycin ointment instilled in his eyes at birth?

✦ Has he had an eye examination before? If so, when was the most recent examination?

✦ Has he passed the normal developmental milestones?

✦ Has he ever had an eye injury?

✦ Does he know how to hold and care for sharp objects such as scissors?

✦ Does he complain of eye pain or headaches?

✦ Does he squint to see objects at a distance?

✦ Does he hold objects close to his eyes to see them?

If your patient is an aging adult, ask him these additional questions:

✦ Have you had any difficulty climbing stairs or driving?

✦ Have you ever been tested for glaucoma? If so, when and what was the result?

✦ If you have glaucoma, has your doctor prescribed eyedrops for you? If so, what kind?

✦ How well can you instill your eyedrops?

✦ Do your eyes ever feel dry? Do they burn? If so, how do you treat the problem?

---

discharge. If visual blurring followed injury, obtain details of the accident, and ask if vision was impaired immediately after the injury. Obtain a medical and medication history.

✦ Have you ever seen spots, floaters, or halos around lights? If yes, is this a sudden change or has it occurred for a while?

 ABNORMAL FINDINGS *A sudden appearance of flashing lights or floaters may indicate a retinal detachment; halos are associated with glaucoma.*

 SPECIAL POINTS *The chronic appearance of spots or floaters is a normal occurrence in elderly patients and those with myopia.*

✦ Do you suffer from frequent eye infections or inflammation?

 ABNORMAL FINDINGS *Frequent infections or inflammation of the eye can indicate low resistance to infection, eyestrain, allergies, or occupational or environmental exposure to an irritant.*

✦ Have you ever had eye surgery? A history of eye surgery may indicate glaucoma, cataracts, or injuries such as detached retina, which may appear as abnormalities on ophthalmoscopic examination.

✦ Have you ever had an eye injury? Injuries, such as those from a penetrating foreign body, can distort the ophthalmoscopic examination.

✦ Do you often have sties? Sties, infected meibomian glands, or glands of Zeis, tend to recur.

✦ Do you have a history of high blood pressure?

 ABNORMAL FINDINGS *Patients with high blood pressure are at risk for arteriosclerosis of the retinal blood vessels and vision disturbances.*

Past health history
(continued)

Abnormal findings

✦ Sudden appearance of flashing lights or floaters indicating retinal detachment; halos (glaucoma)

✦ Frequent infections or inflammation (low resistance to infection, eyestrain, allergies, or occupational or environmental exposure)

✦ High blood pressure (risk for arteriosclerosis of retinal blood vessels and vision disturbances)

Special points

✦ Chronic appearance of spots or floaters is normal in myopic patients and the elderly

Past health history
(continued)

Abnormal findings
✦ In diabetic patients noninflammatory changes in the retina (blindness)

Family history
✦ Myopia
✦ Cataracts
✦ Glaucoma
✦ Loss of vision

Psychosocial history
✦ Finds out about daily habits that affect the eyes
✦ Reveals occupation and work environment
✦ Tells about smoking habits

Assessing the eyes
✦ Inspect the external eye and lids, test visual acuity, assess eye muscle function, palpate the nasolacrimal sac, and examine intraocular structures

---

✦ Do you have a history of diabetes?

ABNORMAL FINDINGS *In patients with diabetes, noninflammatory changes in the retina can lead to blindness.*

✦ Are you taking prescription medications for your eyes? If so, which medications and how often? Ask the patient to describe how he administers his medications, eyedrops, ointments, or gel. Review with the patient how to take his medication. Prescription eye medications should alert you to an eye disorder. For example, a patient who's taking pilocarpine probably has glaucoma.

✦ What other medications are you taking, including prescription drugs, over-the-counter medications, and home remedies? Certain medications can cause visual disturbances.

FAMILY HISTORY
Next, investigate for familial eye disorders. Ask if any member of the patient's family has ever been treated for myopia, cataracts, glaucoma, or loss of vision.

PSYCHOSOCIAL HISTORY
Explore the patient's daily habits that affect the eyes by asking the following questions:

✦ Does your occupation require close use of your eyes, such as long-term reading or prolonged use of a video display terminal? These activities can cause eyestrain or dryness when the person forgets to blink.

✦ Does the air where you work or live contain anything that causes you eye problems? Cigarette smoke, formaldehyde insulation, or occupational materials such as glues or chemicals can cause eye irritation.

✦ Do you wear goggles when working with power tools, chain saws, or table saws, or when engaging in sports that might irritate or endanger the eye, such as swimming, fencing, or playing racquetball? Serious eye irritation or injury can occur with these activities.

✦ Do you smoke or are you exposed regularly to secondhand smoke? Warn the patient that smoking increases the risk of vascular disease, which can damage vision and lead to blindness.

If your patient is visually impaired, ask him how well he can manage activities of daily living. Assess whether he and his family need assistance in learning to use adaptive devices or a referral to an agency that helps visually impaired people.

If your patient is elderly, you'll need to ask additional questions about his ability to perform daily tasks. His answers will help to guide your care.

ASSESSING THE EYES

A complete eye assessment involves inspecting the external eye and lids, testing visual acuity, assessing eye muscle function, palpating the nasolacrimal sac, and examining intraocular structures with an ophthalmoscope.

Before starting your examination, gather the necessary equipment, including a good light source, one or two opaque cards, an ophthalmoscope, vision-test cards, gloves, tissues, and cotton-tipped applicators. Make sure the patient is seated comfortably and that you're seated at eye level with him.

Recognizing common eye disorders

During an eye examination, you may observe any of several abnormalities. These illustrations show some of those abnormal findings.

PERIORBITAL EDEMA

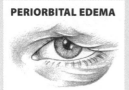

PTOSIS

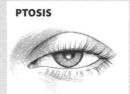

ACUTE HORDEOLUM

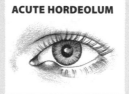

INSPECTING THE EYES

Start your assessment by observing the patient's face. With the scalp line as the starting point, check that his eyes are in a normal position. They should be about one-third of the way down the face and about one eye's width apart from each other. Next assess the conjunctiva, cornea, anterior chamber, iris, pupil, and eyelid.

Eyelids

Each upper eyelid should cover the top quarter of the iris so the eyes look alike. Check for an excessive amount of visible sclera above the limbus (corneoscleral junction). Ask the patient to open and close his eyes to see if they close completely.

 ABNORMAL FINDINGS *If a delay in the downward movement of the patient's upper eyelid in a down gaze is delayed, then the patient has lid lag, which is a common sign of hyperthyroidism. Protrusion of the eyeball, called* exophthalmos *or* proptosis*, is common in patients with hyperthyroidism.*

Assess the lids for redness, edema, inflammation, or lesions. Also, inspect the eyes for excessive tearing or dryness. The eyelid margins should be pink, and the eyelashes should turn outwards. Observe whether the lower eyelids turn inward toward the eyeball, called *entropion,* or outward, called *ectropion.* Examine the eyelids for lumps.

 ABNORMAL FINDINGS *Swelling around the patient's eyes, or periorbital edema, may result from allergies, local inflammation, fluid-retaining disorders, or crying.*

In a patient with ptosis, or a drooping upper eyelid, there may be an interruption in sympathetic innervation to the eyelid, muscle weakness, or damage to the oculomotor nerve.

A patient with acute hordeolum, also called a stye, *has a bacterial infection in a sweat or sebaceous gland on the eyelid. The affected area becomes reddened and painful, and you may observe a green-yellow discharge. (See* Recognizing common eye disorders.*)*

Before palpating the nasolacrimal sac, explain the procedure to the patient. Then put on examination gloves. With the patient's eyes closed, gently palpate the area below the inner canthus, noting tenderness, or swelling, or discharge through the lacrimal point.

 ABNORMAL FINDINGS *If tenderness, swelling, or discharge through the lacrimal point occurs upon palpation, these findings lacrymal puncta could indicate blockage of the naso-lacrimal duct.*

Inspecting the eyes
✦ Assess for normal position
✦ Observe conjunctiva, cornea, anterior chamber, iris, pupil, and eyelid

Eyelids
✦ Check for excessive amount of visible sclera above the limbus
✦ Assess for redness, edema, inflammation, lesions, or lumps
✦ Inspect eyes for excessive tearing or dryness
✦ Observe whether lower eyelids display entropion or ectropion
✦ Palpate nasolacrimal sac, noting tenderness, swelling, or discharge

Abnormal findings
✦ Delaying downward movement of the upper eyelid and protruding eyeball (hyperthyroidism)
✦ Periorbital swelling (allergies, local inflammation, or fluid-retaining disorders)
✦ Drooping upper eyelid (possible damage to the oculomotor nerve)
✦ Reddened, painful area, with green-yellow discharge (acute hordeolum)
✦ Tenderness, swelling, and discharge through lacrimal point (blockage of the nasolacrimal duct)

Tips for assessing corneal sensitivity

◆ Touch a wisp of cotton to the cornea
◆ Absence of blinking indicates damage to cranial nerve

Conjunctiva

◆ Bulbar conjunctiva appears clear and shiny
◆ Sclera's color appears white to buff

Abnormal findings

◆ Excessive redness or exudate
◆ Cobblestone appearance (history of allergies)
◆ Bluish discoloration (scleral thinning)

Special points

◆ In black patients, eye may have flecks of tan

Cornea

◆ Appears clear, without lesions
◆ Test corneal sensitivity, with a wisp of cotton

Tips for assessing corneal sensitivity

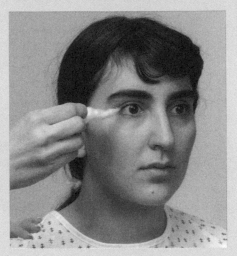

To test corneal sensitivity, touch a wisp of cotton from a cotton ball to the cornea, as shown.

The patient should blink. If there's no response, he may have suffered damage to the sensory fibers of cranial nerve V or to the motor fibers controlled by cranial nerve VI.

Keep in mind that people who wear contact lenses may have reduced sensitivity because they're accustomed to having foreign objects in their eyes.

Remember that a wisp of cotton is the only safe object to use for this test. Even though a 4″ x 4″ gauze pad or tissue is soft, it can cause corneal abrasions and irritation.

Conjunctiva

Next, have your patient look up. Gently pull the lower eyelid down to inspect the bulbar conjunctiva (the delicate mucous membrane that covers the exposed surface of the sclera). It should be clear and shiny.

 ABNORMAL FINDINGS *Note if the patient has excessive redness or exudate of the eye. The palpebral conjunctiva in patients with a history of allergies may have a cobblestone appearance.*

To examine the palpebral conjunctiva (the membrane that lines the eyelids), have the patient look down. Then lift the upper lid, holding the upper lashes against the eyebrow with your finger. The palpebral conjunctiva should be uniformly pink.

With the lid still secured, inspect the bulbar conjunctiva for color changes, foreign bodies, and edema. Also, observe the sclera's color, which should be white to buff.

 SPECIAL POINTS *In a black patient's eye, you may see flecks of tan.*

 ABNORMAL FINDINGS *A bluish discoloration of the patient's eye may indicate scleral thinning.*

Cornea

Examine the cornea by shining a penlight first from both sides and then from straight ahead. The cornea should be clear and without lesions. Test corneal sensitivity by lightly touching the cornea with a wisp of cotton. (See *Tips for assessing corneal sensitivity*.)

Anterior chamber and iris

The eye's anterior chamber is bordered anteriorly by the cornea and posteriorly by the iris. The iris should appear flat, and the cornea should appear convex. The irises should be the same size, color, and shape.

 ABNORMAL FINDINGS *Excess pressure in the patient's eye — such as that caused by acute angle-closure glaucoma — may push the iris forward, making the anterior chamber appear very small.*

Pupils

The pupils should be equal in size, round, and about one-fourth of the size of the irises in normal room light. About one person in four has asymmetrical pupils without disease.

 ABNORMAL FINDINGS *Unequal pupils generally indicate neurologic damage, iritis, glaucoma, or the effect of therapy with certain medications.*

 CLINICAL ALERT A fixed pupil that doesn't react to light can be an ominous neurologic sign.

Test the pupils for direct and consensual response. In a slightly darkened room, hold a penlight about 20″ (50.8 cm) from the patient's eyes, and direct the light at the eye from the side. Note the reaction of the pupil you're testing (direct response) and the opposite pupil (consensual response). They should both react the same way. Note sluggishness or inequality in the response of the patient's pupil.

Repeat the test with the other pupil. *Note:* If you shine the light in a blind eye, neither pupil will respond. If you shine the light in a seeing eye, both pupils will respond consensually.

To test the pupils for accommodation, place your finger approximately 4″ (10 cm) from the bridge of the patient's nose. Ask the patient to look at a fixed object in the distance and then to look at your finger. His pupils should constrict and his eyes converge as he focuses on your finger.

To document that the patient's pupils appear normal, use the abbreviation PERRLA (which stands for pupils equal, round, reactive to light, and accommodation) and the terms direct and consensual.

TESTING VISUAL ACUITY

To test your patient's far, near, and peripheral vision, use a Snellen chart and a near-vision chart. Before each test, ask the patient to remove corrective lenses, if he wears them.

Snellen chart

Have the patient sit or stand 20′ (6.1 m) from the chart, and then cover his left eye with an opaque object. Ask him to read the letters on one line of the chart and then to move downward to increasingly smaller lines until he can no longer discern all of the letters. Have him repeat the test covering his right eye.

Use the "E" chart to test visual acuity in young children and other patients who can't read. Cover the patient's left eye to check the right eye, point to an E on the chart, and ask the patient to point which way the letter faces. Repeat the test with the left eye. (See *Visual acuity charts*, page 356.)

Anterior chamber and iris

✦ Appears flat, with cornea appearing convex
✦ Irises should be equal in size, color, and shape

Abnormal findings
✦ Excess pressure, pushing iris forward (acute-closure glaucoma)

Pupils

✦ Appearing equal in size and round
✦ Test for direct and consensual response and accommodation
✦ Document normal pupils, using PERRLA

Abnormal findings
✦ Unequal pupils (neurologic damage, iritis, glaucoma, or effect of medications)

Alert!

✦ Fixed pupil not reacting to light can be an ominous neurologic sign

Testing visual acuity

✦ Tests far, near, and peripheral vision
✦ Use Snellen chart and near-vision chart
✦ Ask patient to remove corrective lenses

Snellen chart

✦ Requires patient to read letters, with one eye covered, test visual acuity
✦ In young children and in patients who can't read, use "E" chart asking patient to point which way the letter faces

Visual acuity charts

+ Commonly used charts include Snellen and "E" charts
+ Test distance and measure visual acuity
+ Records results as a fraction
+ Normal vision differs with age

Visual acuity charts

The most commonly used charts used for testing vision are the Snellen alphabet chart and the "E" chart, the latter of which is used for young children and adults who can't read. Both charts are used to test distance vision and measure visual acuity. The patient reads each chart at a distance of 20′ (6.1 m).

RECORDING RESULTS
Visual acuity is recorded as a fraction. The top number (20) is the distance between the patient and the chart. The bottom number is the distance from which a person with normal vision could read the line. The larger the bottom number, the poorer the patient's vision.

AGE DIFFERENCES
In adults and children ages 6 and older, normal vision is measured as 20/20. For children younger than age 6, normal vision varies. For children age 3 and younger, normal vision is 20/50; for children age 4, 20/40; and for children age 5, 20/30.

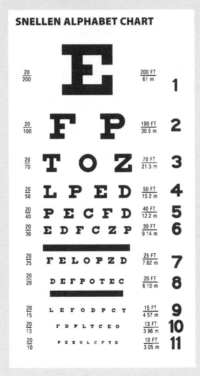

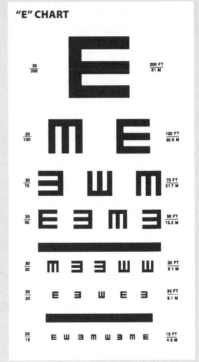

Snellen chart
(continued)

Abnormal findings
+ If test values differ, suspect amblyopia, especially in children

Near-vision chart
+ Test near vision with patient using a special handheld card
+ Have patient read line with smallest distinguishable letters

If the patient wears corrective lenses, have him repeat the test wearing them. Record his vision with and without correction.

 ABNORMAL FINDINGS *If the patient's test values between the two eyes differ by two lines, such as 20/30 in one eye and 20/50 in the other, suspect an abnormality such as amblyopia, especially in children.*

Near-vision chart
To test near vision, cover one of the patient's eyes with an opaque object, and hold a special card (that simulates a Snellen chart) 14″ (35.6 cm) from his eyes. Have him read the line with the smallest letters he can distinguish. Repeat the test with

the other eye. If the patient wears corrective lenses, have him repeat the test while wearing them. Record the visual accommodation with and without lenses.

Any patient who complains of blurring with the card at 14″ or who can't read it accurately needs retesting and then referral to an ophthalmologist, if necessary. Keep in mind that a patient who's illiterate may be too embarrassed to say so. If a patient seems to be struggling to read the type, or stares at it without attempting to read, change to the "E" chart.

Color perception testing

Congenital color blindness is usually a sex-linked recessive trait passed from mothers to male offspring. (Acquired color deficit is pathologic.) People with color blindness can't distinguish among red, green, and blue.

Of the many tests to detect color blindness, the most common involves asking a patient to identify patterns of colored dots on colored plates. The patient who can't discern colors will miss the patterns.

 SPECIAL POINTS *In a child, early detection of color blindness allows him to learn to compensate for the deficit and also alerts teachers to the student's special needs.*

ASSESSING EYE MUSCLE FUNCTION

A thorough assessment of the eyes includes an evaluation of the extraocular muscles. To evaluate these muscles, you'll need to assess the corneal light reflex and the cardinal positions of gaze.

Corneal light reflex

To assess the corneal light reflex, ask the patient to look straight ahead; then shine a penlight on the bridge of his nose from about 12″ to 15″ (30.5 cm to 38 cm) away. The light should fall at the same spot on each cornea.

 ABNORMAL FINDINGS *When assessing the patient's corneal light reflex, if the light doesn't fall at the same spot on each cornea, the eyes aren't being held in the same plane by the extraocular muscles. This finding is common in patients with lack of muscle coordination, a condition called* strabismus.

Cardinal positions of gaze

Cardinal positions of gaze evaluates the oculomotor, trigeminal, and abducent nerves as well as the extraocular muscles. To perform this test, ask the patient to remain still while you hold a pencil or other small object directly in front of his nose at a distance of about 18″ (45.6 cm).

Ask him to follow the object with his eyes, without moving his head. Then move the object to each of the six cardinal positions (right superior, right lateral, right inferior, left superior, left lateral, and left inferior), returning to the midpoint after each movement. The patient's eyes should remain parallel as they move.

 ABNORMAL FINDINGS *In a patient with nystagmus and amblyopia, one eye fails to follow an object.*

Cover-uncover test

The third test to assess extraocular muscles is the cover-uncover test. This test usually isn't done unless you detect an abnormality during one of the two previous tests. To perform a cover-uncover test, have the patient stare at a wall on the other side of the room. Cover one eye and watch for movement in the uncovered eye. Remove the eye cover, and watch for movement again. Repeat the test with the other eye.

Cover-uncover test
(continued)
✦ Eye movement occurring while covering or uncovering eye (cranial nerve impairment)

Peripheral vision testing
✦ Tests optic nerve and measures retina's ability to receive stimuli from periphery of its field
✦ Assumes the health care provider has normal vision; testing can be subjective

Examining intraocular structures
✦ Use ophthalmoscope to directly observe internal structures
✦ Shine light into pupil to elicit a reflection of light off the choroid
✦ Focus on the anterior chamber and lens
✦ Examine retina, vitreous body for clarity, blood vessels, and the optic disc

Abnormal findings
✦ Clouding, foreign matter, or opacities (cataracts, ending examination)

 ABNORMAL FINDINGS *If a patient experiences eye movement while covering or uncovering the eye, this is considered abnormal. It may result from weak or paralyzed extraocular muscles, which may be caused by cranial nerve impairment.*

Peripheral vision testing

Assessment of peripheral vision tests the optic nerve (cranial nerve II) and measures the retina's ability to receive stimuli from the periphery of its field. You can grossly evaluate peripheral vision by assessing visual fields, which compares the patient's peripheral vision with your own. However, because this assumes you have normal vision, the test can be subjective and inaccurate.

To test peripheral visual fields, follow this procedure. Sit facing the patient, about 2′ (61 cm) away, with your eyes at the same level as his. Have him stare straight ahead. Cover one of your eyes with an opaque cover or your hand, and ask him to cover the eye directly opposite your covered eye. Next, bring an object, such as a penlight, from the periphery of the superior field toward the center of the field of vision. The object should be equidistant between you and the patient. Ask him to tell you the moment the object appears. If your peripheral vision is intact, you and the patient should see the object at the same time.

Repeat the procedure clockwise at 45-degree angles, checking the superior, inferior, temporal, and nasal visual fields. When testing the temporal field, you'll have difficulty moving the penlight far enough out so that neither person can see it, so test the temporal field by placing the penlight somewhat behind the patient and out of his visual field. Slowly bring the penlight around until the patient can see it.

EXAMINING INTRAOCULAR STRUCTURES

The ophthalmoscope allows you to directly observe internal structures of the eye. To see those structures properly, you'll need to adjust the lens disc. Use the green, plus numbers on the disc to focus on near objects such as the patient's cornea and lens. Use the red, minus numbers to focus on distant objects such as the retina.

Before the examination, have the patient remove his contact lenses (if they're tinted) or eyeglasses and darken the room to dilate his pupils and make your examination easier. Ask the patient to focus on a point behind you. Tell him that you'll be moving into his visual field and blocking his view. Also, explain that you'll be shining a bright light into his eye, which may be uncomfortable but not harmful. (See *Examining the eye.*)

Set the lens disc at zero, and hold the ophthalmoscope about 4″ (10 cm) from the patient's eye. Direct the light through the pupil to elicit the red reflex, a reflection of light off the choroid. Check the red reflex for depth of color.

Now, move the ophthalmoscope closer to the eye. Adjust the lens disc so you can focus on the anterior chamber and lens.

 ABNORMAL FINDINGS *You may observe clouding, foreign matter, or opacities in the patient's eye. If his lens is opaque, indicating cataracts, you may not be able to complete the examination.*

To examine the retina, start with the dial turned to zero. Rotate the lens-power disc to adjust for your refractive correction and the patient's refractive error. Now, observe the vitreous body for clarity. The first retinal structures you'll see are the blood vessels. Rotating the dial into the negative numbers will bring the blood vessels into focus. The arteries will look thinner and brighter than the veins.

Follow one of the vessels along its path toward the nose until you reach the optic disc, where all vessels in the eye originate.

Examining the eye

This illustration shows the correct position for the examiner and the patient when an ophthalmoscope is used to examine the eye's internal structures.

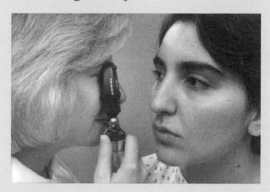

 ABNORMAL FINDINGS *If the patient displays arteriovenous crossings in the eyes, examine for arteriovenous nicking (localized constrictions of the vessels), which might be a sign of hypertension.*

The optic disc is a creamy pink to yellow-orange structure with clear borders and a round-to-oval shape. With practice, you'll be able to identify the physiologic cup, a small depression that occupies about one-third of the disc's diameter. The disc may fill or exceed your field of vision. If you don't see it, follow a blood vessel toward the center until you do. The nasal border of the disc may be somewhat blurred.

Completely scan the retina by following four blood vessels from the optic disc to different peripheral areas. The retina should have a uniform color and be free from scars and pigmentation. (See *Anatomy of the retina,* page 360.) As you scan the patient's eyes, note any lesions or hemorrhages.

Finally, move the light laterally from the optic disc to locate the macula, the part of the eye most sensitive to light. It appears as a darker structure, free from blood vessels. Your view may be fleeting because most patients can't tolerate having a beam of light fall on the macula. If you locate it, ask the patient to shift his gaze into the light.

INTERPRETING YOUR FINDINGS

After you assess the patient, a group of findings may lead you to suspect a particular disorder. (See *The eyes: Interpreting your findings,* page 361.)

EYE DISORDERS

CONJUNCTIVITIS

An inflammation of the conjunctiva, conjunctivitis usually occurs as benign, self-limiting pinkeye. It may also be chronic, possibly indicating degenerative changes or damage from repeated acute attacks. In the Western hemisphere, conjunctivitis is probably the most common eye disorder.

Examining intraocular structures
(continued)

Abnormal findings
✦ Arteriovenous crossings in the eyes (hypertension)

Eye disorders

Facts about conjunctivitis

✦ Inflammation of the conjunctiva
✦ Chronic occurrences indicate degenerative changes or damage

Anatomy of the retina

This illustration shows the retina's complex anatomy and structures.

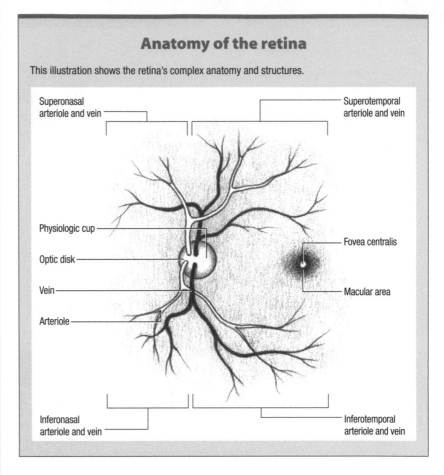

Superonasal arteriole and vein

Superotemporal arteriole and vein

Physiologic cup

Optic disk

Vein

Arteriole

Fovea centralis

Macular area

Inferonasal arteriole and vein

Inferotemporal arteriole and vein

Facts about conjunctivitis
(continued)

✦ Causes including bacterial, viral, and chlamydial infection
✦ Results in hyperemia of the conjunctiva, discharge, and pain

Special points

✦ In children, accompanying sore throat and fever possible

Facts about cataracts

✦ Common cause of vision loss
✦ Gradually developing opacity of the lens or lens capsule
✦ Painless, gradual blurring and loss of vision occur

Special points

✦ In patients over age 70, prevalent part of aging
✦ Surgery improves vision in 95% of cases

Causes include bacterial, viral, and chlamydial infection. Less common causes are allergy, parasitic disease and, rarely, fungal infection, or occupational irritants. Idiopathic causes are associated with certain systemic diseases, such as erythema multiforme and thyroid disease.

Signs and symptoms include hyperemia of the conjunctiva, discharge (mucopurulent with bacterial infection and watery with viral infection), and pain and photophobia with corneal involvement, itching and burning with allergy, and sensation of a foreign body in the eye with acute bacterial infection.

SPECIAL POINTS *In children with conjunctivitis, an accompanying sore throat or fever is possible.*

CATARACTS

A common cause of vision loss, a cataract is a gradually developing opacity of the lens or lens capsule of the eye. Cataracts commonly occur bilaterally, with each progressing independently. Exceptions are traumatic cataracts, which are usually unilateral, and congenital cataracts, which may remain stationary.

SPECIAL POINTS *In patients over age 70, cataracts are prevalent as part of aging. Prognosis is usually good, with surgery improving vision in 95% of cases.*

The eyes: Interpreting your findings

The chart below shows common groups of findings for the signs and symptoms of the eyes, along with their probable causes.

SIGN OR SYMPTOM AND FINDINGS	PROBABLE CAUSE
Visual blurring	
✦ Gradual visual blurring ✦ Halo vision ✦ Visual glare in bright light ✦ Progressive vision loss ✦ Gray pupil that later turns milky white	✦ Cataract
✦ Constant morning headache that decreases in severity during the day ✦ Possible severe, throbbing headache ✦ Restlessness ✦ Confusion ✦ Nausea and vomiting ✦ Seizures ✦ Decreased level of consciousness	✦ Hypertension
✦ Paroxysmal attacks of severe, throbbing, unilateral or bilateral headache ✦ Nausea and vomiting ✦ Sensitivity to light and noise ✦ Sensory or visual auras	✦ Migraine headache
Eye discharge	
✦ Purulent or mucopurulent, greenish white discharge that occurs unilaterally ✦ Sticky crusts that form on the eyelids during sleep ✦ Itching and burning ✦ Excessive tearing ✦ Sensation of a foreign body in the eye	✦ Bacterial conjunctivitis
✦ Scant but continuous purulent discharge that's easily expressed from the tear sac ✦ Excessive tearing ✦ Pain and tenderness near the tear sac ✦ Eyelid inflammation and edema noticeable around the lacrimal punctum	✦ Dacryocystitis
✦ Continuous frothy discharge ✦ Chronically red eyes with inflamed lid margins ✦ Soft, foul-smelling, cheesy yellow discharge elicited by pressure on the meibomian glands	✦ Meibomianitis

Senile cataracts develop in elderly patients, probably because of changes in the chemical state of lens proteins. Congenital cataracts occur in neonates as genetic defects or as a result of maternal rubella during the first trimester. Traumatic cataracts develop after a foreign body injures the lens with sufficient force to allow aqueous or vitreous humor to enter the lens capsule.

Complicated cataracts occur secondary to uveitis, glaucoma, retinitis pigmentosa, or detached retina. They may also occur in the course of a systemic disease (such as diabetes, hypoparathyroidism, or atopic dermatitis), and they can result from ionizing radiation or infrared rays. Toxic cataracts result from drug or chemical toxicity with agents such as ergot or phenothiazine.

Signs and symptoms include painless, gradual blurring and loss of vision. With progression, the pupil whitens. Other possible symptoms include the appearance of halos around lights, blinding glare from headlights at night, and glare and poor vision in bright sunlight.

MACULAR DEGENERATION

Macular degeneration causes loss of central visual acuity and occurs in two forms. The serous (disciform, exudative) form is marked by formation of a mound resulting from serous detachment of the pigment epithelium and invasion of the area by neovascular tissue. Neovascularization may lead to hemorrhage and scar formation, which can sometimes be treated successfully with laser therapy to restore central vision.

The atrophic form involves retinal pigmentary epithelial damage, damage to choriocapillaries, and photoreceptor loss. However, it doesn't usually cause hemorrhaging and may regress spontaneously. Atrophic macular degeneration rarely needs laser therapy or other treatments.

DIABETIC RETINOPATHY

Diabetic retinopathy occurs in two forms: nonproliferative and proliferative. In nonproliferative, or background, retinopathy, microaneurysms and small retinal hemorrhages appear in the macular area. In proliferative retinopathy, new blood vessels leak fluid and lipid along the retinal surface. Fibrous tissue also forms.

Diabetic retinopathy, in its nonproliferative form, may have no symptoms or may cause loss of central visual acuity and diminished night vision from leakage of fluid into the macular region. Signs and symptoms of the proliferative form include sudden vision loss from vitreous hemorrhage, or macular distortion or retinal detachment from scar tissue formation.

GLAUCOMA

The term glaucoma refers to a group of disorders that are characterized by abnormally high intraocular pressure (lOP) and that can damage the optic nerve. It occurs in three primary forms: open-angle (primary), acute angle-closure, and congenital. It may also be secondary to other causes.

Chronic open-angle glaucoma results from overproduction of aqueous humor or obstruction of its outflow through the trabecular meshwork or Schlemm's canal. This form of glaucoma is usually familial and affects 90% of all patients with glaucoma.

Acute angle-closure glaucoma, also called *narrow-angle glaucoma,* results from obstruction to the outflow of aqueous humor from anatomically narrow angles between the anterior iris and the posterior corneal surface. It also results from shallow anterior chambers, a thickened iris that causes angle closure on pupil dilation, or a bulging iris that presses on the trabeculae, closing the angle (peripheral anterior synechiae).

Facts about macular degeneration

+ Causes loss of central visual acuity
+ Occurs in serous and atrophic forms

Facts about diabetic retinopathy

+ Nonproliferative form appears with microaneurysms and small retinal hemorrhages in the macular area
+ Proliferative form appears with new blood vessels leaking fluid and lipid along the retinal surface

Facts about glaucoma

+ A group of disorders characterized by abnormally high IOP
+ Damages optic nerve
+ Occurs as open-angle, acute angle-closure, and congenital
+ Early detection with tonometry and visual field analysis

Tonometry

An effective screen for early detection of glaucoma, tonometry also provides an indirect measurement of intraocular pressure (IOP). A rise in IOP may cause the eyeball to harden and become more resistant to extraocular pressure.

TYPES OF TONOMETRY

Indentation tonometry tests this resistance by measuring how deeply a known weight depresses the cornea. *Applanation tonometry* provides the same information by measuring the amount of force required to flatten a known area of the cornea.

Tonometry
+ Provides an indirect measurement of IOP
+ Indentation tonometry tests resistance of cornea
+ Applanation tonometry tests force required to flatten an area of the cornea

Congenital glaucoma is inherited as an autosomal recessive trait. Secondary glaucoma can result from uveitis, trauma, or drugs such as corticosteroids. Vein occlusion or diabetes can cause neovascularization in the angle.

Patients with IOP within the normal range of 8 to 21 mm Hg can develop signs and symptoms of glaucoma, and patients who have abnormally high IOP may have no clinical effects. Chronic open-angle glaucoma is usually bilateral and slowly progressive. Its onset is insidious. Symptoms appear late in the disease. They include mild aching in the eyes, gradual loss of peripheral vision, seeing halos around lights, and reduced visual acuity, especially at night, that's uncorrectable with glasses.

 CLINICAL ALERT The onset of acute angle-closure glaucoma is typically rapid, constituting an ophthalmic emergency. Unless treated promptly, this glaucoma produces permanent loss of or decreased vision in the affected eye. Signs and symptoms include unilateral inflammation and pain, pressure over the eye, moderate pupil dilation that's nonreactive to light, cloudy cornea, blurring and decreased visual acuity, photophobia, seeing halos around lights, nausea, and vomiting.

Early detection of glaucoma can be accomplished through tonometry and visual field analysis. (See *Tonometry*.)

Strabismus

With strabismus, the absence of normal, parallel, or coordinated eye movement results in eye misalignment. Strabismus affects about 2% of the population, primarily children; incidence is higher in persons with central nervous system disorders, such as cerebral palsy, mental retardation, or Down syndrome. Prognosis for correction varies with the timing of treatment and disease onset.

The cause of strabismus is unknown but may include congenital defect, trauma, high refractive errors, or anisometropia (unequal refractive power).

An obvious indication is misalignment of the eyes — esotropia (eyes deviate inward), exotropia (eyes deviate outward), hypertropia (eyes deviate upward), or hypotropia (eyes deviate downward). This misalignment is evident upon assessment of the six cardinal positions of gaze, the cover-uncover test, or the corneal light reflex test. Diplopia, amblyopia, and other visual disturbances can also indicate strabismus.

Optic atrophy

Optic atrophy, or degeneration of the optic nerve, can develop spontaneously (primary) or follow inflammation or edema of the nerve head (secondary). Some forms may subside without treatment, but optic nerve degeneration is irreversible.

Alert!
+ Acute angle-closure glaucoma onset occurs rapidly
+ Without immediate treatment, glaucoma produces permanent loss of or decreased vision

Facts about strabismus
+ Absence of normal, parallel, or coordinated eye movement resulting in eye misalignment
+ Affects children and persons with CNS disorders
+ Causes eyes to deviate inward, outward, upward, or downward

Facts about optic atrophy
+ Degeneration of the optic nerve develops spontaneously or following inflammation or edema of nerve head

Optic atrophy usually results from central nervous system disorders, such as pressure on the optic nerve from aneurysms or intraorbital or intracranial tumors (descending optic atrophy). Optic neuritis in patients with multiple sclerosis, retrobulbar neuritis, or tabes also can cause optic atrophy. Other causes include retinitis pigmentosa, chronic papilledema and papillitis, congenital syphilis, glaucoma, trauma, and ingestion of toxins, such as methanol and quinine. Central retinal artery or vein occlusion that interrupts the blood supply to the optic nerve can cause degeneration of ganglion cells, a condition called *ascending optic atrophy.*

Painless loss of either visual field or visual acuity, or both, can indicate optic atrophy. Loss of vision may be abrupt or gradual, depending on the cause.

CORNEAL ABRASION

Corneal abrasion, the most common eye injury, is a scratch on the surface epithelium of the cornea. With treatment, prognosis is usually good. However, a corneal scratch produced by a fingernail, a piece of paper, or other organic substance may cause a persistent lesion. Occasionally, the epithelium doesn't heal properly, and a recurrent corneal erosion may develop, with effects more severe than the original injury.

A foreign body causes corneal abrasion. Risk factors include failing to wear protective glasses in hazardous occupations and contact lens use.

Indications include redness, increased tearing, sensation of "something in the eye," pain disproportionate to the size of the injury, possible diminished visual acuity, and photophobia.

UVEITIS

Inflammation of the uveal tract, or uveitis, can occur in any one of several forms: anterior uveitis, which affects the iris (iritis) or both the iris and the ciliary body; posterior uveitis, which affects the choroid (choroiditis), or both the choroid and the retina (chorioretinitis); or panuveitis, which affects the entire uveal tract. Although clinical distinction isn't always possible, anterior uveitis occurs in two forms — granulomatous and nongranulomatous.

Untreated anterior uveitis progresses to posterior uveitis, causing scarring, cataracts, and glaucoma. With immediate treatment, anterior uveitis usually subsides after a few days to several weeks. However, recurrence is likely. Posterior uveitis usually produces some residual vision loss and marked blurring of vision.

Typically, uveitis is idiopathic. It can result from allergy, bacteria, viruses, fungi, chemicals, trauma, surgery, or systemic disease, such as rheumatoid arthritis, ankylosing spondylitis, and toxoplasmosis.

Signs and symptoms of anterior uveitis include moderate-to-severe eye pain, severe ciliary injection, photophobia, tearing, and a small, nonreactive pupil. Other indications are blurred vision and possible deposits on the back of the cornea (seen in the anterior chamber) called *keratic precipitates.*

Signs and symptoms of posterior uveitis include slightly decreased or blurred vision, photophobia, floating spots, or possible posterior synechia.

BLEPHARITIS

A common inflammatory condition of the lash follicles and meibomian glands of the upper or lower eyelids, blepharitis is common in children and is commonly bilateral. It usually occurs as seborrheic (nonulcerative) blepharitis or as staphylococcal (ulcerative) blepharitis. Both types may coexist. Blepharitis tends to recur and become chronic.

Seborrhea of the scalp, eyebrows, and ears generally causes seborrheic blepharitis. Staphylococcus aureus infection causes ulcerative blepharitis. Another cause is pediculosis of the brows and lashes (from *Phthirus pubis* or *Pediculus humanus capitis*), which irritates the lid margins.

Signs and symptoms of blepharitis include redness of the eyelid margins, itching of affected eye, burning of affected eye, foreign-body sensation, and sticky, crusted eyelids on waking. Other indications are unconscious eye rubbing, continual blinking, greasy scales (in seborrheic blepharitis), flaky scales on lashes, loss of lashes, and ulcerated areas on lid margins (in ulcerative blepharitis). Nits on the lashes are a sign of pediculosis.

Facts about blepharitis
(continued)

✦ Signs and symptoms: redness of the eyelid margins, itching and burning of affected eye, foreign-body sensation, and sticky, crusted eyelids on waking

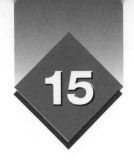

Ears, nose, and throat

A LOOK AT THE EARS, NOSE, AND THROAT

The ability to hear, smell, and taste allows us to communicate with others, connect with the world around us, and take pleasure in life. Because these senses play such vital roles in daily life, you'll need to thoroughly assess a patient's ears, nose, and throat.

Besides revealing impairments in hearing, smell, and taste, your assessment also can uncover important clues to physical problems in the patient's integumentary, musculoskeletal, cardiovascular, respiratory, immune, and neurologic systems.

To perform an accurate physical assessment, you'll need to understand the anatomy and physiology of the ears, nose, and throat.

EARS

The ear is divided into three parts: external, middle, and inner. The anatomy and physiology of each part play separate but important roles in hearing.

Structures of the ear

The ear can be divided into three main parts—the external ear, the middle ear, and the inner ear. (See *Structures of the ear*.)

External ear

The flexible external ear consists mainly of elastic cartilage. This part of the ear contains the ear flap, also known as the *auricle* or *pinna*, and the auditory canal. The outer third of this canal has a bony framework. Although not part of the external ear, the mastoid process is an important bony landmark behind the lower part of the auricle.

Bone covered by thin skin forms the inner two-thirds. The adult's external canal leads inward, downward, and forward to the middle ear. It's lined with glands that

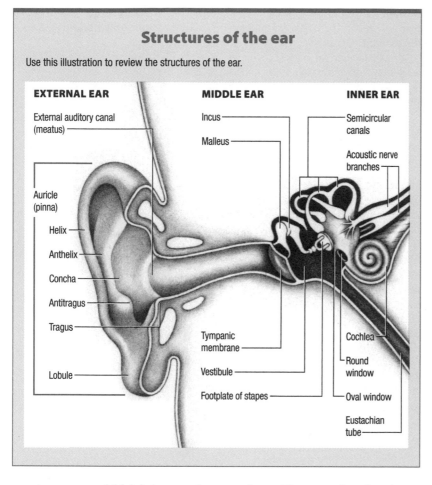

Structures of the ear

Use this illustration to review the structures of the ear.

EXTERNAL EAR

- External auditory canal (meatus)
- Auricle (pinna)
- Helix
- Anthelix
- Concha
- Antitragus
- Tragus
- Lobule

MIDDLE EAR

- Incus
- Malleus
- Tympanic membrane
- Vestibule
- Footplate of stapes

INNER EAR

- Semicircular canals
- Acoustic nerve branches
- Cochlea
- Round window
- Oval window
- Eustachian tube

secrete cerumen, which lubricates and protects the ear. The external ear functions to collect sounds and transmit them to the middle ear.

 SPECIAL POINTS *You may see coarse hair in the ear canal of elderly male patients.*

Middle ear

The tympanic membrane separates the external and middle ear. This pearl gray structure consists of three layers: skin, fibrous tissue, and a mucous membrane. Its upper portion, the pars flaccida, has little support; its lower portion, the pars tensa, is held taut. The center, or umbo, is attached to the tip of the long process of the malleus on the other side of the tympanic membrane.

A small, air-filled structure, the middle ear performs three vital functions.
- It transmits sound vibrations across the bony ossicle chain to the inner ear.
- It protects the auditory apparatus from intense vibrations.
- It equalizes the air pressure on both sides of the tympanic membrane to prevent it from rupturing.

The middle ear contains three small bones of the auditory ossicles: the malleus, or hammer; the incus, or anvil; and the stapes, or stirrup. These bones are linked like a chain and vibrate in place. The long process of the malleus fits into the incus,

External ear
(continued)

Special points
- ✦ In elderly male patients, coarse hair may appear in ear canal

Middle ear

- ✦ Tympanic membrane separates external and middle ear
- ✦ Transmit sound vibrations across bony ossicle chain to inner ear
- ✦ Protects auditory apparatus from intense vibrations
- ✦ Equalizes air pressure to prevent rupture
- ✦ Contains malleus, incus, and stapes
- ✦ Eustachian tube connects middle ear with nasopharynx

Inner ear

+ Consists of closed, fluid filled spaces within temporal bone
+ Contains bony labyrinth, including the vestibule, semicircular canals, and the cochlea
+ Cochlea serves as organ of hearing
+ Vestibule and semicircular canals maintain equilibrium

Functions of the ear

+ Enables hearing and maintains equilibrium

Hearing

+ Structures of external ear transmit sound waves
+ Cochlear branch of acoustic nerve transmits vibrations to brain where it interprets sound
+ Sound waves travel on pathways including air conduction and bone conduction

Equilibrium

+ Cristae respond to body movements
+ Moving releases impulses through the vestibular portion of the acoustic nerve to the brain
+ Pressure of gravity in inner ear maintains equilibrium and balance

Nose

+ Organ of smell
+ Filters, warms, and humidifies inhaled air

forming a true joint, and allows the two structures to move as a single unit. The proximal end of the stapes fits into the oval window, an opening that joins the middle and inner ear.

The eustachian tube connects the middle ear with the nasopharynx, equalizing air pressure on either side of the tympanic membrane. This tube also connects the ear's sterile area to the nasopharynx. The tube is opened during yawning or swallowing.

A normally functioning eustachian tube keeps the middle ear free from contaminants from the nasopharynx. Upper respiratory tract infections and allergies can block the tube, obstructing middle ear drainage, which may cause otitis media or effusion.

Inner ear

The inner ear consists of closed, fluid-filled spaces within the temporal bone. It contains the bony labyrinth, which includes three connected structures: the vestibule, the semicircular canals, and the cochlea. These structures are lined with the membranous labyrinth. A fluid called *perilymph* fills the space between the bony labyrinth and the membranous labyrinth, cushioning these sensitive organs.

The vestibule and semicircular canals help maintain equilibrium. The cochlea, a spiral chamber that resembles a snail shell, is the organ of hearing. The organ of Corti, part of the membranous labyrinth, contains hair cells that receive auditory sensations. The vestibular branch of the acoustic nerve contains peripheral nerve fibers that terminate in the epithelium of the semicircular canals, and the central branch terminates in the medulla at the vestibular nucleus.

Functions of the ear

The ear, a sensory organ, enables hearing and maintains equilibrium.

Hearing

When sound waves reach the external ear, structures there transmit the waves through the auditory canal to the tympanic membrane, causing it to vibrate and sending it to the stapes, through the oval window, producing sound waves of the perilymph. Finally, the cochlear branch of the acoustic nerve (cranial nerve VIII) transmits the vibrations to the temporal lobe of the cerebral cortex, where the brain interprets the sound.

Sound waves travel through the ear by two pathways—air conduction and bone conduction. Air conduction occurs when sound waves travel in the air through the external and middle ear to the inner ear. Bone conduction occurs when sound waves travel through the bone to the inner ear.

Balance

Besides controlling hearing, structures in the middle and inner ear control balance. The semicircular canals of the inner ear contain cristae—hairlike structures that respond to body movements. Endolymph fluid bathes the cristae.

When a person moves, the cristae bend, releasing impulses through the vestibular portion of the acoustic nerve to the brain, which controls balance. When a person is stationary, nerve impulses to the brain orient him to this position, and the pressure of gravity on the inner ear helps him maintain balance.

NOSE

The nose is more than the sensory organ of smell. It also plays a key role in the respiratory system by filtering, warming, and humidifying inhaled air. When you assess the nose, you'll typically assess the paranasal sinuses, too.

The lower two-thirds of the external nose consists of flexible cartilage; the upper one-third is rigid bone. Posteriorly, the internal nose merges with the pharynx. Anteriorly, it merges with the external nose.

The internal and external nose are divided vertically by the nasal septum, which is straight at birth and in early life but becomes slightly deviated or deformed in almost every adult. Only the posterior end, which separates the posterior nares, remains constantly in the midline.

Air entering the nose passes through the vestibule, which is lined with coarse hair that helps filter out dust. Olfactory receptors lie above the vestibule in the roof of the nasal cavity and the upper one-third of the septum. Known as the *olfactory region,* this area is rich in capillaries and mucus-producing goblet cells that help warm, moisten, and clean inhaled air. Kiesselbach's area, the most common site of nosebleeds, is located in the anterior portion of the septum. Because of its rich blood supply, the nasal mucosa is redder than the oral mucosa.

Further along the nasal passage are the superior, middle, and inferior turbinates. Separated by grooves called *meatuses,* the curved bony turbinates and their mucosal covering ease breathing by warming, filtering, and humidifying inhaled air.

Four pairs of paranasal sinuses open into the internal nose, including the:
+ maxillary sinuses, located on the cheeks below the eyes
+ frontal sinuses, located above the eyebrows
+ ethmoidal and sphenoidal sinuses, located behind the eyes and nose in the head.

The sinuses serve as resonators for sound production and provide mucus.

You'll be able to assess the maxillary and frontal sinuses, but the ethmoidal and sphenoidal sinuses aren't readily accessible. (See *Anatomic structure of the nose, mouth, and oropharynx,* page 370.)

The small openings between the sinuses and the nasal cavity can easily become obstructed because they're lined with mucous membranes that can become inflamed and swollen.

THROAT

The throat, or pharynx, is divided into the nasopharynx, the oropharynx, and the laryngopharynx. Located within the throat are the hard and soft palates, the uvula, and the tonsils. The mucous membrane lining the throat is normally smooth and bright pink to light red.

Food travels through the pharynx to the esophagus. Air travels through it to the larynx. The epiglottis diverts material away from the glottis during swallowing and helps prevent aspiration. By vibrating expired air through the vocal cords, the larynx produces sound. Changes in vocal cord length and air pressure affect the voice's pitch and intensity. The larynx also stimulates the vital cough reflex when a foreign body touches its sensitive mucosa. The most important function of the larynx is to act as a passage for air between the pharynx and the trachea.

The neck is formed by the cervical vertebrae and the major neck and shoulder muscles, together with their ligaments. Other important structures of the neck include the trachea, thyroid gland, and chains of lymph nodes.

The thyroid gland lies in the anterior neck, just below the larynx. Its two cone-shaped lobes are located on either side of the trachea and are connected by an isthmus below the cricoid cartilage, which gives the gland its butterfly shape. The largest endocrine gland, the thyroid produces the hormones triiodothyronine (T3) and thyroxine (T4), which affect the metabolic reactions of every cell in the body.

Structures of the nose
+ External nose consists of flexible cartilage and bone
+ Internal nose merges with pharynx and external nose
+ Nasal septum vertically divides internal and external nose
+ Vestibule contains olfactory receptors
+ Kiesselbach's area contains rich blood supply
+ Paranasal sinuses include maxillary, frontal, and ethmoidal and sphenoidal
+ Inflamed and swollen openings between the sinuses and nasal cavity can cause obstruction

Throat
+ Divided into nasopharynx, oropharynx, and laryngopharynx
+ Hard and soft palates, uvula, and tonsils lie within
+ Larynx acts as passage for air between pharynx and trachea
+ Includes neck structures, such as trachea, thyroid gland, and chains of lymph nodes

Anatomic structure of the nose, mouth, and oropharynx

These illustrations show the anatomic structures of the nose, mouth, and oropharynx.

NOSE AND MOUTH

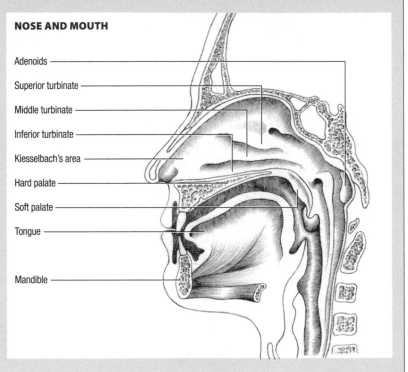

- Adenoids
- Superior turbinate
- Middle turbinate
- Inferior turbinate
- Kiesselbach's area
- Hard palate
- Soft palate
- Tongue
- Mandible

MOUTH AND OROPHARYNX

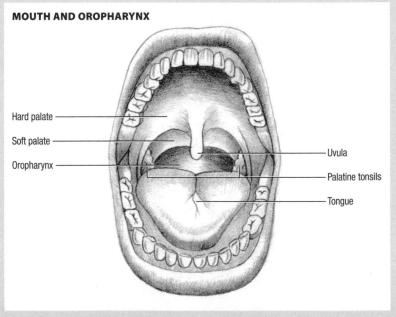

- Hard palate
- Soft palate
- Oropharynx
- Uvula
- Palatine tonsils
- Tongue

OBTAINING A HEALTH HISTORY

To investigate a patient's complaint about the ears, nose, or throat, ask about the onset, location, duration, and characteristics of the symptom as well as what aggravates and relieves it.

ASKING ABOUT THE EARS

The most common ear complaints are hearing loss, tinnitus, pain, discharge, and dizziness.

✦ If the patient reports hearing loss, ask him to describe it fully. Is it unilateral or bilateral? Continuous or intermittent? Ask about a family history of hearing loss. Then obtain the patient's medical history, noting chronic ear infections, ear surgery, and ear or head trauma. Has the patient recently had an upper respiratory infection? After taking a drug history, have the patient describe his occupation and work environment.

✦ Ask the patient to be more specific about complaints of pain such as onset, location, intensity, and associated symptoms.

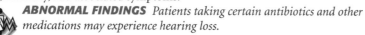 ***ABNORMAL FINDINGS*** *Patients taking certain antibiotics and other medications may experience hearing loss.*

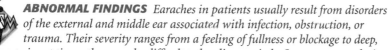 ***ABNORMAL FINDINGS*** *Earaches in patients usually result from disorders of the external and middle ear associated with infection, obstruction, or trauma. Their severity ranges from a feeling of fullness or blockage to deep, boring pain; at times, they may be difficult to localize precisely. Symptoms may be intermittent or continuous and may develop suddenly or gradually.*

Your patient may describe such signs and symptoms as:
✦ *Pain caused by touching or pulling the ear, for instance, usually indicates an external ear infection*
✦ *A deep, throbbing pain indicates a middle ear disorder.*
✦ *A severely inflamed outer ear may result from a swollen or completely blocked ear canal.*
✦ *A feeling of pressure or blockage can stem from a eustachian tube dysfunction that creates negative pressure in the middle ear or from muscle spasm or temporomandibular joint arthralgia.*

SPECIAL POINTS *Common causes of earache in children are acute otitis media and insertion of foreign bodies that become lodged or infected. Be alert for crying or ear tugging in a young child—nonverbal clues to earache.*

✦ Investigate any complaints of discharge. Ask about color and consistency, onset, and any history of head injury.

✦ Ask if the patient has any feelings of abnormal movement or spinning (vertigo). Determine when episodes occur, how often, if they recur, or if nausea, vomiting, or tinnitus accompany them.

✦ Ask the patient if he has allergies.

ABNORMAL FINDINGS *Patients with environmental or seasonal allergies may experience serous otitis media, or inflammation of the middle ear. Otitis externa, or inflammation of the external ear, can be caused by allergic reactions to hair dyes, cosmetics, perfumes, and other personal care products.*

ASKING ABOUT THE NOSE

The most common complaints about the nose include nasal stuffiness, nasal discharge, and epistaxis, or nosebleed. Ask if the patient has had any of these problems. Ask about the color and consistency of any discharge. Also ask about frequent

---

Obtaining a health history

✦ Investigates complaints
✦ Describes onset, location, duration, characteristics, and aggravating factors of symptoms

Asking about the ears

✦ Hearing loss, tinnitus, pain, discharge, and dizziness
✦ Family history of hearing loss
✦ Past medical history
✦ Drug history and occupation

Abnormal findings

✦ Hearing loss (antibiotic intake)
✦ Earaches (infection, obstruction, or trauma)
✦ Pain caused by touching or pulling (external ear infection)
✦ Deep, throbbing pain (middle ear disorder)
✦ Severely inflamed outer ear (blocked ear canal)
✦ Feeling of pressure (eustachian tube dysfunction)
✦ Environmental or seasonal allergies (serous otitis media)
✦ Allergic reactions to personal care products (otitis externa)

Special points

✦ In children, earache possibly caused by acute otitis media and insertion of foreign bodies
✦ Watch for nonverbal cues

Asking about the nose

✦ Nasal stuffiness, nasal discharge, and epistaxis

Asking about the nose
(continued)

Abnormal findings
+ Nasal stuffiness and discharge (environmental allergies)
+ Nasal obstruction (inflammatory, neoplastic, endocrine, or metabolic disorder)

Special points
+ In children, acute nasal obstruction usually results from common cold
+ Between ages 3 and 6, chronic nasal obstruction typically results from large adenoids
+ In neonates, choanal atresia most common congenital cause
+ In children, cystic fibrosis may cause nasal polyps

Alert!
+ Nasal obstruction may signal life-threatening disorders

Asking about the mouth, throat, and neck
+ For mouth, ask about bleeding, mouth or tongue ulcers, bad breath, toothaches
+ For throat, ask about frequent sore throats or hoarseness
+ For neck, ask about pain or tenderness, swelling

Abnormal findings
+ Throat pain, commonly known as *sore throat*, causes discomfort and is typically accompanied by ear pain

colds, hay fever, headaches, and sinus trouble. Ask whether certain conditions or places seem to cause or aggravate the patient's problem. Ask if he has ever had nose or head trauma. Also ask about insertion of a foreign body.

 ABNORMAL FINDINGS *Environmental allergies can cause nasal stuffiness and discharge, and stagnant nasal discharge can act as a culture medium and lead to sinusitis and other infections.*

If the patient's chief complaint is epistaxis and he isn't in any distress, ask the following questions. Does he have a history of recent trauma? How often has he had nosebleeds in the past? Have the nosebleeds been long or unusually severe? Has the patient recently had surgery in the sinus area? Ask about a history of hypertension, bleeding, or liver disorders and other recent illnesses. Ask whether the patient bruises easily. Find out what drugs he uses, especially anti-inflammatories, such as aspirin, and anticoagulants such as warfarin.

If the patient complains of nasal obstruction, ask him about the duration and frequency of the obstruction. Did it begin suddenly or gradually? Is it intermittent or persistent? Unilateral or bilateral? Inquire about the presence and character of drainage. Is it watery, purulent, or bloody? Does the patient have nasal or sinus pain or headaches? Ask about recent travel, the use of drugs or alcohol, and previous trauma or surgery.

 ABNORMAL FINDINGS *Nasal obstruction in a patient may result from an inflammatory, neoplastic, endocrine, or metabolic disorder; a structural abnormality; or a traumatic injury. It may cause discomfort, alter a patient's sense of taste and smell, and cause voice changes.*

 CLINICAL ALERT Although a frequent and typically benign symptom, nasal obstruction may herald certain life-threatening disorders, such as a basilar skull fracture or a malignant tumor.

 SPECIAL POINTS *In children, acute nasal obstruction usually results from the common cold. In infants and children, especially between ages 3 and 6, chronic nasal obstruction typically results from large adenoids. In neonates, choanal atresia is the most common congenital cause of nasal obstruction and can be unilateral or bilateral. Cystic fibrosis may cause nasal polyps in children, resulting in nasal obstruction. However, if the child has unilateral nasal obstruction and rhinorrhea, you should assume a foreign body is lodged in the nose until proven otherwise.*

ASKING ABOUT THE MOUTH, THROAT, AND NECK

Ask the patient if he has bleeding or sore gums, mouth or tongue ulcers, a bad taste in his mouth, bad breath, toothaches, loose teeth, frequent sore throats, hoarseness, or facial swelling. Also, ask whether he smokes or uses other types of tobacco. If the patient is having neck problems, ask if he has neck pain or tenderness, neck swelling, or trouble moving his neck.

Further assess throat pain with the following questions. Ask the patient when he first noticed the pain, and have him describe it. Has he had throat pain before? Is it accompanied by fever, ear pain, or dysphagia? Review the patient's medical history for throat problems, allergies, and systemic disorders.

 ABNORMAL FINDINGS *If a patient experiences throat pain — commonly known as* sore throat *— he has discomfort in any part of the pharynx: the nasopharynx, the oropharynx, or the hypopharynx. This common symptom ranges from a sensation of scratchiness to severe pain. It's typically accompanied by ear pain because cranial nerves IX and X innervate the pharynx as well as the middle and external ear.*

SPECIAL POINTS *In children, sore throat is a common complaint and may result from many of the same disorders that affect adults. Other pediatric causes of sore throat include acute epiglottiditis, herpangina, scarlet fever, acute follicular tonsillitis, and retropharyngeal abscess.*

If the patient complains of dysphagia or difficulty swallowing, ask the patient if swallowing is painful. If so, is the pain constant or intermittent? Have the patient point to where dysphagia feels most intense. Does eating alleviate or aggravate the symptom? Are solids or liquids more difficult to swallow? If the answer is liquids, ask if hot, cold, and lukewarm fluids affect him differently. Does the symptom disappear after he tries to swallow a few times? Is swallowing easier if he changes position? Ask if he has recently experienced vomiting, regurgitation, weight loss, anorexia, hoarseness, dyspnea, or a cough.

 ABNORMAL FINDINGS *In patients with esophageal disorders, dysphagia is the most common — and sometimes only — symptom. However, it may also result from an oropharyngeal, respiratory, neurologic, or collagen disorder or from the effects of toxins and treatments. Dysphagia increases the risk of choking and aspiration and may lead to malnutrition and dehydration.*

Dysphagia is classified by the phase of swallowing it affects:
✦ *Phase 1 dysphagia occurs during the transfer phase when swallowing begins, as the tongue presses against the hard palate to transfer the chewed food to the back of the throat. This phase usually results from a neuromuscular disorder.*
✦ *Phase 2 dysphagia occurs during the transfer phase of swallowing, when the soft palate closes against the pharyngeal wall to prevent nasal regurgitation. This phase usually indicates spasm or cancer.*
✦ *Phase 3 dysphagia occurs during the entrance phase of swallowing, as the food moves through the esophageal sphincter and into the stomach. This phase results from lower esophageal narrowing by diverticula, esophagitis, and other disorders.*

 SPECIAL POINTS *In infants or small children, be sure to pay close attention to sucking and swallowing ability. Coughing, choking, or regurgitation during feeding suggests dysphagia.*

More common in children than adults, corrosive esophagitis and esophageal obstruction by a foreign body are more common causes of dysphagia. However, dysphagia may also result from congenital anomalies, such as annular stenosis, dysphagia lusoria, and esophageal atresia.

In patients older than age 50 with head or neck cancer, dysphagia is usually the first symptom that causes them to seek care. The incidence of such cancers increases markedly in this age-group.

RELATED QUESTIONS

After asking specific questions about the ears, nose, mouth, throat, and neck, ask questions about the patient's general health.

Ask the patient these questions pertaining to signs and symptoms:
✦ Have you noticed changes in the way you tolerate hot and cold weather?
✦ Has your weight changed recently?
✦ Do you have breathing problems or feel as if your heart is skipping beats?
✦ Have you noticed a change in your menstrual pattern?
✦ Do you have a family history of Graves' disease?
✦ Have you noticed any tremors, agitation, difficulty concentrating, or sleeping?

 ABNORMAL FINDINGS *Watch for responses in patients that might indicate a thyroid disorder. Hyperthyroidism can cause heat intolerance, weight loss, and a short menstrual pattern with scant flow. Hypothyroidism can*

cause cold intolerance, weight gain, an increase in menstrual pattern and flow and, in extreme cases, bradycardia and dyspnea from low cardiac output.

ASSESSING THE EARS, NOSE, AND THROAT

Examining the ears, nose, and throat mainly involves using the techniques of inspection, palpation, and auscultation. An ear assessment also requires the use of an otoscope and the administration of hearing acuity tests.

EXAMINING THE EARS

To assess your patient's ears, you'll need to inspect and palpate the external structures, perform an otoscopic examination of the ear canal, and test his hearing acuity.

External observations

Begin by observing the ears for position and symmetry. The top of the ear should line up with the outer corner of the eye, and the ears should look symmetrical, with an angle of attachment of no more than 10 degrees. The face and ears should be the same shade and color.

Auricles that protrude from the head, or "lop" ears, are fairly common and don't affect hearing ability.

 ABNORMAL FINDINGS *Low-set ears commonly accompany congenital disorders, including kidney problems.*

Inspect the auricle for lesions, drainage, nodules or redness. Pull the helix back, and note if it's tender.

 ABNORMAL FINDINGS *If the patient feels pain when you pull the ear back, he may have otitis externa. If the patient has crusted, indurated, or ulcerated lesions that fail to heal, they should be excised and examined. These lesions may indicate a fairly common disorder known as* carcinoma of the auricle, *which may be either basal cell or squamous cell. Advanced lesions are easy to diagnose, but small growths are commonly overlooked.*

Then inspect and palpate the mastoid area behind each auricle.

 ABNORMAL FINDINGS *Assess for tenderness, redness, or warmth. Tenderness behind the ear may be present in otitis media. Redness or warmth could signal a local infection.*

Finally, inspect the opening of the ear canal. Patients normally have varying amounts of hair and cerumen, or earwax, in the ear canal. Cerumen may be flaky and vary in color.

 ABNORMAL FINDINGS *Be alert for discharge, redness, or odor. Also look for nodules or cysts. In acute otitis externa, the ear canal is often swollen, narrowed, moist, pale, tender, and sometimes, reddened. In chronic otitis externa, the ear canal is usually thickened, red, and itchy. Cerumen shouldn't be impacted in the ear canal.*

Temporomandibular joints

Inspect and palpate the temporomandibular joints, which are located anterior to and slightly below the auricle. To palpate these joints, place the middle three fingers of each hand bilaterally over each joint. Then gently press on the joints as the patient opens and closes his mouth. Evaluate the joints for movability, approximation

---

Assessing the ears, nose, and throat

✦ Inspection
✦ Palpation
✦ Auscultation
✦ Use of otoscope
✦ Hearing acuity test

Examining the ears

✦ Inspect and palpate the external structures
✦ Perform an otoscopic examination of ear canal
✦ Test hearing acuity

External observations

✦ Observe for position and symmetry
✦ Note if shading and coloring of face and ears are similar

Abnormal findings

✦ Low-set ears accompanying congenital disorders (kidney problems)
✦ Pain upon ear being pulled back (otitis externa)
✦ Lesions that fail to heal (carcinoma of the auricle)
✦ Tenderness behind the ear (otitis media)
✦ Discharge, redness, or odor (otitis externa)

Temporomandibular joints

✦ Inspect and palpate to evaluate movability, approximation, and discomfort (drawing of bones together), and discomfort. Normally, this process should be smooth and painless for the patient.

 ABNORMAL FINDINGS *The patient shouldn't experience neck pain, vertigo, otalgia, or stuffiness in the ear. Dislocation of the temporomandibular joints may be related to trauma. Arthritis may cause swelling, tenderness, and decreased range of motion. Crepitus or clicking may occur with poor occlusion, meniscus injury, or swelling due to trauma.*

Otoscopic examination

The next part of your ear assessment involves examining the patient's auditory canal, tympanic membrane, and malleus with the otoscope. (See *Using an otoscope,* page 376.)

Before inserting the speculum into the patient's ear canal, check the canal for foreign particles or discharge.

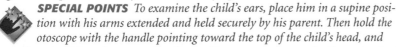 **ABNORMAL FINDINGS** *Obstruction of the ear canal by a foreign body occurs mostly in younger children. often Inanimate objects and vegetables are the most common objects found in a child's ear canal; cotton is the most common object found in an adult's ear canal. Pain and drainage may signal a foreign body, but sometimes no signs or symptoms occur, and the object may be found during a routine examination.*

Then palpate the tragus — the cartilaginous projection anterior to the external opening of the ear — and pull the auricle up.

ABNORMAL FINDINGS *If the tragus in a patient is tender, don't insert the speculum. He could have otitis externa, and inserting the speculum could be painful.*

To insert the speculum of the otoscope, tilt the patient's head away from you. Then grasp the superior posterior auricle with your thumb and index finger and pull it up and back to straighten the canal. Keep your hand along the patient's face to steady the otoscope. Because everyone's ear canal is shaped differently, vary the angle of the speculum until you can see the tympanic membrane.

SPECIAL POINTS *To examine the child's ears, place him in a supine position with his arms extended and held securely by his parent. Then hold the otoscope with the handle pointing toward the top of the child's head, and brace it against him using one or two fingers. Because an ear examination may upset the child with an earache, save it for the end of your physical examination. If your patient is a child younger than age 3, pull the auricle down to get a good view of the membrane.*

Insert the speculum to about one-third its length when inspecting the canal. Make sure you insert it gently because the inner two-thirds of the canal is sensitive to pressure. Note the color of the cerumen. Cerumen that's grayish brown and dry-looking is old. The external canal should be free from inflammation and scaling.

SPECIAL POINTS *The elderly patient may have harder, drier cerumen because of rigid cilia in the ear canal.*

If your view of the tympanic membrane is obstructed by excessive cerumen, don't try to remove it with an instrument or you could cause the patient excessive pain. Instead, use ceruminolytic drops and warm water irrigation, as ordered.

You may need to carefully rotate the speculum for a complete view of the tympanic membrane. The membrane should be pearl gray, glistening, and transparent. The annulus should be white and denser than the rest of the membrane.

Temporomandibular joints *(continued)*

Abnormal findings
- Trauma indicated by dislocation of temporomandibular joints
- Swelling, tenderness, and decreased ROM indicate arthritis
- Crepitus or clicking indicates poor occlusion, meniscus injury, or swelling

Otoscopic examination
- Examine auditory canal, tympanic membrane, and malleus
- Check canal for foreign particles or discharge

Abnormal findings
- Obstruction of the ear canal by foreign body occurs mostly in younger children
- Pain and drainage signals a foreign body
- Tender tragus indicates otitis externa; avoid inserting speculum

Special points
- Examine the child while parent holds him steady
- If patient is under age 3, pull auricle down to view
- In elderly patients, cerumen may appear harder and drier due to rigid cilia in ear canal

Using an otoscope

+ Insert speculum into patient's ear by pulling auricle up and back
+ Position the scope to view tympanic membrane structures

KNOW-HOW

Using an otoscope

The instructions below describe how to use an otoscope to examine the patient's ears.

INSERTING THE SPECULUM

Before inserting the speculum into the patient's ear, straighten the ear canal by grasping the auricle and pulling it up and back, as shown.

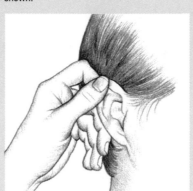

POSITIONING THE SCOPE

To examine the ear's external canal, hold the otoscope with the handle parallel to the patient's head, as shown. Bracing your hand firmly against his head keeps you from hitting the canal with the speculum.

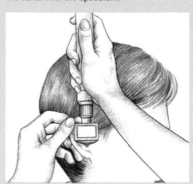

VIEWING THE STRUCTURES

When the otoscope is positioned properly, you should see the tympanic membrane structures shown here.

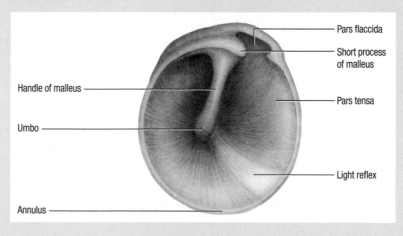

Pars flaccida

Short process of malleus

Handle of malleus

Pars tensa

Umbo

Light reflex

Annulus

Otoscopic examination
(continued)

Abnormal findings

+ Bulging, retraction, bleeding, lesions, or perforations
+ Discharge draining through perforated area
+ If light reflex displaced or absent, tympanic membrane may be bulging, inflamed, or retracted

ABNORMAL FINDINGS *Inspect the patient's tympanic membrane carefully for bulging, retraction, bleeding, lesions, or perforations, especially at the periphery. A perforated tympanic membrane appears as a hole surrounded by reddened tissue. You may see discharge draining through the perforated area.*

SPECIAL POINTS *The elderly patient's eardrum may appear cloudy, a normal finding related to aging.*

Now, examine the membrane for the light reflex. The light reflex in the right ear should be between 4 and 6 o'clock; in the left ear, it should be between 6 and 8 o'clock.

 ABNORMAL FINDINGS *If the light reflex in a patient's ear is displaced or absent, the tympanic membrane may be bulging, inflamed, or retracted.*

Finally, look for the bony landmarks. The malleus will appear as a dense, white streak at the 12 o'clock position. At the top of the light reflex, you'll find the umbo, the inferior point of the malleus.

Hearing acuity tests

The last part of an ear assessment is testing the patient's hearing. Begin by estimating hearing. Ask the patient to occlude one ear, or you can occlude it for him. Insert your finger quickly, but gently in the ear canal. Then stand 1' to 2' (30.5 to 61 cm) away, exhale fully, and whisper softly toward the unoccluded ear. Choose numbers or words that have two syllables that are equally accented such as "nine-four" or "baseball."

If hearing is diminished, use Weber's test and the Rinne test to assess conductive hearing loss, which is impaired sound transmission to the inner ear, and sensorineural hearing loss, which is impaired auditory nerve conduction or inner ear function.

Weber's test

Weber's test is performed when the patient reports diminished or lost hearing in one ear. This test uses a tuning fork to evaluate bone conduction. The tuning fork should be tuned to the frequency of normal human speech, 512 cycles/second.

To perform Weber's test, strike the tuning fork lightly against your hand, and then place the fork on the patient's forehead at the midline or on the top of his head. If he hears the tone equally well in both ears, record this as a normal Weber's test. If he hears the tone better in one ear, record the result as right or left lateralization.

 ABNORMAL FINDINGS *In a patient with conductive hearing loss, during lateralization the tone will sound louder in the ear with hearing loss because bone conducts the tone to the ear. Because the unaffected ear picks up other sounds, it doesn't hear the tone as clearly. In a patient with sensorineural hearing loss, sound is present only in the unaffected ear.*

Rinne test

Perform the Rinne test after Weber's test, to compare air conduction of sound with bone conduction of sound. To do this test, strike the tuning fork against your hand, and then place it over the patient's mastoid process. Ask him to tell you when the tone stops, and note this time in seconds. Next, move the still-vibrating tuning fork to the opening of the ear without touching the ear. Ask him to tell you when the tone stops. Note the time in seconds.

The patient should hear the air-conducted tone twice as long as he hears the bone-conducted tone.

 ABNORMAL FINDINGS *During the Rinne test, if the patient doesn't hear the air-conducted tone longer than the bone-conducted tone, he has a conductive hearing loss in the affected ear.*

Otoscopic examination
(continued)

Special points
+ In elderly patients, eardrum appearing cloudy is a normal finding

Hearing acuity tests
+ Weber's test and Rinne test assess conductive hearing loss

Weber's test
+ For diminished or loss of hearing
+ Tuning fork evaluates bone conduction
+ Hearing tone better in one ear indicates right or left lateralization

Abnormal findings
+ Conductive hearing loss — during lateralization, sound louder in the ear with hearing loss
+ Sensorineural hearing loss — sound present only in unaffected ear

Rinne test
+ Performed after Weber's test
+ Compares air conduction of sound with bone conduction of sound
+ Tuning fork over mastoid process
+ Air-conducted tone should be heard twice as long as bone-conducted tone

Abnormal findings
+ Conductive hearing loss in the affected ear, indicated from inability to hear air-conducted tone longer than bone-conducted tone

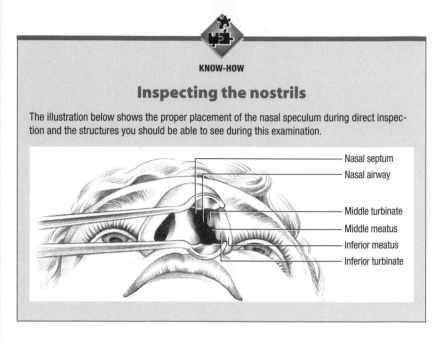

KNOW-HOW

Inspecting the nostrils

The illustration below shows the proper placement of the nasal speculum during direct inspection and the structures you should be able to see during this examination.

- Nasal septum
- Nasal airway
- Middle turbinate
- Middle meatus
- Inferior meatus
- Inferior turbinate

Examining the nose and sinuses

- ✦ Includes checking the sinuses
- ✦ Uses inspection and palpation

Inspecting and palpating the nose

- ✦ Observe for position, symmetry, and color

Abnormal findings

- ✦ Discoloration, swelling, deformity, or skin breakdown
- ✦ Nasal discharge or flaring (respiratory distress)
- ✦ Obstruction (systemic disorders, trauma, allergies, or exposure to irritants)
- ✦ Nasal drainage accompanied by sinus tenderness and fever (acute sinusitis)
- ✦ Bloody discharge, (spontaneous or traumatic epistaxis)
- ✦ Thick, white, yellow, or greenish drainage (infection)
- ✦ Clear, thin drainage (rhinitis or possibly CSF leakage from basilar skull fracture)

EXAMINING THE NOSE AND SINUSES

A complete examination of the nose also includes checking the sinuses. To perform this examination, use the techniques of inspection and palpation.

Inspecting and palpating the nose

Begin by observing the patient's nose for position, symmetry, and color.

ABNORMAL FINDINGS *On inspection and palpation, you may find:*
- ✦ *variations, such as discoloration, swelling, deformity, or skin breakdown (Variations in size and shape are largely due to differences in cartilage and in the amount of fibroadipose tissue.)*
- ✦ *nasal discharge or flaring, which may be normal during quiet breathing in adults and in children (Marked, regular nasal flaring in an adult signals respiratory distress.)*
- ✦ *obstruction of the nasal mucous membranes along with a discharge of thin mucus, which can signal systemic disorders; nasal or sinus disorders such as a deviated septum; trauma, such as a basilar skull or nasal fracture; excessive use of vasoconstricting nose drops or sprays; and allergies or exposure to irritants, such as dust, tobacco smoke, or fumes*
- ✦ *nasal drainage accompanied by sinus tenderness and fever, which suggests acute sinusitis usually involving the frontal or maxillary sinuses*
- ✦ *bloody discharge, which usually results from the patient blowing his nose, but spontaneous or traumatic epistaxis can also occur*
- ✦ *thick, white, yellow, or greenish drainage, which suggests infection*
- ✦ *clear, thin drainage, which may simply indicate rhinitis, but must be monitored closely as it may be cerebrospinal fluid leaking from a basilar skull fracture.*

To test nasal patency and olfactory nerve (cranial nerve I) function, ask the patient to block one nostril and inhale a familiar aromatic substance through the other nostril. Possible substances include soap, coffee, citrus, tobacco, or nutmeg. Ask him to identify the aroma. Then repeat the process with the other nostril, using a different aroma.

KNOW-HOW

Palpating the maxillary sinuses

To palpate the maxillary sinuses, gently press your thumbs on each side of the nose just below the cheekbones, as shown. The illustration also shows the location of the frontal sinuses.

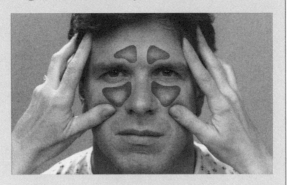

Now, inspect the nasal cavity. Ask the patient to tilt his head back slightly, and then push the tip of his nose up. Use the light from the otoscope to illuminate his nasal cavities.

 ABNORMAL FINDINGS *Check the patient for severe deviation or perforation of the nasal septum. Examine the vestibule and turbinates for redness, softness, and discharge.*

Examine the nostrils by direct inspection, using a nasal speculum and a penlight or small flashlight, or an otoscope with a short, wide-tip attachment. Have the patient sit in front of you with his head tilted back. Put on gloves, and insert the tip of the closed nasal speculum into one nostril to the point where the blade widens. Slowly open the speculum as wide as possible without causing discomfort. Shine the flashlight in the nostril to illuminate the area.

Observe the color and patency of the nostril, and check for exudate. The mucosa should be moist, pink to light red, and free from lesions and polyps. After inspecting one nostril, close the speculum, remove it, and inspect the other nostril. (See *Inspecting the nostrils.*)

 ABNORMAL FINDINGS *In patients with viral rhinitis, the mucosa will appear red and swollen. In patients with allergic rhinitis, the mucosa may be pale, bluish, or red.*

Finally, palpate the patient's nose with your thumb and forefinger, assessing for pain, tenderness, swelling, and deformity.

Examining the sinuses

Next examine the sinuses. Remember, only the frontal and maxillary sinuses are accessible; you won't be able to palpate the ethmoidal and sphenoidal sinuses. However, if the frontal and maxillary sinuses are infected, you can assume that the other sinuses are, too.

Begin by checking for swelling around the eyes, especially over the sinus area. Then palpate the sinuses, checking for tenderness. (See *Palpating the maxillary sinuses.*) To palpate the frontal sinuses, place your thumbs above the patient's eyes just under the bony ridges of the upper orbits, and place your fingertips on his forehead. Apply gentle pressure. Next palpate the maxillary sinuses. If the patient complains of tenderness during palpation of the sinuses, use transillumination to

Palpating the maxillary sinuses

✦ Gently press your thumbs on each side of the nose
✦ Palpate frontal sinuses

Inspecting and palpating the nose
(continued)

Abnormal findings: The nasal septum
✦ Vestibule and turbinate redness, softness, and discharge (severe deviation or perforation)

Abnormal findings: The nasal mucosa
✦ Red and swollen (viral rhinitis)
✦ Pale, bluish, or red (allergic rhinitis)

Examining the sinuses

✦ Examine frontal and maxillary sinuses for swelling and tenderness
✦ Use transillumination to investigate tenderness

Transilluminating the sinuses

+ Detects sinus tumors and obstruction
+ For frontal sinuses, place penlight on supraorbital ring
+ For maxillary sinuses, place penlight on cheekbone just below eye

Examining the sinuses
(continued)

Abnormal findings
+ Local tenderness with pain, fever, and nasal discharge (acute sinusitis)

Examining the mouth, throat, and neck

+ Involves inspection, palpation, and auscultation

Assessing the mouth and throat

+ Involves inspecting the lips, oral mucosa, gums, tongue, mouth floor, and oropharynx; palpating the lips, tongue, and oropharynx; and testing gag reflex

Special points: The lips
+ Bluish hue or flecked pigmentation commonly appear in dark-skinned patients

KNOW-HOW

Transilluminating the sinuses

Transillumination of the sinuses helps detect sinus tumors and obstruction and requires only a penlight. Before you start, darken the room.

FRONTAL SINUSES
Place the penlight on the supraorbital ring, and direct the light upward to illuminate the frontal sinuses just above the eyebrow, as shown.

MAXILLARY SINUSES
Place the penlight on the patient's cheekbone just below the eye, then ask her to open her mouth. The light should transilluminate easily and equally.

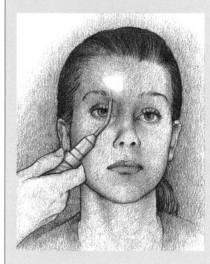
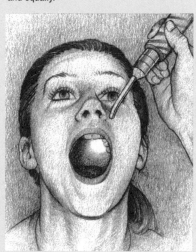

see if the sinuses are filled with fluid or pus. Transillumination can also help reveal tumors and obstructions. (See *Transilluminating the sinuses.*)

 ABNORMAL FINDINGS *If the patient experiences local tenderness and other symptoms such as pain, fever, and nasal discharge, these suggest acute sinusitis.*

EXAMINING THE MOUTH, THROAT, AND NECK

Assessing the mouth and throat requires the techniques of inspection and palpation. Assessing the neck also involves auscultation.

Assessing the mouth and throat

First, inspect the patient's lips. They should be pink, moist, symmetrical, and without lesions. Put on gloves and palpate the lips for lumps or surface abnormalities.

SPECIAL POINTS *A bluish hue or flecked pigmentation of the lips is common in dark-skinned patients.*

Use a tongue blade and a bright light to inspect the oral mucosa. Have the patient open his mouth, and then place the tongue blade on top of his tongue. The oral mucosa should be pink, smooth, moist, and free from lesions and unusual odors.

 SPECIAL POINTS *Increased pigmentation of the oral mucosa is seen in dark-skinned patients.*

Next observe the gingivae, or gums: They should be pink, moist, have clearly defined margins at each tooth, and not be retracted. Inspect the teeth, noting their number, condition, and whether any are missing or crowded. If a patient is wearing dentures, ask him to remove them and then examine the gums.

Finally, inspect the tongue. It should be midline, symmetrical, moist, pink, and free from lesions. The posterior surface should be smooth, and the anterior surface should be slightly rough with small fissures. The tongue should move easily in all directions, and it should lie straight to the front at rest.

 ABNORMAL FINDINGS *Asymmetric protrusion of the patient's tongue suggests a lesion of cranial nerve XII.*

Ask the patient to raise the tip of his tongue and touch his palate directly behind his front teeth. Inspect the ventral surface of the tongue and the floor of the mouth. Next, wrap a piece of gauze around the tip of the tongue and move the tongue first to one side then the other to inspect the lateral borders. They should be smooth and even-textured.

 SPECIAL POINTS *The elderly patient may have varicose veins on the ventral surface of the tongue. The area underneath the tongue is a common site for the development of oral cancers, so be sure to assess it thoroughly.*

Inspect the patient's oropharynx by asking him to open his mouth while you shine the penlight on the uvula and palate. You may need to insert a tongue blade into the mouth and depress the tongue. Place the tongue blade slightly off-center to avoid eliciting the gag reflex. The uvula and oropharynx should be pink and moist, without inflammation or exudates. The tonsils should be pink and shouldn't be hypertrophied. Ask the patient to say "ah," and then observe for movement of the soft palate and uvula.

 ABNORMAL FINDINGS *If your patient has a peritonsillar abscess causing him painful swallowing and a displaced, beefy, red uvula, this is usually caused by acute tonsillitis and is a potential emergency because it can cause airway obstruction. In this condition, a streptococcal infection spreads from the tonsils to the surrounding soft tissue.*
In cranial nerve X paralysis, when the patient says "ah," the soft palate fails to rise and the uvula deviates to the opposite side.

Finally, palpate the lips, tongue, and oropharynx.

 ABNORMAL FINDINGS *Note lumps, lesions, ulcers, or edema of the lips or tongue. Swelling of the lips and tongue could indicate angioedema, which is usually allergic in nature. Lesions and ulcerations on the lips may be related to herpes simplex infection or syphilis. Carcinoma may appear as a scaly plaque, an ulcer, or a nodular lesion—it usually affects the lower lip.*

Assess the patient's gag reflex by gently touching the back of the pharynx with a cotton-tipped applicator or tongue blade. This should produce a bilateral response.

Inspecting and palpating the neck

First, observe the patient's neck. It should be symmetrical and the skin should be intact. Note any scars.

Assessing the mouth and throat (continued)

Special points: The oral mucosa
+ Increased pigmentation normal in dark-skinned patients

Abnormal findings: The tongue
+ Asymmetric protrusion (lesion of CN XII)

Special points: Elderly patients and the tongue
+ In elderly patients, varicose veins may appear on the ventral surface of the tongue
+ Area underneath tongue common site of oral cancers

Abnormal findings: The tonsils
+ Peritonsillar abscess causes painful swallowing and displaced, beefy, red uvula (acute tonsillitis)
+ Deviating uvula (CN X paralysis)

Abnormal findings: The lips and tongue
+ Swelling (angioedema)
+ Lesions and ulcerations on lips (herpes simplex infection or syphilis)
+ Scaly plaque, ulcer, or nodular lesion on lower lip (carcinoma)

Inspecting and palpating the neck
+ Observe for symmetry and intact skin

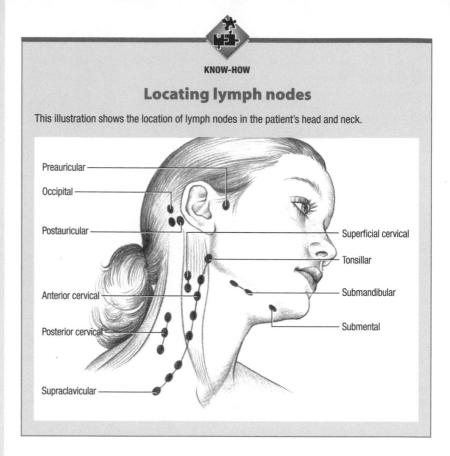

KNOW-HOW

Locating lymph nodes

This illustration shows the location of lymph nodes in the patient's head and neck.

- Preauricular
- Occipital
- Postauricular
- Anterior cervical
- Posterior cervical
- Supraclavicular
- Superficial cervical
- Tonsillar
- Submandibular
- Submental

Inspecting and palpating the neck
(continued)

Abnormal findings

- ✦ Diffusely enlarged thyroid (Graves' disease, Hashimoto's thyroiditis, or endemic goiter)
- ✦ Multiple nodules on thyroid (metabolic disease)
- ✦ Lymph node enlargement (infection)
- ✦ Venous distention (heart failure)

Palpating the lymph nodes

- ✦ Palpating neck gathers further information
- ✦ Assess nodes for size, shape, mobility, consistency, and tenderness

Abnormal findings

- ✦ Enlargement of the supraclavicular node (thoracic or abdominal cancer)
- ✦ Tender nodes (inflammation)
- ✦ Hard or fixed nodes (malignancy)
- ✦ Generalized lymphadenopathy (HIV or AIDS)

ABNORMAL FINDINGS *No visible pulsations, masses, swelling, venous distention, or thyroid or lymph node enlargement should be present. A diffusely enlarged thyroid is commonly related to Graves' disease, Hashimoto's thyroiditis, or endemic goiter. Multiple nodules on the thyroid suggests a metabolic cause; a single nodule may be a benign cyst or a tumor. Lymph node enlargement could indicate infection. Venous distention is seen with heart failure.*

Ask the patient to move his neck through the entire range of motion and to shrug his shoulders. Also, ask him to swallow. Note rising of the larynx, trachea, or thyroid.

Palpate the lymph nodes

Palpate the patient's neck to gather more data. Using the finger pads of both hands, bilaterally palpate the chain of lymph nodes under the patient's chin in the preauricular area; then proceed to the area under and behind the ears. (See *Locating lymph nodes.*) Assess the nodes for size, shape, mobility, consistency, and tenderness, comparing nodes on one side with those on the other.

ABNORMAL FINDINGS *During assessment, you may find:*
- ✦ *Enlargement of a supraclavicular node, especially on the left, which suggests possible metastasis from a thoracic or abdominal cancer.*
- ✦ *Tender nodes, which are indicative of inflammation; hard or fixed nodes, which suggest malignancy.*
- ✦ *Generalized lymphadenopathy, which requires further investigation; human immunodeficiency virus infection or acquired immunodeficiency syndrome may be the cause.*

Structure of the thyroid gland

This illustration shows the structure and location of the thyroid gland.

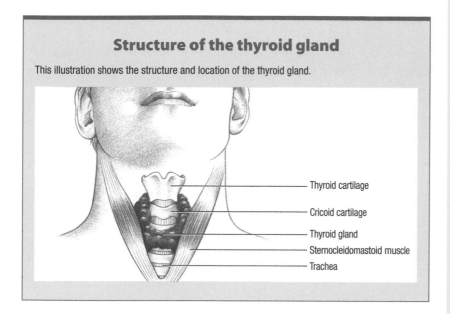

- Thyroid cartilage
- Cricoid cartilage
- Thyroid gland
- Sternocleidomastoid muscle
- Trachea

Palpate the trachea

Next palpate the trachea, normally located midline in the neck. Place your thumbs along each side of the trachea near the lower part of the neck. Check whether the distance between the trachea's outer edge and the sternocleidomastoid muscle is equal on both sides. Note any pain or tenderness.

 ABNORMAL FINDINGS *Tracheal deviation may result from a mass in the neck, or mediastinal mass, atelectasis, or a pneumothorax.*

Palpate the thyroid

To palpate the thyroid, stand behind the patient and put your hands around his neck, with the fingers of both hands over the lower trachea. Ask him to swallow as you feel the thyroid isthmus. The isthmus should rise with swallowing because it lies across the trachea, just below the cricoid cartilage.

Displace the thyroid to the right and then to the left, palpating both lobes for enlargement, nodules, tenderness, a gritty sensation, or a pulsation. (See *Structure of the thyroid gland.*) Lowering the patient's chin slightly and turning toward the side you're palpating helps relax the muscle and facilitate assessment.

 ABNORMAL FINDINGS *If the patient has an enlarged thyroid, this is referred to as a* goiter.

Auscultating the neck

Finally, auscultate the neck. Using light pressure on the bell of the stethoscope, listen over the carotid arteries. Ask the patient to hold his breath while you listen, to prevent breath sounds from interfering with the sounds of circulation.

ABNORMAL FINDINGS *When auscultating the neck, listen for bruits, which signal turbulent blood flow.*

During your assessment, if you detect an enlarged thyroid gland, also auscultate the thyroid area with the bell. Check for a bruit or a soft rushing sound, which indicates a hypermetabolic state.

Palpating the trachea
+ Check that distance between trachea's outer edge and sternocleidomastoid muscle are equal on both sides

Abnormal findings
+ Tracheal deviation (mass in the neck, mediastinal mass, atelectasis, or pneumothorax)

Palpating the thyroid
+ Palpate thyroid isthmus, which should rise with swallowing
+ Displace thyroid, palpating for enlargement, nodules, tenderness, a gritty sensation, or a pulsation

Abnormal findings
+ Goiter (enlarged thyroid)

Auscultating the neck
+ Listen over the carotid arteries with bell of the stethoscope

Abnormal findings
+ Turbulent blood flow (bruits)
+ Bruit or soft rushing sound in enlarged thyroid (hypermetabolic state)

INTERPRETING YOUR FINDINGS

After you assess the patient, a group of findings may lead you to suspect a particular disorder. (See *The ears, nose, and throat: Interpreting your findings.*)

EAR, NOSE, AND THROAT DISORDERS

ACUTE OTITIS MEDIA

Otitis media — or inflammation of the middle ear — may be acute, chronic, or serous. Acute otitis media, which is common in children, appears suddenly and lasts only a short time. Its incidence rises during the winter months, paralleling the seasonal rise in bacterial respiratory tract infections. It results from disruption of eustachian tube patency.

With the acute form, respiratory tract infection, allergic reaction, or positional changes (such as holding an infant in the supine position during feeding) allow reflux of nasopharyngeal flora through the eustachian tube and colonization in the middle ear.

A patient with acute otitis media may be asymptomatic, but the typical signs and symptoms are severe, deep, throbbing pain; upper respiratory tract infection; mild to high fever; hearing loss (usually mild and conductive); lack of response or inattention to spoken word; sensation of blockage in ear; dizziness; obscured or distorted bony landmarks of the tympanic membrane (evident on otoscopy); and nausea and vomiting. Herpetic lesions in the ear canal may be visible. Other possible signs include bulging of the tympanic membrane with concomitant erythema, and purulent drainage in the ear canal from tympanic membrane rupture.

OTITIS EXTERNA

Otitis externa, or inflammation of the external ear canal skin and auricle, may be acute or chronic. It usually occurs in hot, humid, summer weather and is also called *swimmer's ear*. With treatment, the acute form usually subsides within 7 days, although it may become chronic and recurring. Severe chronic otitis externa may reflect underlying diabetes mellitus, hypothyroidism, or nephritis.

Acute otitis externa is characterized by moderate to severe pain. The pain increases when manipulating the auricle or tragus, clenching the teeth, opening the mouth, or chewing. If palpating the tragus or auricle causes pain, the problem is otitis externa, not otitis media.

Other signs and symptoms of acute infection include fever; a foul-smelling aural discharge; partial hearing loss; scaling, itching, inflammation, or tenderness; a swollen external ear canal and auricle, which can be seen on otoscopy; periauricular lymphadenopathy (tender nodes in front of the tragus, behind the ear, or in the upper neck); and, occasionally, regional cellulitis.

Fungal otitis externa may not produce symptoms. However, *Aspergillus niger* produces a black or gray blotting-paper-like growth in the ear canal. The canal lumen is narrowed to one-quarter of the normal size. A thick, red epithelium is visible after the fungal growth is removed.

Ear, nose, and throat disorders

Facts about acute otitis media

+ Inflammation of the middle ear
+ Appears as acute, chronic, or serous
+ Severe, deep, throbbing pain; upper respiratory tract infection; mild to high fever; hearing loss; dizziness, nausea and vomiting
+ Signs include bulging tympanic membrane or drainage from ear canal

Facts about otitis externa

+ Inflammation of the external ear canal skin and auricle
+ Fever, foul-smelling aural discharge, partial hearing loss, inflammation, itching, swelling, tenderness
+ Fungal otitis externa produces black or gray growth in ear canal

The ears, nose, and throat: Interpreting your findings

The chart below shows common groups of findings for the signs and symptoms of disorders of the ears, nose, and throat, along with their probable causes.

SIGN OR SYMPTOM AND FINDINGS	PROBABLE CAUSE
Earache	
✦ Sensation of blockage or fullness in the ear ✦ Itching ✦ Partial hearing loss ✦ Possible dizziness	✦ Cerumen impaction
✦ Mild to moderate ear pain that occurs with tragus manipulation ✦ Low-grade fever ✦ Sticky yellow or purulent ear discharge ✦ Partial hearing loss ✦ Feeling of blockage in the ear ✦ Swelling of the tragus, external meatus, and external canal ✦ Lymphadenopathy	✦ Otitis externa, acute
✦ Severe, deep, throbbing ear pain ✦ Hearing loss ✦ High fever ✦ Bulging, fiery red eardrum	✦ Otitis media, acute suppurative
Hearing loss	
✦ Conductive hearing loss ✦ Ear pain or a feeling of fullness ✦ Nasal congestion ✦ Conjunctivitis	✦ Allergies
✦ Sudden or intermittent conductive hearing loss ✦ Bony projections visible in the ear canal ✦ Normal tympanic membrane	✦ Osteoma
✦ Abrupt hearing loss ✦ Ear pain ✦ Tinnitus ✦ Vertigo ✦ Sense of fullness in the ear	✦ Tympanic membrane perforation
Dysphagia	
✦ Signs of respiratory distress, such as crowing and stridor ✦ Phase 2 dysphagia with gagging and dysphonia	✦ Airway obstruction

(continued)

The ears, nose, and throat: Interpreting your findings *(continued)*

SIGN OR SYMPTOM AND FINDINGS	PROBABLE CAUSE
Dysphagia (continued)	
✦ Phase 2 and 3 dysphagia ✦ Rapid weight loss ✦ Steady chest pain ✦ Cough with hemoptysis ✦ Hoarseness ✦ Sore throat ✦ Hiccups	✦ Esophageal cancer
✦ Painless, progressive dysphagia ✦ Lead line on the gums ✦ Metallic taste ✦ Papilledema ✦ Ocular palsy ✦ Footdrop or wristdrop ✦ Mental impairment or seizures	✦ Lead poisoning
Epistaxis	
✦ Ecchymoses ✦ Petechiae ✦ Bleeding from the gums, mouth, and I.V. puncture sites ✦ Menorrhagia ✦ Signs of GI bleeding, such as melena and hematemesis	✦ Coagulation disorders
✦ Unilateral or bilateral epistaxis ✦ Nasal swelling ✦ Periorbital ecchymoses and edema ✦ Pain ✦ Nasal deformity ✦ Crepitation of the nasal bones	✦ Nasal fracture
✦ Oozing epistaxis ✦ Dry cough ✦ Abrupt onset of chills and high fever ✦ "Rose-spot" rash ✦ Vomiting ✦ Profound fatigue ✦ Anorexia	✦ Typhoid fever
Nasal obstruction	
✦ Watery nasal discharge ✦ Sneezing ✦ Temporary loss of smell and taste ✦ Sore throat ✦ Malaise ✦ Arthralgia ✦ Mild headache	✦ Common cold

The ears, nose, and throat: Interpreting your findings *(continued)*

SIGN OR SYMPTOM AND FINDINGS	PROBABLE CAUSE
Nasal obstruction (continued)	
◆ Anosmia ◆ Clear, watery nasal discharge ◆ History of allergies, chronic sinusitis, trauma, cystic fibrosis, or asthma ◆ Translucent, pear-shaped polyps that are unilateral or bilateral	◆ Nasal polyps
◆ Thick, purulent drainage ◆ Severe pain over the sinuses ◆ Fever ◆ Inflamed nasal mucosa with purulent mucus	◆ Sinusitis
Throat pain	
◆ Seasonal or year-round occurrence ◆ Nasal congestion with a thin nasal discharge and postnasal drip ◆ Paroxysmal sneezing ◆ Decreased sense of smell ◆ Frontal or temporal headache ◆ Pale and glistening nasal mucosa with edematous nasal turbinates ◆ Watery eyes	◆ Allergic rhinitis
◆ Mild to severe hoarseness ◆ Temporary loss of voice ◆ Malaise ◆ Low-grade fever ◆ Dysphagia ◆ Dry cough ◆ Tender, enlarged cervical lymph nodes	◆ Laryngitis
◆ Mild to severe sore throat ◆ Pain may radiate to the ears ◆ Dysphagia ◆ Headache ◆ Malaise ◆ Fever with chills ◆ Tender cervical lymphadenopathy	◆ Tonsillitis, acute

MASTOIDITIS

Mastoiditis, a bacterial infection and inflammation of the mastoid antrum air cells, usually results as a complication of chronic otitis media and, less commonly, of acute otitis media. An accumulation of pus under pressure in the middle ear cavity results in necrosis of adjacent tissue and extension of the infection into the mastoid cells, along with increasing drainage. The infection may lead to cholesteatoma.

Facts about mastoiditis

◆ Bacterial infection and inflammation of the mastoid antrum air cells
◆ Results as a complication of chronic otitis media

Facts about mastoiditis
(continued)

✦ Accumulating pus under pressure in middle ear cavity results in necrosis of adjacent tissue

✦ Causes dull ache and tenderness, fever, and thick, purulent discharge

Facts about pharyngitis

✦ Acute or chronic inflammation of pharyngeal walls

✦ May also include tonsils, palate, and uvula

✦ Causes sore throat and difficulty swallowing

✦ Malaise, fever, headache, and muscle and joint pain

Facts about hearing loss

✦ Cerumen impaction, foreign body, or polyp obstructing ear canal

✦ Otitis media interferes with the transmission of sound

✦ Trauma disrupts middle ear's bony chain

✦ Otosclerosis interferes with transmission of sound vibrations

✦ Toxic drug reaction causes rapid hearing loss

Facts about Ménière's disease

✦ Known as *endolymphatic hydrops*

✦ Causes violent paroxysmal attacks of severe vertigo

✦ Tinnitus, sensorineural hearing loss, nausea, vomiting, sweating, nystagmus

Chronic systemic diseases or immunosuppression may also lead to mastoiditis. The prognosis is good with early treatment.

Signs and symptoms include dull ache and tenderness in the area of the mastoid process; low-grade fever; thick, purulent discharge that gradually becomes more profuse; postauricular erythema and edema (may push the auricle out from the head); conductive hearing loss; and edema, erythema, and perforation of the tympanic membrane. Cholesteatoma of the mastoid may be present as well as lymphosclerosis of the tympanic membrane.

PHARYNGITIS

Pharyngitis is an acute or chronic inflammation of the pharyngeal walls and may include the tonsils, palate, and uvula. It usually occurs among adults who live or work in dusty or dry environments, use their voices excessively, use tobacco or alcohol habitually, or suffer from chronic sinusitis, persistent coughs, or allergies. Acute pharyngitis may precede the common cold or other communicable diseases. Chronic pharyngitis is commonly an extension of nasopharyngeal obstruction or inflammation. Uncomplicated pharyngitis usually subsides in 3 to 10 days.

Signs and symptoms include a sore throat and slight difficulty swallowing (swallowing saliva is usually more painful than swallowing food); sensation of a lump or feeling of fullness in the throat; a constant, aggravating urge to swallow; reddened, inflamed posterior pharyngeal wall; red, edematous mucous membranes studded with white and yellow follicles; and exudate, usually confined to the lymphoid areas of the throat, sparing the tonsillar pillars.

Associated signs and symptoms include malaise, mild fever, headache, and muscle and joint pain, especially in bacterial pharyngitis.

HEARING LOSS

Several factors can interfere with the ear's ability to conduct sound waves. Cerumen, a foreign body, or a polyp may be obstructing the ear canal. Otitis media may have thickened the fluid in the middle ear, which interferes with the vibrations that transmit sound. Otosclerosis may have hardened the bones in the middle ear, or trauma may have disrupted the middle ear's bony chain.

Sensorineural hearing loss also has several causes. The most common cause is loss of hair cells in the organ of Corti. In elderly patients, presbycusis, or progressive hearing loss, results from atrophy of the organ of Corti and the auditory nerve. Hearing loss can also result from trauma to the hair cells caused by loud noise or ototoxicity. (See *Evaluating hearing loss.*)

Also, a toxic reaction to a drug can cause a rapid loss of hearing. If hearing loss is detected, the medication must be discontinued immediately. Drugs that may affect hearing include aspirin, aminoglycosides, loop diuretics, and several chemotherapeutic agents, including cisplatin.

MÉNIÈRE'S DISEASE

Also known as *endolymphatic hydrops*, Ménière's disease affects an estimated 545,000 people in the United States, usually adults between ages 30 and 60. Patients with this condition experience violent paroxysmal attacks of severe vertigo lasting from 10 minutes to several hours. After multiple attacks over several years, this disorder leads to residual tinnitus and hearing loss. A metabolic alteration in the labyrinthine fluid is thought to cause this effect on the vestibular system.

Signs and symptoms of Ménière's disease include severe vertigo, tinnitus, and sensorineural hearing loss. Other signs and symptoms may occur during severe at-

Evaluating hearing loss

Use this chart to review the causes, onset, and associated signs and symptoms of hearing loss.

CAUSE	ONSET	SIGNS AND SYMPTOMS
External ear		
Cerumen impaction	Sudden or gradual	Itching
Foreign body	Sudden	Discharge
Otitis externa	Sudden	Pain, discharge
Middle ear		
Serous otitis media	Sudden or gradual	Fullness, itching
Acute otitis media	Sudden	Pain, fever, upper respiratory tract infection
Perforated tympanic membrane	Sudden	Trauma, discharge
Inner ear		
Presbycusis	Gradual	None
Drug-induced loss (ototoxicity)	Sudden or gradual	Tinnitus, other adverse drug effects
Ménière's disease	Sudden	Dizziness
Acoustic neuroma	Gradual	Vertigo

Evaluating hearing loss

✦ External ear — causes include cerumen impaction, foreign body, or otitis externa
✦ Middle ear — causes include serous otitis media, acute otitis media, or perforated tympanic membrane
✦ Inner ear — causes include ototoxicity, Ménière's disease, or acoustic neuroma

tacks, including nausea, vomiting, sweating, giddiness, nystagmus, and loss of balance and falling to the affected side. Recurring disabling attacks can last 20 minutes to several hours, ending with a sense of unsteadiness and exhaustion. Attacks can occur many times per week.

OTOSCLEROSIS

Also called *hardening of the ear*, otosclerosis is a condition in which spongy bone slowly forms in the otic capsule, particularly at the oval window, impeding normal movement of the stapes.

 SPECIAL POINTS *Otosclerosis — the most common cause of conductive deafness — occurs in at least 10% of whites and is twice as common in females, usually between ages 15 and 30.*

Otosclerosis is the second most common correctable middle-ear disorder. It occurs bilaterally in 75% of cases and, with surgery, the prognosis is good.

Otosclerosis results from a genetic factor transmitted as an autosomal dominant trait. Many patients with this disorder report family histories of hearing loss (excluding presbycusis). Pregnancy may trigger onset.

Facts about otosclerosis

✦ Also called *hardening of the ear*
✦ Spongy bone slowly forms in the otic capsule
✦ Impedes normal movement of the stapes
✦ Results from genetic factor

Special points

✦ Most common form of conductive deafness, especially in whites and females ages 15 to 30

Several signs and symptoms can indicate otosclerosis. They include a slowly progressive unilateral hearing loss, especially for low tones, that may advance to bilateral deafness; tinnitus (low and medium pitch); vertigo; and paracusis of Willis (hearing conversation better in a noisy environment than in a quiet one).

EPISTAXIS

Epistaxis, or nose bleeding, may be primary or secondary.

 SPECIAL POINTS *In children, the bleeding usually originates in the anterior nasal septum and tends to be mild. In adults, the bleeding usually originates in the posterior septum and can be severe. Epistaxis is twice as common in children as in adults.*

Epistaxis usually results from external or internal causes, such as a blow to the nose, nose picking, or insertion of a foreign body. Other causes include hypertension, polyps, inhalation of chemicals that irritate the nasal mucosa, nasal neoplasms, blood coagulation disorders, tumors, and acute or chronic infections, such as sinusitis or rhinitis, which cause congestion and eventual bleeding of the capillary blood vessels.

Signs and symptoms depend on the severity of the bleeding. Bleeding is considered severe if it persists longer than 10 minutes after pressure is applied; severe bleeding may cause blood loss as great as 1 L/hour in adults.

The patient bleeds unilaterally, except when dyscrasia or severe traumatic injury causes epistaxis. Blood oozing from the nostrils usually originates in the anterior nose and is bright red. Blood from the back of the throat originates in the posterior area and may be dark or bright red; it's commonly mistaken for hemoptysis because of expectoration.

With severe epistaxis, blood seeps behind the nasal septum and may enter the middle ear and the corners of the eyes. Other signs and symptoms include lightheadedness, dizziness, slight respiratory distress, and shock. Severe hemorrhage causes a drop in blood pressure, rapid and bounding pulse, dyspnea, pallor, and other indications of progressive shock.

NASAL POLYPS

Nasal polyps are swellings of the sinus mucosa into the cavities of the nose and paranasal sinuses. These benign and edematous growths are usually multiple, mobile, and bilateral. Nasal polyps may become large and numerous enough to cause nasal distention and enlargement of the bony framework, possibly occluding the airway.

 SPECIAL POINTS *Nasal polyps occur more commonly in adults than in children and in more men than women; they also tend to recur. Nasal polyps in children require testing to rule out cystic fibrosis.*

Nasal polyps usually develop as a result of continuous pressure resulting from a chronic allergy that causes mucous membrane edema in the nose and sinuses. They also occur in patients with cystic fibrosis, asthma, disorders of ciliary motility, chronic rhinitis, and chronic sinusitis.

Signs and symptoms include nasal obstruction (primary indication), anosmia, a sensation of fullness in the face, nasal discharge, and shortness of breath. Associated clinical features usually indicate allergic rhinitis.

SEPTAL PERFORATION AND DEVIATION

Perforated septum, a hole in the nasal septum between the two air passages, usually occurs in the anterior cartilaginous septum but may occur in the bony septum. De-

---

Facts about epistaxis

+ Nose bleeding
+ Results from external or internal causes
+ Bleeding severe if lasts longer than 10 minutes
+ Severe epistaxis results in blood seeping behind the nasal septum, entering the middle ear and corners of eyes
+ Light-headedness, dizziness, rapid and bounding pulse indicate progressive shock

Special points

+ More common in children, bleeding originates in anterior nasal septum, tending to be mild; in adults, bleeding originates in posterior septum, tending to be severe

Facts about nasal polyps

+ Swellings of the sinus mucosa
+ Occur as benign and edematous growths; multiple, mobile, and bilateral
+ Becoming larger and numerous, can cause nasal distention, possibly occluding airway

Special points

+ Occur more commonly in adults and men; tend to recur
+ In children, require testing to rule out cystic fibrosis

viated septum, a shift from the midline that commonly occurs in normal growth, is present in most adults. This condition may be severe enough to obstruct the passage of air through the nostrils. With surgical correction, the prognosis for both perforated and deviated septum is good.

Septal perforation can result from several factors, including a traumatic irritation. Most common causes include perichondritis, syphilis, tuberculosis, untreated septal hematoma, inhalation of irritating chemicals, cocaine snorting, chronic nasal infections, nasal carcinoma, granuloma, and chronic sinusitis.

A deviated septum can result from nasal trauma from a fall, a blow to the nose, injury during birth, history of a nasal fracture, or surgery that further exaggerates the deviation that commonly occurs during normal growth.

A septal perforation usually produces no symptoms if it's small, but it may produce a whistle on inspiration. A large perforation can cause rhinitis, epistaxis, nasal crusting, and watery discharge.

Signs and symptoms of a deviated septum include a crooked nose, nasal obstruction (if the deviation is severe), a sensation of fullness in the face, shortness of breath, nasal discharge, recurring epistaxis, headache, and symptoms of infection and sinusitis. A deviated septum alters nasal activity and results in dry mucosa, crusting, bleeding, and changes in the nasal membrane.

SINUSITIS

Acute sinusitis usually results from the common cold and lingers in subacute form in only about 10% of patients. Chronic sinusitis follows persistent bacterial infection. Allergic sinusitis accompanies allergic rhinitis. Hyperplastic sinusitis is a combination of purulent acute sinusitis and allergic sinusitis or rhinitis. Sinusitis can also be viral following an upper respiratory tract infection in which the virus penetrates the normal mucous membrane. Fungal sinusitis is uncommon, but is found more commonly in immunosuppressed or debilitated patients. The prognosis is good for all types of sinusitis.

Signs and symptoms associated with sinusitis include nasal congestion, pressure, pain over the cheeks and upper teeth (in maxillary sinusitis), pain over the eyes (in ethmoid sinusitis), pain over the eyebrows (in frontal sinusitis), and pain behind the eyes (in sphenoid sinusitis). Upon inspection, you may find edematous nasal mucosa and edema of the face and periorbital area.

Other signs and symptoms include fever (in acute sinusitis), nasal discharge (may be purulent in the acute and subacute forms, continuous in the chronic form, watery in the allergic form), nasal stuffiness, and possible inflammation and pus on nasal examination.

LARYNGITIS

Laryngitis is an inflammation of the vocal cords. Acute laryngitis may occur as an isolated infection or as part of a generalized bacterial or viral upper respiratory tract infection. Repeated attacks of acute laryngitis cause inflammatory changes associated with chronic laryngitis.

Acute laryngitis results from infection, excessive use of the voice, inhalation of smoke or fumes, or aspiration of caustic chemicals. Chronic laryngitis results from upper respiratory tract disorders (such as sinusitis, bronchitis, nasal polyps, or allergy), mouth breathing, smoking, gastroesophageal reflux, constant exposure to dust or other irritants, or alcohol abuse.

Facts about septal perforation and deviation

- ✦ Perforated septum — hole in the nasal septum; results from traumatic irritation caused by perichondritis, syphilis, tuberculosis, chronic nasal infections
- ✦ Deviated septum — shift from midline commonly occurring in adults; results from trauma causing crooked nose, nasal obstruction, shortness of breath, symptoms of infection and sinusitis

Facts about sinusitis

- ✦ Acute form results from common cold
- ✦ Lingers as subacute form
- ✦ Chronic form follows persistent bacterial infection
- ✦ Allergic sinusitis accompanies allergic rhinitis
- ✦ Sinusitis signs and symptoms include nasal congestion, pressure, pain over cheeks and upper teeth
- ✦ Fever, nasal discharge, nasal stuffiness, inflammation, and pus

Facts about laryngitis

- ✦ Inflammation of the vocal cords
- ✦ Acute form occurs as an isolated infection and results from infection, excessive use of voice, inhalation of smoke or fumes, or aspiration of caustic chemicals
- ✦ Chronic form results from sinusitis, bronchitis, nasal polyps, allergy, smoking, alcohol abuse

Facts about laryngitis
(continued)
+ Hoarseness, pain, dry cough, fever, malaise

Facts about tonsillitis
+ Inflammation of tonsils occurs in acute and chronic forms
+ Discomfort subsides within 72 hours
+ Mild to severe sore throat, dysphagia, fever, swelling and tenderness of lymph glands, dry throat

Special points
+ Uncomplicated form usually lasts 4 to 6 days; commonly affects children between ages 5 and 10
+ Tonsils tends to hypertrophy during childhood and atrophy after puberty

Look for hoarseness, pain (especially when swallowing or speaking), a dry cough, fever, malaise, dyspnea, shortness of breath, throat clearing, restlessness, and laryngeal edema. Persistent hoarseness is a sign of chronic laryngitis.

TONSILLITIS

Inflammation of the tonsils can be acute or chronic.

 SPECIAL POINTS *The uncomplicated acute form of tonsillitis usually lasts 4 to 6 days and commonly affects children between ages 5 and 10. Tonsils tend to hypertrophy during childhood and atrophy after puberty.*

The discomfort associated with acute tonsillitis usually subsides after 72 hours. Signs and symptoms include mild to severe sore throat (a very young child may stop eating as a result), dysphagia, fever, swelling and tenderness of lymph glands in the submandibular and neck area, muscle and joint pain, chills, malaise, headache, pain (commonly referred to ears), the urge to swallow constantly, dry throat, foul taste in mouth, and a constricted feeling in the back of the throat.

Signs and symptoms of chronic tonsillitis are a recurrent sore throat, yellow or white exudate in tonsillar crypts, and frequent attacks of acute tonsillitis.

Appendices and index

Quick-reference guide to laboratory test results

A

Acetylcholine receptor antibodies, serum
Negative

Acid mucopolysaccharides, urine
Adults: < 13.3 µg glucuronic acid/mg/creatinine/
24 hours

Acid phosphatase, serum
0 to 3.7 U/L (SI, 0 to 3.7 U/L)

Adrenocorticotropic hormone, plasma
< 120 pg/ml (SI, < 26.4 pmol/L)

Alanine aminotransferase
8 to 50 IU/L (SI, 0.14 to 0.85 µkat/L)

Aldosterone, serum
✦ Supine individuals: 3 to 16 ng/dl (SI, 80 to
440 pmol/L)
✦ Upright individuals: 7 to 30 ng/dl (SI, 190 to
832 pmol/L)

Aldosterone, urine
3 to 19 µg/24 hours (SI, 8 to 51 nmol/d)

Alkaline phosphatase, peritoneal fluid
✦ Males > 18 years: 90 to 239 U/L (SI, 90 to 239 U/L)
✦ Females < 45 years: 76 to 196 U/L (SI, 76 to
196 U/L); > 45 years: 87 to 250 U/L (87 to 250 U/L)

Alkaline phosphatase, serum
30 to 85 IU/ml (SI, 42 to 128 U/L)

Alpha-fetoprotein serum
Males and nonpregnant, females: < 15 ng/ml (SI,
< 15 mg/L)

Ammonia, peritoneal fluid
< 50 µg/dl (SI, < 29 µmol/L)

Amniotic fluid analysis
✦ Lecithin-sphingomyelin ratio: > 2
✦ Meconium: absent (except in breech presentation)
✦ Phosphatidylglycerol: present

Amylase, peritoneal fluid
138 to 404 U/L (SI, 138 to 404 U/L)

Amylase, serum
Adults ≥ 18 years: 25 to 85 U/L (SI, 0.39 to
1.45 µkat/L)

Amylase, urine
1 to 17 U/hour (SI, 0.017 to 0.29 µkat/h)

Androstenedione (radioimmunoassay)
✦ Males: 75 to 205 ng/dl (SI, 2.6 to 7.2 nmol/L)
✦ Females: 85 to 275 ng/dl (SI, 3.0 to 9.6 nmol/L)

Angiotensin-converting enzyme
Adults ≥ 20 years: 8 to 52 U/L (SI, 0.14 to
0.88 µkat/L)

Anion gap
8 to 14 mEq/L (SI, 8 to 14 mmol/L)

Antibody screening, serum
Negative

Antidiuretic hormone, serum
1 to 5 pg/ml (SI, 1 to 5 mg/L)

Antiglobulin test, direct
Negative

Antimitochondrial antibodies, serum
Negative

Anti-smooth-muscle antibodies, serum
Negative

Antistreptolysin-O, serum
✦ Preschoolers and adults: 85 Todd units/ml
✦ School-age children: 170 Todd units/ml

Antithrombin III
80% to 120% of normal control values

Antithyroid antibodies, serum
Normal titer < 1:100

Arginine test
+ Human growth hormone levels
  – Males: increase to > 10 ng/ml (SI, > 10 µg/L)
  – Females: increase to > 15 ng/ml (SI, > 15 µg/L)
  – Children: increase to > 48 ng/ml (SI, > 48 µg/L)

Arterial blood gases
+ pH: 7.35 to 7.45 (SI, 7.35 to 7.45)
+ Pao_2: 80 to 100 mm Hg (SI, 10.6 to 13.3 kPa)
+ $Paco_2$: 35 to 45 mm Hg (SI, 4.7 to 5.3 kPa)
+ O_2 CT: 15% to 23% (SI, 0.15 to 0.23)
+ Sao_2: 94% to 100% (SI, 0.94 to 1.00)
+ HCO_3^-: 22 to 25 mEq/L (SI, 22 to 25 mmol/L)

Arylsufatase A, urine
+ Random: 16 to 42 µg/g creatinine
+ 24-hour: 0.37 to 3.60 µ/day creatinine
+ 1-hour test: 2 to 19 µ/1 hour (SI, 2 to 19 µ/h)
+ 2-hour test: 4 to 37 µ/2 hours (SI, 4 to 37 µ/h)
+ 24-hour test: 170 to 2,000 µ/24 hours (SI, 2.89 to 34.0 µkat/L)

Aspartate aminotransferase
+ Males: 8 to 46 U/L (SI, 0.14 to 0.78 µkat/L)
+ Females: 7 to 34 U/L (SI, 0.12 to 0.58 µkat/L)

Aspergillosis antibody, serum
Normal titer < 1:8

Atrial natriuretic factor, plasma
20 to 77 pg/ml

B

Bacterial meningitis antigen
Negative

Bence Jones protein, urine
Negative

Beta-hydroxybutyrate
< 0.4 mmol/L (SI, 0.4 mmol/L)

Bilirubin, amniotic fluid
+ Early: < 0.075 mg/dl (SI, < 1.3 Umol/L)
+ Term: < 0.025 mg/dl (SI, < 0.41 Umol/L)

Bilirubin, serum
+ Adults
  – Direct: < 0.5 mg/dl (SI, < 6.8 µmol/L)
  – Indirect: 1.1 mg/dl (SI, 19 µmol/L)
+ Neonates
  – Total: 1 to 12 mg/dl (SI, 34 to 205 µmol/L)

Bilirubin, urine
Negative

Blastomycosis antibody, serum
Normal titer < 1:8

Bleeding time
+ Template: 3 to 6 minutes (SI, 3 to 6 m)
+ Ivy: 3 to 6 minutes (SI, 3 to 6 m)
+ Duke: 1 to 3 minutes (SI, 1 to 3 m)

Blood urea nitrogen
8 to 20 mg/dl (SI, 2.9 to 7.5 mmol/L)

B-lymphocyte count
270 to 640/µl

C

Calcitonin, plasma
+ Baseline
  – Males: 40 pg/ml (SI, 40 ng/L)
  – Females: 20 pg/ml (SI, 20 ng/L)
+ Calcium infusion
  – Males: 190 pg/ml (SI, 190 ng/L)
  – Females: 130 pg/ml (SI, 130 ng/L)
+ Pentagastrin infusion
  – Males: 110 pg/ml (SI, 110 ng/L)
  – Females: 30 pg/ml (SI, 30 ng/L)

Calcium, serum
+ Adults: 8.2 to 10.2 mg/dl (SI, 2.05 to 2.54 mmol/L)
+ Children: 8.6 to 11.2 mg/dl (SI, 2.15 to 2.79 mmol/L)
+ Ionized: 4.65 to 5.28 mg/dl (SI, 1.1 to 1.25 mmol/L)

Calcium, urine
100 to 300 mg/24 hours (SI, 2.50 to 7.50 mmol/d)

Candida antibodies, serum
Negative

Capillary fragility

Petechiae per 5 cm:	Score:
11 to 20	2 +
21 to 50	3 +
over 50	4 +

Carbon dioxide, total, blood
22 to 26 mEq/L (SI, 22 to 26 mmol/L)

Carcinoembryonic antigen, serum
< 5 ng/ml (SI, < 5 mg/L)

Catecholamines, plasma
+ Supine
  – Epinephrine: undetectable to 110 pg/ml (SI, undetectable to 600 pmol/L)
  – Norepinephrine: 70 to 750 pg/ml (SI, 413 to 4,432 pmol/L)
+ Standing
  – Epinephrine: undetectable to 140 pg/ml (SI, undetectable to 764 pmol/L)
  – Norepinephrine: 200 to 1,700 pg/ml (SI, 1182 to 10,047 pmol/L)

Catecholamines, urine
+ Epinephrine: 0 to 20 µg/24 hours (SI, 0 to 109 nmol/24 h)
+ Norepinephrine: 15 to 80 µg/24 hours (SI, 89 to 473 nmol/24 h)
+ Dopamine: 65 to 400 µg/24 hours (SI, 425 to 2,610 nmol/24 h)

Cerebrospinal fluid
+ Pressure: 50 to 180 mm H_2O
+ Appearance: clear, colorless
+ Gram stain: no organisms

Ceruloplasmin, serum
22.9 to 43.1 g/dl (SI, 0.22 to 0.43 g/L)

Chloride, cerebrospinal fluid
118 to 130 mEq/L (SI, 118 to 130 mmol/L)

Chloride, serum
100 to 108 mEq/L (SI, 100 to 108 mmol/L)

Chloride, urine
+ Adults: 110 to 250 nmol/24 hours (SI, 110 to 250 mmol/d)
+ Children: 15 to 40 nmol/24 hours (SI, 15 to 40 mmol/d)
+ Infants: 2 to 10 mmol/24 hours (SI, 2 to 10 mmol/d)

Cholinesterase (pseudocholinesterase)
204 to 532 IU/dl (SI, 2.04 to 5.32 kU/L)

Coccidioidomycosis antibody, serum
Normal titer < 1:2

Cold agglutinins, serum
Normal titer < 1:64

Complement, serum
+ Total
  – 40 to 90 U/ml (SI, 0.4 to 0.9 g/L)
+ C3
  – Males: 80 to 180 mg/dl (SI, 0.8 to 1.8 g/L)
  – Females: 76 to 120 mg/dl (SI, 0.76 to 1.2 g/L)
+ C4
  – Males: 15 to 60 mg/dl (SI, 0.15 to 0.6 g/L)
  – Females: 15 to 52 mg/dl (SI, 0.15 to 0.52 g/L)

Copper, urine
3 to 35 µg/24 hours (SI, 0.05 to 0.55 µmol/d)

Cortisol, free, urine
< 50 µg/24 hours (SI, < 138 mmol/d)

Cortisol, plasma
+ Morning: 9 to 35 µg/dl (SI, 250 to 690 nmol/L)
+ Afternoon: 3 to 12 µg/dl (SI, 80 to 330 nmol/L)

C-reactive protein, serum
< 0.8 mg/dl (SI, < 8 mg/L)

Creatine kinase
Total
  – Males: 55 to 170 U/L (SI, 0.94 to 2.89 µkat/L)
  – Females: 30 to 135 U/L (SI, 0.51 to 2.3 µkat/L)

Creatinine clearance
+ Males: 94 to 140 ml/min/1.73 m² (SI, 0.91 to 1.35 ml/s/m²)
+ Females: 72 to 110 ml/min/1.73 m² (SI, 0.69 to 1.06 ml/s/m²)

Creatinine, serum
+ Males: 0.8 to 1.2 mg/dl (SI, 62 to 115 µmol/L)
+ Females: 0.6 to 0.9 mg/dl (SI, 53 to 97 µmol/L)

Creatinine, urine
+ Males: 14 to 26 mg/kg body weight/24 hours (SI, 124 to 230 µmol/kg body weight/d)
+ Females: 11 to 20 mg/kg body weight/24 hours (SI, 97 to 177 µmol/kg body weight/d)

Cryoglobulins, serum
Negative

Cyclic adenosine monophosphate, urine
+ 0.3 to 3.6 mg/day (SI, 100 to 723 µmol/d)
or
+ 0.29 to 2.1 mg/g creatinine (SI, 100 to 723 µmol/mol creatinine)

Cytomegalovirus antibodies, serum
Negative

D

D-xylose absorption
+ Blood
  – Adults: 25 to 40 mg/dl in 2 hours
  – Children: > 30 mg/dl in 1 hour
+ Urine
  – Adults: > 3.5 g excreted in 5 hours (age 65 of older, > 5 g in 24 hours)
  – Children: 16% to 33% excreted in 5 hours

E

Epstein-Barr virus antibodies
Negative

Erythrocyte sedimentation rate
+ Males: 0 to 10 mm/hour (SI, 0 to 10 mm/h)
+ Females: 0 to 20 mm/hour (SI, 0 to 20 mm/h)

Esophageal acidity
pH > 5.0

Estrogens, serum
+ Females
  – Menstruating: 26 to 149 pg/ml (SI, 90 to 550 pmol/L)
  – Postmenopausal: 0 to 34 pg/ml (SI, 0 to 125 pmol/L)
+ Males
  – 12 to 34 pg/ml (SI, 40 to 125 pmol/L)
+ Children
  – < 6 years: 3 to 10 pg/ml (SI, 10 to 36 pmol/L)

Euglobulin lysis time
2 to 4 hours (SI, 2 to 4 h)

F

Factor assay, one-stage
50% to 150% of normal activity (SI, 0.50 to 1.50)

Febrile agglutination, serum
+ Salmonella antibody: < 1:80
+ Brucellosis antibody: < 1:80
+ Tularemia antibody: < 1:40
+ Rickettsial antibody: < 1:40

Ferritin, serum
+ Males
  – 20 to 300 ng/ml (SI, 20 to 300 µg/L)
+ Females
  – 20 to 120 ng/ml (SI, 20 to 120 µg/L)
+ Infants
  – 1 month: 200 to 600 ng/ml (SI, 200 to 600 µg/L)
  – 2 to 5 months: 50 to 200 ng/ml (SI, 50 to 200 µg/L)
  – 6 months to 15 years: 7 to 140 ng/ml (SI, 7 to 140 µg/L)
+ Neonates
  – 25 to 200 ng/ml (SI, 25 to 200 µg/L)

Fibrinogen, plasma
200 to 400 mg/dl (SI, 2 to 4 g/L)

Fibrin split products
+ Screening assay: < 10 µg/ml (SI, < 10 mg/L)
+ Quantitative assay: < 3 µg/ml (SI, < 3 mg/L)

Fluorescent treponemal antibody absorption, serum
Negative

Folic acid, serum
1.8 to 9 ng/ml (SI, 4 to 20 nmol/L)

Follicle-stimulating hormone, serum
+ Menstruating females
  – Follicular phase: 5 to 20 mIU/ml (SI, 5 to 20 IU/L)
  – Ovulatory phase: 15 to 30 mIU/ml (SI, 15 to 30 IU/L)
  – Luteal phase: 5 to 15 mIU/ml (SI, 5 to 15 IU/L)
+ Menopausal females
  – 5 to 100 mIU/ml (SI, 50 to 100 IU/L)
+ Males
  – 5 to 20 mIU/ml (5 to 20 IU/L)

Free thyroxine, serum
0.9 to 2.3 ng/dl (SI, 10 to 30 nmol/L)

Free triiodothyronine
0.2 to 0.6 ng/dl (SI, 0.003 to 0.009 nmol/L)

G

Galactose 1-phosphate uridyl transferase
+ Qualitative: negative
+ Quantitative: 18.5 to 28.5 U/g of hemoglobin

Gamma-glutamyl transferase
+ Males ≥ 16 years: 6 to 38 U/L (SI, 0.10 to 0.63 µkat/L)
+ Females 16 to 45 years: 4 to 27 U/L (SI, 0.08 to 0.46 µkat/L); > 45 years: 6 to 38 U/L (SI, 0.10 to 0.63 µkat/L)
+ Children: 3 to 30 U/L (SI, 0.05 to 0.51 µkat)

Gastric acid stimulation
+ Males: 18 to 28 mEq/hour
+ Females: 11 to 21 mEq/hour

Gastric secretion, basal
+ Males: 1 to 5 mEq/hour
+ Females: 0.2 to 3.3 mEq/hour

Gastrin, serum
50 to 150 pg/ml (SI, 50 to 150 ng/L)

Globulin, peritoneal fluid
30% to 45% of total protein

Glucose, amniotic fluid
< 45 mg/dl (SI, < 2.3 mmol/L)

Glucose, cerebrospinal fluid
50 to 80 mg/dl (SI, 2.8 to 4.4 mmol/L)

Glucose, peritoneal fluid
70 to 100 mg/dl (SI, 3.5 to 5 mmol/L)

Glucose, plasma, fasting
70 to 100 mg/dl (SI, 3.9 to 6.1 mmol/L)

Glucose-6-phosphate dehydrogenase
4.3 to 11.8 U/g (SI, 0.28 to 0.76 mU/mol) of hemoglobin

Glucose tolerance, oral
Peak at 160 to 180 mg/dl (SI, 8.8 to 9.9 mmol/L) 30 to 60 minutes after challenge dose

Growth hormone suppression
Undetectable to 3 ng/ml (SI, undetectable to 3 µg/L) after 30 minutes to 2 hours

---

H

Ham test
Negative

Haptoglobin, serum
40 to 180 mg/dl (SI, 0.4 to 1.8 g/L)

Heinz bodies
Negative

Hematocrit
+ Males
  – 42% to 52% (SI, 0.42 to 0.52)
+ Females
  – 36% to 48% (SI, 0.36 to 0.48)
+ Children
  – 10 years: 36% to 40% (SI, 0.36 to 0.40)
+ Infants
  – 3 months: 30% to 36% (SI, 0.30 to 0.36)
  – 1 year: 29% to 41% (SI, 0.29 to 0.41)
+ Neonates
  – At birth: 55% to 68% (SI, 0.55 to 0.68)
  – 1 week: 47% to 65% (SI, 0.47 to 0.65)
  – 1 month: 37% to 49% (SI, 0.37 to 0.49)

Hemoglobin (Hb) electrophoresis
+ Hb A: 95% (SI, 0.95)
+ Hb A_2: 1.5% to 3% (SI, 0.015 to 0.03)
+ Hb F: <2% (SI, <0.02)

Hemoglobin, unstable
+ Heat stability: negative
+ Isopropanol: stable

Hemoglobin, urine
Negative

Hemosiderin, urine
Negative

Hepatitis B surface antigen, serum
Negative

Herpes simplex antibodies, serum
Negative

Heterophil agglutination, serum
Normal titer <1:56

Hexosaminidase A and B, serum
Total: 5 to 12.9 U/L (hexosaminidase A constitutes 55% to 76% of total)

Histoplasmosis antibody, serum
Normal titer <1:8

Homovanillic acid, urine
<10 mg/24 hours (SI, <55 µmol/d)

Human chorionic gonadotropin, serum
<4 IU/L

Human chorionic gonadotropin, urine
Pregnant women
  – First trimester: 500,000 IU/24 hours
  – Second trimester: 10,000 to 25,000 IU/24 hours
  – Third trimester: 5,000 to 15,000 IU/24 hours

Human growth hormone, serum
+ Males: undetectable to 5 ng/ml (SI, undetectable to 5 µg/L)
+ Females: undetectable to 10 ng/ml (SI, undetectable to 10 µg/L)
+ Children: undetectable to 16 ng/ml (SI, undetectable to 16 µg/L)

Human immunodeficiency virus antibody, serum
Negative

Human placental lactogen, serum
+ Males and nonpregnant females: <0.5 µg/ml
+ Pregnant females at term: 9 to 11 µg/ml

17-hydroxycorticosteroids, urine
+ Males
  – 4.5 to 12 mg/24 hours (SI, 12.4 to 33.1 µmol/d)
+ Females
  – 2.5 to 10 mg/24 hours (SI, 6.9 to 27.6 µmol/d)
+ Children
  – 8 to 12 years: <4.5 mg/24 hours (SI, <12.4 µmol/d)
  – <8 years: <1.5 mg/24 hours (SI, <4.14 µmol/d)

5-hydroxyindoleacetic acid, urine
2 to 7 mg/24 hours (SI, 10.4 to 36.6 µmol/d)

Hydroxyproline, total, urine
1 to 9 mg/24 hours (SI, 1.0 to 3.4 IU/d)

I J

Immune complex, serum
Negative

Immunoglobulins (Ig), serum
+ IgG: 800 to 1,800 mg/dl (SI, 8 to 18 g/L)
+ IgA: 100 to 400 mg/dl (SI, 1 to 4 g/L)
+ IgM: 55 to 150 mg/dl (SI, 0.55 to 1.5 g/L)

Insulin, serum
0 to 35 µU/ml (SI, 144 to 243 pmol/L)

Insulin tolerance test
10- to 20-ng/dl (SI, 10- to 20-µg/L) increase over baseline levels of human growth hormone and adrenocorticotropic hormone

Iron, serum
+ Males: 60 to 170 µg/dl (SI, 10.7 to 30.4 µmol/L)
+ Females: 50 to 130 µg/dl (SI, 9 to 23.3 µmol/L)

Iron, total binding capacity, serum
300 to 360 µg/dl (SI, 54 to 64 µmol/L)

K

17-ketogenic steroids, urine
+ Males: 4 to 14 mg/24 hours (SI, 13 to 49 µmol/d)
+ Females: 2 to 12 mg/24 hours (SI, 7 to 42 µmol/d)
+ Children
  − Infants to 11 years: 0.1 to 4 mg/24 hours (SI, 0.3 to 14 µmol/d)
  − 11 to 14 years: 2 to 9 mg/24 hours (SI, 7 to 31 µmol/d)

Ketones, urine
Negative

17-ketosteroids, urine
+ Males: 10 to 25 mg/24 hours (SI, 35 to 87 µmol/d)
+ Females: 4 to 6 mg/24 hours (SI, 4 to 21 µmol/d)
+ Children
  − Infants to 10 years: < 3 mg/24 hours (SI, < 10 µmol/d)
  − 10 to 14 years: 1 to 6 mg/24 hours (SI, 2 to 21 µmol/d)

L

Lactate dehydrogenase (LD)
+ Total: 71 to 207 IU/L (SI, 1.2 to 3.52 µkat/L)
+ LD_1: 14% to 26% (SI, 0.14 to 0.26)
+ LD_2: 29% to 39% (SI, 0.29 to 0.39)
+ LD_3: 20% to 26% (SI, 0.20 to 0.26)
+ LD_4: 8% to 16% (SI, 0.08 to 0.16)
+ LD_5: 6% to 16% (SI, 0.06 to 0.16)

Lactic acid, blood
0.93 to 1.65 mEq/L (SI, 0.93 to 1.65 mmol/L)

Leucine aminopeptidase
+ Males: 80 to 200 U/ml (SI, 80 to 200 kU/L)
+ Females: 75 to 185 U/ml (SI, 75 to 185 kU/L)

Leukoagglutinins
Negative

Lipase, serum
< 160 U/L (SI, < 2.72 µkat)

Lipids, fecal
Constitute < 20% of excreted solids; < 7 g excreted in 24 hours

Lipoproteins, serum
+ High-density lipoprotein cholesterol
  − Males: 37 to 70 mg/dl (SI, 0.96 to 1.8 mmol/L)
  − Females: 40 to 85 mg/dl (SI, 1.03 to 2.2 mmol/L)
+ Low-density lipoprotein cholesterol:
  − In individuals who don't have coronary artery disease: < 130 mg/dl (SI, < 3.36 mmol/L)

Long-acting thyroid stimulator, serum
Negative

Lupus erythematosus cell preparation
Negative

Luteinizing hormone, serum
+ Menstruating women
  − Follicular phase: 5 to 15 mIU/ml (SI, 5 to 15 IU/L)
  − Ovulatory phase: 30 to 60 mIU/ml (SI, 30 to 60 IU/L)
  − Luteal phase: 5 to 15 mIU/ml (SI, 5 to 15 IU/L)
+ Postmenopausal women
  − 50 to 100 mIU/ml (SI, 50 to 100 IU/L)
+ Males
  − 5 to 20 mIU/ml (SI, 5 to 20 IU/L)
+ Children
  − 4 to 20 mIU/ml (SI, 4 to 20 IU/L)

Lyme disease serology
Nonreactive

Lysozyme, urine
0 to 3 mg/24 hours

M

Magnesium, serum
1.3 to 2.1 mg/dl (SI, 0.65 to 1.05 mmol/L)

Magnesium, urine
6 to 10 mEq/24 hours (SI, 3.0 to 5.0 mmol/d)

Manganese, serum
0.4 to 1.4 µg/ml

Melanin, urine
Negative

Myoglobin, urine
Negative

N

5′-nucleotidase
2 to 17 U/L (SI, 0.034 to 0.29 µkat/L)

O

Occult blood, fecal
<2.5 ml

Oxalate, urine
≤40 mg/24 hours (SI, ≤456 µmol/d)

P Q

Parathyroid hormone, serum
✦ Intact: 10 to 50 pg/ml (SI, 1.1 to 5.3 pmol/L)
✦ N-terminal fraction: 8 to 24 pg/ml (SI, 0.8 to 2.5 pmol/L)
✦ C-terminal fraction: 0 to 340 pg/ml (SI, 0 to 35.8 pmol/L)

Partial thromboplastin time
21 to 35 seconds (SI, 21 to 35 s)

Pericardial fluid
✦ Amount: 10 to 50 ml
✦ Appearance: clear, straw-colored
✦ White blood cell count: <1,000/µl (SI, <1.0 × 10⁹/L)
✦ Glucose: approximately whole blood level

Peritoneal fluid
✦ Amount: <50 ml
✦ Appearance: clear, straw-colored

Phenylalanine, serum
<2 mg/dl (SI, <121 µmol/L)

Phosphates, serum
✦ Adults: 2.7 to 4.5 mEq/L (SI, 0.87 to 1.45 mmol/L)
✦ Children: 4.5 to 6.7 mEq/L (SI, 1.45 to 1.78 mmol/L)

Phosphates, urine
<1,000 mg/24 hours

Phospholipids, plasma
180 to 320 mg/dl (SI, 1.80 to 3.20 g/L)

Plasma renin activity
✦ Normal sodium diet: 1.1 to 4.1 ng/ml/hour (SI, 0.30 to 1.14 ng LS)
✦ Restricted sodium diet: 6.2 to 12.4 ng/ml/hour (SI, 1.72 to 3.44 ng LS)

Phosphate, tubular reabsorption, urine and plasma
80% reabsorption

Plasminogen, plasma
Immunologic method: 10 to 20 mg/dl (SI, 0.10 to 0.20 g/L)

Platelet aggregation
3 to 5 minutes (SI, 3 to 5 m)

Platelet count
✦ Adults: 140,000 to 400,000/µl (SI, 140 to 400 × 10⁹/L)
✦ Children: 150,000 to 450,000/µl (SI, 150 to 450 × 10⁹/L)

Potassium, serum
3.5 to 5 mEq/L (SI, 3.5 to 5 mmol/L)

Potassium, urine
✦ Adults: 25 to 125 mmol/24 hours (SI, 25 to 125 mmol/d)
✦ Children: 22 to 57 mmol/24 hours (SI, 22 to 57 mmol/d)

Pregnanediol, urine
✦ Nonpregnant females
 − 0.5 to 1.5 mg/24 hours (during the follicular phase of the menstrual cycle)
✦ Pregnant females
 − First trimester: 10 to 30 mg/24 hours
 − Second trimester: 35 to 70 mg/24 hours
 − Third trimester: 70 to 100 mg/24 hours
✦ Postmenopausal females
 − 0.2 to 1 mg/24 hours
✦ Males
 − 0 to 1 mg/24 hours

Pregnanetriol, urine
✦ Males ≥16 years: 0.4 to 2.5 mg/24 hours (SI, 1.2 to 7.5 µmol/d)
✦ Females ≥16 years: 0 to 1.8 mg/ hours (SI, 0.3 to 5.3 µmol/d)

Progesterone, plasma
+ Menstruating females
  – Follicular phase: < 150 ng/dl (SI, < 5 nmol/L)
  – Luteal phase: 300 to 1,200 ng/dl (SI, 10 to 40 nmol/L)
+ Pregnant women
  – First trimester: 1,500 to 5,000 ng/dl (SI, 50 to 160 nmol/L)
  – Second and third trimesters: 8,000 to 20,000 ng/dl (SI, 250 to 650 nmol/L)

Prolactin, serum
Undetectable to 23 ng/ml (SI, undetectable to 23 µg/L)

Prostate-specific antigen
+ 40 to 50 years: 2 to 2.8 mg/ml (SI, 2 to 2.8 µg/L)
+ 51 to 60 years: 2.9 to 3.8 mg/ml (SI, 2.9 to 3.8 µg/L)
+ 61 to 70 years: 4 to 5.3 mg/ml (SI, 4 to 5.3 µg/L)
+ ≥71 years: 5.6 to 7.2 mg/ml (SI, 5.6 to 7.2 µg/L)

Protein, cerebrospinal fluid
15 to 50 mg/dl (SI, 0.15 to 0.5 g/L)

Protein C, plasma
70% to 140% (SI, 0.70 to 1.40)

Protein, total, peritoneal fluid
0.3 to 4.1 g/dl (SI, 3 to 41 g/L)

Protein, urine
50 to 80 mg/24 hours (SI, 50 to 80 mg/d)

Prothrombin time
10 to 14 seconds (10 to 14 s)

Pulmonary artery pressures
+ Right atrial: 1 to 6 mm Hg
+ Left atrial: approximately 10 mm Hg
+ Systolic: 20 to 30 mm Hg
+ Systolic right ventricular: 20 to 30 mm Hg
+ Diastolic: 10 to 15 mm Hg
+ End-diastolic right ventricular: < 5 mm Hg
+ Mean: < 20 mm Hg
+ Pulmonary artery wedge pressure: 6 to 12 mm Hg

Pyruvate kinase
+ Ultraviolet: 9 to 22 U/g of hemoglobin
+ Low substrate assay: 1.7 to 6.8 U/g of hemoglobin

Pyruvic acid, blood
0.08 to 0.16 mEq/L (SI, 0.08 to 0.16 mmol/L)

R

Red blood cell count
+ Males: 4.5 to 5.5 million/µl (SI, 4.5 to 5.5 × 10^{12}/L)
+ Females: 4 to 5 million/µl (SI, 4 to 5 × 10^{12}/L)
+ Neonates: 4.4 to 5.8 million/µl (SI, 4.4 to 5.8 × 10^{12}/L)
+ 2 months: 3 to 3.8 million/µl (SI, 3 to 3.8 × 10^{12}/L) (increasing slowly)
+ Children: 4.6 to 4.8 million/µl (SI, 4.6 to 4.8 × 10^{12}/L)

Red blood cell survival time
25 to 35 days

Red blood cells, urine
0 to 3 per high-power field

Red cell indices
+ Mean corpuscular volume: 84 to 99 µm³ (SI, 84 to 99 fL)
+ Mean corpuscular hemoglobin: 26 to 32 pg/cell (SI, 0.40 t 0.53 fmol/cell)
+ Mean corpuscular hemoglobin concentration: 30 to 36 g/dl (SI, 300 to 360 g/L)

Respiratory syncytial virus antibodies, serum
Negative

Reticulocyte count
+ Adults: 0.5% to 2.5% (SI, 0.005 to 0.025)
+ Infants (at birth): 2% to 6% (SI, 0.02 to 0.06), decreasing to adult levels in 1 to 2 weeks

Rheumatoid factor, serum
Negative or titer < 1:20

Ribonucleoprotein antibodies
Negative

Rubella antibodies, serum
Titer of 1:8 or less indicates little or no immunity; titer more than 1:10 indicates adequate protection against rubella

S

Semen analysis
+ Volume: 0.7 to 6.5 ml
+ pH: 7.3 to 7.9
+ Liquefaction: within 20 minutes
+ Sperm count: 20 to 150 million/ml

Sickle cell test
Negative

Sjögren's antibodies
Negative

Sodium chloride, urine
110 to 250 mEq/L (SI, 100 to 250 mmol/d)

Sodium, serum
135 to 145 mEq/L (SI, 135 to 145 mmol/L)

Sodium, urine
+ Adults: 40 to 220 mEq/L/24 hours (SI, 40 to 220 mmol/d)
+ Children: 41 to 115 mEq/L/24 hours (SI, 41 to 115 mmol/d)

Sporotrichosis antibody, serum
Normal titers < 1:40

T

Terminal deoxynucleotidyl transferase, serum
+ Bone marrow: < 2%
+ Blood: undetectable

Testosterone, plasma or serum
+ Males: 300 to 1,200 ng/dl (SI, 10.4 to 41.6 nmol/L)
+ Females: 20 to 80 ng/dl (SI, 0.7 to 2.8 nmol/L)

Thrombin time, plasma
10 to 15 seconds (10 to 15 s)

Thyroid-stimulating hormone, neonatal
+ ≤2 days: 25 to 30 µIU/ml (SI, 25 to 20 mU/L)
+ >2 days: < 25 µIU/ml (SI, < 25 mU/L)

Thyroid-stimulating hormone, serum
Undetectable to 15 µIU/ml (SI, undetectable to 15 mU/L)

Thyroid-stimulating immunoglobulin, serum
Negative

Thyroxine-binding globulin, serum
Immunoassay: 16 to 32 µg/dl (SI, 120 to 180 mg/ml)

Thyroxine, total, serum
5 to 13.5 µg/dl (SI, 60 to 165 nmol/L)

T-lymphocyte count
1,500 to 3,000/µl

Transferrin, serum
200 to 400 mg/dl (SI, 2 to 4 g/L)

Triglycerides, serum
+ Males: 44 to 180 mg/dl (SI, 0.44 to 2.01 mmol/L)
+ Females: 11 to 190 mg/dl (SI, 0.11 to 2.21 mmol/L)

Triiodothyronine, serum
80 to 200 ng/dl (SI, 1.2 to 3 nmol/L)

U

Uric acid, serum
+ Males: 3.4 to 7 mg/dl (SI, 202 to 42 µmol/L)
+ Females: 2.3 to 6 mg/dl (SI, 143 to 357 µmol/L)

Uric acid, urine
250 to 750 mg/24 hours (SI, 1.48 to 4.43 mmol/d)

Urinalysis, routine
+ Color: straw to dark yellow
+ Appearance: clear
+ Specific gravity: 1.005 to 1.035
+ pH: 4.5 to 8.0
+ Epithelial cells: 0 to 5 per high-power field
+ Casts: none, except 1 to 2 hyaline casts per low-power field
+ Crystals: present

Urine osmolality
+ 24-hour urine: 300 to 900 mOsm/kg
+ Random urine: 50 to 1,400 mOsm/kg

Urobilinogen, fecal
50 to 300 mg/24 hours (SI, 100 to 400 EU/100 g)

Urobilinogen, urine
+ 0.1 to 0.8 EU/2 hours (SI 0.1 to 0.8 EU/2 h)
or
+ 0.5 to 4.0 EU/24 hours (SI, 0.5 to 4.0 EU/d)

Uroporphyrinogen I synthase
≥7 nmol/second/L

V

Vanillylmandelic acid, urine
1.4 to 6.5 mg/24 hours (SI, 7 to 33 µmol/day)

Venereal Disease Research Laboratory test, cerebrospinal fluid
Negative

Venereal Disease Research Laboratory test, serum
Negative

Vitamin A, serum
30 to 80 µg/dl (SI, 1.05 to 2.8 µmol/L)

Vitamin B$_2$, serum
3 to 15 µg/dl

Vitamin B$_{12}$, serum
200 to 900 pg/ml (SI, 148 to 664 pmol/L)

Vitamin C, plasma
0.2 to 2 mg/dl (SI, 11 to 114 µmol/L)

Vitamin C, urine
30 mg/24 hours

Vitamin D$_3$, serum
10 to 60 ng/ml (SI, 25 to 150 nmol/L)

W X Y

White blood cell count, blood
4,000 to 10,000/µl (SI, 4 to 10 × 10^9/L)

White blood cell count, peritoneal fluid
< 300/µl (SI, < 300 × 10^9/L)

White blood cell count, urine
0 to 4 per high-power field

White blood cell differential, blood
✦ Adults
  – Neutrophils: 54% to 75% (SI, 0.54 to 0.75)
  – Lymphocytes: 25% to 40% (SI, 0.25 to 0.40)
  – Monocytes: 2% to 8% (SI, 0.02 to 0.08)
  – Eosinophils: 1% to 4% (SI, 0.01 to 0.04)
  – Basophils: 0 to 1% (SI, 0 to 0.01)

Z

Zinc, serum
70 to 120 µg/dl (SI, 10.7 to 18.4 µmol/L)

Quick guide to head-to-toe assessment

The chart on the following pages provides guidelines for a systematic head-to-toe assessment. It groups assessment techniques by body region and nurse-patient positioning to make the assessment as efficient as possible and to avoid tiring the patient. The first column describes the assessment technique to use for each body system or region. The second column lists normal findings for adults. The third column reviews special considerations, including the purpose of the technique as well as nursing and developmental considerations.

TECHNIQUE	NORMAL FINDINGS	SPECIAL CONSIDERATIONS
HEAD and NECK		
Inspect the patient's head. Note hair color, texture, and distribution. Palpate from the forehead to the posterior triangle of the neck for the posterior cervical lymph nodes.	Symmetrical, rounded normocephalic head positioned at midline and erect with no lumps or ridges	• This technique can detect asymmetry, size changes, enlarged lymph nodes, and tenderness. • Wear gloves for palpation if the patient has scalp lesions. • Inspect and gently palpate the fontanels and sutures in an infant.
Palpate in front of and behind the ears, under the chin, and in the anterior triangle for the anterior cervical lymph nodes.	Nonpalpable lymph nodes or small, round, soft, mobile, nontender lymph nodes	• This technique can detect enlarged lymph nodes. • Palpable lymph nodes may be normal in a patient under age 12.
Palpate the left and then the right carotid artery.	Bilateral equality in pulse amplitude and rhythm	• This technique evaluates circulation through the carotid pulse.
Auscultate the carotid arteries.	No bruit on auscultation	• Auscultation in this area can detect a bruit, a sign of turbulent blood flow.
Palpate the trachea.	Straight, midline trachea	• This technique evaluates trachea position.
Palpate the suprasternal notch.	Palpable pulsations with an even rhythm	• Palpation in this area allows evaluation of aortic arch pulsations.
Palpate the supraclavicular area.	Nonpalpable lymph nodes	• This technique can detect enlarged lymph nodes.
Palpate the thyroid gland and auscultate for bruits.	Thin, mobile thyroid isthmus; nonpalpable thyroid lobes	• Palpation detects thyroid enlargement, tenderness, or nodules.
Have the patient touch his chin to his chest and to each shoulder, each ear to the corresponding shoulder, then tip his head back as far as possible.	Symmetrical strength and movement of neck muscles	• These maneuvers evaluate range of motion (ROM) in the neck.

TECHNIQUE	NORMAL FINDINGS	SPECIAL CONSIDERATIONS
HEAD and NECK *(continued)*		
Place your hands on the patient's shoulders while the patient shrugs them against resistance. Then place your hand on the patient's left cheek, then the right, and have the patient push against it.	Symmetrical strength and movement of neck muscles	• This procedure checks cranial nerve XI (accessory nerve) functioning and trapezius and sternocleidomastoid muscle strength.
Have the patient smile, frown, wrinkle his forehead, and puff out his cheeks.	Symmetrical smile, frown, and forehead wrinkles; equal puffing out of the cheeks	• This maneuver evaluates the motor portion of cranial nerve VII (facial nerve).
Occlude one nostril externally with your finger while the patient breathes through the other. Repeat on the other nostril.	Patent nostrils	• This technique checks the patency of the nasal passages.
Inspect the internal nostrils using a nasal speculum or an ophthalmoscope handle with a nasal attachment.	Moist, pink to red nasal mucosa without deviated septum, lesions, or polyps	• This technique can detect edema, inflammation, and excessive drainage. • Use only a flashlight to inspect an infant's or toddler's nostrils; a nasal speculum is too sharp.
Palpate the nose.	No bumps, lesions, edema, or tenderness	• This technique assesses for structural abnormalities in the nose. • An infant's nose usually is slightly flattened.
Palpate and percuss the frontal and maxillary sinuses. If palpation and percussion elicit tenderness, assess further by transilluminating the sinuses.	No tenderness on palpation or percussion	• These techniques are used to elicit tenderness, which may indicate sinus congestion or infection. • In a child under age 8, frontal sinuses commonly are too small to assess.
Palpate the temporomandibular joints as the patient opens and closes his jaws.	Smooth joint movement without pain; correct approximation	• This action assesses the temporomandibular joints and the motor portion of cranial nerve V (trigeminal nerve).
Inspect the oral mucosa, gingivae, teeth, and salivary gland openings, using a tongue blade and a penlight.	Pink, moist, smooth oral mucosa without lesions or inflammation; pink, moist slightly irregular gingivae without sponginess or edema; 32 teeth with correct occlusion	• This technique evaluates the condition of several oral structures. • A child may have up to 20 temporary (baby) teeth. • Slight gingival swelling may be normal during pregnancy.

TECHNIQUE	NORMAL FINDINGS	SPECIAL CONSIDERATIONS
HEAD and NECK *(continued)*		
Observe the tongue and the hard and soft palates.	Pink, slightly rough tongue with a midline depression; pink to light red palates with symmetrical lines	• Observation provides information about the patient's hydration status and the condition of these oral structures.
Ask the patient to stick out his tongue.	Midline tongue without tremors	• This procedure tests cranial nerve XII (hypoglossal nerve).
Ask the patient to say "Ahh" while sticking out his tongue. Inspect the visible oral structures.	Symmetrical rise in soft palate and uvula during phonation; pink, midline, cone-shaped uvula; +1 tonsils (both tonsils behind the pillars)	• Phonation ("Ahh"') checks portions of cranial nerves IX and X (glossopharyngeal and vagus nerves). Lowering the tongue aids viewing.
Test the gag reflex using a tongue blade.	Gagging	• Gagging during this procedure indicates that cranial nerves IX and X are intact.
Place the tongue blade at the side of the tongue while the patient pushes it to the left and right with his tongue.	Symmetrical ability to push tongue blade to left and right	• This action tests cranial nerve XII.
Test the sense of smell using a test tube of coffee, chocolate, or another familiar substance.	Correct identification of smells in both nostrils	• This action tests cranial nerve I (olfactory nerve). • Make sure the patient keeps both eyes closed during the test.
EYES and EARS		
Perform a visual acuity test using the standard Snellen eye chart or another visual acuity chart, with the patient wearing corrective lenses if needed.	20/20 vision	• This test assesses the patient's distance vision (central vision) and evaluates cranial nerve II (optic nerve).
Ask the patient to identify the pattern in a specially prepared page of color dots or plates.	Correct identification of pattern	• This test assesses the patient's color perception.
Test the six cardinal positions of gaze.	Bilaterally equal eye movement without nystagmus	• This test evaluates the function of each of the six extraocular muscles and tests cranial nerves III, IV, and VI (oculomotor, trochlear, and abducens nerves).

TECHNIQUE	NORMAL FINDINGS	SPECIAL CONSIDERATIONS
EYES and EARS *(continued)*		
Inspect the external structures of the eyeball (eyelids, eyelashes, and lacrimal apparatus).	Bright, clear, symmetrical eyes free of nystagmus; eyelids close completely; no lesions, scaling, or inflammation	• This inspection allows detection of such problems as ptosis, ectropion (outward-turning eyelids), entropion (inward-turning eyelids), and styes.
Inspect the conjunctiva and sclera.	Pink palpebral conjunctiva and clear bulbar conjunctiva without swelling, drainage, or hyperemic blood vessels; white, clear sclera	• Inspection detects conjunctivitis and the scleral color changes that may occur with systemic disorders.
Inspect the cornea, iris, and anterior chamber by shining a penlight tangentially across the eye.	Clear, transparent cornea and anterior chamber; illumination of total iris	• This technique assesses anterior chamber depth and the condition of the cornea and iris. • An elderly patient may exhibit a thin, grayish ring in the cornea (called *arcus senilis*).
Examine the pupils for equality of size, shape, reaction to light, and accommodation.	Pupils equal, round, reactive to light and accommodation (PERRLA), directly and consensually	• Testing the pupillary response to light and accommodation assesses cranial nerves III, IV, and VI.
Observe the red reflex using an ophthalmoscope.	Sharp, distinct orange-red glow	• Presence of the red reflex indicates that the cornea, anterior chamber, and lens are free from opacity and clouding.
Inspect the ear. Perform an otoscopic examination if indicated.	Nearly vertically positioned ears that line up with the eye, match the facial color, are similarly shaped, and are in proportion to the face; no drainage, nodules, or lesions	• A dark-skinned patient may have darker orange or brown cerumen (earwax); a fair-skinned patient typically will have yellow cerumen.
Palpate the ear and mastoid process.	No pain, swelling, nodules, or lesions	• This assessment technique can detect inflammation or infection. It may also uncover other abnormalities, such as nodules or lesions.
Perform the whispered voice test or the watch-tick test on one ear at a time.	Whispered voice heard at a distance of 1′ to 2′ (30 to 61 cm); watch-tick heard at a distance of 5″ (13 cm)	• This test provides a gross assessment of cranial nerve VIII (acoustic nerve).

TECHNIQUE	NORMAL FINDINGS	SPECIAL CONSIDERATIONS
EYES and EARS *(continued)*		
Perform Weber's test using a 512 or 1024 hertz (Hz) tuning fork.	Tuning fork vibrations heard equally in both ears or in the middle of the head	• This test differentiates conductive from sensorineural hearing loss. • The sound is heard best in the ear with a conductive loss.
Perform the Rinne test using a 512 or 1024 Hz tuning fork.	Tuning fork vibrations heard in front of the ear for as long as they are heard on the mastoid process	• This test helps differentiate conductive from sensorineural hearing loss.
POSTERIOR THORAX		
Observe the skin, bones, and muscles of the spine, shoulder blades, and back as well as symmetry of expansion and accessory muscle use.	Even skin tone; symmetrical placement of all structures; bilaterally equal shoulder height; symmetrical expansion with inhalation; no accessory muscle use	• Observation provides information about lung expansion and accessory muscle use during respiration. It may also detect a deformity that can alter ventilation, such as scoliosis.
Assess the anteroposterior and lateral diameters of the thorax.	Lateral diameter up to twice the anteroposterior diameter (2:1)	• This assessment may detect abnormalities, such as an increased anteroposterior diameter (barrel chest may be as low as 1:1). • Normal anteroposterior diameters vary with age. • Measure an infant's chest circumference at the nipple line.
Palpate down the spine.	Properly aligned spinous processes without lesions or tenderness; firm, symmetrical, evenly spaced muscles	• This technique detects pain in the spine and paraspinous muscles. It also evaluates the muscles' consistency.
Palpate over the posterior thorax.	Smooth surface; no lesions, lumps, or pain	• This technique helps detect musculoskeletal inflammation.
Assess respiratory excursion.	Symmetrical expansion and contraction of the thorax	• This technique checks for equal expansion of the lungs.

TECHNIQUE	NORMAL FINDINGS	SPECIAL CONSIDERATIONS
POSTERIOR THORAX *(continued)*		
Palpate for tactile fremitus as the patient repeats the word "ninety-nine."	Equally intense vibrations of both sides of the chest	• Palpation provides information about the content of the lungs; vibrations increase over consolidated or fluid-filled areas and decrease over gas-filled areas.
Percuss over the posterior and lateral lung fields.	Resonant percussion note over the lungs that changes to a dull note at the diaphragm	• This technique helps identify the density and location of the lungs, diaphragm, and other anatomic structures. • Percussion may produce hyperresonant sounds in a patient with chronic obstructive pulmonary disease or an elderly patient because of hyperinflation of lung tissue.
Percuss for diaphragmatic excursion on each side of the posterior thorax.	Excursion from 1¼" to 2¼" (3 to 6 cm)	• This technique evaluates diaphragm movement during respiration.
Auscultate the lungs through the posterior thorax as the patient breathes slowly and deeply through the mouth. Also auscultate lateral areas.	Bronchovesicular sounds (soft, breezy sounds) between the scapulae; vesicular sounds (soft, swishy sounds about two notes lower than bronchovesicular sounds) in the lung periphery	• Lung auscultation helps detect abnormal fluid or mucus accumulation as well as obstructed passages. • Auscultate a child's lungs before performing other assessment techniques that may cause crying, which increases the respiratory rate and interferes with clear auscultation. • A child's breath sounds are normally harsher or more bronchial than an adult's.
ANTERIOR THORAX		
Observe the skin, bones, and muscles of the anterior thoracic structures as well as symmetry of expansion and accessory muscle use during respiration.	Even skin tone; symmetrical placement of all structures; symmetrical costal angle of less than 90 degrees; symmetrical expansion with inhalation; no accessory muscle use	• Observation provides information about lung expansion and accessory muscle use. It may also detect a deformity that can prevent full lung expansion, such as pigeon chest.
Inspect the anterior thorax for lifts, heaves, or thrusts. Also check for the apical impulse.	No lifts, heaves, or thrusts; apical impulse not usually visible	• Apical impulse may be visible in a thin or young patient.

TECHNIQUE	NORMAL FINDINGS	SPECIAL CONSIDERATIONS
ANTERIOR THORAX *(continued)*		
Palpate over the anterior thorax.	Smooth surface; no lesions, lumps, or pain	• This technique helps detect musculoskeletal inflammation.
Assess respiratory excursion.	Symmetrical expansion and contraction of the thorax	• This technique checks for equal expansion of the lungs.
Palpate for tactile fremitus as the patient repeats the word "ninety-nine."	Equally intense vibrations of both sides of the chest, with more vibrations in the upper chest than in the lower chest	• Palpation provides information about the content of the lungs.
Percuss over the anterior thorax.	Resonant percussion note over lung fields that changes to a dull note over ribs and other bones	• This technique helps identify the density and location of the lungs, diaphragm, and other anatomic structures. • Percussion is unreliable in an infant because of the infant's small chest size. • Percussion may produce hyperresonant sounds in an elderly patient because of hyperinflation of lung tissue.
Auscultate the lungs through the anterior thorax as the patient breathes slowly and deeply through the mouth. Also auscultate lateral areas.	Bronchovesicular sounds (soft, breezy sounds) between the scapulae; vesicular sounds (soft, swishy sounds about two notes lower than bronchovesicular sounds) in the lung periphery	• Lung auscultation helps detect abnormal fluid or mucus accumulation. • Auscultate a child's lungs before performing other assessment techniques that may cause crying. • Breath sounds are normally harsher or more bronchial in a child.
Inspect the breasts and axillae with the patient's hands resting at the sides of her body, placed on her hips, and raised above her head.	Symmetrical, convex, similar-looking breasts with soft, smooth skin and bilaterally similar venous patterns; symmetrical axillae with varying amounts of hair, but no lesions; nipples at same level on chest and of same color	• This technique evaluates the general condition of the breasts and axillae and detects such abnormalities as retraction, dimpling, and flattening. • Expect to see enlarged breasts with darkened nipples and areolae and purplish linear streaks if the patient is pregnant.
Palpate the axillae with the patient's arms resting against the sides of the body.	Nonpalpable nodes	• This technique detects nodular enlargements and other abnormalities.

TECHNIQUE	NORMAL FINDINGS	SPECIAL CONSIDERATIONS
ANTERIOR THORAX *(continued)*		
Palpate the breasts and nipples with the patient lying supine.	Smooth, relatively elastic tissue without masses, cracks, fissures, areas of induration (hardness), or discharge	• This technique evaluates the consistency and elasticity of the breasts and nipples and may detect nipple discharge. • The premenstrual patient may exhibit breast tenderness, nodularity, and fullness. • A pregnant patient may discharge colostrum from the nipple and may exhibit nodular breasts with prominent venous patterns.
Inspect the neck for jugular vein distention with the patient lying supine at a 45-degree angle.	No visible pulsations	• This technique assesses right-sided heart pressure.
Palpate the precordium for the apical impulse.	Apical impulse present in the apical area (fifth intercostal space at the midclavicular line)	• This action evaluates the size and location of the left ventricle.
Auscultate the aortic, pulmonic, tricuspid, and mitral areas for heart sounds.	S_1 and S_2 heart sounds with a regular rhythm and an age-appropriate rate	• Auscultation over the precordium evaluates the heart rate and rhythm and can detect other abnormal heart sounds. • A child or a pregnant woman in the third trimester may have functional (innocent) heart murmurs.
ABDOMEN		
Observe the abdominal contour.	Symmetrical flat or rounded contour	• This technique determines whether the abdomen is distended or scaphoid. • An infant or a toddler will have a rounded abdomen.
Inspect the abdomen for skin characteristics, symmetry, contour, peristalsis, and pulsations.	Symmetrical contour with no lesions, striae, rash, or visible peristaltic waves	• Inspection can detect an incisional or umbilical hernia, or an abnormality caused by bowel obstruction.
Auscultate all four quadrants of the abdomen.	Normal bowel sounds in all four quadrants; no bruits	• Abdominal auscultation can detect abnormal bowel sounds.
Percuss from below the right breast to the inguinal area down the right midclavicular line.	Dull percussion note over the liver; tympanic note over the rest of the abdomen	• Percussion in this area helps evaluate the size of the liver.

TECHNIQUE	NORMAL FINDINGS	SPECIAL CONSIDERATIONS
ABDOMEN *(continued)*		
Percuss from below the left breast to the inguinal area down the left midclavicular line.	Tympanic percussion note	• Percussion that elicits a dull note in this area can detect an enlarged spleen.
Palpate all four abdominal quadrants.	Nontender organs without masses	• Palpation provides information about the location, size, and condition of the underlying structures.
Palpate for the kidneys on each side of the abdomen.	Nonpalpable kidneys or solid, firm, smooth kidneys (if palpable)	• This technique evaluates the general condition of the kidneys.
Palpate the liver at the right costal border.	Nonpalpable liver or smooth, firm, nontender liver with a rounded, regular edge (if palpable)	• This technique evaluates the general condition of the liver.
Palpate for the spleen at the left costal border.	Nonpalpable spleen	• This procedure detects splenomegaly (spleen enlargement).
Palpate the femoral pulses in the groin.	Strong, regular pulse	• Palpation assesses vascular patency.
UPPER EXTREMITIES		
Observe the skin and muscle mass of the arms and hands.	Uniform color and texture with no lesions; elastic turgor; bilaterally equal muscle mass	• The skin provides information about hydration and circulation. Muscle mass provides information about injuries and neuromuscular disease.
Ask the patient to extend his arms forward and then rapidly turn his palms up and down.	Steady hands with no tremor or pronator drift	• This maneuver tests proprioception and cerebellar function.
Place your hands on the patient's upturned forearms while the patient pushes up against resistance. Then place your hands under the forearms while the patient pushes down.	Symmetrical strength and ability to push up and down against resistance	• This procedure checks the muscle strength of the arms.
Inspect and palpate the fingers, wrists, and elbow joints.	Smooth, freely movable joints with no swelling	• An elderly patient may exhibit osteoarthritic changes.
Palpate the patient's hands to assess skin temperature.	Warm, moist skin with bilaterally even temperature	• Skin temperature assessment provides data about circulation to the area.

TECHNIQUE	NORMAL FINDINGS	SPECIAL CONSIDERATIONS
UPPER EXTREMITIES *(continued)*		
Palpate the radial and brachial pulses.	Bilaterally equal rate and rhythm	• Palpation of pulses helps evaluate peripheral vascular status.
Inspect the color, shape, and condition of the patient's fingernails, and test for capillary refill.	Pink nail beds with smooth, rounded nails; brisk capillary refill; no clubbing	• Nail assessment provides data about the integumentary, cardiovascular, and respiratory systems.
Place two fingers in each of the patient's palms while the patient squeezes your fingers.	Bilaterally equal hand strength	• This maneuver tests muscle strength in the hands.
LOWER EXTREMITIES		
Inspect the legs and feet for color, lesions, varicosities, hair growth, nail growth, edema, and muscle mass.	Even skin color; symmetrical hair and nail growth; no lesions, varicosities, or edema; bilaterally equal muscle mass	• Inspection assesses adequate circulatory function.
Test for pitting edema in the pretibial area.	No pitting edema	• This test assesses for excess interstitial fluid.
Palpate for pulses and skin temperature in the posterior tibial, dorsalis pedis, and popliteal areas. Perform the straight leg test on one leg at a time.	Bilaterally even pulse rate, rhythm, and skin temperature	• Palpation of pulses and temperature in these areas evaluates the patient's peripheral vascular status.
Perform the straight leg test on one leg at a time	Painless leg lifting	• This test checks for vertebral disk problems.
Palpate for crepitus as the patient abducts and adducts the hip. Repeat on the opposite leg.	No crepitus; full ROM without pain	• Perform Ortolani's maneuver on an infant to assess hip abduction and adduction.
Ask the patient to raise his thigh against the resistance of your hands. Repeat this procedure on the opposite thigh.	Each thigh lifts easily against resistance	• This maneuver tests the motor strength of the upper legs.
Ask the patient to push outward against the resistance of your hands.	Each leg pushes easily against resistance	• This maneuver tests the motor strength of the lower legs.
Ask the patient to pull backward against the resistance of your hands.	Each leg pulls easily against resistance	• This maneuver tests the motor strength of the lower legs.

TECHNIQUE	NORMAL FINDINGS	SPECIAL CONSIDERATIONS
NERVOUS SYSTEM		
Lightly touch the ophthalmic, maxillary, and mandibular areas on each side of the patient's face with a cotton-tipped applicator and a pin.	Correct identification of sensation and location	• This test evaluates the function of cranial nerve V (trigeminal nerve).
Touch the dorsal and palmar surfaces of the arms, hands, and fingers with a cotton-tipped applicator and a pin.	Correct identification of sensation and location	• This test evaluates the function of the ulnar, radial, and medial nerves.
Touch several nerve distribution areas on the legs, feet, and toes with a cotton-tipped applicator and a pin.	Correct identification of sensation and location	• This test evaluates the function of the dermatome areas randomly.
Place your fingers above the patient's wrist and tap them with a reflex hammer. Repeat on the other arm.	Normal reflex reaction	• This procedure elicits the brachioradialis deep tendon reflex (DTR).
Place your fingers over the antecubital fossa and tap them with a reflex hammer. Repeat on the other arm.	Normal reflex reaction	• This procedure elicits the biceps DTR.
Place your fingers over the triceps tendon area and tap them with a reflex hammer. Repeat on the other arm.	Normal reflex reaction	• This procedure elicits the triceps DTR.
Tap just below the patella with a reflex hammer. Repeat this procedure on the opposite patella.	Normal reflex reaction	• This procedure elicits the patellar DTR.
Tap over the Achilles tendon area with a reflex hammer. Repeat this procedure on the opposite ankle.	Normal reflex reaction	• This procedure elicits the Achilles DTR.
Stroke the sole of the patient's foot with the end of the reflex hammer handle.	Plantar reflex	• This procedure elicits plantar flexion of all toes. • Expect Babinski's sign in children age 2 and under.
Ask the patient to demonstrate dorsiflexion by bending both feet upward against resistance.	Both feet lift easily against resistance	• This procedure tests foot strength and ROM.
Ask the patient to demonstrate plantar flexion by bending both feet downward against resistance.	Both feet push down easily against resistance	• This procedure tests foot strength and ROM.

TECHNIQUE	NORMAL FINDINGS	SPECIAL CONSIDERATIONS
NERVOUS SYSTEM *(continued)*		
Using your finger, trace a one-digit number in the palm of the patient's hand.	Correct identification of traced number	• This procedure evaluates the patient's tactile discrimination through graphesthesia.
Place a familiar object, such as a key or a coin, in the patient's hand.	Correct identification of object	• This procedure evaluates the patient's tactile discrimination.
Observe the patient while he walks with a regular gait, on the toes, on the heels, and heel-to-toe.	Steady gait, good balance, and no signs of muscle weakness or pain in any style of walking	• This technique evaluates the cerebellum and motor system and checks for vertebral disk problems.
Inspect the scapulae, spine, back, and hips as the patient bends forward, backward, and from side to side.	Full ROM, easy flexibility, and no signs of scoliosis or varicosities	• Inspection evaluates the patient's ROM and detects musculoskeletal abnormalities such as scoliosis.
Perform the Romberg test. Ask the patient to stand straight with both eyes closed and both arms extended, with hands palms up.	Steady stance with minimal weaving	• This test checks cerebellar functioning and evaluates balance and coordination.

Laboratory value changes in elderly patients

TEST VALUES AGES 20 TO 40	AGE-RELATED CHANGES	CONSIDERATIONS
SERUM		
Albumin 3.5 to 5 g/dl (SI, 35 to 50 g/L)	Younger than age 65: Higher in males Older than age 65: Equal levels that then decrease at same rate	Increased dietary protein intake needed in older patients if liver function is normal; edema—a sign of low albumin level
Alkaline phosphatase 30 to 85 IU/L (SI, 42 to 128 U/L)	Increases 8 to 10 IU/L	May reflect liver function decline or vitamin D malabsorption and bone demineralization
Beta globulin 0.7 to 1.1 g/dl (SI, 7 to 11 g/L)	Increases slightly	Increases in response to decrease in albumin if liver function is normal; increased dietary protein intake needed
Blood urea nitrogen Men: 10 to 25 mg/dl (SI, 3.6 to 9.3 mmol/L) Women: 8 to 20 mg/dl (SI, 2.9 to 7.5 mmol/L)	Increases, possibly to 69 mg/dl (SI, 25.8 mmol/L)	Slight increase acceptable in absence of stressors, such as infection or surgery
Cholesterol Men: < 205 mg/dl (SI,< 5.30 mmol/L) Women: < 190 mg/dl (SI, < 4.90 mmol/L)	Men: Increases to age 50, then decreases Women: Lower than men until age 50, increases to age 70, then decreases	Rise in cholesterol level (and increased cardiovascular risk) in women as a result of postmenopausal estrogen decline; dietary changes, weight loss, and exercise needed
Creatine kinase 55 to 170 U/L (SI, 0.94 to 2.89 µkat/L)	Increases slightly	May reflect decreasing muscle mass and liver function
Creatinine 0.6 to 1.3 mg/dl (SI, 53 to 115 µmol/L)	Increases, possibly to 1.9 mg/dl (SI, 168 µmol/L) in men	Important factor to prevent toxicity when giving drugs excreted in urine

TEST VALUES AGES 20 TO 40	AGE-RELATED CHANGES	CONSIDERATIONS
SERUM *(continued)*		
Creatinine clearance Men: 94 to 140 ml/min/1.73 m² (SI, 0.91 to 1.35 ml/s/m2) Women: 72 to 110 ml/min/1.73 m² (SI, 0.69 to 1.06 ml/s/m²)	Men: Decreases; formula: ([140 − age]) × kg body weight)/(72 × serum creatinine) Women: 85% of men's rate	Reflects reduced glomerular filtration rate; important factor to prevent toxicity when giving drugs excreted in urine
Hematocrit Men: 45% to 52% (SI, 0.45 to 0.52) Women: 37% to 48% (SI, 0.37 to 0.48)	May decrease slightly (unproven)	Reflects decreased bone marrow and hematopoiesis, increased risk of infection (because of fewer and weaker lymphocytes and immune system changes that diminish antigen-antibody response)
Hemoglobin Men: 14 to 18 g/dl (SI, 140 to 180 g/L) Women: 12 to 16 g/dl (SI, 120 to 160 g/L)	Men: Decreases by 1 to 2 g/dl Women: Unknown	Reflects decreased bone marrow, hematopoiesis, and (for men) androgen levels
High-density lipoprotein Men: 37 to 70 mg/dl (SI, 0.96 to 1.8 mmol/L) Women: 40 to 85 mg/dl (SI, 1.03 to 2.2 mmol/L)	Levels higher in women than in men but equalize with age	Compliance with dietary restrictions required for accurate interpretation of test results
Lactate dehydrogenase 71 to 207 U/L (SI, 1.2 to 3.52 μkat/L)	Increases slightly	May reflect declining muscle mass and liver function
Leukocyte count 4,000 to 10,0000/μl (SI, 4 to 10 × 10⁹/L)	Decreases to 3,100 to 9,000/μl (SI, 3.1 to 9 × 10⁹/L)	Decrease proportionate to lymphocyte count
Lymphocyte count 25% to 40% (SI, 0.25 to 0.4)	Decreases	Decrease proportionate to leukocyte count
Platelet count 140,000 to 400,000/μl (SI, 140 to 400 × 10⁹/L)	Change in characteristics; decreased granular constituents, increased platelet-release factors	May reflect diminished bone marrow and increased fibrinogen levels

TEST VALUES AGES 20 TO 40	AGE-RELATED CHANGES	CONSIDERATIONS
SERUM *(continued)*		
Potassium 3.5 to 5.5 mEq/L (SI, 3.5 to 5.5 mmol/L)	Increases slightly	Requires avoidance of salt substitutes composed of potassium, vigilance in reading food labels, and knowledge of hyperkalemia's signs and symptoms
Thyroid-stimulating hormone 0 to 15 µIU/ml (SI, 15 mU/L)	Increases slightly	Suggests primary hypothyroidism or endemic goiter at much higher levels
Thyroxine 5 to 13.5 µg/dl (SI, 60 to 165 mmol/L)	Decreases 25%	Reflects declining thyroid function
Triglycerides Men: 44 to 180 mg/dl (SI, 0.44 to 2.01 mmol/L) Women: 10 to 190 mg/dl (SI, 0.11 to 2.21 mmol/L)	Increases slightly	Suggests abnormalities at any other levels, requiring additional tests such as serum cholesterol
Triiodothyronine 80 to 220 ng/dl (SI, 1.2 to 3 nmol/L)	Decreases 25%	Reflects declining thyroid function
URINE		
Glucose 0 to 15 mg/dl (SI, 0 to 8 mmol/L)	Decreases slightly	May reflect renal disease or urinary tract infection (UTI); unreliable check for older diabetics because glucosuria may not occur until plasma glucose level exceeds 300 mg/dl
Protein 50 to 80 mg/24 hours (SI, 50 to 80 mg/d)	Increases slightly	May reflect renal disease or UTI
Specific gravity 1.032 (SI, 1.032)	Decreases to 1.024 (SI, 1.024) by age 80	Reflects 30% to 50% decrease in number of nephrons available to concentrate urine

Resources for professionals, patients, and caregivers

General health care Web sites

✦ *www.healthfinder.gov* — from the U.S. government; searchable database with links to Web sites, support groups, government agencies, and not-for-profit organizations that provide health care information for patients

✦ *www.healthweb.org* — from a group of librarians and information professionals at academic medical centers in the midwestern United States; offers a searchable database of evaluated Web sites for patients and health care professionals

✦ *www.medmatrix.org* — includes journal articles, abstracts, reviews, conference highlights, and links to other major sources for health care professionals

✦ *www.mwsearch.com* — named Medical World Search, this site searches thousands of selected medical sites

Organizations

✦ American Academy of Family Physicians — offers handouts and other resources to patients and health care professionals, plus links to other sites: *www.aafp.org*

✦ Joint Commission on Accreditation of Healthcare Organizations: *www.jcaho.org*

Government agencies

✦ Agency for Healthcare Research and Quality: *www.ahcpr.gov*

✦ Centers for Disease Control and Prevention: *www.cdc.gov*

✦ Centers for Medicare & Medicaid Services: *www.cms.hss.gov*

✦ National Center for Complementary and Alternative Medicine: *www.nccam.nih.gov*

✦ National Guideline Clearinghouse: *www.guideline.com*

✦ National Library of Medicine, Specialized Information Services (information resources and services in toxicology, environmental health, chemistry, HIV/AIDS, and specialized topics in minority health): *www.sis.nlm.nih.gov*

✦ U.S. Department of Health & Human Services: *www.dhhs.gov*

✦ U.S. Food and Drug Administration: *www.fda.gov*

Links to Spanish-language sites

✦ Agency for Healthcare Research and Quality: *www.ahcpr.gov* (click on "Información en español")

✦ CANCERCare, Inc.: *www.cancercare.org* (click on "En español")

✦ Healthfinder: *www.healthfinder.gov* (click on "Español")

✦ National Cancer Institute: *www.cancer.gov/espanol*

Condition-specific sites
Aging

✦ American Society on Aging: *www.asaging.org*

✦ National Institute on Aging: *www.nia.nih.gov;* 301-496-1752

✦ U.S. Administration on Aging: *www.aoa.dhhs.gov*

AIDS/HIV/STDs

✦ Centers for Disease Control and Prevention, National Prevention Information Network: *www.cdcnpin.org/scripts/index.asp*

✦ HIV/AIDS Treatment Information Service: *www.sis.nlm.nih.gov/aids/aidstrea.html;* 800-448-0440 (Spanish available); TTY, 800-243-7012

✦ National AIDS Hotline (24 hours): 800-342-AIDS; Spanish, 800-344-7432; TTY, 800-243-7889

✦ Office of AIDS Research: *www.sis.nlm.nih.gov/aids/oar.html*

Allergies and asthma

✦ Allergy & Asthma Disease Management Center: *www.aaaai.org/aadmc*

✦ Allergy & Asthma Network — Mothers of Asthmatics: *www.aanma.org;* 800-878-4403

✦ Allergy, Asthma & Immunology Online: *www.allergy.mcg.edu*

✦ American Academy of Allergy Asthma & Immunology: *www.aaaai.org;* 800-822-2762

✦ Global Initiative For Asthma: *www.ginasthma.com*

✦ Joint Council of Allergy, Asthma and Immunology: *www.jcaai.org*

✦ National Asthma Education and Prevention Program: *www.nhlbi.nih.gov/about/naepp*

✦ National Institute of Allergy and Infectious Diseases: *www.niaid.nih.gov*

Alzheimer's disease

✦ Agency for Healthcare Research and Quality (AHRQ) Early Alzheimer's Disease Clinical Practice Guideline — Patient and Family Guide: *www.ahcpr.gov/clinic/alzcons.htm*

✦ AHRQ's Recognition and Assessment Guideline: *www.ahcpr.gov/clinic/alzover.htm*

✦ Alzheimer's Association: *www.alz.org;* 800-272-3900

✦ Alzheimer's Disease Education & Referral Center: *www.alzheimers.org;* 800-438-4380

✦ Alzheimer Europe: - *www.alzheimer-europe.org*

✦ AlzWell Caregiver Page: *www.alzwell.com*

Arthritis

✦ American Autoimmune Related Diseases Association, Inc.: *www.aarda.org*

✦ American College of Rheumatology: *www.rheumatology.org*

✦ Arthritis Foundation: *www.arthritis.org;* 800-283-7800

✦ National Institute of Arthritis and Musculoskeletal and Skin Diseases: *www.nih.gov/niams*

Attention deficit disorder/hyperactivity

✦ National Attention Deficit Disorder Association: *www.add.org*

Cancer

✦ American Cancer Society: *www.cancer.org;* 800-ACS-2345

✦ CANCERCare, Inc.: *www.cancercare.org*

✦ Cancer News on the Net: *www.cancernews.com*

✦ National Breast Cancer Awareness Month: *www.nbcam.org*

✦ National Cancer Institute: *www.cancer.gov*

✦ National Cancer Institute, Cancer Information Service: 800-4-CANCER

✦ National Cancer Institute, Cancer Literature Search: *www.cancer.gov/search/pubmed*

✦ National Cancer Institute, Cancer Trials: *www.cancer.gov/clinicaltrials*

✦ National Center for Chronic Disease Prevention and Health Promotion: *www.cdc.gov/nccdphp*

✦ National Comprehensive Cancer Network: *www.nccn.org*

✦ Susan G. Komen Breast Cancer Foundation: *www.komen.org*

✦ Y-Me National Breast Cancer Organization: *www.y-me.org*; 800-221-2141; 800-986-9505 (Español)

Cardiac

✦ American Heart Association: *www.americanheart.org*; 800-242-8721

✦ Mayo Heart Center: *www.mayohealth.org* (click on "Heart")

✦ National Heart, Lung, and Blood Institute: *www.nhlbi.nih.gov*

✦ National Stroke Association: *www.stroke.org*

Diabetes

✦ American Association of Diabetes Educators: *www.aadenet.org*; 800-338-3633

✦ American Diabetes Association: *www.diabetes.org*

✦ Diabetes self-care equipment for the visually impaired: Palco Labs, Inc.: *www.palcolabs.com*; 800-346-4488

✦ Joslin Diabetes Center: *www.joslin.harvard.edu*

✦ National Institute of Diabetes & Digestive & Kidney Diseases: *www.niddk.nih.gov*

Disabilities

✦ University of Virginia: General Resources About Disabilities: *www.curry.edschool.virginia.edu/go/cise/ose/resources/general.html*; Assistive Technology Resources: *www.curry.edschool.virginia.edu/go/cise/ose/resources/asst_tech.html*

Elder abuse

✦ National Center for Victims of Crime: *www.ncvc.org*

✦ National Center on Elder Abuse: *www.elderabusecenter.org*

Gastrointestinal

✦ American Liver Foundation: *www.liverfoundation.org*

✦ National Institute of Diabetes & Digestive & Kidney Diseases: *www.niddk.nih.gov*

✦ National Kidney Foundation: *www.kidney.org*; 800-622-9010

Musculoskeletal

✦ American College of Foot and Ankle Surgeons: *www.acfas.org*

✦ Amputee Coalition of America: *www.amputee-coalition.org*; 888-AMP-KNOW (267-5669)

✦ National Institue of Arthritis and Musculoskeletal and Skin Disorders: *www.niams.nih.gov*

✦ National Osteoporosis Foundation: *www.nof.org*

Neurology

✦ ALS Association: *www.alsa.org;* 818-880-9007

✦ American Brain Tumor Association: *www.abta.org;* 800-886-2282

✦ Association of Late-Deafened Adults, Inc.: *www.alda.org*

✦ EAR Foundation/Meniere's Network: *www.theearfoundation.org*

✦ National Association of the Deaf: *www.nad.org*

✦ National Federation of the Blind: *www.nfb.org*

✦ National Institute of Neurological Disorders and Stroke: *www.ninds.nih.gov*

✦ National Institute on Deafness and Other Communication Disorders: *www.nidcd.nih.gov*

Pediatrics

✦ Children with Diabetes: *www.childrenwithdiabetes.com*

✦ Cystic Fibrosis Foundation: *www.cff.org;* 800-FIGHT CF (344-4823)

✦ Cystic Fibrosis Mutation Data Base: *www.genet.sickkids.on.ca/cftr*

✦ Cystic Fibrosis USA: *www.cfusa.org*

✦ Down's Heart Group: *www.downs-heart.downsnet.org*

✦ Emory University Sickle Cell Information Center: *www.emory.edu/PEDS/SICKLE/newweb.htm*

✦ Families of Spinal Muscular Atrophy: *www.fsma.org;* 800-886-1762

✦ Growth Charts for Children with Down Syndrome: *www.growthcharts.com*

✦ Internet Resource for Special Children: *www.irsc.org*

✦ National Down Syndrome Society: *www.ndss.org*

✦ National Institute of Child Health & Human Development: *www.nichd.nih.gov*

✦ National Pediatric AIDS Network: *www.npan.org*

✦ Spina Bifida Association of America: *www.sbaa.org;* 800-621-3141

✦ United Cerebral Palsy: *www.ucpa.org;* 800-872-5827

Psychiatry

✦ American Psychological Association: *www.apa.org;* 800-374-2721

✦ Depressive and Bipolar Support Alliance: *www.dbsalliance.org*

✦ National Alliance for the Mentally Ill: *www.nami.org;* 800-950-NAMI (950-6264)

✦ National Mental Health Association: *www.nmha.org;* 800-969-6642

Respiratory

✦ American Heart Association (smoking cessation information): 800-242-8721

✦ American Lung Association: *www.lungusa.org;* 800-LUNG-USA (local affiliates answer)

✦ National Emphysema Foundation: *www.emphysemafoundation.org*

Skin

✦ National Pressure Ulcer Advisory Panel: *www.npuap.org*

✦ Wound Care Information Network: *www.medicaledu.com*

✦ Wound Care Institute, Inc.: *www.woundcare.org;* 305-919-9192

✦ Wound, Ostomy and Continence Nurses Society: *www.wocn.org;* 888-224-WOCN

Substance abuse

✦ Al-Anon & Alateen (including Spanish and French language options): *www.al-anon.alateen.org*

✦ Alcoholics Anonymous (including Spanish and French language options): *www.alcoholics-anonymous.org*

✦ Narcotics Anonymous World Services: *www.wsoinc.com*

✦ National Centers for Disease Control and Prevention, Tobacco Information and Prevention Source: *www.cdc.gov/tobacco*

✦ National Council on Alcoholism and Drug Dependence: *www.ncadd.org;* 800-NCA-CALL (622-2255)

✦ National Institute on Alcohol Abuse and Alcoholism: *www.niaaa.nih.gov*

✦ Substance Abuse & Mental Health Services Administration: *www.samhsa.gov*

Women's health

✦ American College of Cardiology: *www.acc.org*

✦ American Heart Association: *www.women.americanheart.org*

✦ American Medical Women's Association: *www.amwa-doc.org*

✦ JAMA Women's Health Information Center: *www.amaassn.org/special/womh/womh. htm*

✦ Johns Hopkins Intelihealth: *www.intelihealth.com* (click on "Women's health")

✦ Office on Women's Health (U.S. Department of Health & Human Services): *www.4women.gov/owh*

✦ Womens' Health Initiative: *www.nhlbi.nih.gov/whi*

Index

i refers to an illustration; t refers to a table; **boldface** refers to a full-color illlustration.

425

i refers to an illustration; t refers to a table; **boldface** refers to a full-color illlustration.

i refers to an illustration; t refers to a table; **boldface** refers to a full-color illlustration.

i refers to an illustration; t refers to a table; **boldface** refers to a full-color illustration.

i refers to an illustration; t refers to a table; **boldface** refers to a full-color illlustration.

i refers to an illustration; t refers to a table; **boldface** refers to a full-color illustration.

---

i refers to an illustration; t refers to a table; **boldface** refers to a full-color illustration.

i refers to an illustration; t refers to a table; **boldface** refers to a full-color illlustration.

i refers to an illustration; t refers to a table; **boldface** refers to a full-color illustration.

i refers to an illustration; t refers to a table; **boldface** refers to a full-color illlustration.